Understanding the Nature of
SENSORY INTEGRATION
WITH DIVERSE POPULATIONS

Editors

Susanne Smith Roley, M.S., OTR

Erna Imperatore Blanche, Ph.D., OTR, FAOTA

Roseann C. Schaaf, M.Ed., OTR/L, FAOTA

Foreword by
Florence Clark, Ph.D., OTR, FAOTA

pro·ed
An International Publisher

8700 Shoal Creek Boulevard
Austin, Texas 78757-6897
800/897-3202   Fax 800/397-7633
www.proedinc.com

(2001)

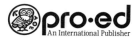
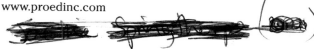

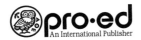

© 2001 by PRO-ED, Inc.
8700 Shoal Creek Boulevard
Austin, Texas 78757-6897
800/897-3202   Fax 800/397-7633
www.proedinc.com

Cover photo and photos on pages 250, 255, 260, 367, 369, 371, 375, and 376 by Shay McAtee.

ISBN-13: 978-141640332-6
ISBN-10: 141640332-9

Previously published by Therapy Skill Builders, a division of
The Psychological Corporation, under ISBN 0761615156.

Printed in the United States of America

2   3   4   5   10   09

Contributing Authors

Marie Anzalone, Sc.D., OTR, FAOTA
Assistant Professor of Clinical
  Occupational Therapy
Columbia University
New York, New York

Erna Imperatore Blanche, Ph.D., OTR,
FAOTA
Co-owner and co-director, Therapy West
Adjunct Instructor, Department
  of Occupational Science and Therapy
University of Southern California
Los Angeles, California

Janice P. Burke, Ph.D., OTR/L, FAOTA
Associate Professor and Chairman
Department of Occupational Therapy
College of Health Professions
Thomas Jefferson University
Philadelphia, Pennsylvania

Sharon A. Cermak, Ph.D., OTR, FAOTA
Professor, Department of Occupational Therapy
Sargent College of Health and
  Rehabilitation Sciences
Boston University
Boston, Massachusetts

Florence Clark, Ph.D., OTR, FAOTA
Professor and Chair
Department of Occupational Science
  and Occupational Therapy
University of Southern California
Los Angeles, California

Clare Giuffrida, Ph.D., FAOTA, OTR/L
Assistant Professor, Department of
  Occupational Therapy
University of Florida
Gainesville, Florida

Essie Jacobs, Ph.D., OTR
When this chapter was written, Essie Jacobs,
  Ph.D., OTR, was Assistant Professor in the
  Occupational Therapy Program, Department
  of Kinesiology, University of Wisconsin-
  Madison, Wisconsin. She currently resides
  in Seattle, Washington.

Lois Hickman, M.S., OTR, FAOTA
Private Practice
Lyons, Colorado

Gary W. Kraemer, Ph.D., OTR
Professor, Department of Kinesiology
  and Occupational Therapy
Medical Sciences Center
University of Wisconsin-Madison

Daniel N. McIntosh, Ph.D.
(University of Michigan)
Associate Professor, Department of Psychology
University of Denver
Denver, Colorado

Zoe Mailloux, M.A., OTR, FAOTA
Director of Administration,
  Pediatric Therapy Network
Torrance, California

Lucy Jane Miller, Ph.D., OTR
Occupational therapist and research scientist
University of Colorado Health Sciences Center
and the Departments of Pediatrics and
  Rehabilitation Medicine
Director, Sensory Integration Dysfunction
  Treatment And Research (STAR) Center
The Children's Hospital
Denver, Colorado

Teresa A. May-Benson, M.S., OTR/L
Research Director,
  Occupational Therapy Associates
Watertown, Massachusetts
MCH Fellow, Doctoral Program
  for Therapeutic Studies
Boston University
Boston, Massachusetts

Bonnie Nakasuji, M.A., OTR
  Co-owner and co-director, Therapy West
  Los Angeles, California

Diane Parham, Ph.D., OTR, FAOTA
  Associate Professor, Department
    of Occupational Science and Therapy
  University of Southern California
  Los Angeles, California

Gretchen Reeves, Ph.D., OT, FAOTA
  Assistant Professor, Medical College of Ohio
  Toledo, Ohio

Susanne Smith Roley, M.S., OTR
  Project Director, Comprehensive Program
    in Sensory Integration
  University of Southern California
  Coordinator of Education and Research
  Pediatric Therapy Network
  Los Angeles, California

Roseann C. Schaaf, M.Ed., OTR/L, FAOTA
  Vice Chairman, Department of
    Occupational Therapy
  Thomas Jefferson University
  Philadelphia, Pennsylvania

Jodie Simon, Ph.D.
  Post-doctoral fellow, Developmental Psychobiology
  University of Colorado Health Sciences Center
  Denver, Colorado

Colleen M. Schneck, Sc.D., OTR/L, FAOTA
  Professor, Department Occupational Therapy
  Eastern Kentucky University
  Richmond, Kentucky

Mary Schneider, Ph.D., OTR
  Professor, Occupational Therapy
    in the Department of Kinesiology
  University of Wisconsin-Madison
  Madison, Wisconsin

Judith Reisman, Ph.D., OTR, FAOTA
  Director, Occupational Therapy Program
  University of Minnesota
  Minneapolis, Minnesota

Clare A. Summers, M.A., OTR
  Sensory Integration Specialist
  Children's Hospital
  Denver, Colorado

Susan L. Spitzer, Ph.D. (Cand.), OTR
  Doctoral Candidate
  University of Southern California
  School Occupational Therapist
  Los Angeles Unified School District
  Los Angeles, California

Stacey Szklut, M.S., OTR/L
  Clinical Director, Occupational Therapy Associates
  Watertown, Massachusetts

Mary-Margaret Windsor, Sc.D., OTR/L
  Visiting Assistant Professor, Towson University
  Towson, Maryland

Dedication

This book is dedicated to our children:
Aja, Brooks, Dana, Dominique, Dylan,
Genevieve, Ian, Laura, Lisa and Sean;

To our mentor, A. Jean Ayres;

And to the loving memory of Paul E. Smith.

About the Authors

Susanne Smith Roley, M.S., OTR has specialized in the application of sensory integration within occupational therapy throughout her more than 20 years of practice. She received a bachelor of science degree in Occupational Therapy at Indiana University and master of science in Allied Health Sciences at Boston University. She subsequently trained with Dr. A. Jean Ayres and participated in the re-standardization of the *Sensory Integration and Praxis Tests*. Susanne is the project director for the Comprehensive Program in Sensory Integration in the Department of Occupational Science and Occupational Therapy at the University of Southern California. She is in private practice in Orange County and is Coordinator of Education and Research at Pediatric Therapy Network. She is an internationally recognized author and lecturer on the theory and application of sensory integration.

Erna Imperatore Blanche, Ph.D., OTR, FAOTA has been an occupational therapist for more than 20 years. She graduated from the University of Chile as an occupational therapist, has a masters degree in Special Education from Teacher's College Columbia University, and a doctorate in Occupational Science from the University of Southern California. She studied with Dr. A. Jean Ayres through OT610, the clinical training program at the University of Southern California, and is a primary instructor for this ongoing program. Erna is co-owner of Therapy West, a pediatric center in Los Angeles and is an adjunct faculty member at the Department of Occupational Science and Occupational Therapy at the University of Southern California. She has published and lectured extensively on the topics of sensory integration, neurodevelopmental treatment, play, and occupational science in the United States and abroad.

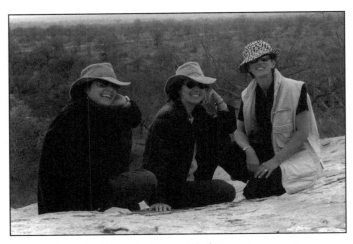

The authors/editors (left to right) Erna Imperatore Blanche, Susanne Smith Roley, and Roseann Schaaf in Kruger National Park, South Africa.

Roseann C. Schaaf, M.Ed., OTR/L, FAOTA is the vice chairman and director of graduate programs in the Department of Occupational Therapy at Thomas Jefferson University. She earned her bachelor's degree in Occupational Therapy and master's degree in Education from Temple University and is completing her doctorate in Neural and Behavioral Sciences at Bryn Mawr College. Roseann implements the theoretical principles of sensory integration throughout her clinical practice, research, and teaching. She is the author of numerous articles and chapters on various aspects of sensory integration theory and practice, and has lectured extensively in the United States and abroad. Currently, Roseann is working with Dr. Lucy Jane Miller to investigate the neuro-physiologic substrates of sensory modulation dysfunction, a sub-type of sensory integrative dysfunction.

Contents

Foreword

FLORENCE CLARK, PH.D., OTR, FAOTA

Occupations are the activities that we do that make life worth living. They range from the routine activities we must do to maintain health and hygiene to the types of engagement that express our loves and passions. Wilcock (1998) has defined occupational deprivation as a state in which a person does not have the opportunity to engage in occupations that develop capacities, sustain health or contribute to happiness. Along with her colleagues in the newly formed International Society of Occupational Scientists, she embraces the principle of occupational justice—that in a truly humane world all people should be helped to live a life filled with engagement in meaningful and health-promoting occupation.

One of the key barriers to occupational justice for children, as well as for some adults, is sensory integration dysfunction. Children and adults with this condition typically experience some degree of occupational deprivation, not because of poverty or social injustice, but because neural mechanisms within their bodies are malfunctioning. Unable to adequately interpret the sensations that arise from experience, these individuals tend to refrain from engagement in activity. Fortunately, more than 20 years ago A.J. Ayres, PhD, identified this previously neglected disorder and spent the rest of her life developing the science necessary to explain its neural substrates, which stimulated a powerful therapeutic approach. Consequently, occupational therapists and other health practitioners who have studied and applied the theory in practice have helped scores of individuals who would have otherwise suffered from occupational deprivation to engage in activities that stretch their capacities, improve sensory processing, and ultimately promote health.

Since the time of her death in 1988, the influence of Dr. Ayres' intellectual legacy has continued to grow. In this new millennium, the next generation of researchers, scholars, and practitioners are moving forward with the scientific research that Dr. Ayres initiated.

The editors of this volume, Susanne Smith Roley, Erna Imperatore Blanche and Roseann Schaaf, as well as those who have contributed chapters, are among this group. The editors in particular are to be commended for possessing the motivation and foresight to assemble into a single volume, chapters on state-of-the-art current research and clinical insights on sensory integration theory and practice. The scope and depth of the content included in these chapters is, in a sense, a treasure chest filled to its rim with a diverse array of precious jewels and pearls.

Current reviews of the relevant literature as synthesized in this volume demonstrate that Dr. Ayres' original theoretical formulations are not outmoded. For example, she strongly endorsed the view that experience shapes brain development, and that brain development and neural mechanisms, in turn, influence behavior. This position is strongly supported in the respective chapters in this volume by Jacobs and Schneider, and by Kraemer. Kraemer, for example, cites studies that indicate that the impact of experience on brain development and behavior is greater than previously thought. Far from refuting initial tenets of sensory integration theory, such recent research has refined and enhanced our understanding of them. For example, Miller, Reisman, McIntosh, and Simon hypothesize the existence of a new syndrome of sensory integration dysfunction called sensory modulation dysfunction, which exists in addition to those initially described by Ayres. Likewise, Giuffrida introduces an information processing model to refine our understanding of praxis, and Blanche and Parham expand upon Ayres' notion of the ways in which sensory integration impacts behavioral organization by introducing a perspective that incorporates the orchestration of activities in space and time. Other contributions synthesize state-of-the-art research on topics that Dr. Ayres considered of great import, such as the chapters on ideation by May-Benson, proprioception by Blanche and Schaaf, and attention and arousal by Reeves. These chapters integrate Ayres' perspective with the most recent discoveries in sensory integration. Categorically, advances in science today seem to be corroborating Ayres' initial formulations concerning the essential nature of sensory integrative dysfunction.

In reviewing the chapters devoted to intervention in this volume, I was struck by their comprehensiveness and complexity, as well as by the extent to which they epitomize the linkage of theory to practice. Hoshmand and Polkinghorne (1992) have warned that in professions there is a danger of theory becoming irrelevant to practice, along with a corresponding danger of practitioners doing their work without reference to theory. However, the chapters in this book indicate that theory and practice in sensory integration are reciprocally related. Through a careful consideration of these chapters, we can extract the clinical puzzles to which theoretical work must be directed and observe the detailed applications of theory to practice. The two chapters on assessment illustrate this kind of reciprocity. Burke's narrative approach to clinical assessment complements the standardized testing procedures Dr. Ayres developed, incorporating Ayres' theoretical framework while adding practical information that would not be ascertained without a fluid, open, clinical reasoning process. Windsor, Roley, and Szklut propose an assessment approach that draws upon sensory integration theory to provide a richer understanding of clients' participation in their social world. In both assessment approaches, constructs from sensory integration theory provide the basis for understanding the client's status. Additionally, in that they suggest links between sensory integrative dysfunction and other parameters of the client's life, they underscore the need for systematic research on these hypothetical relationships.

Another highly significant contribution of this volume is its emphasis on the application of sensory integration theory and practice to diverse populations. During her lifetime, Dr. Ayres concentrated on extending her theory to aphasic, learning disabled and autistic children. Continuing in this tradition, this volume contains carefully constructed chapters on the application of the theory to high-risk infants and young children (Schaaf and Anzalone, chapter 14), children with visually impairment and blindness (Roley and Schneck, chapter 15), children with cerebral palsy (Blanche and Nakasuji, chapter 16), children with autism (Mailloux, chapter 17), institutionalized occupationally deprived children (Cermak, chapter 18), Fragile X Syndrome (Hickman, chapter 19), and Down Syndrome (Giuffrida, chapter 8). These chapters illustrate what sensory integration theory and practice add beyond the knowledge and practices of other orientations.

One theme that consistently emerges from the chapters in this volume is that although sensory integration theory was intended to be a scientific theory, it has given rise to an intervention approach with a particular philosophy. The core of this philosophy is that intervention should occur in a context characterized by playfulness and compassion in which provision of sensory experiences is carefully monitored by a trained therapist. For example, in her chapter on regulation, arousal, and attention, Reeves describes intervention as creating opportunities to facilitate appropriate adaptive responses. And in her chapter on autism, Mailloux describes the importance of a safe and comfortable environment in which a variety of sensations can be experienced and interpreted. No matter where or with which population the sensory integration approach is being practiced, what one should witness is a person engaged in challenging activities that are neither stressful nor boring, that are satisfying and fun, and from which confidence and competence are built.

Given this philosophy, and based on her dissertation research, Blanche applies sensory integration theory to the more general concern of lifestyle redesign for all people. Blanche reports that she found that adults naturally pursue occupations that nourish their sensory needs. Her work suggests that creative applications of sensory integration theory to human existence in general may result in healthier and happier individuals. Individuals who are able to assess their sensory needs and develop a customized plan of activity are enabled to develop their capacities, reduce stress, and transform their lives in positive ways. This volume takes sensory integration theory to a new level of excellence and positions it to have a significant impact on much of humanity.

References

Ayres, J. Sensory Integration and Learning Disorders. (1972). Los Angeles, California: Western Psychological Services.

Ayres, J. Sensory Integration and the Child. (1979). Los Angeles, California: Western Psychological Services.

Hoshmand, L. T., & Polkinghorne, D. E. (1992). Redefining the Science-Practice Relationship and Professional Training. American Psychologist, 47, 55-65.

Wilcock, A. A. An Occupational Perspective of Health. (1998). Thorofare, New Jersey: SLACK Incorporated.

Preface

Susanne Smith Roley, M.S., OTR

Erna Imperatore Blanche, Ph.D., OTR, FAOTA

Roseann C. Schaaf, M.Ed., OTR/L, FAOTA

Dr. A. Jean Ayres, founder of sensory integration as used in occupational therapy, applied the theory of sensory integration to a variety of diagnostic groups throughout her career (1972a, 1979). The classic promotional film on sensory integration, *Help Me Be Me* (Brown, 1974), contains a memorable scene in which an adult woman with developmental disabilities is unable to crack an egg. The narration identifies this woman as having dyspraxia and poor integration of vestibular/proprioceptive sensations necessary for postural control and insecurity with movement against gravity. Also featured in this film are children with Autistic Disorder, learning disabilities, and attention-deficit disorders. Ayres recognized that many individuals with developmental, physical, socioemotional, and/or cognitive disabilities demonstrate inabilities to process, integrate, and utilize sensory information adequately. This film graphically displays the applicability of sensory integration theory and practice to diverse populations of individuals with disabilities.

Sensory integration became best known and used with children experiencing learning and behavior problems during the time Ayres was developing the *Southern California Sensory Integration Tests* (SCSIT; 1972b) and their revision, the *Sensory Integration and Praxis Tests* (SIPT; 1989), largely because research funding was available to study learning disabilities in the 1970s. Ayres designed the SCSIT and subsequently the SIPT not only to detect and determine the nature of an individual's hidden deficits in sensory integration but also to validate her theory of sensory integration (1980, 1989). In the SCSIT manual dated 1980, Ayres pointed out that individuals with learning disabilities constituted the main population on which she had based the development of sensory integration theory. However, she recognized that her theory and intervention principles extended beyond children with learning disabilities (1989). Many children with developmental disabilities exhibit dysfunction in sensory integration, and these deficits in sensory integration often interfere with these children's abilities to function even more than their primary diagnoses. Accordingly, this book not only documents the current state of practice using sensory integration theory but also challenges practitioners and researchers to move beyond its traditional use and applications.

The interrelationship between the process of sensory integration and daily life is apparent to those who have lived with the consequences of disability and sensory integrative deficits. One of the editors of this book grew up with two brothers with Fragile X syndrome. The debilitating effects of sensory integrative dysfunction have been obvious in her brothers. Both of Susanne's brothers, Keith and Paul, were labeled educable mentally retarded. Not until 1989 were their disabilities diagnosed as Fragile X syndrome, a genetically-based disorder characterized by mental retardation, generalized low tone, anxiety, poor eye contact, difficulty coping with social situations, and sensitivity to sensory stimuli (Hagerman, 1996).

As children, Keith and Paul received special education. Unfortunately, they did not qualify for any therapy services because their tested cognitive level was equivalent to their functioning level. Following high school, Keith and Paul lived independently and worked full time, capable of routine activities of daily living. Although their ability to follow rote routines allowed independence, they had very little social contact and were unable to alter their routine without assistance. Complications in daily life, such as a malfunctioning water softener or missing the bus, were overwhelming for them. At one point when Paul and Keith were harassed by a group of young teenage boys, they became so distressed that they refused to open the window shades of their house ever again.

When Paul died unexpectedly, Keith became depressed and disoriented and was unable to continue working. He could not manage time or carry out his activities of daily living. The grieving process amplified Keith's deficits in self-regulation, praxis, sensory modulation, and social language. He required hospitalization for depression. The professionals providing treatments for Keith's depression failed to realize the extent of his preexisting self-regulatory difficulties. The changes in routine, hospitalization, and novelty of contexts following Paul's death added to his feelings of anxiety and loss of control. Consequently, Keith lost not only his best and only friend, his job, and his home, but all of his independence.

Keith, not unlike most individuals without disabilities, had chosen a daily occupation (bus boy) that gave him a sense of mastery, nourished his sensory needs, and provided stability to his life. However, when he most needed this daily occupation to meet the stresses encountered in his present state, it was no longer available to him. From a sensory point of view, he no longer reaped the calming and organizing benefits of carrying heavy trays for 8 hours a day, 6 days a week. Rather than living and working as part of his neighborhood community, Keith's participation in typical contexts decreased, and he required maximum supports from the social service community. It was only after crisis that he became eligible to receive a wide variety of services that had not previously been available to him.

The questions are ever-present and plentiful in hindsight: What would have been the outcome if Keith had received sensory integrative intervention? Could he have developed a broader base of social support? Could he have maintained his self-regulatory abilities in the midst of a life-altering event? With minimal modifications, could he have recovered more quickly to regain the independent lifestyle that he had created? Although more research is necessary to further validate and replicate the effects of a sensory integrative approach, anecdotal and case-study evidence is abundant (Blanche, Botticelli, & Hallway, 1995; Daems, 1994; Parham, 1998; Parham & Mailloux, 1996; Schaaf, 1990; Schaaf, Merrill, & Kinsella, 1987). Individuals like Paul and Keith who have functional deficits physically, socially, and emotionally, not only because of their diagnosis but also because of the resulting sensory integrative dysfunction, cannot wait for the labors of research and the politics of funding to catch up with the theoretical and practical advances.

This book continues the discussion and development of the therapeutic use of sensory integration theory and the application of sensory integration principles to diverse populations. To support the clinical reasoning process, researchers, theoreticians, and practitioners explore and expand sensory integration theory. The authors of the theoretical section of this text (chapters 1 through 10) include data and literature from diverse fields such as occupational science, psychobiology, psychology, neuroscience, and child development to support and extend the theoretical principles of sensory integration and their application to diverse populations. The clinical section (chapters 11 through 20) presents a combination of qualitative and quantitative data-gathering, clinical-reasoning strategies and intervention principles that guide examination of the impact of sensory integration function and dysfunction in individuals with developmental disabilities. These clinical chapters present the application of sensory integration theory and intervention principles to children with known developmental delays (visual impairment, cerebral palsy, Autistic Disorder, and Fragile X syndrome) and children who have not necessarily been identified with developmental delays (children with sensory modulation disorders, high-risk infants, and children exposed to environmental deprivation).

The information provided by the scholars, researchers, and clinicians contributing to this book is a significant step forward in the understanding of the difficulties, possibilities, and strategies for individuals with disabilities. It is our hope that this project will be a foundation that furthers advancements in the understanding and application of sensory integration.

References

Ayres, A.J. (1972a). *Sensory integration and learning disorders*. Los Angeles: Western Psychological Services.

Ayres, A.J. (1972b). *Southern California Sensory Integration Tests*. Los Angeles: Western Psychological Services.

Ayres, A.J. (1979). *Sensory integration and the child*. Los Angeles: Western Psychological Services.

Ayres, A.J. (1980). *Southern California Sensory Integration Tests Manual—Revised*. Los Angeles: Western Psychological Services.

Ayres, A.J. (1989). *Sensory Integration and Praxis Tests*. Los Angeles: Western Psychological Services.

Blanche, E.I., Botticelli, T.M., & Hallway, M.K. (1995). *Combining neuro-developmental treatment and sensory integration principles: An approach to pediatric therapy*. Tucson, AZ: Therapy Skill Builders.

Brown, D. (Writer & Director). (1975). *Help me be me* [Film]. (Available from Earth Links, 519 Seabright Avenue, Suite #103, Santa Cruz, CA 95062)

Daems, J. (Ed.). (1994). *Reviews of research in sensory integration*. Torrance, CA: Sensory Integration International.

Hagerman, R.J. (1996). Physical and behavioral phenotype. In R.J. Hagerman & A. Cronister (Eds.), *Fragile X syndrome: Diagnosis, treatment and research* (2nd ed., pp. 3–87). Baltimore, MD: The Johns Hopkins University Press.

Parham, L.D. (1998). The relationship of sensory integrative development to achievement in elementary students: Four-year longitudinal patterns. *Occupational Therapy Journal of Research, 18*(3), 105–127.

Parham, L.D., & Mailloux, Z. (1996). Sensory integration. In J. Case-Smith, A.S. Allen, & P.N. Pratt (Eds.), *Occupational therapy for children* (3rd ed., pp. 307–355). St. Louis: Mosby-Year Book, Inc.

Schaaf, R. (1990). Play behavior and occupational therapy. *American Journal of Occupational Therapy, 44*, 68–75.

Schaaf, R., Merrill, S., & Kinsella, N. (1987). Sensory integration and play behavior: A case study of the effectiveness of occupational therapy using sensory integrative techniques. *Occupational Therapy in Health Care, 4*(2), 61–75.

Acknowledgments

We wish to extend sincere appreciation to all of our mentors, co-workers, colleagues, students, and others who have contributed to our professional growth and who have supported this project. We especially want to thank all of the children and families. You have taught us the importance of sensory integration in everyday life and made this book possible.

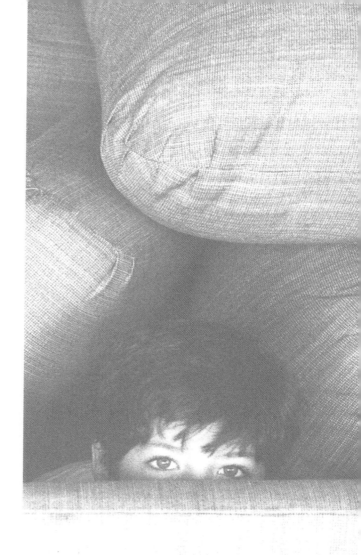

Sensory Integration Revisited:

A Philosophy of Practice

Susan Spitzer, M.A., OTR

Susanne Smith Roley, M.S., OTR

Dr. A. Jean Ayres originated the theory of sensory integration and was responsible for bringing to consciousness a way of looking at children that had not been done before (Kovalenko, in Roley & Wilbarger, 1994). Sensory integration has uncovered complex neurological processes that are foundational for an individual's participation in meaningful daily occupations. Although this theory and its application have flourished and developed since Dr. Ayres' original work, it is a frame of reference that continues to reflect the heart, mind, and soul of this remarkable woman. It is her original work that defines the philosophy of sensory integration and sets it apart from other types of interventions utilized within the field of occupational therapy.

Dr. A. Jean Ayres

The groundwork done by Dr. Ayres throughout her professional life has remained as both the infrastructure and the authority for theory development in sensory integration. Dr. Ayres epitomizes the archetype of the wounded healer (L. Kovalenko, in Roley & Wilbarger, 1994). Anna Jean Ayres was a frail child (Sieg, 1988) who suffered from her own "hidden disorders," which undoubtedly influenced her choice of a vocation, her practice, and her research. She was driven to investigate the hidden disorders that interfered with learning and behavior. Dr. Ayres became a scholar, investigating and acquiring knowledge of the neurophysiologic underpinnings of behavior. She studied the literature in neurology, psychology, and ontogenetic and phylogenetic development. She utilized her keen analytic abilities to create a remarkably detailed and sophisticated series of tests that could assess and document hidden disabilities. She created intervention strategies and equipment based on her understanding of typical development, believing that the child's innate drive to develop emerged through play.

Her deep understanding of hidden sensory integration disorders shaped Dr. Ayres' empathic intervention with her clients. For example, determining that a child was becoming suddenly unruly because of tactile defensiveness, she stated, "Sometimes that type of touch can be bothersome" (Brown, 1975). She invited children into an activity, asking questions and making comments such as, *Would you like the handles? What a marvelous idea to pick up those beanbags! What might happen if you put them in your pockets while you climbed the ladder?* If a child "misbehaved," she validated and acknowledged the difficulty of an activity with a comment such as, *That must have been very difficult for you. Perhaps you might try again next time.* She anticipated the sensory and praxis needs of a child, noting, *You've had enough of that swing? Let me help you like this. You figure out how to put your leg over while I stand here and hold the tire.* She motivated voluntary participation by tapping the child's innate drive to learn and play. Children bonded with her and depended on her quiet, consistent presence. She provided only enough assistance to ensure their success while introducing just a small additional challenge. She called the relationship between clients and the therapist utilizing sensory integration principles the "art of therapy" (Ayres, 1972a).

Dr. Ayres exhibited enormous respect for the children whom she served. Her style of intervention demonstrated a philosophy of compassion and respect for the individual's drive to develop his or her own nervous system through self-motivated interaction with the environment. Based on this compassion and respect, the therapist must probe beyond the obvious and investigate the subtleties underlying the child's presenting issues of sleepiness, overstimulation, inattention, fear, clumsiness, lack of motivation, antisocial attitude, or depression. The therapist cares whether the child is happy or knows how to play, and enjoys a child's unique person whatever his or her range of age-appropriate functional skills.

Dr. Ayres' work was ahead of the consciousness of her time (Kovalenko, in Roley & Wilbarger, 1994). Currently, most pediatric texts in occupational therapy reference sensory integration principles. The concepts have spread well beyond the profession of occupational therapy and are now commonplace, evident in natural settings in every city in the United States in such places as Gymborees and other play gyms. Participants in school meetings commonly discuss such sensory integrative terms as "tactile defensiveness." However, despite the widespread use of sensory integration, debates about the validity of sensory integrative concepts and interventions continue. This level of passionate discussion informally validates sensory integration as a theory worthy of debate (Kielhofner, 1992).

Much of the passion for sensory integration springs from its core philosophy as well as the variance between individual experiences with this approach. Its gentle, child-led, playful, yet intellectually demanding nature tends to generate intense emotions and commitment on the part of those who utilize it. The sensory integration frame of reference was developed within, and continues to be suited ideally for, the profession of occupational therapy. Sensory integration theory provides a scientific foundation for techniques that support the arousal, affect, and motivation of children and that result in experiencing a sense of well being, engagement, and mastery.

Clients who are the direct recipients of this approach perceive the intervention as pleasurable and anticipate the sessions with enthusiasm. Parents and other caregivers often feel awe and relief at finding an intervention that contributes to the health and well being of their child and family. The comments of one mother in comparing another therapeutic approach with the sensory integrative approach illustrate this point:

> I could not stand to watch my child cry every time we drove into the parking lot for therapy. One time my child was screaming and the therapist said that they just had to work through my child's resistance. It turned out that the therapist had stretched my child's tendon until it had torn. I never went back [to that first therapist]. It seems like this sensory integrative approach has the same goals, but you were also concerned that my daughter was happy. You played with her and made her smile. She was relaxed and easy to handle when we left therapy. You looked beyond her spasticity. You accepted her and liked her the way she was (Mother of a child with cerebral palsy, personal communication, 1986).

Sensory Integration: A Foundation for Occupation

Sensory integration is "the organization of sensory input for use" (Ayres, 1979, p. 184). Sensory integration is the foundation for adaptive responses to challenges imposed by the environment and learning. As such, it is a natural outcome of typical development (Turkewitz, 1994). Normal sensory integrative abilities provide the foundation that enables meaningful and purposeful participation in a full range of daily occupations (see Figure 1.1). Sensory integration theory considers the dynamic interactions between the person's abilities or disabilities and how they act or interact with their environment.

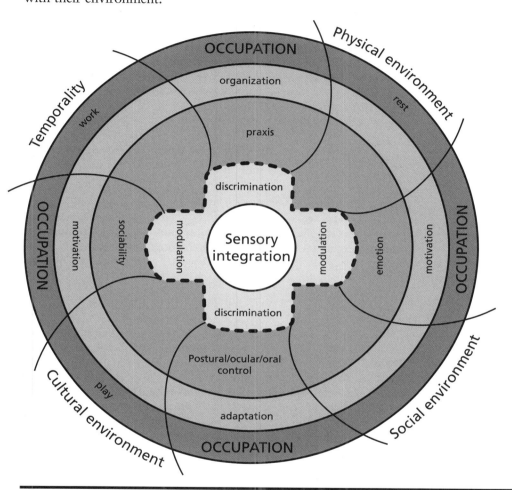

Figure 1.1. Dynamic process of sensory integration

The relationship of sensory integration to engagement in daily occupations resembles a rolling wheel. In this case, sensory integration is the hub. The spokes are sensory modulation, supporting social engagement and emotional well being, and sensory discrimination, supporting praxic skills and postural, ocular, and oral control. These spokes link to a rim of adaptation, motivation, and organization. The wheel supports the tier of occupations— work, play, leisure, and rest. This wheel spins in an occupational context of the physical, social, and cultural environments. The wheel (in its entirety and in its parts) and the environment are in constant interaction, exerting forces on each other. In the case of the sensory integrative wheel, the degree of flexibility and interaction with the occupational context can be much greater than that of a literal wheel rolling through physical space.

The core theoretical components of sensory integration are (a) the necessity of integrated sensation, (b) the adaptive response and self-direction, (c) the dynamic process of sensory integration, and (d) the role of sensory integration in typical development. Review of these components helps explain the contributions of sensory integration to health, well being, and occupation.

Necessity of Integrated Sensation

The literature on environmental enrichment and deprivation provides evidence that healthy individuals require salient interactions with the environment that provide accurate sensory information to their central nervous systems (Lane, 1997). Ayres originally described sensation as food that "nourish(es) the brain" (1979, p. 7), a metaphor elaborated upon by Wilbarger (1995), who coined the phrase "sensory diet." The individual's abilities to register and process the type, quantity, and intensity of sensation provided by the environment result in behaviors and feeling states that are either organized or disorganized. Physical environmental factors such as prenatal stress can cause sensory integrative deficits (see chapter 14, Sensory Integration for High-Risk Infants and Young Children, by Schaaf & Anzalone). Interactions with a child in care-giving activities can influence a child's physiological functioning (i.e., arousal and self-regulation) (Holloway, 1997). Relationships also influence physiological regulation (Hofer, 1995). Psychobiological research indicates that the mother-infant interactions and individual biological regulation influence an infant's activity level (New York State Psychiatric Institute, 1996). When assessing regulatory abilities or optimum level of sensory nourishment, it is important, therefore, not to examine the individual out of context. Rather, the focus of assessment must be the types of sensation that the individual processes within the ever-changing sociocultural and physical environments in which his or her occupations occur.

Most people in today's western society discuss the "five senses" of sight, touch, hearing, smell, and taste as the gateway to sensual life experiences. Sensory integration theory has recognized a more encompassing view of sensation that includes the various aspects of touch (including pain, temperature, deep pressure, and vibration) as well as other sensory systems (such as perception of movement, gravity, muscle tension, joint position, and tendon stretch). Recent studies have acknowledged the influence of other types of sensations such as those received by the viscera (i.e., interoceptors) (Porges, 1993) and those generated by electrical, chemical, vibratory, barometric pressure, and electromagnetic energy (Gallagher, 1993; Sandyk, 1996).

A brief review of one of the most widely researched sensations, pain, illustrates the complexity of sensation. Melzack and Wall (1973) demonstrated that pain is not attached to any specific skin or tissue site, although damage to skin or tissue frequently triggers pain. Damaged tissue does not always yield pain: some individuals feel pleasure in conditions that damage tissue, and some do not register any sensation at all even with life-threatening wounds. Individuals can experience and perceive pain to emanate from limbs that no longer exist (phantom pain), as well as from many locations on the body, such as a stomachache, headache, backache, general body aches, etc. The intensity with which an individual perceives pain varies depending on the individual's threshold, past experience, anticipation of the experience, self-control, breathing techniques, and medication (Montegue, 1978). Emotional pain unrelated to personal physical injury can be devastating to occupational performance and health. All sensations most likely are as complex as pain, and researchers have yet to examine them as thoroughly as pain.

Researchers frequently study sensory systems in isolation (e.g., the role of vision in depth perception or the role of the vestibular system in the detection of movement and gravity). This "single-systems" approach lends depth to the understanding of each specific system. Functionally, however, the integration of sensation from various sensory modalities is essential for interpreting typical multisensory contexts. Ayres' factor analyses suggested that certain sensory systems function together to facilitate perception (Ayres, 1965, 1966a, 1966b, 1969, 1971, 1972a, 1972b, 1972c, 1972d, 1976, 1977, 1986, 1989b). For example, the proprioceptive and tactile systems typically work together to provide a basis for body awareness and praxis, and the visual and auditory systems work together in the perception of written and verbal language (Ayres, 1989b). These same data indicate that children with sensory integrative dysfunction might use different sensory combination strategies to perform tasks than do children without sensory integrative dysfunction. For example, a child with sensory integrative dysfunction might combine vision with proprioception, or vestibular with auditory processing. Clinically, frequent observation of children with sensory integrative dysfunction indicates that children with sensory processing deficits rely more heavily on visual data to perform skilled actions than do children who are developing typically. Therefore it is important not only to examine how the sensory systems function together but also to consider how children with sensory integration problems use their sensory systems to compensate for deficits.

Ayres (1972a) cited neuroscientific evidence to support the view that "multisensory stimuli are more effective than messages from one modality only" (p. 30). That is, the individual is more likely to detect an event that provides multisensory input and to respond more quickly (Streri, 1993). Neuroscientific research continues to support the importance of convergence of multisensory input and the interrelatedness of the sensory systems (Wallace, Wilkinson, & Stein, 1996). Neuroscientists also have researched how sensory integration occurs in the brain. They have attempted to identify the location, incidence, and properties of neurons that respond to multisensory cues (e.g., Blair & Thompson, 1995; Regan, He, & Regan, 1995; Wallace et. al.). Others have explained how specific types of sensory input are integrated and involved in cognitive functions such as the abstract representation of space and intention (Anderson, 1995). Interestingly, this relatively recent neuroscientific research supports the original theory developed by Ayres in 1972. She noted that "[it is not] appropriate to think in terms of isolated sensory modality development or function...[because this] is not the major means by which the brain functions" (1972a, p. 31).

According to sensory integration theory, the tactile/proprioceptive and vestibular/proprioceptive systems interact routinely with the auditory and visual systems to supply the multimodal sensory information needed to make a meaningful motor response. From a sensory integrative perspective, the investigation of multimodal processing relationships is of greatest importance. The factor analyses of the *Southern California Sensory Integration Tests* (SCSIT; Ayres, 1972c) and later the *Sensory Integration and Praxis Tests* (SIPT; Ayres, 1989a) provide evidence of consistent relationships between specific sensory areas. Ayres demonstrated relationships between these senses and other systems related to cognitive and motor functions (Ayres, 1965, 1966a, 1966b, 1972b, 1972d, 1974, 1977, 1986, 1989b). See Table 12.2 in Chapter 12: Assessment of Sensory Integration and Praxis, by Windsor, Smith Roley, and Szklut.

Turkewitz and Kenny (1982) proposed that during development, the timing of the onset of the interactions between the sensory systems is instrumental in determining the relationships between systems and in shaping the nature of functioning within a single modality. "Exposure to similar [sensory] circumstances at different stages of development can have radically different consequences" (Turkewitz, 1994, p. 11). Earlier-than-normal introduction of visual input can have a negative influence on the processing capabilities of other sensory modalities, specifically auditory attention in premature children (Turkewitz, 1994). He proposed that auditory attention deficits are mediated by a sensory threshold mechanism rather than or in addition to an attentional one.

The Adaptive Response and Self-Direction

Although the integration of sensations is critical to function, it is of minimal use to the organism without the capacity to react to those sensations in a meaningful way. The individual must have self-motivated, purposeful, and increasingly adaptive responses in order to continue to grow as an individual. Dr. Ayres believed that this drive to be adaptive in an ever-changing environment is innate and that, given the appropriate level of challenge, the nervous system would present itself with opportunities for increased neuronal growth through an adaptive response.

One of the most common misinterpretations made by those unfamiliar with the theory of sensory integration is an overemphasis on sensation. Sensory stimulation, as opposed to sensory integration, does not have the concomitant focus on the integration of that sensation, the organization of the information for a future plan of behavior, action, or reaction, and the monitoring of the action plan in motion. Although sensation is indeed an important feature, SI theory does not approach the individual as the passive recipient of environmentally imposed stimuli. The individual not only processes sensation but also organizes and integrates it to form a meaningful outcome.

A meaningful outcome occurs through what Ayres called the adaptive response, an adjustment to some environmental demand (Ayres, 1972a, 1979). Adaptive behaviors include but are not restricted to motor, or action-oriented, responses. A physical adaptive response might be an increase in postural control, a more sustained tonic support of a position, or moving one's eyes in the direction of the mother's voice. An adaptive response might be a more organized autonomic nervous system reaction that can have physiological correlates (such as improved respiration and heart rates, digestive functions, and sleep/wake cycles) that are not all easily observable. An affective adaptive response might be increased emotional stability under stressed conditions (such as the absence of a primary caregiver, slightly less sleep, or an unfamiliar transition). An adaptive response also might mean a more organized response to a given routine, such that the temporal-spatial sequencing of the response is more rhythmic and fluid, such as being able to run and kick a moving soccer ball.

Implicit in the concept of the adaptive response is the active participation of the individual, who thereby actively processes and organizes responses to the changing environment. Adaptive response is, in effect, a measure of the individual's ability to cope and successfully meet an environmental challenge. Whether the individual's response is adaptive or not depends on the individual, his or her developmental level, the level of previously acquired skill, and his or her degree of sensory integration (Ayres, 1972a). The more highly integrated the individual, the more complex, age-appropriate adaptive responses are expected. Less complex actions would constitute an adaptive response for an individual with less mature sensory integration. Habitual action or behavioral patterns require no adaptive capacities unless there is a change in the demand from the environment. In order to raise the adaptive response level of the individual, elements of both the social and physical environment must tax the individual's capacity for coping at least slightly. The child must be responding more adaptively, more effectively than he or she was able to do previously (Ayres, 1972a). The adaptive response is moment-by-moment specific. What is adaptive in one minute might be habitual the next. The adaptive response encompasses diverse systems that support occupational performance, including homeostatic mechanisms, affective states, cognitive and attention components, as well as action and motor-related systems.

One of the most confusing aspects of the adaptive response concept is its apparently circular definition in sensory integration theory. An adaptive response is both an indicator of and a promoter of sensory integration—an indicator of the degree of sensory integration because "the effectiveness of the response is dependent upon the accuracy of the sensory feedback" during the response (Ayres, 1972a, p. 127), and a promoter of sensory integration because "[w]hen the muscles work together to form an adaptive body movement, those muscles and joints send well-organized sensations to the brain" (Ayres, 1979, p. 143). The concept of an adaptive response is elusive, at best. An individual's precise adaptive response is not predictable (Ayres, 1972a; Spitzer, 1999).

The Dynamic Process of Sensory Integration

Spitzer (1999) has characterized sensory integration as a dynamic process. As a dynamic process, sensory integration is a self-organizing activity of the individual interacting within an environmental context. The individual gains and organizes sensory information through interactions with the environment. "Sensory integration sorts, orders, and eventually puts all of the individual sensory inputs together into a whole brain function" (Ayres, 1979 p. 28). What emerges from this process is increasingly complex behavior, the adaptive response, and occupational engagement. "When the functions of the brain are whole and balanced, body movements are highly adaptive, learning is easy, and good behavior is a natural outcome" (Ayres, 1979, p. 28). In fact, Lewkowicz and Lickliter (1994) assert that the interactions between the sensory systems enable development. It is the complexity and comprehensiveness of sensory integration theory that allows therapists to examine the interactions of these processes as well as to create strategies for enhancing adaptive behavior (see Table 1.1).

The consideration of sensory integration as a dynamic system helps therapists to look beyond a single-system view of sensory analysis with the clients. For example, individuals with visual impairment often have concomitant difficulties in the areas of fine and gross motor functions, sensory modulation, praxis, language, and social and cognitive skills (Chen & Dote-Kwan, 1995). Frequently, it is assumed that the deficits are related to the visual impairment. But observations of typically developing individuals with blindness indicate wide variability in their functional abilities. From a sensory-integrative perspective, it is important to consider the potential multisensory ramifications of a single system loss. See Chapter 15: Sensory Integration and Visual Deficits, Including Blindness, by Roley and Schneck.

Ayres' theoretical development in the area of dynamic systems was ahead of her time. Other theorists did not propose dynamic systems models until the 1980s. The theoretical paradigms in use at the time, such as general systems theory, simply could not account for emergent phenomena. More recent theoretical developments in dynamic systems theory might help explicate the complexity of emergent behavior in sensory integration (Spitzer, 1999) (see Table 1.2). Dynamic systems theory originated in physics, and researchers in biology and human development now are applying it to their fields of study. It is the currently and increasingly accepted model for studying the complexity of emergent behavior, replacing general systems theory. It appears that the recent theoretical developments of dynamic systems theory might, in certain respects, better support and lend credibility to sensory integration than have previous theoretical paradigms. However, it is important to be cautious in making any applications of dynamic systems theory to sensory integration without further investigation (Spitzer, 1999; Streri, 1993).

The complexity of sensory integration as a dynamic process is at the crux of frequent misunderstandings for new therapists, students, parents, and other professionals. On the surface, without a deep knowledge of sensory integration, it can be difficult to see how therapy relates to the child's goals and objectives. Consider, for example, a child who has anencephaly with subsequent cerebral palsy and global developmental delays. The therapist creates functional mobility, eating, and feeding goals and objectives with the family. The child comes for therapy. The child screams if anyone tries

Table 1.1. Analysis of Sensory Experience

Impulse	Modalities	Arousal	Memory	Perception	Effort	Action
internal sensory event	temperature	—	—	—	—	—
	pain	registration	—	significance	motivation	—
	vibration	—	habituation	—	attention	—
	vestibular	orientation	—	associations	—	goal-oriented management of time and activity
	proprioception	modulation	internal motor maps	synthesis	motor skills	exploring and manipulating the environment
external stimulus event	tactile	emotion	—	—	selection/organization of behavior	participating member of society/culture
	taste	—	internal sensory maps	—	responding adaptively	—
	smell	—	—	—	—	—
	auditory	—	sensory recognition	discrimination	—	engaging in occupation
	visual	—	feedforward	feedback	praxis	reflection and lifestyle adjustments

Experiencing sensation is a hidden process of complex nonlinear relationships that support effort and action. The person both generates and experiences sensation from a variety of modalities that are modulated, matched with existing memories, synthesized into perceptions, and utilized for all aspects of interaction and occupation. The very act of experiencing sensation alters the nature of the individual and the way in which the individual experiences sensation.

Table 1.2. The Relationship of Dynamic Systems Theory to Sensory Integration and Resulting Implications

Key Concepts in Dynamic Systems Theory	Comparison to Sensory Integration Theory	Issues and Opportunities Raised
Emergence of Behavior: occurs through an interaction of factors; nonlinear; not predetermined or programmed	SI (intersensory integration) is the foundation for more complex behaviors to emerge (Ayres, 1972a).	Difficult to predict the precise result of therapy (practice or research); we cannot "know" a priori (Ayres, 1972a; Cool, 1995). Need to develop better ways to measure outcomes/effectiveness.
Environmental Interaction: open system must interact with the environment or it dies; behavior emerges in particular environmental and task contexts (Thelen & Ulrich, 1991)	A rich sensory environment is critical to the development of sensory integration (Ayres, 1979; Merrill, 1990).	Reinforces the importance of context (intervention context and context of daily life).
Self-Organization: only the person can organize itself; a spontaneous process of finding new solutions when the old solutions no longer work (Kamm, Thelen, & Jensen, 1990)	Child-directed therapy; the child is encouraged to be an active participant in own therapy (Ayres, 1972a, 1979).	Reinforces the centrality of the child's active role in therapy.
Attractor States: a relatively stable state or pattern of behaviors to which the system is drawn (Thelen & Ulrich, 1991) **Phase Shifts:** the transitions from one attractor state to another	Increasingly complex patterns of behavior are called an adaptive response (Ayres, 1972a, 1979). Intervention baseline and outcomes (targeted behavior/skill) can be conceptualized as attractor states.	A therapeutic or naturally occurring "push" can be necessary to help a child move from one pattern of behaviors (level of participation in occupations) to another, more complex level of participation in occupations.
Control Parameter: the primary factor responsible for a phase shift; its role differs in significance with each phase shift (heterarchy model)	Sensory input and the adaptive response can be conceptualized as control parameters in SI. Nervous system can be conceptualized as a control parameter in occupation. SI emphasizes role of the nervous system, primarily using a modified hierarchy model.	Need to consider other control parameters (outside the nervous system) in assessment and intervention. Might want more research/theory development on more specifically identifying control parameters. When is the nervous system (or sensory integration) the control parameter for engagement in occupation? How should the nervous system be conceptualized?
Disorganization: phase shifts occur through initial disorganization (control parameter destabilizes system, prompting the system to reorganize itself)	Formal theory suggests SI as an increasingly ordered process (Ayres, 1972a) SI also has a spiral quality (Ayres, 1972a; Fisher & Murray, 1991) Some level of anxiety/risk is present in the "just-right challenge" (Dunkerley, Tickle-Degnen, & Coster, 1997; Koomar, 1997)	What is the role of disorganization during intervention? how much? when? (more information is needed to guide clinical reasoning)

to handle him. The therapist spends three sessions holding the child, wrapped tightly, and bouncing gently on a swing, which is the only interaction the child will tolerate. At the end of this time, the mother reports that the child is using gestures and sounds to ask for juice for the first time and is happier. The hidden complexity for this child was that he had difficulty tolerating moving in space and an upright posture.

The therapist stabilized posture and helped the child to tolerate an upright position, and the child was able to sit up, decrease his anxiety level, and begin to socialize with his mother. Although the intervention might look like simple sensory stimulation to the untrained observer, the complexities of these outcomes demonstrate that the dynamic process of sensory integration is anything but simple.

The therapist must feel comfortable in his or her role providing this gentle, nurturing form of therapy. Skilled intervention emerges with increased knowledge of the theoretical foundations along with respect for the child's affective communication, reading autonomic nervous system signs, and making inferences about sensory processing. Sensory integrative procedures help organize the child before and during the work on more action-oriented goals potentially utilizing another frame of reference in conjunction with sensory integration. Improved social communication is a functional outcome that one might not have been able to predict initially from working on the general goal of modulating arousal levels.

This example illustrates how difficult it is to predict a one-to-one cause-and-effect relationship between intervention and outcomes. The "determination of the amount of increased integration resulting from therapy is particularly difficult, for it appears in behavior apparently unrelated to the activity" (Ayres, 1972a, p. 262). Instead, the outcomes *emerge* from the intervention. In a strict sensory integrative approach, the therapist seldom works directly on acquiring a specific skill but works rather on the foundation necessary to build that skill. For example, in order to promote attention for tabletop activities, a therapist might offer the child a variety of gross motor activities that provide proprioceptive-vestibular input to help the child modulate arousal level rather than focus intervention on attention per se.

Furthermore, a therapist cannot simply provide more vestibular input and expect a proportional increase in balance reactions. An example of the nonlinear outcomes might be that the child responds to intervention with improved auditory comprehension without further changes in balance reactions.

The Role of Sensory Integration in Development

Sensory integration occurs throughout development (see Table 1.3). The theory assumes that maturation is the process of the unfolding of the genetic coding in conjunction with the interaction of the individual with the physical and social environment (see chapter 14, Sensory Integration for High-Risk Infants and Young Children, by Schaaf & Anzalone). As a result of experience, there are changes within the nervous system (see chapter 2, Neuroplasticity and the Environment: Implications for Sensory Integration, by Jacobs & Schneider). Experience is the dynamic interaction between the individual and the environment. The dynamic interactions create structural and functional nervous system changes in the "ecological brain" (Shore, 1996). The role of the nervous system is critical in the integration of information and expression of the individual's potential.

Sensory integration theory proposes that, by providing an optimal sensory environment and inviting active participation of the individual, both structural and functional growth occurs within central nervous system. Studies of environmental enrichment support this proposition (Diamond, 1988; Rakic, Bourgeois, & Goldman-Rakic, 1994). Participation in an optimal sensory environment improves the child's ability to

Table 1.3. The Role of Sensory Integration in Development

Prenatal Period	Neonatal Period	1 to 6 Months	6 to 12 Months	Second Year	3 to 7 Years
5.5 weeks gestation: response to tactile stimuli: avoidant reaction	Tactile sensations: maternal-infant bond uses touch for comfort uses touch for feeding	Tactile-visual exploration Three-dimensional perception Tactile proprioceptive Differentiating self/nonself Exploration of caregiver as extension of self	Tactile skills refined: developing hand skills Vision maps to leg muscles	Tactile guiding skills with fine motor and general praxis	Developing skilled tool use Somatosensory dominance for postural control
9 weeks gestation: approach reaction head to chest: proprioceptive reaction	Proprioception: molding to caregiver's body Phasic movements of limbs provide proprioception and continue development of body scheme	Vestibular-proprioceptive-visual integration provides beginning postural control Weight bearing on forearms and hands Tactile maps to neck	Beginning bilateral motor control, crawling, creeping, pull to stand	Body scheme developing well and contributing to body concept and image	Gauges own strength and size for hugs, pouring, sitting in a group
Reflexes such as rooting, sucking, Babkin, grasp, flexor withdrawal, Galant, and neck righting Last 6–8 weeks gestation: integrating inverted position	Vestibular maps to neck used to modify arousal Beginning neck control	Increasing mastery of posture against gravity Transitional movements Multisensory mapping for head control	Moving through space, postural control of movements, including those against gravity	Improving balance and postural control while holding still and moving	Good balance Coordinated during simple active sports such as soccer Bike riding
After about 28 weeks gestation: sees light hears and remembers familiar sounds and voices	Visual and auditory systems immature Recognizes familiar sounds from in utero Likes to look at high-contrast images and faces	Primarily receptive to visual and auditory information; beginning discrimination of location and distance Visual system maps to neck	Repetitive sounds and later dissimilar sounds Putting gestures with words	Use of language Creating feelings of control over the environment	Complex auditory discrimination and language interpretation Reduced visual guidance of posture
		Beginning motor planning: mouth and facial movements, then eye and hand	Increasingly complex motor planning, including limbs and body and use of tools	Ideation becomes creative and imaginative	Can cooperate in a group, take turns, and create and follow complex play

use environmental data more appropriately. It is this focus on the "use" of the neurological processing of sensory input that is the unique focus and research application within occupational therapy (Parham & Mailloux, 1996).

Building Occupational Performance

Although many components of activities and participation might be influenced by sensory integration, there are several key performance components that rely extensively on sensory integration. These performance components are sensory registration, modulation, discrimination, and praxis. Registration of sensation is the detection of stimuli from the body and or the environment. It is essential for all later processing and attention to environmental stimuli. Modulation of sensation is fundamental to functioning because it enables a child to match his or her arousal, attention, and activity level to the demands of the environment without being distracted by irrelevant sensory input. Discrimination of sensation is essential for the development of skilled function, including postural background adjustments and tone, projected action sequences, and skilled motor function. Praxis is a complex process that requires developing a motor program that the person then carried out in a logical fashion for interactions with people and things in the environment. (See chapter 7, The Evolution of the Concept of Praxis in Sensory Integration, by Blanche, for a detailed description of theoretical constructs and their relation to occupation.)

Sensory Integration and Daily Occupations

Research has confirmed the relationship of sensory integration to functioning in various daily occupations (Spitzer, Roley, Clark, & Parham, 1996). Parham (1998) has correlated sensory integrative functioning with arithmetic and reading achievement in school-age children. Other studies have related sensory integrative functioning to play skills in preschoolers (Schaaf, 1990; Schaaf, Merrill, & Kinsella, 1987), although some children compensate better for their deficits than others (Bundy, 1989; Clifford & Bundy, 1989). Sensory integrative dysfunction might contribute to delinquency in adolescents (Fanchiang, Snyder, Zobel-Lachiusa, Loeffler, & Thompson, 1990). Baranek, Foster, and Berkson (1997) have correlated tactile defensiveness with rigid or inflexible behaviors, repetitive verbalizations, visual stereotypes, and abnormal focused affections in children with developmental disabilities, including autism. Kinnealey, Oliver, and Wilbarger (1995) have linked sensory defensiveness with negative emotions such as annoyance, frustration, and fear when encountering occupations that involve various sensory stimuli. Sensory integrative deficits can influence an individual's vocational choices and satisfaction with those choices because the individual might adaptively select those vocations that satisfy the person's sensory needs or, alternatively, be frustrated by vocations that fail to meet his or her sensory needs (Fanchiang, 1996). This research supports Ayres' early contentions that sensory integrative functioning is related to academic achievement (Ayres, 1972a, 1972b, 1972d, 1975, 1979) and emotional well being (Ayres, 1979).

Assessing Sensory Integrative Functioning: A Guide to Intervention

Clinicians assess sensory integration within the context of a thorough evaluation of the child, the child's supports, and environment. The assessment is critical to planning and implementing effective intervention (see chapter 12, Assessment in Sensory Integration, by Windsor, Roley, & Szklut, for details on evaluations and assessments of sensory integrative functioning). Determining the aspects of sensory integrative contributions is challenging, particularly with the diversity of the populations defined as developmentally disabled. Identifying these subtle, hidden deficits requires skills in, experience with, and knowledge of sensory integration as well as typical and atypical development.

Two primary issues are paramount in evaluating sensory integrative deficits in the population of children with developmental disabilities. The first issue is identifying the impact of inadequate sensory processing and praxis on the child's functional abilities. The second issue is to put into perspective the contributions of the sensory integrative disorders with the complexity of factors that are contributing to the developmental delay.

To identify the extent and impact of sensory integrative dysfunction, the therapist must consider the spectrum of disorders, including problems related to sensory modulation, sensory discrimination, postural control, and praxis (Parham & Mailloux, 1996). The therapist looks for convergence and patterns that form a cohesive picture regarding sensory integrative functioning and its influence on the child's problems in daily life activities at the time of referral. The therapist must gain perspective on the extent to which sensory processing affects the individual's ability to engage in age-appropriate play and role behaviors. The therapist analyzes the child's efforts not only in terms of sensory processing for improved perception but also in terms of the child's ability to utilize postural control and praxis in order to meet the spatial temporal requirements in his or her interactions. Frequently, this analysis provides a unifying explanation for seemingly unrelated behavioral difficulties such as late bowel and bladder control, difficulty calming once upset, fatiguing quickly when waiting somewhere, mouthing nonfood objects incessantly, irregular sleep patterns, and poor spontaneous speech.

To put sensory integrative dysfunction into perspective with other factors contributing to occupational performance deficits, the therapist weighs the severity of the sensory integrative issues against other identified factors such as neuromotor deficit or medical condition. For example, David, a first-born child, was referred for evaluation of a fine motor deficit. Other professionals had previously diagnosed speech and language difficulties, particularly with contextual language. David had scored in the 80s on the *Wechsler Intelligence Scale for Children-Revised* (WISC-R; Wechsler, 1974). His parents' perception was that David was a typically developing child with fine motor deficits. The SIPT (Ayres, 1989a) revealed deficiencies in all sensory motor areas tested, but the SIPT was not able to account for the persistent and pervasive difficulties in academic and social areas. The occupational therapist recommended a neuropsychological evaluation that resulted in a diagnosis of Fragile X. David received occupational therapy utilizing primarily a sensory integrative approach and made notable progress, but his team of professionals also adjusted his total educational and medical programming to meet this child's multiple needs more effectively.

The results of the occupational therapy evaluation provide the base for determining the most appropriate intervention approach for the individual child. The intervention plan also takes into consideration the personal, physical, social, and environmental factors that might be affecting the child's engagement in his or her occupations. Once the therapist has determined that a child has sensory integrative issues that are interfering with his or her daily occupations and that occupational therapy is necessary, the SI approach is useful as one part of the intervention plan. The intervention plan considers the potential impact of a sensory integrative approach along with other appropriate frames of reference in concert with the multidisciplinary focus by the family and other professionals. Based on these considerations, the occupational therapist may elect to use a sensory integrative approach as the primary intervention approach or to use some sensory integrative principles in conjunction with another or other treatment approach(es).

Using a Sensory Integrative Approach
for Children With Developmental Disabilities

Building on Ayres' original work, therapists have applied sensory integrative principles for individuals across the lifespan and with various diagnoses (Spitzer et al., 1996). Therapists have used a sensory integrative approach with a variety of developmental disabilities such as:

- autism (Ayres & Tickle, 1980; see also chapter 17, Sensory Integrative Principles in Intervention With Children With Autism, by Mailloux)

- cerebral palsy (Blanche, Botticelli, & Hallway, 1995; Chee, Kreutzberg, & Clark, 1978; see also chapter 16, Sensory Integration and the Child With Cerebral Palsy, by Blanche & Nagasuchi)

- Fragile X Syndrome (Stackhouse, 1994; see also chapter 19, Sensory Integration and Fragile X, by Hickman)

- hearing impairment (Schaffer-Pullan, Polatajko, & Sansom, 1991)

- mental retardation (Clark, Miller, Thomas, Kucherawy, & Azen, 1978)

- premature birth (Anderson, 1986)

- prenatal drug exposure (Stallings-Sahler, 1993)

- visual impairment (Roley, 1995a, 1995b, 1995c; see also chapter 15, Sensory Integration and Visual Deficits, Including Blindness, by Roley & Schneck).

Therapists use sensory integrative principles within the framework of an overall occupational therapy intervention plan (Roley, 1993–1994; Spitzer et al., 1996). Key constructs of this approach include the therapist's maintenance of his or her own artful vigilance while adjusting sensory qualities of the environment; promoting self-direction; enabling a playful context; facilitating adaptive responses in motor, affective, social, and cognitive areas; creating the "just-right challenge"; and tapping the child's inner drive (Ayres, 1972a; Clark, Mailloux, Parham, & Bissell, 1989). Sensory integration can serve as the primary intervention approach, or the therapist can use it in conjunction with other approaches in occupational therapy.

Therapists apply the principles of sensory integration through a continuum of service delivery models (American Occupational Therapy Association, 1997). The classical form of sensory integrative intervention provides therapy through direct service in a specialized setting. A therapist also can provide direct services when treating a child at home, on the playground, or in the context of the classroom. Consultation models might be necessary for altering programs, environments, or approaches for an individual child.

Sensory Alchemy

Typically, children are sensory seeking (Dunn, 1996). Through play, children seek out opportunities to take in body-centered sensory information through the tactile, proprioceptive, and vestibular systems. Despite their parents' best efforts at stopping them, children commonly jump into mud puddles, play with their food, climb on the furniture, and jump on the beds. The multisensory nature of their play provides the ingredients necessary for the alchemy that promotes development. Children with disabilities do not always have the same opportunities for this type of play. They might be limited by their physical capabilities to get onto the beds, let alone jump. They might require specialized equipment for standing and have limited opportunities for safe climbing. They might never get into a mud puddle because well-intentioned caregivers do not want them to get dirty.

Compounding these factors are the neurological impairments that contribute to inadequate sensory processing. Children with developmental delays might be tactually averse to eating food, let alone playing with it. They might have extreme sensitivities to temperature variations and be unable to tolerate playing in a cold puddle. Insecurity with moving through space might limit their capacity to climb or jump without severe emotional anxiety and fear. Children might be unable to discriminate sensation well enough to guide their bodies to climb and negotiate objects. They might be unable to participate in a range of occupations because they engage in extreme sensory seeking by participating in potentially dangerous activities (such as climbing and jumping from high places). They might be at risk for being excluded from social occupations such as play because they are too rough or physical.

Intervention emphasizing a sensory integrative approach addresses the sensory needs of the child in order for the child to make adaptive and organized responses to a variety of circumstances and environments. In its classic form, intervention occurs in a clinic with specialized devices such as suspended equipment, trampolines, barrels, brushes, and big soft pillows (Clark et al., 1989; Koomar & Bundy, 1991; Parham & Mailloux, 1996; Sieg, 1988). In this setting, the therapist utilizes a controlled environment to offer experiences that meet each child's unique sensory needs and enhance the child's processing and organizational abilities.

In natural settings, the varying processing demands necessitate varying the intervention within these different contexts. The demands might be lower, for example, at home in a predictable routine, or higher at school, where there is much noise, many children, and high academic and behavioral demands. For some children, it might be appropriate to address natural occupational contexts first by using the clinic as an experimental area to find the child's balance of sensory data and organizational techniques that are effective in facilitating learning. The therapist and other caregivers then can transfer this knowledge into the typical context, to adapt both the conditions in which the child functions and the child's ability to function in those conditions (Parham & Mailloux, 1996).

Sensory integration is specifically *not* prescriptive. The occupational therapist strives to create a more harmonious match between the child's sensory needs and the typical context in which the child is asked to operate. Consultation and collaboration with the child, the child's family, and professionals involved with the child are important in identifying activities for the child to access appropriate types, combinations, and intensities of sensations while reading the child's cues and positive reactions. The therapist provides suggestions to restructure the physical environment, such as creating safe places to climb and jump, or making a swing or hammock tied to a tree in the backyard. The therapist might aid in organizing the daily schedule so that the child receives sensory opportunities at the most optimal times to promote the child's best performance in other occupations such as class work. The therapist makes recommendations for leisure activities such as jumping on a trampoline, swimming, and visiting water-slide parks that might not have been considered previously.

For example, Nick, a child with multiple sensory and motor impairments, arrived at school after a 45-minute bus ride consistently unable to come out of a deep and restless sleep without extreme irritation, crying, and biting. Upon Nick's arrival at school, an occupational therapist provided activities utilizing deep pressure and proprioceptive input for calming. When Nick began calming, the therapist conducted linear vestibular activities in conjunction with deep pressure until Nick was posturally and emotionally stable. At this point, the therapist elicited more active social and motor involvement through play with balls and favorite toys. Once Nick was able to engage happily, both socially and motorically, he was capable of transitioning to the classroom setting with the occupational therapist for work during language, cognitive, and fine-motor activities. The therapist communicated the success of this routine to the teachers and parents, who then utilized the routine throughout the school day and at home.

Play and Self-Direction

A playful interaction is one of the most critical components of sensory integration (Mailloux & Burke, 1997; Tickle-Degnen & Coster, 1995). Therapists who are most successful in eliciting the active participation of the child's play celebrate the child as an occupational being, authentically honor the child's spirit, enjoy his or her company, and recognize the unique contribution of this child. The therapist invites a child to play together in the play activity in order to facilitate joyful and challenging interactions with the physical, social, and emotional environment. It is through the medium of play that the therapist finds the unique key to unlock the interest and motivation of the child for engaging in appropriate and meaningful activities (Kimball, 1993). The child's inner drive emerges as play progresses.

Tapping the child's innate drive for mastery is one of the primary goals of therapy (Ayres, 1972a). It is this dynamic playful interaction that makes this form of intervention child-led. Tapping into a child's self-direction is especially challenging when working with children who have limited capabilities to communicate their interests. The therapist monitors the child's positive emotional responses as signs that the child wants to continue the activity. For example, a child with autism might have difficulty registering sensory input and, as a result, fail to enjoy typical play activities. The therapist follows the interests of the child to determine what will motivate that child and encourage the child's self-direction towards purposeful and meaningful activities. For example, Cathy had difficulty with transitions. Frequently, when making transitions, she would have tantrums, scream, and become aggressive. A behavioral approach had yielded little success. The occupational therapist strategized to provide Cathy with verbal cues that the transition was going to happen, then allowed her to take what she had been playing with to the next station. Cathy particularly liked the stretchy swing, so the therapist allowed her to make all her transitions carrying this swing, but only if she indicated that she wanted it. With this strategy, Cathy made four transitions in school that day without screaming or running away. Such strategies can be helpful as an initial step toward promoting improved registration and awareness of the environment, thus activating the inner drive to engage in an activity (Ayres, 1979).

Children who seem to lack an inner drive might require a more hands-on approach than is typical in classic sensory integration intervention. Passive sensory stimulation sometimes works with children who might not be able to provide the appropriate type or intensity on their own. A more directed strategy might be necessary initially to promote improved registration and awareness of the environment, thus activating the child's inner drive to engage in an activity and self-direct (Ayres, 1979). In the case of hands-on guidance and passive stimulation, monitoring the adaptive responses requires even greater vigilance because the responses might be quite subtle. The adaptive response is always the guidepost for continuing or discontinuing a given activity and is why the therapy continues to be child-directed.

Children who can follow their innate drive independently and provide their own optimal sensory environment for environmental mastery do not need therapy. Some children avoid following their inner drive due to some fearfulness such as gravitational insecurity. In these cases, "the therapist must encourage, cajole, lure, and manipulate the child into choosing the activities that will help his or her brain develop" (Ayres,

1979, p. 140). When there is a need for more structure and direction, the therapist directs and structures the physical and social environment rather than ordering or directing the child. Clinicians cannot force integration, they can only cultivate it (Ayres, 1972a).

Meeting Challenges Successfully: The Adaptive Response

Facilitating the adaptive response is the role of the occupational therapist, who shapes the environment to elicit ever-more-complex adaptive responses. Therapists use themselves (their voices, facial expressions, body language, attitude, and so forth) as well as activities to help children modulate their responses. Scaffolding is a concept that describes how an adult bridges the gaps in a child's abilities in order to facilitate the child's successful problem-solving, skill acquisition, or engagement in an activity that would be beyond the child's efforts if unassisted (Wood, Bruner, & Ross, 1976). *Occupational scaffolding* describes the way parents structure and support a child's engagement in household occupations (Primeau, 1995). The occupational therapist facilitates an adaptive response through a similar scaffolding process (Dunkerley et al., 1997; Tickle-Degnen & Coster, 1995). The therapist continuously supports involvement in the activity by constantly grading the activity. At all times, the therapist adds, removes, and makes other changes to the environment based on careful observation of the child's responses. The therapist allows the child to practice and refine sensory integrative-based behaviors, providing another scaffolding on which to build more complex adaptive responses. The therapist adds challenges when the child indicates readiness to meet them successfully (see Table 1.4).

Therapists grade activities based on the temporal and spatial demands of the sensory motor environment and the necessity to act within that environment. The occupational therapist examines the child's spatial requirements in body-centered space, near space, and far space (Roley, 1993–1994). The therapist also must examine the temporal components (e.g., the timing or amount of time available) for actions involving movement of the child and the physical objects on which the child is acting (Koomar & Bundy, 1991). Therapists consider the spatial context as well as the temporal context relative to the demand and the observed adaptive response, and make adjustments in either the spatial context and/or the temporal context of any activity in order to grade it to obtain a more skilled, successful, appropriate response.

For example, Eric was having difficulty in the clinic selecting an activity. The therapist recommended throwing balls, manipulating a music toy on a swing, and swinging with another child. None of these activities was enticing to Eric, and the therapist was not observing any adaptive responses. When the therapist analyzed a videotape of this session, it was apparent that Eric was unable to work outside of his immediate body-centered space with any degree of effectiveness. He also was unable to meet the temporal demands of being on moving equipment while engaged in a social or motor activity. During the next session, the therapist graded the tasks to work on activities that were more body-centered in space with a stable environment. By allowing him more stability, a smaller field to have to monitor, and less postural challenge, he was able to begin to show adaptive responses and manifest his inner drive to participate.

Using Sensory Integration in Conjunction With Other Approaches

Children with developmental disabilities have complex needs that require a well-rounded therapy program. Combining sensory integrative principles with other approaches allows for the greatest flexibility in accommodating the specific needs of the child. It is now common to combine several theoretical frames of reference, such as biomechanic, skills training, sensory integration, and neurodevelopmental

Table 1.4. Scaffolding: Eliciting Adaptive Responses
Through the Application of Sensory Integration Theory

Area of Focus	Therapeutic Adjustments	Outcomes
Arousal	Begin interactions with analysis of the child's status here. Decide if interactions need to be excitatory or inhibitory.	Improved attention to relevant aspects of people and things in the environment; readiness to interact
Sensory Modulation	Adjust intensity, duration, and variety of environmental stimuli.	Improved self-regulation of behaviors, emotions, and interactions
Sensory Discrimination	Alter temporal/spatial sensory qualities.	Enhanced perception of broader perceptual field
Skill	Grade challenge in fine and gross motor areas.	Ease of challenging gravity; refinement of learned interactions with objects and people
Praxis	Alter demand relative to creative ideas, sequence of steps, and adjustments based on novelty.	More automatic and dynamic planning of adaptive and complex interactions with objects and people
Organization of Behavior	Adjust responsibility for increasingly complex tasks in time and space	Organizing sequences of multiple interactions both under current circumstances and in the future

The therapist utilizes sensory integrative intervention strategies while facilitating an optimal level of arousal and providing appropriate and meaningful challenges. If arousal, modulation, and discrimination of information are maladaptive, it is difficult to work at the level of skill, praxis, and organization of behavior. When the client obtains or regains an optimal level of arousal, the therapist then can increase demands for adaptive responses in the areas of skill, praxis, and organization of behavior. When demands for organization of behavior, praxis or skill are too difficult, the therapist adjusts the sensory environment, alters the level of challenge, and strives to elicit a comfortable yet alert level of arousal. The therapist elicits the highest level of adaptive response by challenging all levels successfully.

intervention principles in one intervention session. For example, a therapist might use a sensory integrative approach for the first half of the session to help the child become organized and better able to attend, then use the rest of the session to develop particular skills such as fine motor or self-care. Or, one activity might combine the principles of several different approaches. Occupational therapy goals center on building functional skills as appropriate for the child's individual needs although sensory integrative interventions might not use those skills directly in the therapeutic process.

Outcomes and Effectiveness of Intervention

Due to the emergent nature of sensory integration, it has been difficult to predict specific outcomes that will result from intervention utilizing this approach. Yet, this is precisely what is expected of occupational therapists who usually must set specific, measurable objectives prior to initiating therapy. As the pressure of third-party payors continues to increase, continued intervention might hinge on whether the child meets these objectives. This presents a formidable challenge for occupational therapists to predict the exact course of intervention and outcome especially when utilizing approaches that focus on dynamically interacting systems. Documentation of effectiveness is critical to justify intervention convincingly.

Although precise outcomes can be difficult to predict, there are general areas in which occupational therapists can expect outcomes from intervention utilizing a sensory integrative approach. Parham and Mailloux (1996) listed six general areas in which children can experience increases or improvements: the frequency or duration of adaptive responses; the complexity of adaptive responses; self-confidence and self-esteem; gross and fine motor skills; daily living and personal-social skills; and cognitive, language, or academic performance.

Efficacy Research

The efficacy of sensory integrative procedures has been difficult to measure. Effectiveness research generally supports the efficacy of a sensory integrative approach (Spitzer et al., 1996). Most studies have looked at individuals with learning disabilities, but researchers have conducted over two dozen studies on the efficacy of sensory integration-related treatments for individuals with developmental disabilities (Daems, 1994).

Studies examining the effectiveness of a sensory-integrative-based intervention approach for individuals with developmental disabilities generally have supported the effectiveness of the approach with this population:

- **Mental retardation:** With children, a therapeutic sensorimotor program was more effective than a developmental physical education program in improving gross motor, fine motor, and perceptual motor abilities (Montgomery & Richter, 1977). For three young children with profound mental retardation and multiple handicaps, a combined sensory integration and neurodevelopmental treatment approach was effective in increasing postural reactions and interaction with people and objects (Norton, 1975). For adults with profound mental retardation, sensory integration-based intervention helped improve eye contact, vocalizations, and postural control (Clark et al., 1978). Close, Carpenter, and Cibiri (1986) also found sensory integration to be effective in improving acceptance of vestibular stimulation, balance, use of protective reflexes and body awareness, fine motor skills, visual tracking, and attention.

- **Autism:** With preschoolers, weekly occupational therapy with a sensory integration emphasis promoted decreased frequency of nonengaged behavior and increased frequency of mastery (goal-directed) play during classroom free-play time (Case-Smith & Bryan, 1999). With children, occupational therapy using a sensory integrative approach promoted language, awareness of the environment, engagement in purposeful activity, and social and emotional behavior, and decreased self-stimulatory behavior, especially for children who were hyper-responsive to tactile and vestibular input (Ayres & Tickle, 1980).

- **Developmental delay:** Working with a 4-year-old boy, Schaaf et al. (1987) found that 8 weeks of individual occupational therapy using sensory integrative procedures were effective in promoting play, with greatest gains in increased interactions with objects and people, tolerance for vestibular/proprioceptive input, and sensory exploration of the environment.

Most of the studies related to sensory integration and individuals with developmental disabilities have assessed the effects of sensory stimulation, primarily externally imposed stimulation. Although sensory stimulation alone is not a sensory integrative-based approach, the positive findings of these studies do support the use of a sensory integrative approach with individuals who have developmental disabilities. Research has shown that sensory stimulation:

- decreases self-injurious, stereotypic, and self-stimulatory behaviors in adults and children with developmental delays and mental retardation (Bonadonna, 1981; Bright, Bittick, & Fleeman, 1981; Brocklehurst-Woods, 1990; Dura, Mulick, & Hammer, 1988; Iwasaki & Holm, 1989; MacLean & Baumeister, 1982; Reisman, 1993; Storey, Bates, McGhee, & Dycus, 1984; Wells & Smith, 1983)

- improves motor skills in young children with cerebral palsy, Down syndrome, and developmental delay (Chee et al., 1978; Kantner, Clark, Allen, & Chase, 1976; MacLean & Baumeister, 1982)

- increases verbalizations and language development in children with mental retardation and autism (Kantner, Kantner, & Clark, 1982; Magrun, Ottenbacher, McCue, & Keefe, 1981; Ray, King, & Grandin, 1988)

- increases eye contact in an adult with profound mental retardation (Resman, 1981)

As in all fields of research on interventions with humans, continued research is necessary to refine this approach for more effective intervention. Such research must meet increasingly rigorous methodological requirements and creatively and comprehensively assess the range of potential intervention outcomes (Spitzer et. al., 1996). Such research is especially difficult when working with hugely diverse populations such as individuals with developmental disabilities, for whom the calculation of group means sometimes obscures their unique individual differences.

Conclusion

Sensory integration is a theory and a frame of reference in occupational therapy from which to begin the clinical reasoning process. Sensory integration provides alternative explanations for behaviors, deviations in function, and disorganized learning patterns. Reframing the issues in light of the sensory and organizational needs of the individual aids not only the individual's sense of self and purpose but also the family's ability to cope. Sensory integration supports development and occupational engagement through organizing the individual's nervous system. Its philosophy is one of compassion, value, and respect for the inner nature of the individual. Sensory integration theory honors the child as an occupational being and understands intervention to be a part of what will help this child and his or her family to participate meaningfully in the contexts within which they live and thrive.

Works Cited

References

American Occupational Therapy Association. (1997). Sensory integration evaluation and intervention in school-based occupational therapy. *American Journal of Occupational Therapy, 51,* 861–863.

Anderson, J. (1986). Sensory intervention with the preterm infant in the neonatal intensive care unit. *American Journal of Occupational Therapy, 40,* 19–26.

Anderson, R.A. (1995). Encoding of intention and spatial location in the posterior parietal cortex. *Cerebral Cortex, 5,* 457–469.

Ayres, A.J. (1965). Patterns of perceptual-motor dysfunction in children: A factor analytic study. *Perceptual and Motor Skills, 20,* 335–368.

Ayres, A.J. (1966a). Interrelationships among perceptual-motor functions in children. *American Journal of Occupational Therapy, 20*(2), 68–71.

Ayres, A.J. (1966b). Interrelationships among perceptual-motor abilities in a group of normal children. *American Journal of Occupational Therapy, 20*(6), 288–292.

Ayres, A.J. (1969). Deficits in sensory integration in educationally handicapped children. *Journal of Learning Disabilities, 2(3),* 44–52.

Ayres, A.J. (1971). Characteristics of types of sensory integrative dysfunction. *American Journal of Occupational Therapy, 25*(7), 329–334.

Ayres, A.J. (1972a). *Sensory integration and learning disorders.* Los Angeles: Western Psychological Services.

Ayres, A.J. (1972b). Improving academic scores through sensory integration. *Journal of Learning Disabilities, 5,* 336–343.

Ayres, A.J. (1972c). *Southern California Sensory Integration Tests.* Los Angeles: Western Psychological Services.

Ayres, A.J. (1972d). Types of sensory integrative dysfunction among disabled learners. *American Journal of Occupational Therapy, 26*(1), 13–18.

Ayres, A.J. (1974). *The development of sensory integrative theory and practice. A collection of the works of A. Jean Ayres.* Dubuque, IA: Kendall/Hunt Publishing Co. [Original work published in 1960.]

Ayres, A.J. (1975). Sensorimotor foundations of academic ability. In W. M. Cruickshank & D. P. Hallahan (Eds.), *Perceptual and learning disabilities in children: Vol. 2* (pp. 301–358). Syracuse, NY: Syracuse University Press.

Ayres, A.J. (1976). The effect of sensory integrative therapy on learning disabled children. Pasadena, CA: Center for the Study of Sensory Integrative Dysfunction.

Ayres, A.J. (1977). Cluster analyses of measure of sensory integration. *American Journal of Occupational Therapy, 31*(6), 362–366.

Ayres, A.J. (1979). *Sensory integration and the child.* Los Angeles: Western Psychological Services.

Ayres, A.J. (1986). Sensory integrative dysfunction: Test score constellations. Part II of a final project report. Torrance, CA: Sensory Integration International.

Ayres, A.J. (1989a). *Sensory Integration and Praxis Tests.* Los Angeles: Western Psychological Services.

Ayres, A.J. (1989b). *Sensory Integration and Praxis Tests manual.* Los Angeles: Western Psychological Services.

Ayres, A.J., & Tickle, L.S. (1980). Hyper-responsivity to touch and vestibular stimuli as a predictor of positive response to sensory integration procedures by autistic children. *American Journal of Occupational Therapy, 34,* 375–381.

Baranek, G.T., Foster, L.G., & Berkson, G. (1997). Tactile defensiveness and stereotyped behaviors. *American Journal of Occupational Therapy, 51,* 91–95.

Blair, R.W., & Thompson, G.M. (1995). Convergence of multiple sensory inputs onto neurons in the dorsolateral medulla in cats. *Neuroscience, 67,* 721–729.

Blanche, E.I., Botticelli, T.M., & Hallway, M.K. (1995). *Combining neuro-developmental treatment and sensory integration principles: An approach to pediatric therapy.* Tucson, AZ: Therapy Skill Builders.

Bonadonna, P. (1981). Effects of a vestibular stimulation program on stereotypic rocking behavior. *American Journal of Occupational Therapy, 35,* 775–781.

Bright, T., Bittick, K., & Fleeman, B. (1981). Reduction of self-injurious behavior using sensory integrative techniques. *American Journal of Occupational Therapy, 35,* 167–172.

Brocklehurst-Woods, J. (1990). The use of tactile and vestibular stimulation to reduce stereotypic behaviors in two adults with mental retardation. *American Journal of Occupational Therapy, 44,* 536–541.

Brown, D. (Writer & Director). (1975). *Help me be me* [Film]. (Available from Earth Links, 519 Seabright Avenue, Suite #103, Santa Cruz, CA 95062).

Bundy, A.C. (1989). A comparison of the play skills of normal boys and boys with sensory integrative dysfunction. *Occupational Therapy Journal of Research, 9,* 84–100.

Case-Smith, J., & Bryan, T. (1999). The effects of occupational therapy with sensory integration emphasis on preschool-age children with autism. *American Journal of Occupational Therapy, 53,* 489–497.

Chee, F.K. W., Kreutzberg, J.R., & Clark, D.L. (1978). Semicircular canal stimulation in cerebral palsied children. *Physical Therapy, 58,* 1071–1075.

Chen, D., & Dote-Kwan, J. (1995). *Starting points: Instructional practices for young children whose multiple disabilities include visual impairment.* Los Angeles: Blind Children's Center.

Clark, F., Mailloux, Z., Parham, D., & Bissell, J.C. (1989). Sensory integration and children with learning disabilities. In P.N. Pratt & A.S. Allen (Eds.), *Occupational therapy for children* (2nd ed., pp. 457–507). St. Louis: C.V. Mosby.

Clark, F.A., Miller, L.R., Thomas, J.A., Kucherawy, D.A., & Azen, S.P. (1978). A comparison of operant and sensory integrative methods on developmental parameters in profoundly retarded adults. *American Journal of Occupational Therapy, 32,* 86–92.

Clifford, J.M., & Bundy, A.C. (1989). Play preference and play performance in normal boys and boys with sensory integrative dysfunction. *Occupational Therapy Journal of Research, 9,* 202–217.

Close, W., Carpenter, M., & Cibiri, S. (1986). An evaluation study of sensory motor therapy for profoundly retarded adults. *Canadian Journal of Occupational Therapy, 53,* 259–264.

Cool, S.J. (1995). Does sensory integration work? *Sensory Integration Quarterly, 23*(1), 1, 5–9.

Daems, J. (Ed.). (1994). *Reviews of research in sensory integration.* Torrance, CA: Sensory Integration International.

Diamond, M.C. (1988). The significance of enrichment. In *Enriching heredity.* New York: The Free Press.

Dunkerley, E., Tickle-Degnen, L., & Coster, W.J. (1997). Therapist-child interaction in the middle minutes of sensory integration treatment. *American Journal of Occupational Therapy, 51,* 799–805.

Dunn, W. (1996, October). *The Sensory Profile.* Workshop conducted at the annual practice conference of the American Occupational Therapy Association, St. Louis, MO.

Dura, J., Mulick, J., & Hammer, D. (1988). Rapid clinical evaluation of sensory integrative therapy for self-injurious behavior. *Mental Retardation, 26*(2), 83–87.

Fanchiang, S. (1996). The other side of the coin: Growing up with a learning disability. *American Journal of Occupational Therapy, 50,* 277–285.

Fanchiang, S., Snyder, C., Zobel-Lachiusa, J., Loeffler, C.B., & Thompson, M.E. (1990). Sensory integrative processing in delinquent-prone and non-delinquent-prone adolescents. *American Journal of Occupational Therapy, 44,* 630–639.

Fisher, A.G., & Murray, E.A. (1991). Introduction to sensory integration theory. In A.G. Fisher, E.A. Murray, & A.C. Bundy (Eds.), *Sensory integration: Theory and practice* (pp. 3–26). Philadelphia: F.A. Davis.

Gallagher, W. (1993). *The power of place: How our surroundings shape our thoughts, emotions, and actions.* New York: HarperPerennial.

Hofer, M.A. (1995). Hidden regulators: Implications for a new understanding of attachment, separation, and loss. In S. Goldberg, R. Huir, & J. Kerr (Eds.), *Attachment theory: Social development and clinical perspectives.* Hillsdale, NJ: The Analytic Press.

Holloway, E. (1997). Fostering parent-infant playfulness in the neonatal intensive care unit. In L. D. Parham & L.S. Fazio (Eds.), *Play in occupational therapy for children* (pp. 171–183). St. Louis: C.V. Mosby.

Iwasaki, K., & Holm, M. (1989). Sensory treatment for the reduction of stereotypic behaviors in persons with severe multiple disabilities. *Occupational Therapy Journal of Research, 9*(3), 170–183.

Kamm, K., Thelen, E., & Jensen, J.L. (1990). A dynamical systems approach to motor development. *Physical Therapy, 70,* 763–775.

Kantner, R., Clark, D., Allen, L., & Chase, M. (1976). Effects of vestibular stimulation on nystagmus response and motor performance in the developmentally delayed infant. *Physical Therapy, 56,* 414–421.

Kantner, R., Kantner, B., & Clark, D. (1982). Vestibular stimulation effect on language development in mentally retarded children. *American Journal of Occupational Therapy, 36,* 36–41.

Kielhofner, G. (1992). *Conceptual foundations of occupational therapy.* Philadelphia: F.A. Davis Company.

Kimball, J. (1993). Sensory integrative frame of reference. In P. Kramer & J. Hinojosa (Eds.), *Frames of reference for pediatric occupational therapy* (pp. 87–167). Baltimore: Williams and Wilkins.

Kinnealey, M., Oliver, B., & Wilbarger, P. (1995). A phenomenological study of sensory defensiveness in adults. *American Journal of Occupational Therapy, 49,* 444–451.

Koomar, J. (1997). Clinical interpretation of "Therapist-child interaction in the middle minutes of sensory integration treatment." *American Journal of Occupational Therapy, 51,* 806–807.

Koomar, J.A., & Bundy, A.C. (1991) . The art and science of creating direct intervention from theory. In A.G. Fisher, E.A. Murray, & A.C. Bundy (Eds.), *Sensory integration: Theory and practice* (pp. 251–315). Philadelphia: F.A. Davis.

Lane, S. J. (1997). Nurture: Environmental influences on central nervous system functions. In C.B. Royeen (Ed.), *Neuroscience and occupation: Links to occupation* (pp. 1–276). Bethesda, MD: The American Occupational Therapy Association.

Lewkowicz, D.J., & Lickliter, R. (Eds.) (1994). *The development of intersensory perception: Comparative perspectives.* Hillsdale, NJ: Lawrence Erlbaum and Associates, Publishers.

MacLean, W., & Baumeister, A. (1982). Effects of vestibular stimulation on motor development and stereotyped behavior of developmentally delayed children. *Journal of Abnormal Child Psychology, 10,* 229–245.

Magrun, W.M., Ottenbacher, K., McCue, S., & Keefe, R. (1981). Effects of vestibular stimulation on spontaneous use of verbal language in developmentally delayed children. *American Journal of Occupational Therapy, 35,* 101–104.

Mailloux, Z., & Burke, J.P. (1997). Play and the sensory integrative approach. In L. D. Parham & L. S. Fazio (Eds.), *Play in occupational therapy for children* (pp. 112–125). St. Louis: C.V. Mosby.

Melzack, R., & Wall, P.D. (1973). *The challenge of pain.* New York: Basic Books.

Merrill, S.C. (Ed.). (1990). *Environment: Implications for occupational therapy practice—A sensory integrative perspective.* Rockville, MD: American Occupational Therapy Association.

Montegue, A. (1978). *Touching: The human significance of the skin.* New York: Harper and Row.

Montgomery, P., & Richter, E. (1977). Effect of sensory integrative therapy on the neuromotor development of retarded children. *Physical Therapy, 57,* 799–806.

New York State Psychiatric Institute. (1996, September). Exploring the mother-infant relationship for clues to future health. *New York State Psychiatric Institute Newsletter* [On-line], *15(3).* Available: http://156.111.80.209/Newsletter1/mother.htm.

Norton, Y. (1975). Neurodevelopment and sensory integration for the profoundly retarded multiply handicapped child. *American Journal of Occupational Therapy, 29,* 93–100.

Parham, L.D. (1998). The relationship of sensory integrative development to achievement in elementary students: Four-year longitudinal patterns. *Occupational Therapy Journal of Research, 18*(3), 105–127.

Parham, D., & Mailloux, Z. (1996). Sensory integration. In J. Case-Smith, P.N. Pratt, & A.S. Allen (Eds.), *Occupational therapy for children* (3rd ed., pp. 307–356). Portland, OR: Mosby.

Porges, S.W. (1993). The infant's sixth sense: Awareness and regulation of bodily processes. *Zero to Three, 14*(2), 12–16.

Primeau, L.A. (1995). *Orchestration of work and play within families*. Unpublished doctoral dissertation, University of Southern California, Los Angeles.

Rakic, P., Bourgeois, J.P., and Goldman-Rakic, P. (1994). Synaptic development of the cerebral cortex: Implications for learning, memory, and mental illness. *Progress in Brain Research, 102,* 227–243.

Ray, T., King, L., & Grandin, T. (1988). The effectiveness of self-initiated vestibular stimulation in producing speech sounds in an autistic child. *Occupational Therapy Journal of Research, 8*(3), 186–190.

Regan, M.P., He, P., & Regan, D. (1995). An audio-visual convergence area in the human brain. *Experimental Brain Research, 106,* 485–487.

Reisman, J. (1993). Using a sensory integrative approach to treat self-injurious behavior in an adult with profound mental retardation. *American Journal of Occupational Therapy, 47,* 403–411.

Resman, M. (1981). Effect of sensory stimulation on eye contact in a profoundly retarded adult. *American Journal of Occupational Therapy, 35,* 31–35.

Roley, S.S. (1993-1994, Winter). OT is the profession, SI is the tool. *Sensory Integration Quarterly, 21*(4), 7.

Roley, S.S. (1995a). Occupational therapy for young children with multiple disabilities. In D. Chen & J. Dote-Kwan (Eds.), *Starting points: Instructional practices for young children whose multiple disabilities include visual impairments* (pp. 98–106). Los Angeles: Blind Children's Center.

Roley, S.S. (1995b, September). Visual impairments: Issues reflected through four children and their families, Part 1. *Sensory Integration Special Interest Section Newsletter, 18*(3), 2–4.

Roley, S.S. (1995c, December). Visual impairments: Issues reflected through four children and their families, Part 2. *Sensory Integration Special Interest Section Newsletter, 18*(4), 1–7.

Roley, S.S., & Wilbarger, J. (1994, June). What is sensory integration? A series of interviews on the scope, limitations, and evolution of sensory integration theory. *Sensory Integration Special Interest Section Newsletter, 17*(2), 1–7.

Sandyk, R. (1996). Application of weak electromagnetic fields facilitates sensory-motor integration in patients with multiple sclerosis. *International Journal of Neuroscience, 85,* 101–110.

Schaaf, R. (1990). Play behavior and occupational therapy. *American Journal of Occupational Therapy, 44,* 68–75.

Schaaf, R., Merrill, S., & Kinsella, N. (1987). Sensory integration and play behavior: A case study of the effectiveness of occupational therapy using sensory integrative techniques. *Occupational Therapy in Health Care, 4*(2), 61–75.

Schaffer-Pullan, A., Polatajko, H.J., & Sansom, L. (1991). A sensory integrative approach for children with hearing impairment: A case study. *Canadian Journal of Occupational Therapy, 58,* 196–200.

Shore, B. (1996). *Culture in mind: Cognition, culture, and the problem of meaning*. New York: Oxford University Press.

Sieg, K.W. (1988). A. Jean Ayres. In B.R.J. Miller, K.W. Sieg, F.M. Ludwig, S.D. Shortridge, & J. Van Deusen (Eds.), *Six perspectives of theory for the practice of occupational therapy* (pp. 95–142). Rockville, MD: Aspen Publishers, Inc.

Spitzer, S.L. (1999, June). Dynamic systems theory: Relevance to the theory of sensory integration and the study of occupation. *Sensory Integration Special Interest Section Quarterly, 22*(2), 1–4.

Spitzer, S., Roley, S.S., Clark, F., & Parham, D. (1996). Sensory integration: Current trends in the United States. *Scandinavian Journal of Occupational Therapy, 3,* 123–138.

Stackhouse, T.M. (1994, March). Sensory integration concepts and Fragile X syndrome. *Sensory Integration Special Interest Section Newsletter, 17*(1), 2–6.

Stallings-Sahler, S. (1993, September). Prenatal cocaine exposure and infant behavioral disorganization. *Sensory Integration Special Interest Section Newsletter, 16*(3), 1–4.

Storey, K., Bates, P., McGhee, N., & Dycus, S. (1984). Reducing the self-stimulatory behavior of a profoundly retarded female through sensory awareness training. *American Journal of Occupational Therapy, 38*, 510–516.

Streri, A. (1993). *Seeing, reaching, touching: The relations between vision and touch in infancy.* Cambridge, MA: MIT Press.

Thelen, E., & Ulrich, B.D. (1991). Hidden skills: A dynamic systems analysis of treadmill stepping during the first year [Serial No. 223]. *Monographs of the Society for Research in Child Development, 56*(1).

Tickle-Degnen, L., & Coster, W. (1995). Therapeutic interaction and the management of challenge during the beginning minutes of sensory integration treatment. *Occupational Therapy Journal of Research, 15*, 122–141.

Turkewitz, G. (1994). Sources of order for intersensory functioning. In D. J. Lewkowicz & R. Lickliter (Eds.), *The development of intersensory perception: Comparative perspectives* (pp. 3–17). Hillsdale, NJ: Lawrence Erlbaum and Associates, Publishers.

Turkewitz, G., & Kenny, P.A. (1982). Limitations on input as a basis for neural organization and perceptual development. A preliminary theoretical statement. *Developmental Psychology, 15*, 357–368.

Wallace, M.T., Wilkinson, L.K., & Stein, B.E. (1996). Representation and integration of multiple sensory inputs in primate superior colliculus. *Journal of Neurophysiology, 76*, 1246–1266.

Wechsler, D. (1974). *Wechsler Intelligence Scale for Children—Revised.* San Antonio, TX: The Psychological Corporation.

Wells, M., & Smith, D. (1983). Reduction of self-injurious behavior of mentally retarded persons using sensory-integrative techniques. *American Journal of Mental Deficiency, 87*, 664–666.

Wilbarger, P. (1995, June). The sensory diet: Activity programs based on sensory processing theory. *Sensory Integration Special Interest Section Newsletter, 18*(2), 1–4.

Wood, D., Bruner, J.S., & Ross, G. (1976). The role of tutoring in problem solving. *Journal of Child Psychology and Psychiatry, 17*, 89–100.

Neuroplasticity and the Environment:

Implications for Sensory Integration

S. Essie Jacobs, Ph.D., OTR

Mary L. Schneider, Ph.D., OTR

More than 25 years ago, Dr. A. Jean Ayres published her seminal papers (1964, 1965, 1966, 1969, 1972a), providing a unique contribution to the understanding of childhood developmental disorders. In her overview of the sensory integration model, Ayres (1972b) stated that the theoretical framework from which she developed her treatment procedures included basic science experiments as well as human and animal behavioral research. Treatment was key in this model, and Ayres felt strongly that, based on the research existing at that time and her strong sense of responsibility to provide treatment to the child during a critical time of development, she should not wait for certainty about treatment procedures (Scardina, 1986). Ayres established a treatment approach that sought to modify the underlying neurological dysfunction rather than simply treat the symptoms. She was well aware that with advances in the knowledge base in the behavioral and neural sciences, sensory integration theory and treatment procedures would continue to evolve.

One of the basic principles upon which Ayres' theoretical model for treatment rests pertains to plasticity of neural function. She stated that "it is upon this capacity to alter the central nervous system of each child's brain that the success of the sensory integrative approach to remediation of learning disabilities rests" (Ayres, 1972b, p.16). She based this premise on studies showing that the brain could reorganize after certain portions were lesioned. She recognized that this reorganizational ability of the developing brain was a normally occurring process and a likely mechanism by which therapy might influence performance on tasks of learning and perception.

This chapter examines the basic research on plasticity in brain development and function that has implications for sensory integration, in order to bridge the gap from basic science research on neural plasticity to sensory integration theory and practice. The authors also describe several of their own studies that suggest biological-environmental interactions begin early in fetal life, reviewing relevant findings from two perturbation studies to date, chronic psychological stress and alcohol exposure during pregnancy.

The Organism-Environment Interaction

From Ayres' exploration of the scientific literature, she gained a deep respect for the importance of the organism-environment interaction and its role in brain development and function (1972b). Ayres cited Harlow's work on deprivation as a demonstration of the effects of the environment on the organism.

Harlow's work provided foundational evidence regarding deprivation. In rhesus monkeys separated from their mothers at birth, deprivation of tactile, olfactory, thermal, vestibular, auditory, and visual stimulation usually provided by the mother produced profound deficits in social behavior (Harlow, 1958; Harlow, Harlow, & Suomi, 1971). Subsequent studies demonstrated that early postnatal rearing environments exert a significant influence on brain and behavior. For example, a series of studies with rodents showed that environmental influences could actually change the brain's cytoarchitecture. Compared to rats reared in impoverished environments, rats reared in enriched environments demonstrated an increased thickness of the occipital cortex as a consequence of increased cell-body size, increased numbers of support (glial) cells, greater dendritic branching, and increased dendritic spine density (Diamond, Rosenzweig, Bennett, Lindner, & Lyon, 1972; Greenough, 1975; for review see Rosenzweig & Bennett, 1996). Along similar lines, Cooper and Zubek (1958) selectively bred rats for their ability to navigate mazes, producing maze-bright and maze-dull animals. Surprisingly, when animals from either of these groups were reared in single cages with little sensory stimulation, all performed in the dull range, even the offspring of maze-bright animals.

More recent studies have focused on the mechanisms underlying biological-environmental interactions. For example, Meaney and colleagues examined specific neural receptors in certain brain areas of handled rodents. They reported an enduring increase in the concentration of glucocorticoid receptors in the hippocampus of handled rats compared to their nonhandled counterparts (for review see Meaney et al., 1994). Recently, others have expanded on Meaney's work to demonstrate that the catalyst for the glucocorticoid receptor up-regulation is the increase in maternal licking and grooming that handled rat pups receive from their mothers upon being returned to the home cage (Liu et al., 1997). Moreover, an increase in glucocorticoid receptors is adaptive when the organism experiences a stressful situation. Under stressful conditions, glucocorticoid release results in fight-or-flight responses and other stress reactions (see Figure 2.1). The up-regulation of glucocorticoid receptors means that there are more receptors available to take up the released glucocorticoids, and more rapid uptake of the glucocorticoids attenuates the organism's stress responses. Concomitant with the neural changes, the handled rats showed decreased behavioral reactivity to environmental stressors. These studies elucidate the reciprocal nature of the organism-environment interaction and illustrate a recently formulated notion that aspects of the environment actually become incorporated into the biology of the organism via altered neural processes. Such neural changes then influence the way the organism subsequently interacts with the environment (Boyce et al., 1998).

A review of neurobiological principles of neuroplasticity must precede any discussion of environmental influences on development and behavior. Some of the basic science reported here served as a basis upon which Ayres developed her theory of

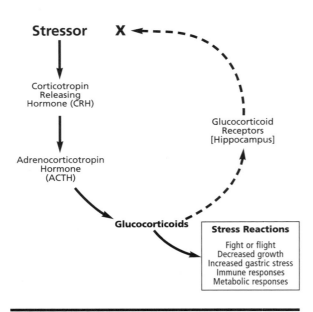

Figure 2.1. Simplified schematic diagram of the pathway through which a stressor triggers glucocorticoid release.

A stressor activates release of corticotrophin releasing hormone (CRH), which causes release of adrenocorticotrophic hormone (ACTH). This results in glucocorticoid release and resulting stress reactions (solid line). Glucocorticoid receptors in the hippocampus take up the released glucocorticoids, which leads to a dampening of the stress reactions (X; dotted line).

sensory integration. This discussion also draws from research that is quite current, exploring how some of the recently proposed mechanisms of action might influence sensory integration.

Brain Growth: A Protracted Process

The ability to make an adaptive response to one's environment is a hallmark of central nervous system function. To achieve this ability, the brain must go through a complex and dynamic developmental process involving a precise sequence of anatomical, functional, and organizational changes (Chugani, 1994). Initially, researchers believed that, except for myelination of subcortical structures, the process ended by 3 years of age. Researchers now know, however, that major changes in the structure of cortical connections continue well into childhood (Huttenlocher, 1994) and adulthood (for review see Buonomano & Merzenich, 1998; Kaas, 1991).

Brain development involves the formation of neurons (neurogenesis) and the establishment of their connections (synaptogenesis). At birth, the human brain is only about one-fourth the size of the adult brain. Although the number of neurons one has is remarkably constant throughout life, the brain becomes larger because neurons grow larger, and the number and extent of connections of their processes (axons and dendrites) increase (Shatz, 1992). For most species, including humans, brain development involves not only synaptic overgrowth but also synapse elimination or pruning, which serves to facilitate sensory information processing in the mature brain. The section on Synaptogenesis and Synapse Elimination, later in this chapter, describes the key mechanisms of neuroplasticity, which support a basic premise of sensory integration that input from the environment has the potential to affect brain (and subsequent behavioral) functions.

Genes and Environment

Neurobiologists generally agree that genes enable axons to establish the basic wiring circuits of the brain. However, because of the sheer number of synaptic contacts in the brain (10^{14} in the adult brain), genetic information by itself cannot specify the total number of neuronal interconnections that occur (Huttenlocher, 1994; Kandel, Schwartz, & Jessell, 1991). The circuitry of the nervous system probably arises from genetically specified instructions that enable detection of the correct pathways and targets in the brain. However, genes do not specify the patterns of connections among neurons explicitly. Edelman (1992) stated that connections shift and reassemble as a result of a dynamic series of events. Influences on the final wiring include the other cells in the vicinity and whether these cells that share proximity engage in correlated activity (see the section on Neural Activity later in this chapter).Consequently, the brain reflects a self-organizing system (Edelman) because the wiring of the brain is not strictly prespecified and the developmental driving forces, although similar from individual to individual, are not identical.

Another important contribution to the final circuitry is the information received from the environment through the sensory systems during childhood. In this way, the mature structure and function of the nervous system reflect bidirectional interactions between biological and environmental influences (Hann, 1998). Investigators have yet to determine the exact way in which these influences vary across development and what specific biological mechanisms and environmental experiences come into play.

Synaptogenesis and Synapse Elimination

The overproduction of neuronal processes and their synaptic contacts in the human cerebral cortex begins early in gestation. Most synaptogenesis, however, occurs in the postnatal period, with a rapid increase of synaptic development occurring between birth and 6 months of age (Huttenlocher, 1979; Huttenlocher & de Courten, 1987). Axons establish contact with their target neurons by branching out and synapsing with dendrites or other receptive regions on selected target cells. An axon can make contact with numerous cells, and these cells in turn receive input not only from that one axon but also from many others (Kalil, 1989). Over time, refinement of these patterns of connections occurs.

Not all of the numerous contacts formed during early development persist in the mature state. Although growth of connections is the hallmark of infancy, synapse elimination begins at about 1 year of age and, for most brain regions, is complete by about 10 years (Huttenlocher, 1994). It is important to note that this pruning of connections in childhood might be necessary for efficient cortical processing to emerge. Pruning might increase synapse efficiency. Furthermore, the fine-tuning of remaining synapses that occurs at the molecular level could also increase synaptic efficiency. These two processes—synapse elimination and fine-tuning—therefore seem related not only to brain maturation but also to behavioral competence (Rakic, Bourgeois, Eckenhoff, Zecevic, & Goldman-Rakic, 1986).

The Role of Neural Activity in Synapse Connectivity

To appreciate fully the profound influence of childhood sensory experience on synapse connectivity, it is necessary to review two neural mechanisms, the Hebb synapse and long-term potentiation. Elements of these proposed neural processes support the notion that activity or use of a synapse strengthens the connectivity and also suggest that sensory input is a primary mode through which this strengthening occurs.

Hebb Synapse

How is it that molecular events contribute to the strengthening or elimination of synapses? In 1949, Donald O. Hebb proposed that a presynaptic cell's repeated or persistent success in activating a postsynaptic cell strengthens and retains the synapse contact between the pre- and postsynaptic neurons. That is, neurons that fire together, wire together; and the effectiveness of an excitatory synapse will increase if input activity to this synapse consistently correlates with the activity of the postsynaptic neuron (Hebb, 1949). Conversely, asynchronous activity between pre- and postsynaptic neurons selectively eliminates synaptic contacts between those neurons (Constantine-Paton, Cline, & Debski, 1990). Although some activity-dependent shaping of connections occurs prenatally in response to spontaneous neuronal discharges, *activity-dependent modifications result primarily from sensory experience throughout childhood.* This suggests that neuronal activity is necessary to complete brain development and that, within limits, experience itself can modify and fine-tune the maturing nervous system, giving the brain a certain degree of adaptability (Shatz, 1992).

This experience-dependent adaptability is extremely relevant to the therapist using a sensory integrative approach. Ayres referred to the importance of correlated neural activity, noting that neurons grow and become interconnected in relation to the kind of electrical and chemical impulses that are directed over them (1972b). She further stated that use of a neural synapse increases the ease by which the fundamental connection takes place; disuse of a synapse reduces the probability that the connection will occur. In addition, ongoing neural activity is a critical component of normal development because it is self-organizing, as noted earlier (Edelman, 1992). For most people, the unfolding neural development enables individuals to interpret the environment and to respond appropriately to it (Ayres, 1972b). For a child whose brain demonstrates poor self-organizing mechanisms, intervention designed to modify these mechanisms might be helpful.

Understanding how behavioral experience alters the functional circuitry of the neocortex and consequently modifies the way it processes information has been a longstanding challenge for neuroscientists. It is not unreasonable to assume that understanding such changes will help clarify the knowledge of adaptive processes that engage the neocortex (e.g., perception, learning, and memory) (Cruickshank & Weinberger, 1996). *Sensory integration therapy, by providing specific sensory input to and eliciting a related adaptive response from the young child, could influence the Hebb synapse (the intercellular interactions that lead to synaptic strengthening or weakening of pre- and postsynaptic connectivity), which in turn enhances the organization of the brain.*

Long-Term Potentiation (LTP)

Evidence for the proposed Hebb synapse has emerged from studies of long-term potentiation (LTP) in the hippocampus, a part of the brain that is critical to learning and memory. Investigators first described LTP in the 1960s when studies showed that controlled bursts of stimulation across synapses produced long-lasting increases in synaptic efficiency (Bliss & Lomo, 1970).

It is relevant at this point to discuss LTP because it might serve as an important mechanism underlying effective sensory integration treatment. Although not addressing learning and memory per se, sensory integration might be inducing synaptic modification—or synaptic plasticity—a reported functional consequence of LTP.

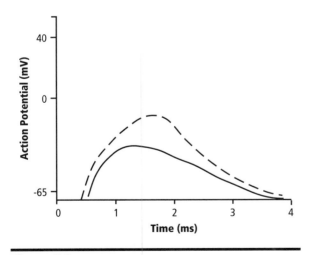

Figure 2.2.

A small excitatory postsynaptic potential (EPSP; solid line) occurs as a result of an action potential in the presynaptic neuron. A burst of high-frequency stimulation (tetanus) to the presynaptic neuron potentiates the EPSP (dashed line).

Properties of LTP

The initial experiments to induce LTP relied on giving a bundle of presynaptic axons a tetanus (a brief burst of high-frequency stimulation), then measuring the resulting excitatory postsynaptic potential (EPSP) in the postsynaptic neuron (Bear, Connors, & Paradiso, 1996). (Remember, one neuron can receive input from many axons.) An EPSP in the postsynaptic cell indicates that the cell membrane has depolarized, or become less negative, as a result of the presynaptic inputs. The early experiments demonstrated that, following the tetanus, stimulation of the presynaptic axons evoked an EPSP much greater than had been measured previously (Figure 2.2). The stimulus burst had, in fact, caused a modification of the activated synapses (synaptic plasticity) such that there was an increased postsynaptic response to the same level of presynaptic stimulation (Bear et al.).

More recently, researchers have clarified that it is not the tetanic stimulation that induces LTP. Rather, the essential element is activation of the converging presynaptic neurons *at the same time* that the postsynaptic neuron depolarizes strongly. This potentiates, or modifies, the active synapses such that the presynaptic neurons are more effective in their effect on the postsynaptic neuron. This point becomes important in a subsequent example of the use of controlled sensory input during sensory integration treatment. The underlying concept is that several presynaptic cells converge on and simultaneously depolarize a postsynaptic cell, not only enhancing the EPSP because of the summated input (Figure 2.2) but also making it possible for the presynaptic cells to depolarize the postsynaptic neuron more effectively. Other synaptic inputs onto the same neuron that are not part of this activation-depolarization coupling (i.e., are not simultaneously transmitting depolarizing input) will not show LTP. A remarkable feature of LTP is the fact that this increased effectiveness of the presynaptic neuron is long-lasting. Bear et al. (1996) showed that LTP induced in awake animals lasts many weeks and possibly even a lifetime.

The role of LTP in sensory integration might be as follows. Consider as an example the child who cannot tolerate much vestibular stimulation but seeks proprioceptive input. A typical therapeutic activity for such a child couples limited vestibular input (e.g., straddling a hammock swing with feet close to the ground) with strong proprioceptive input (such as pulling on a rope) to elicit an adaptive response (e.g., making the hammock move). Imagine that neither the vestibular nor proprioceptive input alone is capable of evoking an action potential in a postsynaptic neuron on which they converge, but that their coupled activation is capable of firing the postsynaptic neuron (Figure 2.3). Based on the principles of LTP, each of these simultaneously activated inputs becomes more effective in its ability to activate the postsynaptic neuron. LTP, therefore, could be one mechanism by which the active synapses are potentiated so that *either* vestibular *or* proprioceptive input might activate the postsynaptic neuron. That is, LTP allows a weak input to be potentiated, and in the above activity, the association of weak vestibular input with strong proprioceptive input could have a potentiating effect on the weak vestibular input. The speculation is that the potentiation occurring during this activity enhances the function of the vestibular system.

Although investigators have yet to resolve the underlying mechanisms of synaptic connectivity and plasticity, the fundamental feature is that the neural activity between the pre- and postsynaptic neurons cannot be random. Indeed, the timing of action potentials at both sites is essential in determining which synaptic connections are strengthened and retained and, conversely, which are weakened and eliminated. Indeed, Ayres (1972b) drew on her knowledge of Hebb's work regarding convergent afferent impulses when she stated that summation of stimuli, all relevant to the same aspect of environment, can produce a response not elicited by one source of stimulus alone. It is in this respect that the proposed Hebb synapse and the research into LTP provide support for sensory integration theory and treatment.

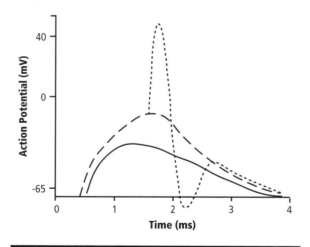

Figure 2.3.

According to the principles of LTP, a weak vestibular input (solid line) coupled with a more robust proprioceptive input (dashed line) elicits an action potential (dotted line) in the neuron on which the inputs converge. This results in both the vestibular and proprioceptive inputs becoming more effective in their ability to activate the postsynaptic neuron in the future.

A small excitatory postsynaptic potential (EPSP; solid line) occurs as a result of an action potential in the presynaptic neuron. A burst of high-frequency stimulation (tetanus) to the presynaptic neuron potentiates the EPSP (dashed line).

The Role of Behavior on Synapse Modification

Hebb synapses and LTP address events at the molecular level of neuroplasticity and brain development. At the behavioral level, there also is evidence that the brain must be stimulated in some way during development in order to achieve the precision of the adult pattern. An extensive amount of evidence suggests that behavioral factors play a crucial role in neural plasticity in that a synaptic connection undergoes significant modification when its activation connects with outcomes *important* to the animal's behavior. In other words, neural activity associated with meaningful behavioral responses is more likely to promote synaptic modifications or neuroplasticity.

Ahissar et al. (1992) recently examined whether and how general behavioral factors such as attention, motivation, and reinforcement affect functional plasticity. From electrophysiological recordings of auditory cortex neurons in adult monkeys, these investigators observed that the changes in neuronal functional plasticity were always greater in the presence of relevant behavior than when behavior was either not present or not relevant. And although Ayres (1972b) did not discuss the neural mechanisms of the adaptive response specifically, she gave numerous examples of how motivation for and emotional investment in an activity influenced a child's progress in therapy. The child who becomes involved in purposeful activity and is willing to put forth effort to make a response of a greater complexity of adaptivity is the child who usually responds well to treatment. Accordingly, this concept of relevant engagement supports the adaptive response that Ayres so strongly encouraged.

Experience-Dependent Cortical Plasticity

Certain types of sensory input early in life actually encourage the formation of neural connections. One additional support for neuroplasticity comes from research on the development of the visual system in cats. There are certain benefits in studying the cat's visual system in the effort to understand the relationship between sensory input and neural connectivity, the most important being the fact that the cat's visual system is not mature until 2 months after birth. This maturational period makes it possible for researchers to control visual experience during the final stages of development and observe the animal's physiological, anatomical, and behavioral responses.

Several of the most significant early studies showed that normal visual experience is critical to the development of primary visual cortex. Conducted in the 1960s and 1970s by David Hubel and Torsten Wiesel, these studies were an outgrowth of their examination of the effects of childhood cataracts. Clinicians had noted that failure to treat a child's condition promptly led to permanent blindness in the obstructed eye. From Hubel and Wiesel's research, for which they received the Nobel Prize, emerged the understanding of critical periods of development (see sidebar on page 36).

Hubel and Wiesel reproduced the effect of a cataract in animals by limiting the activity of one eye for periods ranging from weeks to months, an experimental manipulation called monocular deprivation. They produced monocular deprivation by either placing an opaque lens over one of the animal's eyes or suturing one lid closed. The physiological consequence of this deprivation was asymmetry of synaptic connections. Electrophysiological recordings showed that the open, seeing eye activated cortical neurons typically driven by inputs from the deprived eye. Furthermore, the cortical neurons associated with the open eye elaborated new terminal branches into the cortical territory, carrying information from the deprived eye (Wiesel & Hubel, 1963). Moreover, the degree of domination by the open eye correlated to the duration of visual deprivation. Even short exposures during a brief, most sensitive period produced pronounced changes in eye dominance (Constantine-Paton et al., 1990; Olson & Freeman, 1975). This was not the case when deprivation began later in life. The latter finding is consistent with the experience of adult humans who develop cataracts that are corrected surgically and do not cause lasting blindness. This lack of alteration of the brain's wiring following a cataract in adulthood is likely due to the critical period having ended years earlier. These observations suggest that cortical connectivity forms as a result of use early in development.

Critical Periods of Development

There are critical (or sensitive) periods during sensory cortical development when adequate stimulation of the infant is necessary for the brain ultimately to achieve its normal adult characteristics (Harwerth, Smith, Duncan, Crawford, & von Noorden, 1986). Absence of minimal stimulation (touch, speech, visual images, etc.) during the first year of a baby's life significantly delays development in motor, sensory, social, and cognitive domains. Adverse environments can disrupt normal response properties of sensory system neurons during the early postnatal period. Therefore, the quality of the sensory environment during this critical period of development has a significant impact on performance of mature sensory systems.

Anatomical studies later supplemented the early electrophysiological data. In the mature visual cortex of cats, monkeys, and humans, input from each eye is arranged into separate, alternating vertical columns of neurons called ocular dominance columns. In the newborn, ocular dominance columns have not formed yet and input to the visual cortex is therefore diffuse rather than neatly segregated into eye-specific columns. Monocular deprivation during the critical period prevents the ocular dominance columns from forming properly (Hubel, Wiesel, & LeVay, 1977; Wiesel, 1982). These studies demonstrated that the anatomy of the eye-specific cortical regions also depends on intact visual input. A likely means for the normally occurring columnar formation is selective retraction (pruning) of asynchronously activated inputs from one eye, while correlated activity in specific regions of the visual cortex strengthens and maintains synaptic contacts from the other eye.

Although the focus of this book is the child with developmental disabilities, it is important to appreciate fully that the end of critical periods of development does not signal the end of plasticity in the brain. Adults exhibit experience-dependent plasticity in some higher cortical areas that is as robust as the plastic changes noted in the sensory cortical regions of developing brains (Bear et al., 1996). Recent research on monkeys and other animals shows that the brain continually and dynamically reorganizes itself. Understanding the brain's ability for dynamic reorganization in adulthood helps explain how patients sometimes recover brain functions damaged by injury or disease. Although researchers have recognized for years that new neuronal connections can emerge with surprising speed following injury even in adulthood (Schmid, Rosa, & Calford, 1995), recent research has demonstrated that specific regions of the adult mammalian central nervous system generate new neurons continuously (Johansson et al., 1999). Of great importance is the finding that the proliferation rate of new neurons increases dramatically in response to central nervous system injury. This provocative new research could prove valuable in understanding the mechanisms of neuroplasticity throughout the life span.

The Effects of Prenatal Stress on Function

Prenatal stress and fetal alcohol exposure are two areas of research that demonstrate the effects of environment, specifically the prenatal environment, on nervous system development and function. Recent studies by Schneider and others have shown that neuroplasticity and environmental programming of neural systems are important not only in the postnatal period but in fact begin in the prenatal period. Indeed, a large body of literature exists indicating that the fetal brain is especially vulnerable to damage from toxins and malnourishment. The studies reviewed here provide a model for understanding how the prenatal environment can mold or modify the developing neural system. Furthermore, these studies have important implications for sensory integration because they demonstrate that the nervous system is changeable and can be altered by environmental influences. Understanding environmental risk factors associated with stress, violence, toxins, and malnutrition and their impact upon development is important for highlighting key prevention issues and developing prevention strategies.

Schneider and colleagues have been studying important changes that occur in the postnatal behavior and physiology of rhesus monkeys born to mothers that experienced mild, chronic, unpredictable psychological stress during pregnancy. These studies provide evidence that stressful events occurring in the mother's environment before the birth of the infant can change the behavioral expression of the infant and cause long-lasting effects on the individual's behavior and physiology as development unfolds.

In the first study, the animals experienced 10-minute stressors (removal from home cage and exposure to three random loud noises) that modelled recurrent, episodic stress on gestational days 90 to 145 of a 165-day gestation period. The prenatally stressed monkey offspring were lower in birth weight, delayed in independent self-feeding, more distractible, lower on an evaluation of muscle tone (Schneider, 1992b), and showed decreased postrotary nystagmus (Schneider & Coe, 1993; Schneider, Roughton, Koehler, & Lubach, 1999). As they matured, they showed evidence of delayed cognitive development (Schneider, 1992a), increased stress reactivity (Clarke & Schneider, 1993; Schneider, 1992c), altered social and adaptive behavior (Clarke, Soto, Bergholz, & Schneider, 1996), impaired stress hormone regulation (Clarke, Wittwer, Abbott, & Schneider, 1994), and differences in concentrations of dopamine and norepinephrine neurotransmitters in cerebral spinal fluid (Schneider et al., 1999). These studies clearly underscore not only the vulnerability of the prenatal infant's nervous system but also the short- and long-term effects of stress on development, learning, and levels of brain neurotransmitters.

These results led to an important question: Is there a critical period during fetal development when the brain is most vulnerable to prenatal stress effects and, if so, is there a time when prenatal stress has its most significant effects? A second study compared the offspring of mothers who were stressed during early gestation (gestational days 45 to 90) to those whose mothers were stressed during mid-late gestation (days 90 to 145) and controls. Infants born to mothers exposed to stress in early pregnancy weighed less and had more pronounced and more pervasive motor impairments compared to those from the other two groups. Specifically, the early pregnancy stress group demonstrated decreased muscle tone, coordination, balance, righting responses, and postrotary nystagmus response in comparison to the mid-late gestation stress and the control groups. On measures of attention and motor maturity, animals from both experimental groups scored lower than those monkeys whose mothers had undisturbed pregnancies (Schneider et al., 1998).

These findings suggest that excess maternal stress can induce attention and neuro-motor deficits in offspring. However, from a critical or sensitive period perspective, the results fail to support the notion that a sensitive period exists for these effects. A sensitive period implies that when particular events occur during but not outside of a specific stage of development, they induce altered structure or function (Sillito, 1983). Offspring from mothers stressed during either early or mid-late gestation had attention and neuromotor deficits, although monkeys stressed during early gestation also had low birth weights, decreased postrotary nystagmus, and more severe motor impairments. In light of the conceptualizations of the sensitive period by Bornstein (1989) and Hinde (1962), it is perhaps more helpful to view the sensitive period not as constant but rather as a peak, skewed to the onset, followed by a plateau that gradually tapers off. In this light, the data from these studies suggest that sensitivity to prenatal stress peaks in early gestation and tapers off in mid-late gestation.

Alcohol and Stress During the Prenatal Period

A second issue addressed by the research of Schneider and others is whether prenatal stress exacerbates the effects of other prenatal perturbations known to affect neuro-development of the offspring adversely, such as exposure to alcohol. To deal with the question of whether prenatal stress exacerbates the effects of known teratogens, the researchers randomly assigned pregnant monkeys to one of four groups: a group that received stress alone, a group that received stress and alcohol, a group that received alcohol alone, and a control group that received a sucrose solution (Schneider, Roughton, & Lubach, 1997).

The findings indicated that alcohol (the teratogen) accompanied by stress during gestation resulted in increased fetal losses and birth weight reductions in males compared to stress alone, alcohol alone, or controls. Infants from both the alcohol alone and alcohol-plus-stress conditions demonstrated lower scores on measures of attention and motor maturity than controls (Schneider et al., 1997). Finally, infants that were exposed in utero either to alcohol alone or alcohol plus stress showed increased glucocorticoid responsivity to stress (Schneider & Koehler, 1997).

Neuroimaging studies are currently underway to establish the linkage between these findings and actual alterations in neural systems, such as dopamine receptors in the striatum. In addition, the authors are conducting correlative studies of neurotransmitter function and behavioral measures in an effort to elucidate the relationship between brain function and the behavioral profile associated with prenatal stress and/or prenatal alcohol exposure.

Implications for Sensory Integration

Research has shown that prenatal stress and/or fetal alcohol exposure can affect a number of behavioral and physiological systems in the developing offspring. These studies provide a model for understanding how the prenatal environment can mold or modify the developing neural system and have important implications for sensory integration.

Another interesting focus of these studies concerns the notion of adaptability. Malleability of certain neural systems allows individuals to adapt to the unique demands of their environment. As noted earlier, environmental events become incorporated into the biology of the individual in the form of altered neural processes. These alterations then come into play when the organism encounters new experiences

(Boyce et al., 1998). For example, the infants from the prenatal stress group showed high levels of stress hormones under challenging conditions. Because individuals whose mothers experienced stress during pregnancy are also likely to be born into a stressful environment, increased release of glucocorticoids in response to stress might enable more rapid mobilization of energy resources and might promote changes in cognitive processes necessary to deal with a high-stress environment. However, the bulk of the evidence supports the hypothesis that animals (including humans) from prenatally stressed pregnancies show alterations in neuronal functioning that are similar to those occurring in depression in humans (Meijer, 1985; Wadhwa, Dunkel-Schetter, Chicz-DeMet, Porto, & Sandman, 1996).

Other researchers have suggested a model for fetal programming of human disease based on the concept of a set point determined during intrauterine life (Barker, 1995). Additional research hopefully will elucidate some of the processes through which prenatal stress transforms neural development. Moreover, researchers have yet to determine how the postnatal environment interacts to attenuate or exacerbate prenatal stress effects.

Further studies need to examine glucocorticoid reactivity to stress in individuals with sensory integrative dysfunction. It is interesting to note that Ayres described children with sensory integrative disorders as fearful and anxious, which suggests enhanced or unmodulated stress responsivity. Additionally, she stated that they tend to be "emotionally labile, . . . less well prepared to cope, . . . and emotionally fragile" (1972b, p. 210). She also described a now well-known syndrome in which children respond to tactile stimulation with anxiety and discomfort and subsequently either withdraw or display overt hostility (Ayres, 1972b).

In a more recent study, Koomar (1996) studied 5- to 13-year-old children whom occupational therapists had identified as dyspraxic. She reported two relationships in these children: one between anxiety and gravitational insecurity and another between anxiety and dyspraxia. This important study lends support to Ayres' hypothesis that some children with sensory integrative dysfunction are prone to anxiety and provides further suggestion of increased responsivity in these children.

If children with sensory integrative dysfunction show this increased responsivity to stressful or challenging events, might this hyperresponsivity to stress be alerting the individual to potential danger and helping to mobilize energy? If so, could reduction in stress reactivity produce more desirable behavioral responsivity? Further studies by occupational therapy researchers need to examine the hormonal responses to environmental stress or challenge in children with sensory integrative dysfunction.

Summary

Central to many of the theories describing mechanisms by which the infant's nervous system produces an adaptive response to environmental changes and challenges is the concept of neural plasticity and the way in which the nervous system organizes and reorganizes relative to experiences with the environment. This provides important and significant support for sensory integration therapy and practice in that:

1. Sensory input appears capable of enhancing neural connectivity through LTP and the Hebb cell.

2. Activity that is meaningful to the individual, or what Ayres called the adaptive response, promotes this neural activity.

3. There is clear evidence of plasticity in the visual system, and it is likely that plasticity also occurs in other sensory systems.

4. Environment and biology interact in a bidirectional manner, and this begins early in fetal life.

Works Cited

References

Ahissar, E., Vaadia, E., Ahissar, M., Bergman, H., Arieli, A., & Abeles, M. (1992). Dependence of cortical plasticity on correlated activity of single neurons and on behavioral context. *Science, 257,* 1412–1415.

Ayres, A.J. (1964). Tactile functions: Their relation to hyperactive and perceptual motor behavior. *American Journal of Occupational Therapy, 18,* 83–95.

Ayres, A.J. (1965). Patterns of perceptual-motor dysfunction in children: A factor analytic study. *Perceptual and Motor Skills, 20,* 335–368.

Ayres, A.J. (1966). Interrelationships among perceptual-motor functions in children. *American Journal of Occupational Therapy, 20,* 288–292.

Ayres, A.J. (1969). Deficits in sensory integration in educationally handicapped children. *Journal of Learning Disabilities, 2,* 160–168.

Ayres, A.J. (1972a). Improving academic scores through sensory integration. *Journal of Learning Disabilities, 5,* 338–343.

Ayres, A.J. (1972b). *Sensory integration and learning disorders.* Los Angeles: Western Psychological Services.

Barker, D.J. (1995). The fetal and infant origins of disease. *European Journal of Clinical Investigation, 25,* 457–463.

Bear, M.F., Connors, B.W., & Paradiso, M.A. (1996). *Neuroscience: Exploring the brain.* Baltimore: Williams and Wilkins.

Bliss, T.V., & Lomo, T. (1970). Plasticity in a monosynaptic cortical pathway. *Journal of Physiology, 207,* 61P.

Bornstein, M.H. (1989). Sensitive periods in development: Structural characteristics and causal interpretations. *Psychological Bulletin, 105,* 179–197.

Boyce, W.T., Frank, E., Jensen, P.S., Kessler, R.C., Nelson, C.A., & Steinberg, L. (1998). Social context in developmental psychopathology: Recommendations for future research from the MacArthur Network on psychopathology and development. *Development and Psychopathology, 10,* 143–164.

Buonomano, D.V., & Merzenich, M.M. (1998). Cortical plasticity: From synapses to maps. *Annual Review of Neuroscience, 21,* 149–186.

Chugani, H.T. (1994). Development of regional brain glucose metabolism in relation to behavior and plasticity. In G. Dawson & K.W. Fischer (Eds.), *Human behavior and the developing brain* (pp. 153–175). New York: Guilford Press.

Clarke, A.S., & Schneider, M.L. (1993). Prenatal stress has long-term effects on behavioral responses to stress in juvenile rhesus monkeys. *Developmental Psychobiology, 26,* 293–304.

Clarke, A.S., Soto, A., Bergholz, T., & Schneider, M.L. (1996). Maternal gestational stress alters adaptive and social behavior in adolescent rhesus monkey offspring. *Infant Behavior and Development, 19,* 453–463.

Clarke, A.S., Wittwer, D.J., Abbott, D.H., & Schneider, M.L. (1994). Long-term effects of prenatal stress on HPA axis activity in juvenile rhesus monkeys. *Developmental Psychobiology, 27,* 257–269.

Constantine-Paton, M., Cline, H.T., & Debski, E. (1990). Patterned activity, synaptic convergence, and the NMDA receptor in developing visual pathways. *Annual Review of Neuroscience, 13,* 29–54.

Cooper, R.M., & Zubek, J.P. (1958). Effects of enriched and restricted early environments on the learning ability of bright and dull rats. *Canadian Journal of Psychology, 12,* 159–164.

Cruickshank, S.J., & Weinberger, N.M. (1996). Evidence for the Hebbian hypothesis in experience-dependent physiological plasticity of neocortex: A critical review. *Brain Research Reviews, 22,* 191–228.

Diamond, M.C., Rosenzweig, M.R., Bennett, E.L., Lindner, B., & Lyon, L. (1972). Effects of environmental enrichment and impoverishment on rat cerebral cortex. *Journal of Neurobiology, 3,* 47–64.

Edelman, G.M. (1992). *Bright air, brilliant fire: On the matter of the mind.* New York: Harper Collins.

Greenough, W.T. (1975). Experiential modification of the developing brain. *American Scientist, 63,* 37–46.

Hann, D.M. (1998). Developmental plasticity conference: Introduction. In D.M. Hann, L.C. Huffman, I.I. Lederhendler, & D. Meinecke (Eds.), *Advancing research on developmental plasticity: Integrating the behavioral science and neuroscience of mental health* (pp. 1–8). Bethesda, MD: National Institutes of Health.

Harlow, H.F. (1958). The nature of love. *American Psychologist, 13,* 673–685.

Harlow, H.F., Harlow, M.K., & Suomi, S.J. (1971). From thought to therapy: Lessons from a primate laboratory. *American Scientist, 59,* 538–549.

Harwerth, R.S., Smith, E.L., Duncan, G.C., Crawford, M.L.J., & von Noorden, G.K. (1986). Multiple sensitive periods in the development of the primate visual system. *Science, 232,* 235–238.

Hebb, D.O. (1949). *The organization of behavior: A neuropsychological theory.* New York: Wiley.

Hinde, R.A. (1962). Sensitive periods and the development of behavior. *Little Club Clinic in Developmental Medicine, 7,* 25–36.

Hubel, D.H., Wiesel, T.N., & LeVay, S. (1977). Plasticity of ocular dominance columns in monkey striate cortex. *Philosophical Transactions of the Royal Society of London (Series B), 278,* 377–407.

Huttenlocher, P.R. (1979). Synaptic density in human frontal cortex: Developmental changes and effects of aging. *Brain Research, 163,* 195–205.

Huttenlocher, P.R. (1994). Synaptogenesis in human cerebral cortex. In G. Dawson & K.W. Fischer (Eds.), *Human behavior and the developing brain* (pp. 137–157). New York: Guilford Press.

Huttenlocher P.R., & de Courten, C. (1987). The development of synapses in striate cortex in man. *Human Neurobiology, 6,* 1–9.

Johansson, C.B., Momma, S., Clarke, D.L., Risling, M., Lendahl, U., & Firsén, J. (1999). Identification of a neural stem cell in the adult mammalian central nervous system. *Cell, 96,* 25–34.

Kaas, J.H. (1991). Plasticity of sensory and motor maps in adult mammals. *Annual Review of Neuroscience, 14,* 137–167.

Kalil, R.E. (1989). Synapse formation in the developing brain. *Scientific American, 260,* 76–85.

Kandel, E.R., Schwartz, J.H., & Jessell, T.M. (1991). *Principles of neural science* (3rd ed.). Norwalk, CT: Appleton & Lange.

Koomar, J.A. (1996). Vestibular dysfunction and dyspraxia associated with anxiety rather than behavioral inhibition. *Sensory Integration Special Interest Newsletter, 19,* 1–4.

Liu, E., Diorio, J., Tannenbaum, B., Caldji, C., Francis, D., Freedman, A., Sharma, S., Pearson, D., Plotsky, P.M., & Meaney, M.J. (1997). Maternal care, hippocampal glucocorticoid receptors, and hypothalamic-pituitary-adrenal responses to stress. *Science, 277,* 1659–1662.

Meaney, M.J., O'Donnell, D., Viau, V., Ghatnagar, S., Sarrieau, A., Smythe, J.W., Shanks, N., & Walker, D. (1994). Corticosteroid receptors in rat brain and pituitary during development and hypothalamic-pituitary-adrenal (HPA) function. In P. McLaughlin & I. Zagon (Eds.), *Receptors and the developing nervous system* (pp. 163–202). London: Chapman & Hall.

Meijer, A. (1985). Child psychiatric sequelae of maternal war stress. *Acta Psychiatry Scandinavia, 72,* 505–511.

Olson, C.R., & Freeman, R.D. (1975). Progressive changes in kitten striate cortex during monocular vision. *Journal of Neurophysiology, 38,* 26–32.

Rakic, P., Bourgeois, J.P., Eckenhoff, M.F., Zecevic, N., & Goldman-Rakic, P.S. (1986). Concurrent overproduction of synapses in diverse regions of the primate cerebral cortex. *Science, 232,* 232–234.

Rosenzweig, M.R., & Bennett, E.L. (1996). Psychobiology of plasticity: Effects of training and experience on brain and behavior. *Behavioral Brain Research, 78,* 57–65.

Scardina, V. (1986, Fall). Scardina presentation featured at SII Symposium 1986. *Sensory Integration International News, 14,* 1–10.

Schmid, L.M., Rosa, M.G.P., & Calford, M.B. (1995). Retinal detachment induces massive immediate reorganization in visual cortex. *Neuroreport, 6,* 1349–1353.

Schneider, M.L. (1992a). Delayed object permanence development in prenatally stressed rhesus monkey infants (*Macaca mulatta*). *Occupational Therapy Journal of Research, 12,* 96–110.

Schneider, M.L. (1992b). The effect of mild stress during pregnancy on birth weight and neuromotor maturation in rhesus monkey infants (*Macaca mulatta*). *Infant Behavior and Development, 15,* 389–403.

Schneider, M.L. (1992c). Prenatal stress exposure alters postnatal behavioral expression under conditions of novelty challenge in rhesus monkey infants. *Developmental Psychobiology, 25,* 141–152.

Schneider, M.L., Clarke, A.S., Kraemer, G.W., Roughton, E.C., Lubach, G., Rimm-Kaufman, S., Schmidt, D., & Ebert, M. (1998). Prenatal stress alters brain biogenic amine levels in primates. *Development and Psychopathology, 10,* 427–440.

Schneider, M.L., & Coe, C.L. (1993). Repeated social stress during pregnancy impairs neuromotor development of the primate infant. *Journal of Developmental and Behavioral Pediatrics, 14,* 81–87.

Schneider, M.L., & Koehler, A. (1997, June). The effect of moderate alcohol consumption and/or stress during pregnancy on offspring behavior and neuroendocrine responses. *Neurobehavioral Teratology Society Twenty-first Annual Meeting (Neurotoxicology and Teratology), 19*(3), 243–244.

Schneider, M.L., Roughton, E.C., Koehler, A.J., & Lubach, G.R. (1999). Growth and development following prenatal stress exposure in primates: An examination of ontogenetic vulnerability. *Child Development, 70,* 263–274.

Schneider, M.L., Roughton, E., & Lubach, G. (1997). Moderate alcohol consumption and psychological stress during pregnancy induces attention and neuromotor impairments in primate infants. *Child Development, 68,* 747–759.

Shatz, C. J. (1992). The developing brain. *Scientific American, 267,* 60–67.

Sillito, A.M. (1983). Plasticity in the visual cortex. *Nature, 303,* 477–478.

Wadhwa, P.D., Dunkel-Schetter, C., Chicz-DeMet, A., Porto, M., & Sandman, C.A. (1996). Prenatal psychosocial factors and the neuroendocrine axis in human pregnancy. *Psychosomatic Medicine, 58,* 432–446.

Wiesel, T.N. (1982). Postnatal development of the visual cortex and the influence of environment. *Nature, 299,* 583–591.

Wiesel, T.N., & Hubel, D.H. (1963). Single cell responses in striate cortex of kittens deprived of vision in one eye. *Journal of Neurophysiology, 26,* 1003–1007.

Developmental Neuroplasticity:
A Foundation for Sensory Integration

GARY W. KRAEMER, PH.D., OTR

Prenatal stress, as discussed in chapter 2, might lead to changes in neural plasticity of the newborn. Another significant factor in the postnatal period is discussed in this chapter. The mother's stress level will also affect the development and expression of the infant's nervous system. This chapter focuses on maternal stress and how this affects mothering behavior, and subsequently the infant's development. It will also help provide a framework for postnatal plasticity that may be applied to clinical practice. The material in this chapter focuses specifically on the dynamic relations between environment, stress, genetics, and infant development, highlighting the long-term effects of prenatal stress on future generations. This information supports sensory integration theory by demonstrating that inadequate sensory experiences, such as those that an infant reared by a stressed mother would receive, affect infant development and behavior, not only in utero but also in future generations. This knowledge is of value to sensory integration theory and practice because it establishes a framework for appreciation of the critical role that early sensory experiences play in later behavior and development.

Mammalian Mothers and Infants as Dynamic Systems

The mammalian literature provides some evidence and clues about mother-infant relationships and the effects of these relationships on development. For example, the stressed mother who is typically involved in care of the stressed newborn serves as a model for viewing the interactions of the mother's and the infant's systems. First, in looking back toward the underlying causes of prenatal stress, it is important to consider how the pregnant mother herself developed and learned to adapt to stressors or succeeded in minimizing her exposure to stressors. How she learned to mother her newborn and buffer postnatal environmental stressors to which the infant might be exposed is also an issue.

Looking forward, the female offspring of thriving mammalian species typically become parents themselves and therefore are affected by the experiences they had with their mothers. The issue of how early environment affects postnatal sensory integration can be critical. In other words, how the mother performs the task of mothering can relate to integrative experiences that the new mother had with her own mother. This begins a dynamic interaction between experience, integration, and future behavior.

To examine this issue, it is helpful to place a "time window" over a mother-infant system that extends both backward and forward in time and has as the minimum players the mother and her infant. The window shifts in time, showing the mother as once an infant, the infant grown and a mother, and the interrelationship of the two as dynamic, interactive systems.

The current view of development as the interaction of dynamic systems is significantly different from past developmental theories and has relevance to this discussion. The old view of development saw the genetic code as a plan or blueprint for the structure of the individual that ultimately determines the individual's behavior. The more recent developmental perspective proposes that changes in many biological systems are and must be promoted by an interaction with the environment (Hofer, 1987; Kraemer, 1992b; Thelen & Smith, 1994).

This chapter refers to biological systems that are dependent on environmental interactions to determine many aspects of their functional structure as *dynamic* systems. In the present context, *plasticity* refers to the ability of the nervous system to change its functional structure and parameters of function in relation to environmental stimuli. The expression of plasticity (the ability to change) depends upon an interaction between the genetic code, past and ongoing experience, and an ability of biological dynamic systems to develop models or internal representations of both probable and preferred future states (also referred to as attractor states). Research in psychobiology indicates that learning is much more important for animal maternal and infant behaviors than previously thought (Fleming, Morgam, & Walsh, 1996).

Study of the neurobiological basis of mother-young interactions in nonhuman mammals has revealed three principles that apply to species-characteristic behaviors in animals and to some aspects of human behavior (Fleming, Morgam, et al., 1996).

1. Behavior patterns considered to be preprogrammed are not necessarily expressed automatically or autonomously. Interactions that the infant usually has with its mother promote typical neurobiological development and the expression of innate behavior.

2. Learning in infancy and adulthood can bring about substantial modification in innate behavior patterns, often considered to be stereotyped once they have been expressed.

3. Developing the ability to modify stereotyped behaviors also appears to depend on early experiences.

Consistent with these principles, the expression of maternal behavior in reproductive maturity and the ability to modify this behavior in relation to environmental contingencies depend on experiences that the mother had with her own mother (Fleming, O'Day, & Kraemer, 1999).

The literature cited in the following section illustrates these principles. The first objective is to describe how maternal care influences infant neurobiological development in ways that are enduring and that can, in turn, affect the infant's subsequent adult social and maternal behavior. The second objective is to describe how experiences that the mother has with offspring modify her own sensory, neural, endocrine, and neurochemical mechanisms that mediate learning and plasticity. These experience-based changes tune the expression of hormonally primed innate maternal behavior and alter the responsiveness of the mother to present and future offspring. Such effects then play out in neurobiological development of offspring and their subsequent maternal behavior. A final objective is to consider the role of learning and plasticity in human development and in developmental pathology.

The Mother-Young Relationship in Animals

The way a mother cares for her young influences not only the infant's neurobiology but also the infant's later social and maternal behaviors. Nonhuman mammalian mothers typically display a stereotyped set of behavioral responses to their newborns. They show species-typical ways of transporting, holding, feeding, and grooming the young and of protecting them from predators and other dangers (Rosenblatt & Snowdon, 1995). Maternal behaviors enabling the young to suckle promote the infant's physiological and immunological resilience and physical maturation. Adequate maternal behavior also influences appropriate social and emotional development in the young that enhances their later reproductive success. In return, mammalian neonates exhibit behavior that is even more stereotyped and rigid than maternal behavior. This includes orchestrated orienting responses towards the mother, seeking of teats or nest sites, and emission of sound signals that elicit maternal responses (crying, squealing, and so forth). Ultimately, the reciprocal exhibition of maternal behaviors and newborn signaling increases the probability that young will survive and, beyond survival, will mate and rear their own offspring successfully. It might seem puzzling, then, that what is perceived as relatively rigidly dictated behavior ultimately relates to mechanisms of sensory integration and neural plasticity.

The Infant Becomes Experienced Through the Mother

The behavioral effects of early experiences within the context of the maternal nest are mediated by neurochemistry and neuroanatomy that have altered substantially in response to the early experiences (Fleming et al., 1999). Rat pups develop specific recognition of the mother's odor as the mother licks the pups. The formation of this association between licking and maternal odor depends on licking-induced activation of the developing brain's norepinephrine neurons that project to the olfactory bulbs (Wilson & Sullivan, 1994). Recognition of maternal odor by offspring depends on neural plasticity, that is, molecular, neurochemical, and cytoarchitectural changes in the olfactory bulb of the brain. Consequently, there is a clear relationship between sensory input and changes in the nervous system.

Early experiences with the mother also affect developing young in more diffuse ways that affect their emotional lability, cognitive style, and responsiveness to stress. For example, maternal licking and touching of the rat pup produce long-term reductions in emotional reactivity to novelty and stress (Francis et al., 1996). Natural variations in mothering behavior produce these decreases and can affect the way individuals interact socially and, subsequently, with their own offspring.

Mothers Learn About and From Their Infants: Behavioral Effects

Experiences acquired during adulthood facilitate and modify the expression of species-characteristic patterns of adult behavior that increase the survival chances of young (Fleming, Corter, & Steiner, 1996). For example, sheep mothers (ewes) will initially nurse any lamb, but soon after parturition, a ewe learns to recognize its own lamb by its odor. Once the ewe has smelled her lamb's odor (usually the mother's own amniotic fluid), she butts away all alien-smelling lambs and permits only hers to nurse. This is a change from the behaviors she exhibited earlier, caused by a change in her nervous system precipitated by the perception of her own lamb's odors (Poindron & Levy, 1990).

In ewes, a variety of neuropeptides, including oxytocin and corticotrophin-releasing hormone, increase in concentration at parturition and act in synergy with cervical stimulation (which occurs during the birth of the lamb) to enhance recognition and subsequent learning of the new lamb's odors (Poindron & Levy, 1990). Consolidation of the association between the mother's birthing stimuli (cervical dilation) and attraction to the lamb's odor appears to include neurochemical changes in the olfactory bulb and the brain (Keverne, 1995). Development of specific odor recognition involves changes in olfactory bulb mechanisms (Levy, Kendrick, Keverne, Porter, & Romeyer, 1996). This recognition of and then attraction to the lamb, which is an example of neural plasticity in adulthood, occurs within hours of giving birth and requires only a few minutes of exposure to the lamb to form (Poindron & Levy).

Human mothers experience a similar phenomenon when they come to recognize their own infant's odors, cries, and touch characteristics (Fleming, Morgam, et al., 1996). They are able to do so even with very brief exposure to these features on the first few postpartum days. Mothers who nurse their infants sooner after birth and/or who keep their faces in close proximity to their infants while holding them (hence acquiring more olfactory experience?) are more attracted to their infant's body odors and come to recognize them more easily (Fleming, Steiner, & Corter, 1997). Moreover, in many primate species (including humans), prior experiences of caring for young either during adolescence (with siblings) or after a previous birth can have profound effects on how competent or motivated mothers are in caring for their own offspring (Fleming, Ruble, Flett, & Shaul, 1988).

Transgenerational Integration

Many psychobiological systems exhibit "loops" in maternal-infant relationships such as the one described previously. Recognition of the mother by the infant and the infant by the mother involves the formation of an olfactory recognition in association with somatic stimulation (cervical stimulation in the ewe, being licked in the pup). This process in both mother and infant involves somatosensory activation of the brain sympathetic nervous system. Such activation promotes formation of cytoarchitectural and synaptic changes leading to increased discrimination of odors and association of odor information with somatosensory stimulation provided either by birthing (in the case of the mother) or by maternal grooming or cleaning (in the case of the offspring). These processes occur within the olfactory bulb itself, and they are transported across time windows and generations.

It is likely that the experience of associating maternal odors with behavioral responses (i.e., licking) in infancy lays the foundation for rapid expression of maternal behavior in adulthood. Stated another way, the development of the rat pup's ability to discriminate maternal odor means that the neural machinery from receptor mechanisms to more central processing has changed. This is likely to determine how this rat will process and discriminate pup odors when the pup becomes a mother herself (Fleming et al., 1999). Thus, one might be interested in how mothering prospectively affects infant behavior, or how the mothering the infant received as a pup retrospectively accounts for adult behavior. In either case, there are numerous factors that affect how the mother responds to her own offspring.

Maternal Deprivation

One of the ways to determine how experiences with the mother affect the offspring's behavior is to contrast the behavior of individuals who were mothered with those who had no mother. In mammals, this obviously does not mean that individuals with no mother were not cared for at all, otherwise they would not be alive. For animals, having no mother means though that the infant was fed, cleaned, and provided for, the infant did not have the experiences typically provided by a biological mother. Other research has found that maternally deprived (peer-reared) monkeys demonstrate high stress reactivity and that maternal deprivation in primates produces deficits in subsequent mothering behavior (Clarke, 1993; Harlow, Harlow, & Hansen, 1963; Kraemer, 1992a; Suomi & Ripp, 1983).

Although investigators have not studied the neurobiological effects of complete maternal deprivation in humans, studies of children reared in orphanages in Romania indicate that these children exhibit disrupted physiological, sensorimotor, emotional, and cognitive development that is remarkably similar to that observed in isolated rhesus monkeys (Carlson & Earls, 1997). Other findings reported by these researchers include dysregulation of the hypothalamic-pituitary-adrenocortical axis and performance on the *Bayley Scales of Infant Development* (Bayley, 1993) that is strikingly below the norm.

There is also substantial evidence that infants who experienced abusive or neglectful parenting exhibit difficulty parenting their own offspring (Knutson, 1995). This is an intergenerational effect in which children who have been abused develop personalities as adults lacking in self-knowledge and empathy for their own children's pain and misfortune (Werner, 1989). Given the effects of experience on the brain in other animals, it is quite possible that these children have experienced neurologic changes that result in altered affective, perceptual, and cognitive function during development (Kraemer, 1997). Such changes are more than likely to affect how they perceive and respond maternally to their own offspring, how they approach maternal care responsibilities, and how they are able to learn or modify maternal care practices (Fleming et al., 1999).

These data demonstrate that learning and plasticity mechanisms are critical in the regulation of transactional relationships, of which the mother-young relationship is but one example. In mammals, olfactory and somatosensory experiences play a role in the attraction between mother and young and in their mutual recognition. These experiences permit the young to maintain proximity to their own mothers and enable them to respond appropriately to their own offspring when they grow up. Mothers, in turn, depend on postpartum experiences with their young to sustain their responsiveness in the absence of hormonal effects that can play a role at birth.

Experiences with offspring earlier in life or after a previous birth also enhance, refine, or tune responsiveness towards subsequent offspring. **Experience with one another profoundly changes brain neurochemistry, structure, and function in both mother and young. Such effects are usually adaptive in a positive way: they promote survival of offspring and enhance their later ability to rear their own offspring.** On the other hand, these same plasticity mechanisms can operate negatively. Adverse experiences such as maternal deprivation, abuse, or neglect can affect neurobiological development in ways that promote developmental psychopathology and limit the ability of individuals to care adequately for their offspring. Why this should be this way is unknown. Perhaps the major theoretical and clinical problems to be faced are why is it that changes in plastic systems can be persistent or even permanent?

The Bridge Between Science and Practice

How can a theory of development involving multiple levels of analysis (social, behavioral, and biological), multiple aspects of central nervous system function (sensory, motor, endocrine, emotional, cognitive), and multiple sources of probable causation of change serve both basic scientists and clinicians? One possibility is to develop a theory that focuses on the interactions and integration of systems in addition to the cause-and-effect mechanisms within systems. Such theories should not be foreign to the reader. Sensory integration theory is one such example. This section of the chapter puts sensory integration theory into the broader context of contemporary developmental psychobiology, first taking a historical perspective that outlines multiple systems theory, which is more akin to medical models of development and clinical reasoning, then using this foundation to outline a holistic model that is ultimately more compatible with current trends in psychobiology and clinical occupational therapy.

Holistic Versus Multiple Systems

Figure 3.1 graphically portrays a multiple-systems view of the development of the human individual from conception to maturity. Conceptually distinct subsystems of the neonate must change over time, and in concert, in order to comprise a typically developed mature individual. In this way, it is possible to characterize the whole human as having somatic, neurophysiological, psychosocial, emotional, and cognitive aspects. These components themselves contain many subcomponents. For example, the nervous system consists of peripheral and central nervous systems. Within the central nervous system (CNS), further subdivisions include structural, metabolic support, neurotransmitter, and neuroendocrine subsystems, and so on.

According to this view, one explanation for typical development is that genes express multiple codeveloping systems (i.e., CNS, skeletal anatomy, physiology) beginning at conception, and these systems change over time. These changes might

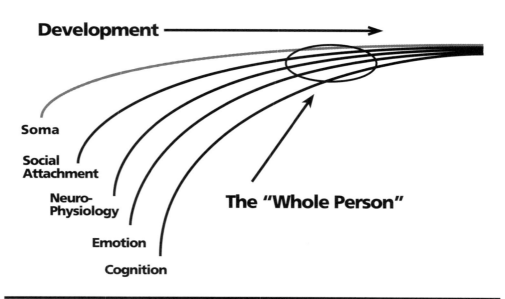

Figure 3.1. Multiple-systems view of development

run in parallel, in a preprogrammed or autonomous fashion. A human infant is born with a brain approximately one-fourth the volume of the typical adult brain. The brain increases in size because of increased neuronal arborization and concurrent proliferation of support cells. The cranium is also expanding postpartum. It could be that the brain (neural and support tissue) and cranium (bone) are set genetically to grow at a certain rate. In typical development, the processes determining brain and cranial growth would not have to interact because volume needed (brain) versus volume encompassed (cranium) would be predetermined. The critical idea here is that much of what is considered "typical physiological development" does not necessarily include the provision that developing systems interact with one another.

If one or more systems fail, what might occur is a divergence from typical development, with many systems being functionally intact but constrained by the lack of development in other systems (see Figure 3.2). Hence, a disorder that limited neural plasticity, for example, would have an impact on the development of the brain (a system with many subcomponents).

In general terms, a genetic defect, disease, poisoning, or trauma might affect one system in the brain and, consequently, constrain the development of other intact and "healthy" systems. According to this view, the goal of problem identification (diagnosis) is to locate the root or most basic problem. Intervention then targets the failing or deficient system. If intervention is successful, hopefully the symptoms would regress and typical developmental processes would resume.

The problem with this "medical-model" view of basing diagnosis and treatment of developmental disorders on the idea that pathology can be localized to one or more subsystems is that it seems to apply to only a small proportion of developmental disorders. To see why this is true requires a review of some terminology and concepts of development and developmental pathology from a psychobiological and holistic viewpoint.

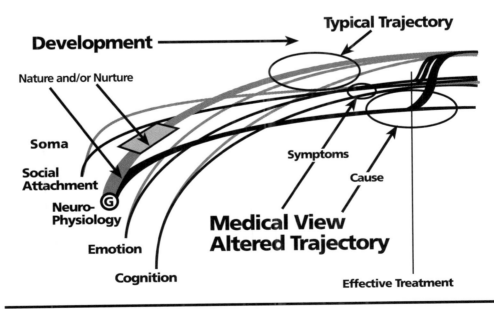

Figure 3.2. Medical diagnosis and treatment

The Psychobiological or Holistic View: Developmental Trajectory

Interaction and Integration

The preceding example of brain and bone growth involved only two systems, brain and bone, and was restricted in that these were the only two systems interacting. Furthermore, there was a presumption that although bone growth might constrain brain development, solving the bone growth problem presumably could allow the brain to resume its development where it left off. After all, there was nothing wrong with this system in the first place. It is important to consider the reasons why this view does not work for many developmental disorders.

There are mechanisms that act as an interface between internal (self) and external regulation. A number of "interface" mechanisms provide for communication between systems. Multiple systems of the individual interact with one another; they do not run in parallel, and their actions must be integrated.

One might suppose that at a most basic or physiological level, genetics determines the integration of biological systems. However, as noted in the preceding sections, interactions with the environment affect the biology of the individual and have implications for understanding developmental disorders.

A genetic defect or exposure to disease, trauma, or some kind of physiological insult produces a localized effect on one system, and, consequently, that system is now set on a different trajectory (Figure 3.3). The system will not develop at the same rate and with the same characteristics nor will it reach the same optimal mature state of function as the unchallenged system. The hypothesis is that because of the interrelatedness of the multiple systems, the trajectories of the codeveloping systems follow this change. They do not remain unaffected in their own function.

Many biological systems do not have predetermined states of function that they autonomously seek. Instead, they change or adapt their function in relation to interactions with other systems. They are plastic in the sense of maximum adaptability, but they must preserve their own base functions. Figure 3.3 shows the

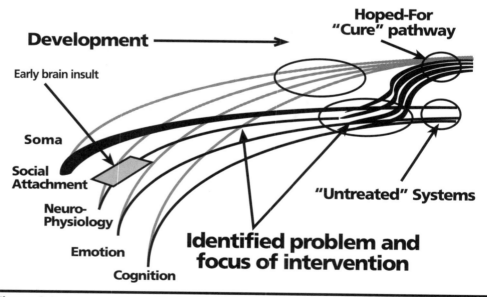

Figure 3.3. Intervention effects

hoped-for effect of treatment, that is, when the affected system is put right, other systems follow a return to a typical developmental trajectory.

Another implication is that even if the malfunctioning system were corrected, (a) the system now sits in a set of systems that have been altered themselves, and (b) all of the systems, not just the one that was repaired, have to have some means of returning to the original/typical trajectory. In order for recovery from a trajectory deflection to occur, altered systems must remain plastic enough to change back to what would have been their usual modes of interaction. Clearly the issues center on how adaptive various systems might be. That is, what are the limits on how much they can change and still sustain the function of the whole? What might the limits be on returning to the typical trajectory once disruption to the initial modes of interaction has occurred?

Adaptive Plasticity and Trajectories

One System

Chapter 2 presented a synopsis of how development in the visual system is plastic early on, enabling the full development of binocular vision, then fixed beyond a certain point in development. That the development of the visual system is determined in part by experience is an example of adaptive plasticity.

Strabismus is a vision disorder in which children cannot fuse the images produced by both eyes, so they begin to favor one eye and neglect input from the other. At the behavioral and neuronal level, strabismus leads to dominance by one eye and a loss of vision in the other. If the child's vision problem is not corrected by age 8 or 9 years, the child will lose use of the neglected eye permanently (Kandel, Schwartz, & Jessell, 1991). This is an example of a cause of trajectory deflection (strabismus) on an initially plastic system. Once the cause has been in place too long, however, correction of the original problem does not allow the visual system to return to its typical binocular trajectory. Effects of this sort indirectly affect development in many other systems.

Many Systems

It is likely that the child with vision in only one eye will interact with his or her environment differently from children with typical vision. Certainly, this visual deficit would have an impact on performance of life tasks heavily dependent on binocular vision, and could affect how development of other abilities and capacities occurs. From a holistic view, it is important to understand how trajectory deflections at one stage of development—and perhaps in only one system (visual)—might affect the development of the individual as a whole.

Trajectories and Stages of Development

It is possible to view development as having a trajectory. However, the typical trajectory is not linear. Humans and most other multicellular organisms develop in stages. In typical development there are periods of continuous, quantitative, incremental change, punctuated by periods of relatively rapid qualitative change. Theorists refer to passing from one stage of development to another as a *discontinuity*, at the end of which one generally has moved to a qualitatively different level. Developmental stages usually build sequentially, and there seem to be critical periods during which discontinuities usually (or must) take place.

One view of passage through each stage (discontinuity) attributes these discontinuities to integration of quantitative changes in many systems to produce a qualitative change in the performance and abilities of the individual. In the preceding section on adaptive plasticity, a child's response to strabismus was an example of viewing altered development as a trajectory deflection. In this section, however, it is helpful to consider discontinuities as predetermined and necessary trajectory deflections involving the whole individual, such as when infants begin to seek hidden objects (evidence of object permanence), make the transition from crawling to walking, display fear of strangers, and shift from babbling to using words. Experience with objects ultimately affects how infants express their representations of objects using language. Therefore, perception, movement, and cognitive development are not separate aspects of the individual; they are interactive aspects. This interaction has implications for subsequent development, demonstrating how alterations in the infant's processing of and response to sensation can alter abilities that typically develop later.

It is evident that visual deprivation or much more global insults to development (e.g., prenatal stress) during the child's early developmental stages can affect infants' abilities, such as how they perceive their environment, how they move about, and how they express themselves.

Accordingly, there are two implications of "stage theory." One is that there are points in chronology and in relation to the environment when the individual is typically plastic and there is a discontinuity in development. The second implication is that something can go wrong at these transitions and the individual does not make the change. The latter counts as a trajectory deflection at a holistic level because these developmental stages appear to be hierarchical. If an infant fails to make a transition during a presumably critical or sensitive period, then it is unlikely that the infant will make any of the subsequent transitions that are higher in the hierarchy. Clearly, this view does not hold much hope for therapists, especially those working with older children and adults. Fortunately, there are no biological constraints underlying stage theory; rather, the theory itself is constraining. The next section of this chapter offers an alternative perspective.

Plasticity of the Whole Individual

The dynamic-systems explanation of development proposes that subsystems of the individual have a genetically preferred trajectory and that these subsystems are continuously plastic. In the typical case, a set of environmental factors common to most developing individuals guides the organization of these subsystems. For example, mammalian infants usually are reared by their mothers. The mother typically presents a certain pattern and sequence of stimuli (tactile, visual, gustatory, etc.) to the infant. From this viewpoint, the organization of the physiological systems of the infant occurs in relation to stimuli that a mother usually presents. To the degree that maternal behavior itself is orchestrated in species-typical patterns, most infants of the species will experience a common pattern and sequence of maternal rearing.

In this view, a discontinuity occurs when the codevelopment of multiple systems reaches a point where there is a shift from one pattern of interaction to another relative to past development and what the individual is doing in the prevailing environment. For example, mammalian mothers usually wean their infants at what seems to be a particular stage in development. In the dynamic view, what causes weaning are adaptive changes in many systems driven by the changing transactions between mother and infant. These changes are dependent in some measure upon behavioral and physical maturation of the infant and, in other aspects, upon changes in maternal behavior. At some point the quantitative changes allow a further integration that produces a qualitative change in behavior that the infant is able to initiate and perform. This discontinuity is also marked by qualitative changes in the way the infant interacts with other members of the species and maintains its own metabolic homeostasis apart from the mother. In this bottom-up view, the development of the infant looks like it might be preprogrammed because it occurs in a particular chronology. However, this is a side effect of the fact that there is a common set of environmental circumstances in which the genetically mandated development and weaning of the infant usually occur.

There are three important implications of the dynamic systems view. The first is that plasticity in multiple codeveloping systems is constantly in play and is not turned off and on according to a genetic program or blueprint for typical development. The second implication is that interactions with the environment are critical and necessary factors in development. Third, dynamic systems both generate and accommodate to an environmental surround. In other words, the actions of the infant produce changes in the surrounding environment, and part of what the infant must accommodate to are the effects of its own actions.

What drives a typical qualitative change, then, is a pattern of integrated development that eventually adds up to a new way of perceiving and responding to the environment. What maintains a qualitative change is that the integrated system/individual in its new configuration is not able to process information/sensation in the way that it did prior to the qualitative change.

In the example of weaning, the infant experiencing sensory defensiveness is not likely to respond in the same way to the common set of stimuli to which most infants are exposed. Adaptive plasticity changes occur, to be sure, but they are not orchestrated in the typical way. Such an infant might wean early, and depending on the infant's discomfort during feedings, the mother might begin to prop the bottle. In this case, early in development the transactions between mother and infant are apparently different from what is typical. Presumably there will be discontinuities, but these most likely will be atypical, reflecting a different trajectory.

This perspective is quite fitting for therapists working with such children. It supports efforts to work toward qualitative changes, whether these children are developing along a typical trajectory or one that is different. Therapists provide the building blocks to guide clients to new discontinuities on a trajectory that is closer to typical. The challenge is to identify what is truly plastic and therefore able to adapt. An understanding of the underlying mechanisms by which plastic changes occur will allow for more effective goal setting.

Conclusions and Implications

This chapter, as well as the previous one, offers evidence that plasticity in the mammalian nervous system is taking place constantly and is affected largely by the experiences that the organism has with the environment. Based on research at the University of Wisconsin, this chapter proposes a conceptual framework for describing and understanding neural plasticity as it might apply to sensory integration theory. This framework appreciates the fundamental role that the organism-environment interaction plays in neural plasticity, and that this can begin even before birth. Organism-environment interactions include the nature and quality of maternal care, the social environment in which the child grows up, and the number and severity of stressors, each of which can contribute to the course of sensory integrative development. This chapter also puts forth the argument that an individual's own actions have important developmental consequences as these actions, in turn, produce changes in the environment to which the individual must accommodate.

The study of development is clearly a difficult task, although not an intractable one. Repeated observations of the quality of maternal care and the nature of the social environment should help researchers determine how these factors interact and contribute to sensory integrative development in children. Parallel studies are currently underway with nonhuman primates. These systematic studies elucidate how manipulations of the pre- and postnatal environment influence development. Researchers can implement therapeutic procedures or prevention strategies at various developmental time points. Studies with infants who differ in sensory integrative functioning would also be helpful.

Understanding neural plasticity and its application to sensory integration theory is of paramount importance in extending current developmental knowledge in sensory integration theory. It seems clear that this theoretical model must go beyond single-factor models to address accurately the complex issues at hand. The degree to which the investigators are successful will depend upon the degree to which occupational therapists understand and use these complex models. Recognition of the complexity should serve as a challenge to occupational therapy researchers and clinicians—a challenge that will be of value in furthering sensory integration theory and development as well as advancing clinical practice.

References

Bayley, N. (1993). *The Bayley Scales of Infant Development* (2nd ed.). San Antonio, TX: The Psychological Corporation.

Carlson, M., & Earls, F. (1997). Psychological and neuroendocrinological sequelae of early social deprivation in institutionalized children in Romania. *Annals of the New York Academy of Sciences, 807,* 419–428.

Clarke, A.S. (1993). Social rearing effects on HPA axis activity over early development and in response to stress in young rhesus monkeys. *Developmental Psychobiology, 26,* 433–447.

Fleming, A.S., Corter, C., & Steiner, M. (1996). Sensory and hormonal control of maternal behavior in rat and human mothers. In C. Pryce and R. Martin (Eds.), *Motherhood in human and nonhuman primates: Biosocial determinants* (pp. 106–114). New York: Karger.

Fleming, A.S., Morgam, H.D., & Walsh, C. (1996). Experiential factors in postpartum regulation of maternal care. In J.S. Rosenblatt & C.T. Snowdon (Eds.), *Parental care: Evolution, mechanisms, and adaptive significance* (pp. 385–422). New York: Academic Press.

Fleming, A., O'Day, D.H., & Kraemer, G.W. (1999). Neurobiology of mother-infant interactions: Central nervous system plasticity and intergenerational affiliation. *Neuroscience and Biobehavioral Reviews, 23,* 673–685.

Fleming, A.S., Ruble, D.N., Flett, G.L., & Shaul, D. (1988). Postpartum adjustment in first-time mothers: Relations between mood, maternal attitudes and mother-infant interactions. *Developmental Psychology, 24,* 77–81.

Fleming, A.S., Steiner, M., & Corter, C. (1997). Cortisol, hedonics, and maternal responsiveness in human mothers. *Hormones and Behavior, 32(2),* 85–98.

Francis, D., Diorio, J., LaPlante, P., Weaver, S., Seckl, J.R., & Meaney, M.J. (1996). The role of early environmental events in regulating neuroendocrine development. Moms, pups, stress, and glucocorticoid receptors. *Annals of the New York Academy of Sciences, 794,* 136–152.

Harlow, H.F., Harlow, M.K., & Hansen, E.W. (1963). The maternal affectional system of rhesus monkeys. In H.L. Rheingold (Ed.), *Maternal behavior in mammals* (pp. 254–281). New York: Wiley.

Hofer, M.A. (1987). Early social relationships: A psychobiologist's view. *Child Development, 58,* 633–647.

Kandel, E.R., Schwartz, J.H., & Jessell, T.M. (1991). *Principles of neural science* (3rd ed.). Norwalk, CT: Appleton & Lange.

Keverne, E.B. (1995). Olfactory learning. *Current Opinion in Neurobiology, 5,* 482–488.

Knutson, J.F. (1995). Psychological characteristics of maltreated children: Putative risk factors and consequences. *Annual Review of Psychology, 46,* 401–431.

Kraemer, G.W. (1992a). Psychobiological attachment theory (PAT) and psychopathology. *Behavioral and Brain Sciences, 15*(3), 525–534.

Kraemer, G.W. (1992b). A psychobiological theory of attachment. *Behavioral and Brain Sciences, 15*(3), 493–511.

Kraemer, G.W. (1997). Psychobiology of early social attachment in rhesus monkeys: Clinical implications. *Annals of the New York Academy of Sciences, 807,* 401–418.

Levy, F., Kendrick, K.M., Keverne, E.B., Porter, R.H., & Romeyer, A. (1996). Physiological, sensory, and experimental factors in sheep. In J.S. Rosenblatt & C.T. Snowdon (Eds.), *Parental care: Evolution, mechanisms, and adaptive significance* (pp. 385–422). New York: Academic Press.

Poindron, P., & Levy, F. (1990). Physiological, sensory and experiential determinants of maternal behavior in sheep. In N.A. Krasnegor & R.S. Bridges (Eds.), *Mammalian parenting: Biochemical, neurobiological and behavioral determinants* (pp. 133–157). New York: Oxford University Press.

Rosenblatt, J., & Snowdon, C. (1995). *Parental care: Evolution, mechanisms, and adaptive significance.* New York: Academic Press.

Suomi, S.J., & Ripp, C. (1983). A history of motherless monkey mothering at the University of Wisconsin Primate Laboratory. In M. Reite & N. Caine (Eds.), *Child abuse: The non-human primate data* (pp. 49–78). New York: Alan R. Liss.

Thelen, E., & Smith, L.B. (1994). *A dynamic systems approach to the development of cognition and action.* New York: Academic Press.

Werner, E.E. (1989). High risk children in young adulthood: A longitudinal study from birth to 32 years. *American Journal of Orthopsychiatry, 59*(1), 72–81.

Wilson, D.A., & Sullivan, R.M. (1994). Neurobiology of associative learning in the neonate: Early olfactory learning. *Behavioral & Neural Biology, 61,* 1–18.

Additional Readings

Clarke, A.S., & Schneider, M.L. (1993). Prenatal stress has long-term effects on behavioral responses to stress in juvenile rhesus monkeys. *Developmental Psychobiology, 26,* 293–304.

Clarke, A.S., Soto, A., Bergholz, T., & Schneider, M.L. (1996). Maternal gestational stress alters adaptive and social behavior in adolescent rhesus monkey offspring. *Infant Behavior and Development, 19,* 453–463.

Clarke, A.S., Wittwer, D.J., Abbott, D.H., & Schneider, M.L. (1994). Long-term effects of prenatal stress on HPA axis activity in juvenile rhesus monkeys. *Developmental Psychobiology, 27,* 257–269.

Fleming, A.S., & Luebke, C. (1981). Timidity prevents the virgin female rat from being a good mother: Emotionality differences between nulliparous and parturient females. *Physiology and Behavior, 27,* 863–868.

Harlow, H.F. (1958). The nature of love. *American Psychologist, 13,* 673–685.

Harlow, H.F., Harlow, M.K., & Suomi, S.J. (1971). From thought to therapy: Lessons from a primate laboratory. *American Scientist, 59,* 538–549.

Hubel, D.H., Wiesel, T.N., & LeVay, S. (1977). Plasticity of ocular dominance columns in monkey striate cortex. *Philosophical Transactions of the Royal Society of London* (Series B), *278,* 377–407.

Kraemer, G.W., & Clarke, A.S. (1996). Social attachment, brain function, and aggression. *Annals of the New York Academy of Sciences, 794*, 121–135.

Kraemer, G.W., Ebert, M.H., Schmidt, D.E., & McKinney, W.T. (1989). A longitudinal study of the effect of different social rearing conditions on cerebrospinal fluid norepinephrine and biogenic amine metabolites in rhesus monkeys. *Neuropsychopharmacology, 2*, 175–89.

Schneider, M.L., Clarke, A.S., Kraemer, G.W., Roughton, E.C., Lubach, G., Rimm-Kaufman, S., Schmidt, D., & Ebert, M. (1998). Prenatal stress alters brain biogenic amine levels in primates. *Development and Psychopathology, 10*(3), 427–440.

Schneider, M.L., Roughton, E.C., Koehler, A.J., & Lubach, G.R. (1999). Growth and development following prenatal stress exposure in primates: An examination of sensitive periods. *Child Development, 70*(2), 263–274.

An Ecological Model of Sensory Modulation:

Performance of Children With Fragile X Syndrome, Autistic Disorder, Attention-Deficit/Hyperactivity Disorder, and Sensory Modulation Dysfunction

Lucy Jane Miller, Ph.D., OTR

Judith E. Reisman, Ph.D., OTR, FAOTA

Daniel N. McIntosh, Ph.D.

Jodie Simon, Ph.D.

Defining Sensory Modulation

The term *sensory modulation* references both physiological reactions and behavioral responses. Behaviorally, the term refers to the ability of an individual to regulate and organize responses to sensations in a graded and adaptive manner, congruent with situational demands (Ayres, 1972; Parham & Mailloux, 1996; Royeen & Lane, 1991). Physiologically, the term refers to cellular mechanisms of habituation and sensitization that alter the structure and/or function of nerve cells, affecting synaptic transmission (Kandel, 1991). Occupational therapists should be aware of the difference between the two uses of the term and carefully indicate the process to which they are referring. Most critical is the distinction between neurophysiological and neuropsychological views on sensory integration processes and use of the terms in occupational therapy to discuss behaviors related to sensory integration function and dysfunction (Miller & Lane, 2000). In particular, differentiating the terminology that describes *processes* that are not observable (i.e. occurring at the cellular and/or nervous system level) from the terminology that describes *behavioral manifestations* of these processes that are observable in sensory integrative functions and dysfunctional patterns is essential. Occupational therapists must begin to differentiate clearly between what they **observe** and what they **infer** occurs in the central nervous system (Miller & Lane). Clinicians can **infer** that dysfunctional behavior patterns in sensory modulation dysfunction relate to underlying *neurophysiologic processes*, but empirical research proving this hypothesis does not exist at the current time (Hanft, Miller, & Lane, 2000). (See Appendix 4-A for a glossary of definitions.)

Recently, a group of occupational therapists with extensive knowledge of sensory integration theory and practice collaborated to define sensory modulation processes, sensory modulation abilities, and sensory modulation dysfunction (SMD). Sensory modulation ability was defined as the "capacity to regulate and organize the degree, intensity, and nature of responses to sensory input in a graded and adaptive manner. This allows the individual to achieve and maintain an optimal range of performance and to adapt to challenges in daily life" (Miller & Lane, 2000). Dysfunction in sensory modulation (SMD) was defined as a problem in regulating and organizing the degree, intensity, and nature of responses to sensory input in a graded manner. SMD disrupts an individual's ability to achieve and maintain an optimal range of performance, and to adapt to challenges in daily life. SMD includes hyperresponsivity, hyporesponsivity and fluctuating responsivity (Lane, Miller, & Hanft, 2000). The behavioral and physiological processes that occur in SMD might be related, but empirical evidence demonstrating that common mechanisms underlie both is lacking. Those using the term SMD should specify "physiological modulation" or "behavioral modulation."

Is Sensory Modulation Dysfunction a Valid Syndrome?

Several occupational therapy researchers (Ayres, 1972; Fisher, Murray, & Bundy, 1991) have hypothesized that sensory modulation dysfunction (SMD) is a syndrome. To be a syndrome, SMD must have documented convergent and divergent validity, demonstrating that characteristics within a group found to have SMD occur reliably, and that this exact pattern of symptoms is not replicated in any other diagnostic group (e.g., AD/HD, Mood Disorders) (Pennington, 1991). The underlying hypothesis of this chapter is that SMD is a syndrome that can occur either with other disorders such as Fragile X syndrome, Autistic Disorders, Obsessive Compulsive Disorders, Mood Disorders, and Attention Deficit Disorders, or as a separate condition. Researchers need to conduct additional research to clarify the comorbidities between SMD and other disorders before stating with certainty that SMD is a valid, separate syndrome from other recognized disorders (e.g., AD/HD and Anxiety Disorders), research must confirm the comorbidity vs. differentiation of SMD and other disorders.

Though anecdotal and theoretical discussions suggest the validity of SMD as a separate diagnostic condition (Fisher & Murray, 1991; Kimball, 1993), little empirical research exists validating this theory. Miller and colleagues have implemented a program of research (1995 to 2000) to evaluate this and other related questions about SMD. This chapter summarizes the ongoing research and presents

1. a new model of SMD, including definitions of four *external dimensions* and three *internal dimensions* in SMD

2. physiological and behavioral data on five cohorts of children with Fragile X syndrome (FXS), Autistic Disorder (Aut), Attention Deficit Hyperactivity Disorders (AD/HD), sensory modulation dysfunction (SMD), and typical development (Typ)

3. the physiological methods and behavioral scales used to research the group differences

4. preliminary empirical data for each group

This chapter relates the observed data to the theoretical model and suggests directions for additional research.

Behavioral Symptoms of Dysfunction in Sensory Modulation

Individuals with SMD demonstrate hyperresponsivity, hyporesponsivity, or lability in response to sensory stimuli (Dunn, 1997; Parham & Mailloux, 1996; Royeen & Lane, 1991) and exhibit unusual patterns of sensation seeking or avoiding (e.g., "fight or flight" reactions to non-noxious sensations) (Ayres, 1979). Accompanying emotional states include anxiety, depression, anger, hostility, and lability. Attentional concomitants include distractibility, disorganization, impulsivity, and hyperactivity. Children with SMD frequently have problems with functional performance in such activities as dressing, play, mealtime, bath time, and social interactions (McIntosh, Miller, Shyu, & Hagerman, 1999). Parents of children with SMD report concerns related to poor social participation, insufficient self-regulation, and inadequate perceived competence and self-esteem (Cohn & Miller, 2000). Some symptoms overlap with behaviors observed in Attention Deficit and Anxiety Disorders.

Physiological Symptoms of Sensory Modulation Dysfunction

Empirical research on the physiological manifestations of SMD is limited. Individuals with FXS almost always evidence symptoms of sensory hyperreactivity as measured by electrodermal reactivity (EDR) (Hagerman, 1996) and have atypical EDR after sensation (Belser & Sudhalter, 1995; Miller et al., 1999). Like children with FXS, children with SMD and no identified comorbid disorder also demonstrate increased magnitude, higher frequency, and less habituation in response to sensory stimuli as measured by EDR (McIntosh, Miller, Shyu, et al., 1999). Children with AD/HD have widely disparate sensory modulation capacities as measured by EDR (Mangeot, 1999).

The New Theoretical Model

The literature suggests that SMD is associated with both physiological abnormalities and behavioral deficits. It is a widely held belief that contextual factors play a vital role in mediating responsivity in SMD (Parham & Mailloux, 1996). The complexity of considering all these factors led to the development of a new conceptual model to help focus research questions and interpret results.

The new theoretical model, the *Ecological Model of Sensory Modulation* (EMSM), elaborates both contextual factors and individual symptoms. The four contextual *external dimensions* (culture, environment, relationships, and tasks) influence the three personal *internal dimensions* (sensation, emotion, and attention). This model builds on two earlier working models of SMD:

- Royeen and Lane (1991) suggested a linear continuum of SMD from hyperreactive to hyporeactive.

- Dunn (1997) later proposed a categorical model with two dimensions: one axis represented *behavioral response* varying from "Responds in Accordance with Threshold" to "Responds to Counteract the Threshold"; the other axis depicted neurological threshold varying from high to low.

The EMSM highlights the external contextual factors interacting with internal characteristics to create SMD. In addressing the importance of ecological factors in understanding human performance, numerous theoreticians have considered the effect of context and task on behavior (Banaji & Prentice, 1994; Cohn & Cermak, 1998; Dunn, Brown, & McGuigan, 1994; Moen, Elder, & Luscher, 1995; Rogoff, 1982; Vygotsky, 1962). However, the occupational therapy literature has not previously emphasized the importance of ecological factors in SMD. Previous discussions of SMD tended to focus on performance components, such as sensory and motor responses, instead of more contextual factors, such as the effect of sensory responsivity at home, in school, and in community life. The EMSM embodies the belief that the responses of individuals with SMD can be understood **only** within the context of their external life. Accordingly, it is the *interaction between the internal and external factors* that produces SMD.

Elements of the Ecological Model of SMD

The Four External Dimensions

The occupational therapy literature, particularly literature related to sensory integration dysfunction, frequently overlooks the four *external dimensions*—culture, environment, relationships, and task (see Figure 4.1)—particularly in relation to sensory integration theory and practice. In SMD, however, referrals for occupational therapy come from a person's inability to interact appropriately with the environment.

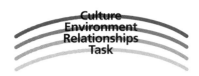

Figure 4.1. External dimensions of the Ecological Model of Sensory Modulation

Culture: The societal mores and expectations that surround the person.

Environment: The physical and sensory milieu in which the individual finds him- or herself.

Relationships: The interactions and connections that one has with other people.

Task: The occupations (roles and "jobs") of the individual. For children, this includes activities of daily living, play, school, sleep, and social relating.

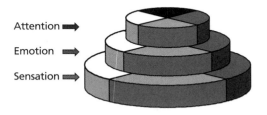

Figure 4.2. Internal dimensions of the Ecological Model of Sensory Modulation

Attention: The ability to sustain performance for tasks and relationships, including controlling impulses and activity level.

Emotion: The ability to perceive emotional stimuli and regulate affective and behavioral responses.

Sensation: The ability to receive and manage the sensory information that comes into the nervous system from the outside world.

In the EMSM, *each* external dimension interacts with *each* internal dimension, either to support or to challenge responses in a specific situation. A "just-right match" between internal and external dimensions occurs when there is a good fit between (a) the supports or demands of task, relationships, environment, and culture and (b) the individual's capacity for processing sensation, emotion, and attention. A good fit results in adaptive performance (e.g., completed tasks or processes). When the external dimensions do not provide the appropriate "scaffolding" or impede performance, problems occur.

When there is good fit between external dimensions and occupational roles and tasks, the situation provides a "just-right challenge" and adaptive responses are maximized. Adaptive responses occur when the child is engaged and challenged and has the structures and supports needed for activity or action completion. For example, a *culture* with good fit has the right mix of permissiveness and structure to match the child's needs. An *environment* with good fit provides interesting but not overwhelming stimulation. A *relationship* with good fit can help mitigate the fear that certain sensations can induce. Finally, a *task* with a good fit provides a balance between structure and freedom that "fits" the needs of the individual.

Sometimes the demands of task, relationships, environment, and/or culture can cause dysregulation in the individual. For example, the demands for quiet in a certain *culture* might pressure a child who is active to fit into that *cultural* milieu. Similarly, the presence of too complex or too simple an *environment* can produce severe disorganization. The demand for direct eye contact and maintenance of personal space in *relationships* can exacerbate anxiety. The *task* of coloring inside the lines can be either too easy or too hard for a child, resulting in poor performance.

The Three Internal Dimensions

The *internal dimensions*—sensation, emotion, and attention—constitute aspects of enduring differences among individuals, varying with learned or constitutional individual difference. The *internal dimensions* are affected by input from the four *external dimensions*. For example, one's perception of the sound of footsteps differs according to whether one is walking on a dark night on an unfamiliar, deserted street or walking on a sunny day in a familiar, crowded market. The perception also likely varies depending on whether one is typically anxious or carefree.

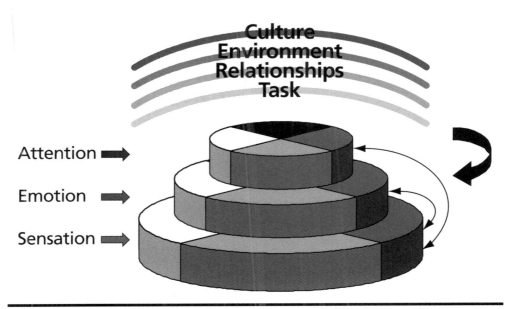

Figure 4.3. The Ecological Model of Sensory Modulation

    light shading = underresponsivity
medium shading = normal responsivity
                (a match between the external and internal dimensions)
    dark shading = overresponsivity
            black = lability, severe overresponsivity alternating with severe underresponsivity

Figure 4.2 depicts the three *internal dimensions* with stacked rings. Each ring rotates independently but can affect the revolution of other rings. Each ring is multidimensional, consisting of several factors. For example, sensation consists of seven subdivisions: tactile, vestibular, proprioceptive, visual, auditory, olfactory, and gustatory stimuli. For the purposes of simplicity in this chapter, subdivisions in internal dimensions are embedded within the three main rings.

The three rotating *internal dimensions* are circular rather than linear. Figure 4.3 depicts each internal dimension with shading to delineate responsivity: hyporesponsivity, normal responsivity, hyperresponsivity, and lability in responsivity.

The literature suggests that pushing an individual beyond the overreactive end of the continuum can result in hypoactive (or "shutdown") responses. For example, Chapman (1966) described a phenomenon in persons with schizophrenia who experienced severe sensory hyperreactivity and shut down both physiologically and behaviorally in what he termed a "blocking reaction." Kimball (1993) cautioned that some children might react in a dangerous way with quick fluctuations from overarousal to physiological "shutdown." She noted that severe physiological reactions might include changes in respiration, cardiac function, blood pressure resulting in decreased consciousness, and shock. This form of severe reaction has been documented medically in at least two cases (Kimball), although she described the more typical "shutdown" pattern as "shut[ting] off input and appear[ing] to be underaroused" (p. 98). Further empirical evidence related to this phenomenon is needed to ascertain with assurance whether extreme sensory overresponsivity *causes* shutdown responses.

When there is an imbalance between the supports and demands of the external dimensions and the adaptive capacities of the internal dimensions, the result is maladaptive behaviors. See Table 4.1 for some of the observable behaviors associated with unmodulated responses in the three internal dimensions.

Table 4.1. Observable Behaviors in Sensory Modulation Dysfunction

Internal Dimensions	Underresponsive	Overresponsive
Attention	Perseveration Unaware	Hyperactivity Impulsivity/Disinhibition Inattention
Emotion	Flat affect Lack of empathy	Hostility, anger Tearfulness Withdrawal
Sensation	Responds slowly Poor discrimination	Responds quickly Intense responses Poor habituation Fight-fright-flight responses

Figure 4.3 depicts the Ecological Model of Sensory Modulation with arrows designating hypothesized directions of effects in SMD. The arrows in the SMD model illustrate the hypothesis that SMD is driven by poor processing of sensation, affecting both emotion and attention.

The hypothesis of the SMD model is that children with this disorder have a core deficit in sensory reception, integration, regulation, or some combination of these. A further hypothesis is that these sensory abnormalities can cause emotional and attentional problems.

This model has a different central focus from other models that attempt to explain childhood disorders. For example, Barkley (1998) hypothesized that children with attention deficits might have a core deficit in the attention dimension. Other researchers hypothesized that people with Autistic Disorder have a core deficit in emotion regulation (Dawson & Lewy, 1989; Dawson, Meltzoff, Osterling, & Rinaldi, 1998). Thus, despite sometimes overlapping symptoms, individual syndromes can have different underlying core deficits in the three internal dimensions.

Study Protocol

Descriptions of the Five Cohorts in This Study

Children Who Are Typically Developing (Typical)

Sources of referral for the 46 typically developing children, ages 3 to 13 years, included parents, faculty, neighbors, and staff of the project. Parents completed a screening regarding potential risk factors at birth (low birth weight, prematurity, other complications) and current status (e.g., school, emotional or medical problems), which had to be negative for a child to be included in this sample.

Children With Fragile X Syndrome (FXS)

Twenty-three children, ages 3 to 12 years, were identified with FXS at The Fragile X Treatment and Research Center at The Children's Hospital in Denver, Colorado, and the diagnoses were confirmed by molecular studies. Most of the children in this group

(~70%) were on medications at the time of this study (~20% on stimulants, ~67% on selective serotonin reuptake inhibitors, and ~13% on anticonvulsants). The average IQ in this group was 70.

Children With Autistic Disorder (Autistic)

These eight children, ages 5 to 13 years, were found to have Autistic Disorder using scales and clinical tests (ADOS, Lord et al., 1989, and ADI-R, Lord, Rutter, & LeCouteur, 1994) to confirm *Diagnostic and Statistical Manual of Mental Disorders* (4th ed.) (*DSM-IV;* American Psychiatric Association, 1994) criteria: impaired social interactions and communication and a markedly restricted, repetitive, or stereotyped repertoire of behavior with restricted interests and activities. Referral sources included The Autism Treatment Center at the University of Colorado Health Science Center and The Child Development Unit at The Children's Hospital in Denver.

Children With Attention Deficit Disorders (AD/HD)

Forty children, ages 5 to 13 years, were referred by several centers in Denver (The Attention and Behavior Center, The Child Development Unit at The Children's Hospital) and by pediatricians and psychologists in private practice. Children's diagnoses were based on *DSM-IV* criteria and include all three Types: Inattentive, Hyperactive-Impulsive, and Combined. The average IQ in this group was 94.

Children With Symptoms of SMD and No Other Disorder (SMD)

Thirty-two children, ages 3 to 9 years, were identified as exhibiting SMD symptoms during occupational therapy assessment at The Children's Hospital in Denver. The criteria included observations during testing and atypical responses on the *Leiter-R Examiner Rating Scale* (Leiter-R; Roid & Miller, 1997) and confirmation by a detailed clinical interview of parents by the first author of this chapter (see Cohn & Miller, 2000, for interview protocol). The average IQ in this group was 108. Table 4.2 provides sample descriptions.

Table 4.2. Description of Samples

Group		N	Mean Age (years)	Age Range (years)
Typical		46	7.6	3–13
	Females	16		
	Males	30		
FXS		23	8.78	3–12
	Females	7		
	Males	16		
Autistic Disorder		8	8.5	5–13
	Females	1		
	Males	7		
AD/HD		40	8.27	5–13
	Females	9		
	Males	31		
SMD		32	5.87	3–9
	Females	11		
	Males	21		

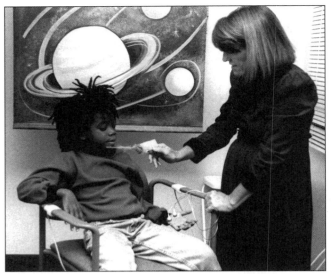

Figure 4.4. Kalisha and experimenter during the Sensory Challenge Protocol.

Instrumentation

The Sensory Challenge Protocol

Electrodermal reactivity provides quantifiable data about the extent of physiological reactions to sensory stimuli. EDR measures changes in electrical conductance of the skin associated with eccrine sweat gland activity (Andreassi, 1989; Fowles, 1986). EDRs occur in the presence of startling or threatening stimuli or aggressive or defensive feelings (Fowles) and during positive and negative emotional events (Andreassi). An absence of electrodermal habituation to repeated stimuli might be related to defensive reactions to stimuli (Boucsein, 1992).

Previous research has demonstrated that individuals with certain medical or behavioral diagnoses exhibit atypical EDRs:

- Down syndrome (Clausen, Lidsky, & Sersen, 1976; Martinez-Selva, Garcia-Sanchez, & Florit, 1995; Wallace & Fehr, 1970)
- Schizophrenia (Kim, Shin, Kim, Cho, & Kim, 1993)
- Attention Deficit Disorders (Fowles & Furuseth, 1994; Rosenthal & Allen, 1978; Satterfield & Dawson, 1971)
- Conduct Disorder (Zahn & Kruesi, 1993)
- Autistic Disorder (Bernal & Miller, 1970; Stevens & Gruzelier, 1984; van Engeland, 1984)
- Fragile X syndrome (Belser & Sudhalter, 1995; Miller et al., 1999)

Because EDR provides a physiological marker of responses to stimuli, the *Sensory Challenge Protocol* (Appendix 4-B) was designed specifically to measure sensory reactivity in a controlled laboratory paradigm (see Miller et al., 1999, for a full description). The protocol gauges responsivity in a "pretend spaceship" presenting 50 sensory stimuli—ten trials in each of five sensory domains (olfactory, auditory, visual, tactile, and vestibular)—for 3 seconds each. The EDR is recorded at a sample rate of 1000 Hz. throughout the session.

The sample profiles in Figure 4.5a–c demonstrate three types of EDRs. In each figure, the vertical lines represent the administration of a 3-second stimulus (e.g., a 3-second bell sound). The oscillating tracings in Figures 4.5a, b, and c depict the person's EDR. The segments in Figures 4.5a, b, and c are small portions of an individual's full reactions during a Sensory Challenge Protocol lab. For example, in Figure 4.5a there are six vertical lines representing six of the ten movement stimuli presented to one individual.

The typical reaction (Figure 4.5a) shows a large peak after the first stimulus, with only one peak after each stimulus, and habituation by the fifth stimulus. In contrast, hyperreactivity (Figure 4.5b) produces large peak magnitudes, more than one peak after some stimuli, and no habituation. Hyporeactivity (Figure 4.5c) produces very small magnitudes of EDR and almost no peaks.

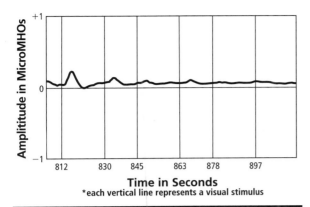

Figure 4.5a. Typical reaction

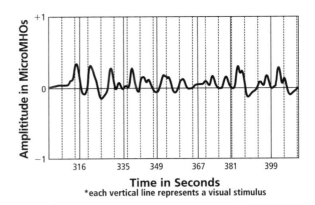

Figure 4.5b. Hyperreactivity

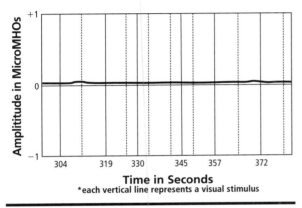

Figure 4.5c. Hyporeactivity

Between each of the vertical lines (i.e., administration of a sensory stimulus) on an EDR tracing, thousands of skin conductance data points occur. Computerized data reduction produced three variables: amplitude of reactions, frequency of reaction, and the number of stimuli administered before habituation occurs. The three variables are highly correlated (see McIntosh, Miller, Shyu, et al., 1999; Miller et al., 1999); therefore, for simplicity, this chapter reports only magnitude of reactions. Magnitude refers to the amplitude of the reaction after the stimulus. High scores represent "more" reactivity (magnitudes are presented in log transformation units). (See previous publications by Miller and McIntosh for more detail on EDR measurement.)

Parent Report Scales

In addition to the EDR measurements of physiologic reactivity, three norm-referenced standardized parent-report scales (described below) were administered to measure behavioral symptoms associated with sensory responses. (See Tables 4.3, 4.4, and 4.5 for content areas of each subtest on rating scales.) These scales have excellent reliability and good validity for measuring the processes of interest in this study. Raw scores have been converted to standardized z-scores, with more Typical performance indicated by higher z-scores.

Sensation

The *Short Sensory Profile* (SSP; McIntosh, Miller, & Shyu, 1999) is a 38-item measure of responses to common events that have sensory components. The subtests are Tactile Sensitivity, Taste/Smell Sensitivity, Visual/Auditory Sensitivity, Movement Sensitivity, Auditory Filtering, Low Energy/Weak, and Under-Responsive/Seeks Sensation. The *Leiter-R* (Roid & Miller, 1997) provides an additional subtest in this dimension, Sensitivity and Regulation.

Emotion

The Leiter-R provides additional measures for the emotion dimension with subtests in Energy and Feelings (measuring depression), Adaptation, Moods and Confidence (measuring anxiety), and Social Abilities. The *Child Behavior Checklist* (CBCL;

Table 4.3. Description of Content Areas
Measured by the *Short Sensory Profile* (SSP)

Subtest	Description of Domain Measured	Sample Item
Tactile Sensitivity	Responses to textures	Responds emotionally or aggressively to touch
Taste/Smell Sensitivity	Overresponsive to tastes and smells	Picky eater regarding textures
Under-Responsive/ Seeks Sensation	Tendency to seek out movement stimulation	Seeks all kinds of movement and this interferes with daily routines
Auditory Filtering	Ability to filter out background noise	Is distracted or has trouble functioning if there is a lot of background noise
Visual/Auditory Sensitivity	Overresponsive to visual stimuli and sounds	Responds negatively to unexpected or loud noises (i.e., vacuum, dog-barking, hairdryer)
Low Energy/Weak	Tendency to become tired and have weakness	Poor endurance/tires easily
Movement Sensitivity	Overresponsive to vestibular stimuli	Becomes anxious or distressed when feet leave ground

Table 4.4. Description of Content Areas
Measured by the *Leiter-R Parent Rating Scale* (Leiter-R)

Subtest	Description of Domain Measured	Sample Item
Attention	Ability to focus, concentrate and remember	Focuses even if noisy outside
Activity Level	Ability to remain calm and regulated	Appropriate amount of moving
Impulsivity	Ability to wait appropriately	Waits to get your attention; plays alone
Adaptation	Ability to adapt and transition	Transitions between places/activities easily
Moods and Confidence	Ability to regulate fear, worries, moods and anxiety	Confident, steady, and calm
Energy and Feelings	Ability to modulate depressed, melancholic or pessimistic feelings	Feels that can not succeed at anything
Social Abilities	Ability to attain and sustain relationships with peers and adults	Cooperative, agreeable and respectable
Sensitivity and Regulation	Ability to modulate reactions to sensation and regulate ideas and thoughts	"Fight or flight" reaction when hugged

Table 4.5 Description of Content Areas
Measured by the *Child Behavior Checklist* (CBCL)

Subtest	Description of Domain Measured	Sample Item
Withdrawn	Behaviors related to isolating oneself	Fears going to school
Somatic Complaints	Issues related to physical problems that do not have a diagnosable cause	Has stomachaches or cramps
Anxious/Depressed	Feelings of worry or extreme sadness	Unhappy, sad or depressed
Social Problems	Interactions with peers and adults	Clings to adults or too dependent
Thought Problems	Propensity toward obsessive or odd ideation	Sees things that are not there
Attention Problems	Difficulty with sustained attention and hyperactivity	Cannot concentrate, cannot pay attention for long
Delinquent Behavior	Behaviors related to destructive or disobedient actions	Steals outside the home
Aggressive Behavior	Externalized symptoms of anger and hostility	Physically attacks people
Sex Problems	Issues related to gender identity or sexuality	Wishes to be of opposite sex

Achenbach, 1991) assesses social and emotional behaviors with the following sub-tests: Social Problems, Aggressive Behavior, Thought Problems, Anxiety and Depression, Somatic Complaints, Withdrawn, Delinquent, and Sex Problems.

Attention
The Leiter-R has Attention, Activity Level, and Impulsivity subtests, and the CBCL includes an Attention Problems subtest.

SMD in Children With Developmental Disabilities

Relation of Findings to Ecological Model of Sensory Modulation

This section presents findings related to the *internal dimensions* of the EMSM. Findings related to *external dimensions* will be published elsewhere.

The discussion begins with descriptive data, synthesizing results for each clinical group on the three internal dimensions and presenting subtest scores (Figures 4.6–4.8, 4.10–4.12). The figures compare two clinical cohorts to children who are typically developing, first comparing children with Fragile X syndrome (FXS) and children with Autistic Disorder (Autistic) to typically developing children (Typical), then comparing children with Attention Deficit Disorders (AD/HD) and children with sensory modulation dysfunction (SMD) to typically developing children (Typical). The results for each group cover each *internal dimension*: sensation, emotion, and attention. To analyze data, the researchers used analyses of variance (ANOVA), with trial as a within-subjects factor and group as a between-subjects factor.

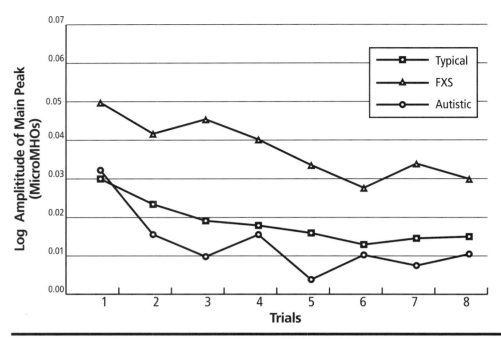

Figure 4.6. Electrodermal reactivity results for children developing Typically compared to children with Fragile X syndrome and children with Autistic Disorder

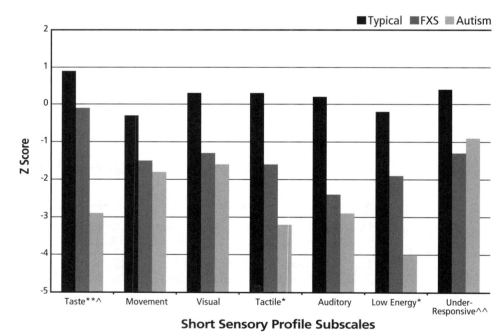

* Subtest differentiates between FXS and Autistic at a significant level (*p* < .01).
** Subtest differentiates between FXS and Autistic at a highly significant level (*p* < .001)
^ Subtest does not differentiate between Autistic and Typical at a significant level.
^^ Subtest does not differentiate between either Autistic or FXS and Typical at a significant level.

Figure 4.7. *Short Sensory Profile* ratings for children with Fragile X syndrome, children with Autistic Disorder, and children developing Typically

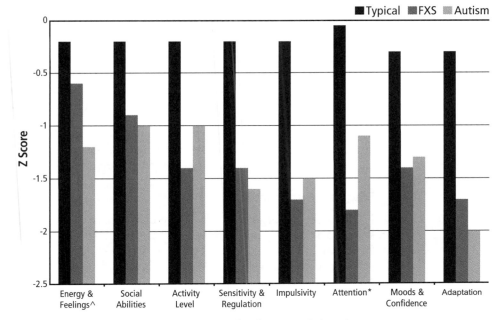

Figure 4.8. *Leiter-R* parent ratings for children with Fragile X syndrome, children with Autistic Disorder, and children developing Typically

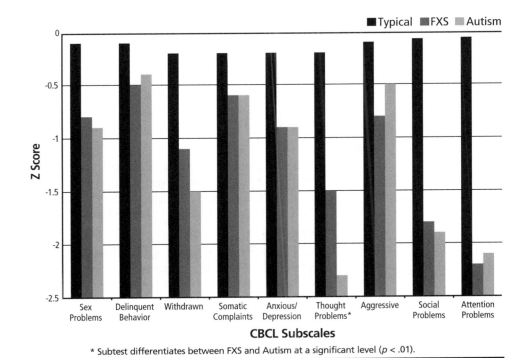

Figure 4.9. *Child Behavior Checklist* results for children with Fragile X syndrome, children with Autistic Disorder, and children developing Typically

After presenting the findings, the discussion moves to the relative role of sensation, compared to emotion and attention, in each disorder and hypothesizes an EMSM model depicting the *internal dimensions* for each disorder based on the preliminary data in this study. The discussion compares children with a diagnosis of FXS to children with a diagnosis of Autistic Disorder, then compares children with AD/HD to those with SMD. These data are preliminary and should form the basis for hypothesis generation and cross-validation only, rather than for drawing definitive conclusions.

Findings: Fragile X Syndrome and Autistic Disorder Compared to Children Who Are Typically Developing

Fragile X Syndrome

FXS is a genetic disorder, and children with this disorder have significant overresponsivity to sensory stimuli (Scharfenaker et al., 1996), attention deficits (Hagerman, 1996), and social-emotional difficulties (Sobesky, 1996). The authors hypothesize that severe difficulties with sensation in FXS might affect both emotion regulation and attention.

Sensation

Physiologically, the FXS group displayed higher magnitudes of EDR than any other group across all sensory domains (see Figure 4.6).The FXS group were behaviorally highly responsive to sensation, significantly different from Typ in all areas except taste/smell sensitivity. Symptoms of SMD were reflected in low scores on Auditory Filtering, Tactile Sensitivity, Movement Sensitivity, and Visual/Auditory Sensitivity (SSP) and on Sensitivity and Regulation (Leiter-R). FXS also had moderately low Under-Responsive/Seeks Sensation scores (SSP), suggesting that some children with FXS are movement seekers whereas others are movement avoiders (see Figure 4.7). Scores in sensation were a bit higher than attention but about the same as emotion.

Emotion

FXS was significantly different from Typical in all areas of emotion except depression (Energy and Feelings; Leiter-R) and Anxious/Depressed (CBCL). Five problem areas were Moods and Confidence (anxiety) and Adaptation (Leiter-R), and Social Problems, Thought Problems, and Withdrawn (CBCL) (see Figures 4.8 and 4.9). Scores in emotion were similar to sensation and higher (better performance) than attention.

Attention

FXS scores were lowest on Auditory Filtering (SSP) and Attention (Leiter-R and CBCL) and, though slightly better on Impulsivity and Activity Level (Leiter-R), still in the moderately impaired range (see Figures 4.7–4.9). Scores on the attention subtests were lower than on the sensation and emotion subscales.

FXS Relation to EMSM

This preliminary information suggests that children with FXS have significant attention regulation difficulties, sensory overresponsivity behaviorally, and sensory hyperreactivity physiologically. In addition, they display emotion regulation problems, particularly in socialization, adaptation, and thought problems. Based on this study, the performance of the children with FXS is not different from typically developing children in Taste/Smell sensitivity or Feelings and Energy (depression).

The extreme deficits in attention and sensation dimensions suggest that these could be core deficits in FXS. Figure 4.10 provides a visual representation of FXS on the internal dimensions of the EMSM. Children with FXS are overresponsive in all three *internal dimensions,* depicted by the dark quadrant of each ring facing forward in

Findings: AD/HD and SMD Compared to Typical

AD/HD

The defining mark of AD/HD is impaired attention, with three subtypes in the *DSM-IV*: Predominately Inattentive Type, Predominately Hyperactive-Impulsive Type, and Combined Type.

Attention

This study confirmed the hypothesis that children with AD/HD would have deficits in the attention dimension. The AD/HD group exhibited more severe deficits in Auditory Filtering (SSP) than any other group, along with significant difficulties in Attention, Impulsivity, and Activity Level (Leiter-R), and Attention Problems (CBCL) (see Figures 4.12–4.14). In addition, the low scores on Under-Responsive/Seek Sensation (SSP) might be related to hyperactivity. Of note is a subgroup within the AD/HD sample that had Low Energy (SSP), indicating that some children in this sample were movement avoiders.

Emotion

The AD/HD group had significant problems in Adaptation (Leiter-R) and moderate problems with Social Problems and Aggressive Behavior (CBCL). Difficulties with Thought Problems (CBCL), Moods and Confidence (Leiter-R), and Anxious/Depression (CBCL) occurred to a lesser degree (see Figures 4.13 and 4.14). Scores in emotion were similar to scores in sensation, with many in the moderately impaired range.

Sensation

Physiologically, the AD/HD group had intriguing results. Children demonstrated an extremely large orienting reaction on the first trial of each sensory domain, followed by an immediate and significant decrease in reactivity almost to the reaction level of the Typical group for subsequent trials. Though the orienting reaction was larger than typically developing children's, clear habituation to sensory input was evident (see Figure 4.15).

Behaviorally, the AD/HD group displayed significant overresponsivity in Tactile and Visual Sensitivity (SSP) but almost normal scores on Movement Sensitivity (SSP). Both a movement-seeking subgroup (SSP, Under-Responsive/Seeks Sensation) and a movement-avoiding subgroup (SSP, Low Energy/Weak) were distinguishable (see Figure 4.12). The sensation and emotion domains exhibited about the same level of function, with sensation scores less impaired than attention scores.

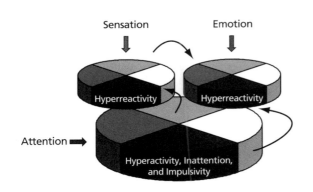

Figure 4.16. Ecological Model of Sensory Modulation in AD/HD

AD/HD Relation to EMSM

The children with AD/HD showed significant problems in subtests measuring attention, impulsivity, and activity level. Excessive sensory responsivity was especially notable in tactile and visual domains, with a tendency toward either movement seeking or avoiding. Although these children demonstrated a large orienting response physiologically, they quickly habituated. Emotion problems were notable in adaptation and sociability.

In a visual representation of AD/HD on the *internal dimensions* of EMSM (Figure 4.16), attention is the core deficit with arrows from attention toward sensation and emotion. Because sensation is more impaired than emotion, the arrow from

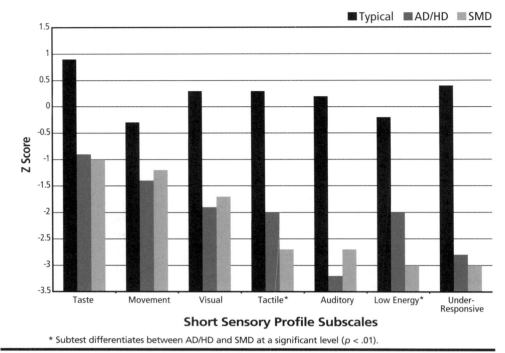

Figure 4.12. *Short Sensory Profile* ratings for children with AD/HD, children with SMD, and children developing Typically

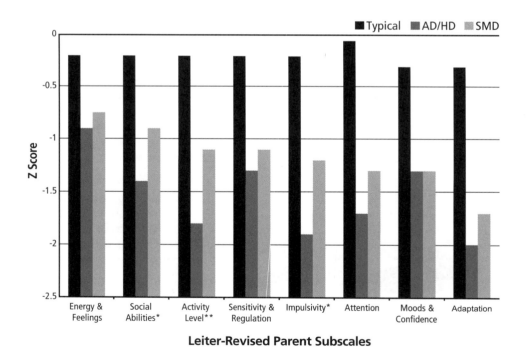

Figure 4.13. *Leiter-R* parent ratings for children with AD/HD, children with SMD, and children developing Typically

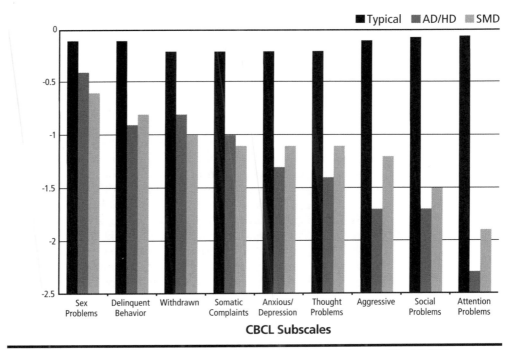

Figure 4.14. *Child Behavior Checklist* ratings for children with AD/HD, children with SMD, and children developing Typically

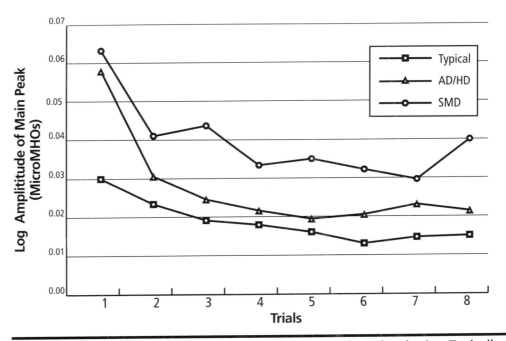

Figure 4.15. Electrodermal reactivity results for children developing Typically compared to children with AD/HD and children with SMD

sensation points toward emotion. The children with AD/HD demonstrate hyperresponsivity (dark shading) in all three dimensions.

Sensory Modulation Dysfunction

Scores less than −3.0 SD on SSP and the assessing occupational therapist's referral of SMD were the criteria for inclusion of children in the SMD group.

Sensation

Children in the SMD group showed extreme hyperresponsivity on behavioral measures, particularly on subtests of Tactile and Visual sensitivity (SSP). In addition, this group demonstrated a pattern of Under-Responsiveness/Seeks Movement sensation and Low Energy (movement avoiding) (SSP). Although the literature identifies "gravitational insecurity" (Fisher, 1991) as a potential concomitant of SMD, few children in this sample exhibited symptoms of overresponsivity to movement stimuli (SSP) (see Figure 4.12). Physiologically, children with SMD demonstrated extreme hyperreactivity, with high magnitudes of responses, multiple peaks, and poor habituation (see also McIntosh, Miller, Shyu, et al., 1999). The EDR responses of the SMD group appeared more hyperreactive than any other group except FXS.

Attention

The children in the SMD group showed impairment in attention, particularly on the Auditory Filtering subtest (SSP) and Attention Problems (CBCL), though less impairment than the AD/HD group. Moderate levels of inattention were evident (Leiter-R and CBCL), and Impulsivity and Activity were significantly impaired compared to the Typical group (Leiter-R) (see Figures 4.13 and 4.14).

Emotion

In the emotion dimension, moderate problems occurred in Adaptation and Social Abilities (Leiter-R) and Social Problems (CBCL), with lesser impairments in Moods and Confidence (depression) (Leiter-R), and Aggressive Behavior, Thought Problems, and Anxious/Depression (CBCL) (see Figures 4.13 and 4.14).

SMD Relation to EMSM

These data suggest that sensation might be the core deficit in children with SMD, including extreme physiological hyperreactivity after sensation, and extreme behavioral overresponsivity to sensation, particularly in tactile and visual domains (see Figure 4.12). Significant problems occurred in Auditory Filtering (SSP), probably related to attention deficits, which were in the moderate range (often without hyperactivity or impulsivity). Children demonstrated difficulty with adaptation and socialization in the emotion dimension. This preliminary evidence suggests that sensory problems might be the core deficit in SMD, contributing to both the attentional and the emotional problems. Because attention scores were lower than emotion scores, the arrows point from sensation toward emotion and attention, with another arrow from attention to emotion (Figure 4.17).

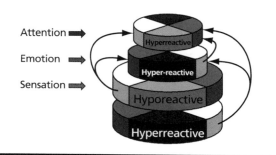

Figure 4.17. Ecological Model of Sensory Modulation in SMD

Comparison of AD/HD and SMD

Several domains differentiate these two clinical groups. Physiologically, the SMD group had more severe hyperreactivity with poor habituation, whereas the AD/HD group had a large initial orienting reaction, then habituated quickly. Overall mean sensory responsivity scores showed greater impairment for SMD than for AD/HD, with a significant difference on Low Energy (avoiding movement). The SMD group also displayed more impairment in movement seeking (Under-Responsive/Seeks Sensation), though not significantly more impaired (see Figure 4.12).

In the attention dimension, the AD/HD group showed greater impairment, with significantly more impairment on Activity Level, Impulsivity, and Social Abilities (see Figure 4.13) than the SMD group. In the emotion dimension, there were no clear differences, although the AD/HD group had lower scores, but not significantly lower, in Aggressive Behavior and Thought Problems than did the SMD group. Both groups had extremely impaired Auditory Filtering scores (~ -3 SD below the mean).

Moving From Data Back to Model

With preliminary data providing a baseline about the *internal dimensions* of these five groups of children, a plethora of research questions arise related to the model. These questions can help shape future research. The overarching question for each group is, Considering the three dimensions hypothesized in the model, does a **core deficit** exist in one *internal dimension* of each clinical disorder that directly affects function in the other two dimensions, and if so, in which internal dimensions does the deficit occur? The answer to this question will have a direct affect on intervention. Is a sensation deficit core in SMD and Autistic Disorder? Is an attention deficit core in AD/HD? Are both sensation and attention core deficits in FXS?

Because so little is known about sensory modulation dysfunction, the EMSM model can help guide future questions. However, a determination of whether SMD is a valid syndrome will be possible only after numerous studies describe the etiology, brain mechanisms, neuropsychological features, and behavioral symptoms of SMD and evaluate the degree of similarity with and difference from other disorders (e.g., AD/HD and anxiety disorders).

Limitations of This Study and Additional Questions

An important limitation to this study was the sample. The FXS sample was the most defined, given that FXS is a genetic disorder confirmed with molecular tests. The Autistic Disorder sample was quite specific because all participants met the criteria for Autistic Disorder specified in the *DSM-IV* and were tested using the ADOS and ADI. However, because the Autistic Disorder criteria are behavioral rather than genetic, subjective judgments form the basis of diagnosis. The evaluators were experienced professionals at The Autism Center at the University of Colorado who used standardized tests to classify the sample; therefore confidence exists that children in the sample did have Autistic Disorder, though the sample size was too small for generalization of results.

The AD/HD and SMD samples are more problematic. The *DSM-IV* describes three Types of attentional disorders, and this sample contained all three subtypes. Because an objective genetic marker of AD/HD does not exist, the accuracy of diagnosis depends on the diagnostic skills of the referring sources. The children with SMD were identified by master occupational therapy clinicians and had no other diagnosis at the time of referral. It is possible that some members of the SMD sample had undiagnosed AD/HD or Anxiety Disorders and that some members of the AD/HD sample had undiagnosed SMD. Future studies will need clear markers to construct nonoverlapping AD/HD and SMD groups. Perhaps poor habituation, using EDR as a dependent measure, can serve as a marker for SMD, and a large orienting response with good habituation can demarcate AD/HD. Empirical investigation of the comorbidity of SMD and AD/HD using standard diagnostic criteria for both groups is essential.

Current research in AD/HD supports the proposition that the core deficit in AD/HD is impulsivity (Barkley, 1998). These data support this suggestion. Is it possible to differentiate AD/HD from SMD by objective tests of impulsivity and sustained attention? To evaluate this, scales such as Logan's Stop Task (Logan, 1994), and the Attention Sustained and Attention Divided subtests from the Leiter-R might be helpful. Will these objective performance-based measures provide the clarity for subject inclusion needed to study the difference between AD/HD and SMD? Additional empirical evidence is certainly requisite before more definitive conclusions are possible.

Questions raised by this study include: Are there two groups of children within AD/HD, one with SMD and one without? Might it be possible to discriminate the groups within AD/HD based on EDR patterns after sensory stimulation? Would the two types of AD/HD groups (with and without sensory dysfunction) respond differently to medication and to OT using a sensory integration framework?

Another interesting finding was the significant difference physiologically between the FXS and Autistic Disorder groups. Children in the FXS group were extremely hyperreactive to sensory stimulation; individuals in the Autistic Disorder group were hyporeactive. These preliminary findings raise interesting theoretical questions. Clearly, the presence and impact of sensory processing disorders in both groups need further study.

Conclusion

This program of research in SMD is continuing, addressing questions of syndrome validity and intervention effectiveness as well as issues related to the underlying neurological, physiological, and biochemical mechanisms that could be disordered in SMD. The studies described in this chapter have not proven that SMD is a disorder; however, preliminary empirical evidence suggests that this might be true. Occupational therapy literature persistently discusses SMD as a syndrome. Because, as yet, syndrome validation is unproven, the use of a more conservative label such as "sensory modulation dysfunction" (SMD) would probably be more appropriate. Until additional evidence with cross-validation from different laboratories comes forth that demonstrates convergence (e.g., reliable characteristics in SMD) and divergence (e.g., differences in SMD and other disorders), it is premature to label SMD a syndrome.

In a larger venue, the field of occupational therapy is replete with articles, chapters, and newsletter columns discussing sensory integration theory and practice. Dozens of workshops elucidate components of sensory integration intervention. Ongoing controversy abounds related to intervention effectiveness.

One of the issues demonstrated by the studies discussed in this chapter is how little is known about SMD. The data raise profound questions about the nature of the dysfunction, including whether it is in fact a discrete syndrome, and highlight the importance of additional **empirical** research. Researchers **must** examine the effectiveness of treating children who receive their diagnoses based upon reliable, operationally defined methods, use specific and replicable interventions, and utilize relevant outcome measures that are tied to predicted hypotheses. Studies that address questions related to the neurological, physiological, and biochemical mechanisms and processes in children who manifest symptoms of SMD are crucial. Compelling research that links deficits at the neurophysiological or biochemical level to problems in meaningful occupations and quality of life is fundamental.

This research is complex, time-consuming, and expensive. It requires a committed and knowledgeable multidisciplinary team including therapists and scientists. Limited professional resources should be used **not** to argue about the effectiveness of sensory integration intervention or the "best" methods of assessment and intervention of these complex disorders but rather to <u>collaborate</u> in defining critical research questions and in funding and implementing scientific studies to answer those questions. Only in this way will the therapeutic disciplines best serve the children and families affected by sensory integrative dysfunction.

Acknowledgments

We would like to acknowledge the tremendous support of Dr. Marshall Haith, who reviewed this manuscript and provided consultation on the constructs. In addition, the lab director and lab assistants Jude McGrath, Kelly Church, Julie Bonnell, and Todd Ognibene devoted countless hours gathering data for this chapter. Dr. Randi Hagerman provided leadership on issues related to Fragile X syndrome and Dr. Sally Rogers on issues related to Autistic Disorder. This complex work could not be completed without the dedication of the treating occupational therapists: Clare Summers, Sharen Trunnell, Nicki Pine, Robin Seger, Lisa Waterford, Becky Greer, and Julie Butler. The administrative support of Dr. Dennis Matthews, director of Pediatric Rehabilitation at The Children's Hospital in Denver, Colorado, is also gratefully acknowledged. Finally, we appreciate the contributions of Judy Benzel, who provided administrative support, and Kimberley Dohren and the Photography/Computer Graphics Department at The Children's Hospital in Denver for assistance with figures.

Primary funding for this work was provided by the Wallace Research Foundation. Additional support has been provided by a NIH Career Award to the first author (# 1 K01 HD01183-01). The overhead expenses were supported in part by a grant from Maternal and Child Health (MCH grant # MC J 08941301).

References

Achenbach, T.M. (1991). *Manual for the Child Behavior Checklist/4–18 and 1991 Profile.* Burlington, VT: University of Vermont, Department of Psychiatry.

American Psychiatric Association. (1994). *Diagnostic and statistical manual of mental disorders* (4th ed.). Washington, DC: Author.

Andreassi, J.L. (1989). *Psychophysiology: Human behavior and physiological response.* Hillsdale, NJ: Lawrence Erlbaum Associates.

Ayres, A.J. (1972). *Sensory integration and learning disorders.* Los Angeles: Western Psychological Services.

Ayres, A.J. (1979). *Sensory integration and the child.* Los Angeles: Western Psychological Services.

Banaji, M.R., & Prentice, D.A. (1994). The self in social contexts. *Annual Reviews in Psychology, 45,* 297–332.

Barkley, R.A. (1998). *Attention deficit hyperactivity disorder: A handbook for diagnosis and treatment* (2nd ed.). New York: Guilford Press.

Belser, R.C., & Sudhalter, V. (1995). Arousal difficulties in males with Fragile X syndrome: A preliminary report. *Developmental Brain Dysfunction, 8,* 270–279.

Bernal, M.E., & Miller, W.H. (1970). Electrodermal and cardiac responses of schizophrenic children to sensory stimuli. *Society for Psychophysiological Research, 7*(2), 155–168.

Boucsein, W. (1992). *Electrodermal activity.* New York: Plenum Press.

Bryson, S.E., Wainwright-Sharp, J.A., & Smith, I.M. (1990). Autism: a developmental spatial neglect syndrome? In J.T. Enns (Ed.), *The development at attention: Research and Theory* (pp. 405–419). North-Holland: Elsevier Science Publishers B.V.

Buchsbaum, M.S., Siegel, B.V., Jr., Wu, J.C., Hazlett, E., Sicotte, N., Haier, R., Tanguay, P., Asarnow, R., Cadorette, T., Donoghue, D., Lagunas-Solar, M., Lott, I., Paek, J., & Sabalesky, D. (1992). Brief report: Attention performance in autism and regional brain metabolic rate assessed by positron emission tomography. *Journal of Autism and Development Disorders, 22*(1), 115–125.

Chapman, J. (1966). The early symptoms of schizophrenia. *British Journal of Psychiatry, 112*, 225–251.

Clausen, J., Lidsky, A., & Sersen, E.A. (1976). Measurement of autonomic functions in mental deficiency. In R. Karrer (Ed.), *Developmental psychophysiology of mental retardation* (pp. 39–91). Springfield, IL: Thomas.

Cohn, E., & Cermak, S.A. (1998). Including the family perspective in sensory integration outcomes research. *American Journal of Occupational Therapy, 52*(7), 540–546.

Cohn, E., & Miller, L.J. (2000). Parental hopes for therapy outcomes: Children with sensory modulation disorders. *American Journal of Occupational Therapy, 54*(1), 1–8.

Dawson, G., & Lewy, A. (1989). Arousal, attention, and the socioemotional impairments of individuals with autism. In G. Dawson (Ed.), *Autism: Nature, diagnosis, and treatment* (pp. 49–74). New York: Guilford.

Dawson, G., Meltzoff, A., Osterling, J., & Rinaldi, J. (1998). Neuropsychological correlates of early symptoms of autism. *Child Development, 69*(5), 1276–1285.

DiPietro, J., & Porges, S.W. (1991). Vagal responsiveness to gavage feeding as an index of preterm status. *Pediatric Research, 29*(3), 231–236.

Dunn, W. (1997). The impact of sensory processing abilities on the daily lives of young children and their families: A conceptual model. *Infants & Young Children, 9*(4), 23–35.

Dunn, W., Brown, C., & McGuigan, A. (1994). The ecology of human performance: A framework for considering the effect of context. *American Journal of Occupational Therapy, 48*(7), 595–607.

Fisher, A.G. (1991). Vestibular-proprioceptive processing and bilateral integration and sequencing deficits. In A.G. Fisher, E.A. Murray, & A.C. Bundy (Eds.), *Sensory integration: Theory and practice* (pp. 71–107). Philadelphia: F.A. Davis Company.

Fisher, A.G., & Murray, E.A. (1991). Introduction to sensory integration theory. In A.G. Fisher, E.A. Murray, & A.C. Bundy (Eds.), *Sensory integration: Theory and practice* (pp. 3–26). Philadelphia: F.A. Davis Company.

Fisher, A.G., Murray, E.A., & Bundy, A.C. (1991). *Sensory integration: Theory and practice.* Philadelphia: F.A. Davis Company.

Fowles, D.C. (1986). The eccrine system and electrodermal activity. In M.G.H. Coles, E. Donchin, & S.W. Porges (Eds.), *Psychophysiology: Systems, processes, and applications* (pp. 51–96). New York: Guilford Press.

Fowles, D.C., & Furuseth, A.M. (1994). Electrodermal hypo-reactivity and antisocial behavior. In D.K. Routh (Ed.), *Disruptive behavior disorders in childhood* (pp. 181–205). New York: Plenum Press.

Hagerman, R.J. (1996). Physical and behavioral phenotype. In R.J. Hagerman & A. Cronister (Eds.), *Fragile X syndrome: Diagnosis, treatment, and research* (2nd ed., pp. 3–87). Baltimore, MD: The John Hopkins University Press.

Hanft, B.E., Miller, L.J., & Lane, S.J. (2000). Toward a consensus in terminology in sensory integration theory and practice: Part 3: Observable behaviors: Sensory integration dysfunction. *Sensory Integration Special Interest Section, 23*(3), 1–4.

Kandel, E.R. (1991). Cellular mechanisms of learning and the biological basis of individuality. In E.R. Kandel, J.H. Schwartz, & T.M. Jessell (Eds.), *Principles of neural science* (3rd ed., pp. 1009–1031). East Norwalk, CT: Appleton & Lange.

Kim, D.K., Shin, Y.M., Kim, C.E., Cho, H.S., & Kim, Y.S. (1993). Electrodermal responsiveness, clinical variables, and brain imaging in male chronic schizophrenics. *Biological Psychiatry, 33,* 786–793.

Kimball, J.G. (1993). Sensory integrative frame of reference. In P. Kramer & J. Hinajosa (Eds.), *Frames of reference for pediatric occupational therapy* (pp. 87–167). Baltimore, MD: Williams and Wilkins.

Lane, S.J., Miller, L.J., & Hanft, B.E. (2000) Toward a consensus in terminology in sensory integration theory and practice: Part 2: Sensory integration patterns of function and dysfunction. *Sensory Integration Special Interest Section, 23*(2), 1–3.

Logan, G.D. (1994). On the ability to inhibit thought and action: A user's guide to the stop signal paradigm. In D. Dagenbach & T.H. Carr (Eds.), *Inhibitory processes in attention, memory, and language* (pp. 189–239). San Diego, CA: Academic Press.

Lord, C., Rutter, M., Goode, S., Heemsbergen, J., Jordan, H., Mawhood, L., & Schopler, E. (1989). Autism Diagnostic Observation Schedule: A standardized observation of communicative and social behavior. *Journal of Autism and Developmental Disorders, 19,* 185–212.

Lord, C., Rutter, M., & LeCouteur, A. (1994). Autism Diagnostic Interview—Revised: A revised version of a diagnostic interview for caregivers of individuals with possible pervasive developmental disorders. *Journal of Autism and Developmental Disorders, 24,* 659–685.

Mangeot, S.D. (1999). *The relationship between disruptions in sensory modulation and attention deficit hyperactivity disorder in children.* Unpublished doctoral paper, University of Denver, Denver, CO.

Martinez-Selva, J.M., Garcia-Sanchez, F.A., & Florit, R. (1995). Electrodermal orienting activity in children with Down syndrome. *American Journal on Mental Retardation, 100*(1), 51–58.

McIntosh, D.N., Miller, L.J., & Shyu, V. (1999). Overview of the Short Sensory Profile (SSP). In W. Dunn (Ed.), *The Sensory Profile: Examiner's manual* (pp. 59–73). San Antonio, TX: The Psychological Corporation.

McIntosh, D.N., Miller, L.J., Shyu, V., & Hagerman, R. (1999). Sensory-modulation disruption, electrodermal responses, and functional behaviors. *Developmental Medicine and Child Neurology, 41,* 608–615.

Miller, L.J. (1988, 1982). *Miller Assessment for Preschoolers (MAP).* San Antonio, TX: The Psychological Corporation.

Miller, L.J., & Lane, S.J. (2000). Toward a consensus in terminology in Sensory Integration theory and practice: Part 1: Taxonomy of neurophysiological processes. *Sensory Integration Special Interest Section, 23*(1), 1–4.

Miller, L.J., McIntosh, D.N., McGrath, J., Shyu, V., Lampe, M., Taylor, A.K., Tassone, F., Neitzel, K., Stackhouse, T., & Hagerman, R. (1999). Electrodermal responses to sensory stimuli in individuals with Fragile X syndrome: A preliminary report. *American Journal of Medical Genetics, 83*(4), 268–279.

Mini Mitter Company. (1999). *Mini-Logger Series 2000.* Sunriver, OR: Author.

Moen, P., Elder, G.H., & Luscher, K. (1995). *Examining lives in context: Perspectives on the ecology of human development.* Washington, DC: American Psychological Association.

Parham, L.D., & Mailloux, Z. (1996). Sensory integration. In J. Case-Smith, A.S. Allen, & P.N. Pratt (Eds.), *Occupational therapy for children* (3rd ed., pp. 307–355). St. Louis: Mosby-Year Book, Inc.

Pennington, B.F. (1991). Issues in syndrome validation. In B.F. Pennington (Ed.), *Diagnosing learning disorders: A neuropsychological framework* (pp. 23–31). New York: Guilford Press.

Porges, S.W. (1985). *Method and apparatus for evaluating rhythmic oscillations in aperiodic physiological response systems.* U.S. Patent #4,510,944.

Porges, S.W. (1992). Vagal tone: A physiologic marker of stress vulnerability. *Pediatrics, 90,* 498–504.

Porges, S.W. (2000). *MX Edit (Version 2.19).* Bethesda, MD: Delta Biometrics, Inc.

Rogoff, B. (1982). Integrating context and cognitive development. *Advances in Developmental Psychology, 2,* 125–170.

Roid, G.H., & Miller, L.J. (1997). *Leiter International Performance Scale—Revised.* Wood Dale, IL: Stoelting Company.

Rosenthal, R.H., & Allen, T.W. (1978). An examination of attention, arousal, and learning dysfunctions of hyperkinetic children. *Psychological Bulletin, 75,* 689–715.

Royeen, C.B., & Lane, S.J. (1991). Tactile processing and sensory defensiveness. In A.G. Fisher, E.A. Murray, & A.C. Bundy (Eds.), *Sensory integration: Theory and practice* (pp. 108–136). Philadelphia: F.A. Davis.

Satterfield, J.H., & Dawson, M.E. (1971). Electrodermal correlates of hyperactivity in children. *Psychophysiology, 8,* 191–197.

Scerbo, A.S., Freedman, L.W., Raine, A., Dawson, M.E., & Venables, P.H. (1992). A major effect of recording site on measurement of electrodermal activity. *Psychophysiology, 29*(2), 241–246.

Scharfenaker, S., O'Connor, R., Stackhouse, T., Braden, M., Hickman, L., |& Gray, K. (1996). An integrated approach to intervention. In R.J. Hagerman & A. Cronister (Eds.), *Fragile X syndrome: Diagnosis, treatment, and research* (2nd ed., pp. 349–411). Baltimore: The Johns Hopkins University Press.

Sobesky, W.E. (1996). The treatment of emotional and behavioral problems. In R.J. Hagerman & A. Cronister (Eds.), *Fragile X syndrome: Diagnosis, treatment, and research* (2nd ed., pp. 332–348). Baltimore: The Johns Hopkins University Press.

Stevens, S., & Gruzelier, J. (1984). Electrodermal activity to auditory stimuli in autistic, retarded, and normal children. *Journal of Autism and Developmental Disorders, 14*(3), 245–260.

van Engeland, H. (1984). The electrodermal orienting response to auditive stimuli in autistic children, normal children, mentally retarded children, and child psychiatric patients. *Journal of Autism and Developmental Disorders, 14*(3), 261–279.

Vygotsky, L.S. (1962). *Thought and language.* Cambridge, MA: MIT Press.

Wallace, R.M., & Fehr, F.S. (1970). Heart rate, skin resistance, and reaction time of mongoloid and normal children under baseline and distraction conditions. *Psychophysiology, 6,* 722–731.

Zahn, T.P., & Kruesi, M.J.P. (1993). Autonomic activity in boys with disruptive behavior disorders. *Psychophysiology, 30,* 605–614.

Definitions of Terms

Magnitude of electrodermal response: A measure (from high to low) of the amount of response to sensory stimuli in the Sensory Challenge Protocol. An extremely high magnitude might correspond to hyperreactivity; an extremely low magnitude might correspond to hypo-reactivity.

Attention: One of the three *internal dimensions* of the Ecological Model of Sensory Modulation; refers to an individual's ability to sustain performance for task completion or interpersonal relationships, including impulse control and activity level.

Behavioral sensory modulation: The ability of an individual to regulate and organize reactions to sensations in a graded and adaptive manner, congruent with situational demands.

Culture: One of the four *external dimensions* of the Ecological Model of Sensory Modulation; refers to the societal mores and expectations surrounding the person.

Electrodermal response (EDR): A physiological measurement that provides quantifiable data about the extent of response to sensory stimuli by measuring changes in electrical conductance of the skin associated with eccrine sweat gland activity. It is an index of sympathetic nervous system activity.

Emotion: One of the three *internal dimensions* of the Ecological Model of Sensory Modulation; refers to an individual's ability to accurately perceive emotional stimuli and regulate affective and behavioral responses.

Environment: One of the four *external dimensions* of the Ecological Model of Sensory Modulation; refers to the physical and sensory milieu in which the individual finds himself or herself.

External Dimensions: One of the two major divisions of the Ecological Model of Sensory Modulation; refers to the effect of context and task on behavior.

Good fit: Results in adaptive performance (e.g., completed tasks or processes) that occurs when the external dimensions provide the appropriate supportive "scaffolding" for the child and if the external dimensions do not interfere with performance.

Internal Dimensions: One of the two major divisions in the Ecological Model of Sensory Modulation; refers to an individual's temperamental and capability characteristics that vary with learned or constitutional individual differences.

Just-right match: Occurs when there is a good fit between the supports or demands of: task, relationships, environment, and culture, and the individual's capacity for sensory processing and emotional and attentional responses.

Just-right challenge: Occurs when there is good fit between external dimensions and internal dimensions, that is, the individual is engaged and challenged and the structures and supports needed for activity or action completion are not too much or too little.

Physiological sensory modulation: Cellular mechanisms of habituation and sensitization used to alter the structure and/or function of nerve cells, affecting synaptic transmission.

Relationships: One of the four *external dimensions* of the Ecological Model of Sensory Modulation; refers to the interactions and connections that one has with other people.

Scaffolding: The "just-right" support that encourages an individual to attempt a task or activity that is a little hard for the person.

Sensory Challenge Protocol: A controlled laboratory paradigm that gauges an individual's responsivity to 50 sensory stimuli (10 trials in five sensory domains) by continuously sampling the individual's electrodermal reactivity.

Sensory Processing: One of the three *internal dimensions* of the Ecological Model of Sensory Modulation; refers to the individual's ability to receive and manage the sensory information that comes into the nervous system from the outside world.

Task: One of the four *external dimensions* of the Ecological Model of Sensory Modulation; refers to the occupations in which the individual engages. For children, this includes activities of daily living, play, school, sleep, and social relating.

Sensory Challenge Protocol

The Sensory Challenge Protocol uses measurements of electrodermal reactivity and vagal tone to gauge individuals' physiological reactions to sensory stimulation. The Sensory Challenge Protocol uses two rooms. The first room is the "spaceship" lab (8 by 9.5 feet) in which the experimenter, a lab technician (e.g., a graduate student, project staff member, clinician who is working to obtain research experience, or an occupational therapist who receives special technical training and who is not involved in treatment of children in the study) administers the stimuli to the child. Figure 4-B.1 depicts the exact lab setup for the Sensory Challenge Protocol.

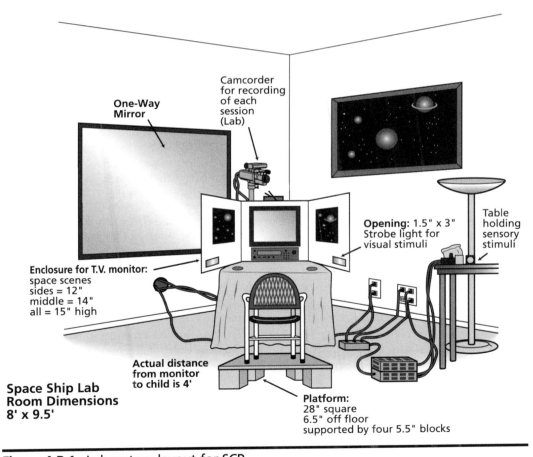

One-Way Mirror

Camcorder for recording of each session (Lab)

Opening: 1.5" x 3"
Strobe light for visual stimuli

Table holding sensory stimuli

Enclosure for T.V. monitor:
space scenes
sides = 12"
middle = 14"
all = 15" high

Actual distance
from monitor
to child is 4'

Space Ship Lab
Room Dimensions
8' x 9.5'

Platform:
28" square
6.5" off floor
supported by four 5.5" blocks

Figure 4-B.1. Laboratory layout for SCP

The second room (4 by 5 feet or larger) contains the computer, all physiological equipment, and the computer operator. The rooms are connected visually either by a one-way mirror into the spaceship or by a video camera in the lab that connects to a monitor in the computer room. The experimenter and the operator can communicate through headsets (Radio Shack Plantronics telephone headset PLX 500) that are hooked up through existing telephone lines in both rooms and are not audible to the child. Consequently, halting or adjusting the proceedings is easy for either the experimenter or the operator with a minimum of disruption to the session. Experimenters and computer operators should be blind to participants' diagnoses.

Introduction

The experimenter greets the child and the parent in the waiting room and explains to the child that he or she is going on a pretend "spaceship" trip. (Previous explanation via phone encourages the parents to prepare the child for this "fun time.") The parent and the child (if he or she is 8 or older) sign an informed consent. The experimenter slowly and gently transitions the child to the laboratory, the pretend spaceship. The lights in the lab are low, and two walls are painted to look like three-dimensional spaceship control panels. A third wall contains a one-way mirror through which the computer operator (and parents) can observe the session and make appropriate notations and adjustments on the electronic record, if needed. (Alternatively, the operator can use the video camera in the spaceship lab that feeds to a monitor in the computer room.) A small wooden frame painted to look like a spaceship control panel (approximately 14 inches wide and hinged on the left and the right sides to 12-inch-wide arms; all three pieces are 15 inches high) sits on a 12-inch-deep table approximately 4 feet in front of the child. A hole in the control panel allows the child to see the screen of a 13-inch video monitor directly ahead. A strobe light is visible through a cutout hole (1.5 by 3 inches) on the right side of the frame.

The experimenter conducts the child into the room and asks the child to step up onto a 28-inch-square board 6.5 inches off the floor. The child sits in a sturdy armchair that is permanently fastened to the board (actually a tilt board that rests on four 4-inch-square by 5.5-inch high wooden cubes). The ambient light in the room remains at a low level throughout the protocol. The child watches a section of the *Apollo 13* video depicting astronauts being "hooked up" as the experimenter attaches the child's electrodes. The specific segment of *Apollo 13* was selected to be entertaining while not emotionally charged. The segment helps the children to be involved, interested, and comfortable with the application of the electrodes.

Instrumentation

Autogenics 5-mm diameter electrodes, filled with electrode paste before the child arrives, are applied to the thenar and hypothenar eminences of the palm of the left hand (Scerbo, Freedman, Raine, Dawson, & Venables, 1992). The experimenter secures the electrodes with a 1.5-inch standard electrode collar.

A Coulbourn Isolated Skin Conductance Coupler (S71-23) applies a constant 0.5 V potential across the electrode pair to condition the electric signal. Because reactions to each stimulus (EDR) are of interest, not the changes in the slower fluctuating tonic skin conductance level, the coupling is AC (alternating current), which corrects for drifts in baseline conductance level over the extended time of the presentation of stimuli (see Boucsein, 1992). A low-cut filter set to 0.2 Hz passes signals above 0.2 Hz without distortion in amplitude. A computer samples the signals at 50 Hz, then digitizes and stores the data.

On-line monitoring of interbeat cardiac output using the Mini-Mitter polar XR (Mini Mitter Company, 1999), a small unit attached to the child's chest with a band, collects vagal tone variables. A separate unit, the Mini-Logger, collects the data and must be located within 18 inches of the Mini-Mitter to detect peak R waves for each cardiac cycle. Collection of time-sequential R-to-R intervals to the nearest millisecond follows the recommendations of Porges (1992). The procedure is noninvasive and painless. A computer (located in the adjacent room) continually amplifies, displays, and records the ECG data for later analysis. This procedure produces an estimate of heart period by minimizing confounding influences and is sensitive to small increments of change over short time periods (DiPietro & Porges, 1991).

Researchers later download the Mini-Logger data into the computer program (Mini Mitter Company, 1999) and manually edit each vagal tone file for artifact by (a) comparing long or short R-R intervals to adjacent values, to identify R-waves that might be errors, and (b) performing integer division of the long intervals and sequential addition of the short intervals. Cardiac vagal tone is estimated according to the patented procedure (DiPietro & Porges, 1991; Porges, 1985) using MX-Edit Software (Porges, 2000):

- converting heart periods to time-based data by sampling during successive 250 ms intervals

- detrending time-based data using a 21-point moving polynomial to remove the trend and periodicities of heart rates slower than the respiratory sinus arrhythmia

- processing the detrended data using a band-pass filter to remove sources of variance of heart period outside the frequency band characteristic of spontaneous breathing for the child (i.e., 0.24 to 1.04 Hz or approximately 15 to 60 breaths per minute) and calculating the natural logarithm of the band-pass variance

When the team has tested the equipment and the computer operator has set the skin conductance sensitivity so that the child's baseline is at 0, the operator signals the experimenter to begin the protocol and records a 2-minute baseline. Then 10 contiguous trials occur in each of 5 sensory systems. The experimenter presents the stimuli for 3 seconds each according to a standard, pseudorandom schedule 15 or 19 seconds apart, with 20 seconds between each sensory modality. A recorded set of instructions to which both the experimenter and the computer operator listen simultaneously through earphones directs the presentation of all stimuli. To control for possible order effects, two audiotapes alternate the order in which the sensory stimuli are presented. The order for tape one is olfactory, auditory, visual, tactile, and vestibular; the order for tape two is tactile, visual, auditory, olfactory, and vestibular. Both tapes present vestibular stimuli last in case the vestibular stimuli disrupt the child to the extent that he or she is not able to complete the protocol.

Presentation of Sensory Stimuli

The experimenter says to the child, "Now we are going to go on a pretend spaceship trip. You are going to smell some funny things, hear and see some funny things, and feel some funny things. Here we go! The first thing is a smell. Take a big breath and smell in now!" The experimenter times the word *now* to correspond with the first olfactory trial on the experimenter's audiotape.

Olfactory: The olfactory stimulus is wintergreen oil kept about half an inch deep in a small vial with a cotton ball. The wintergreen is commercially available in the extract sections of grocery and drug stores (e.g., Walgreen's wintergreen oil, synthetic methyl salicylate n.f.). Wearing a sterile glove, thumb covering the opened vial, the experimenter times his or her movements so that as the tape says "Ready, set, go," the experimenter is ready to uncover the vial and place it about 1 inch from the participant's nose, centered between nose and lips. The experimenter then moves the vial in a 1-inch path from the child's left (on 1), to the child's right (on 2), and to the child's left (on 3) with 1 second for each excursion from side to side. The experimenter tells the child to "smell in" with each excursion. The experimenter then places a thumb over the top of the vial to try to retain any lingering odors in the bottle and drops the vial to his or her side. At the conclusion of the 10 olfactory stimuli, the experimenter turns the glove inside out to trap odors inside the glove before discarding it and reseals the vial.

Auditory: After the 20-second wait period following olfactory stimulation, the experimenter says, "Now we are going to hear some funny things" and starts a tape recorder beginning the series of audio presentations. The stimuli are professionally recorded fire engine siren sounds played at 90 decibels. The tape presents 10 stimuli 8 or 12 seconds apart.

Visual: After the 20-second wait period following auditory stimulation, the experimenter says, "Now we are going to see some funny things." A commercially available 20-watt strobe light set at 10 flashes per second is built into the right "arm" of the spaceship console slightly below eye level. The strobe connects to an Able-Net Incorporated power link so that the experimenter, using a foot pedal, can turn the strobe on and off as directed by the audiotape. The strobe is on for 3 seconds, then remains off until the next trial.

Tactile: After the 20-second wait period following visual stimulation, the experimenter says, "Now we are going to feel some funny things." The experimenter uses the "Mr. Thumbuddy" cloth finger puppet with a 2.5-inch feather (*Miller Assessment for Preschoolers*; Miller, 1982, 1988) for the tactile stimuli. The experimenter gently places the feather outside the participant's right ear canal, then gently draws the feather along the chin line to the bottom of the chin, and finally raises the feather to the child's left ear canal. The experimenter times each movement to correspond with the "1-2-3" on the audiotape.

Vestibular: The participant's chair is securely fastened to the top surface of a 28-inch-square tilt board (Achievement Products, Inc., Canton, Ohio) supported by a 5.5-inch cube at each corner. A 4 inch high board rests under the back of the tilt board so that when the examiner tilts the chair backwards, the chair goes back 30 degrees before gently touching the board on the floor. After the 20-second wait period following tactile stimulation, and before administering the movement stimuli, the experimenter removes the two blocks located behind the participant's seat while holding the platform steady. Then the experimenter smoothly and slowly tips the child backward until the platform touches the board on the floor. The entire tip back occurs over 3 seconds and the return to upright also takes 3 seconds, both in time to the "1-2-3" on the audiotape, one continuous smooth and gentle movement. Children are often startled by the first tip, but typically developing children experience the movement as "fun." After the first tip back, the experimenter says, "[Child's name], I'm here and I will be here the whole time." After the 10 excursions of the chair are complete, the experimenter replaces the blocks under the platform so it becomes a stable surface once again. Then the experimenter starts a short cartoon videotape that plays for 2 minutes, during which the operator records "recovery" data for EDR and vagal tone.

If at any point the child experiences severe discomfort or verbally indicates that he or she wishes to stop, the experimenter terminates the particular stimulus but then makes every reasonable effort to coax the child to complete the remaining stimuli in the session. At the end of the session, the experimenter thanks the child and the parent for participating, and the child chooses a gift. The parent receives a small stipend for participating.

From Neuron to Behavior:

Regulation, Arousal, and Attention as Important Substrates for the Process of Sensory Integration

GRETCHEN DAHL REEVES, PH.D., OT/L, FAOTA

This chapter examines the mechanisms and systems of the brain that regulate behavior and the role that sensory input can play in regulation. Regulation is an internal process of adjustment that ensures order and accuracy in physiological responses (Porges, 1996). Regulation implies that intrinsic mechanisms maintain internal control and sustain the basic operations of the nervous system as well as other organ systems (Derryberry & Reed, 1996). The coordination and balance of central nervous system responses as the brain assimilates and organizes information from ongoing sensory experiences are essential to sensory integration. Regulation provides an important foundation for all behaviors, whether automatic or voluntary. It is an inherent feature of biological systems that maintains internal order and underlies the ability to adapt to new situations (Porges, 1996; Schore, 1997). Because sensory integration intervention creates therapeutic opportunities that facilitate appropriate adaptive responses, an understanding of neural regulation and its relationship to arousal levels and attention can enhance intervention planning. Although researchers continue to investigate the precise way in which the brain assimilates all the right things at the right time to support behavior and performance, the neuroscience literature provides information that is helpful in the process of clinical reasoning.

Processes of Regulation

Neural Regulation

neural regulation: a process by which the CNS controls the timing and sequencing of neuron firing while monitoring internal and external events

All biological systems of the human body are dependent on operations of the central nervous system (CNS). The CNS controls the timing and sequencing of responses of all organs of the body and constantly monitors ongoing internal and external events (Schore, 1997). This constant monitoring is essential to the survival and integrity of the individual and is the essence of neural regulation. The brain uses the information it receives from multiple sources to establish internal order as a basis for adaptive behavior. When needed, the brain can mobilize internal physical resources during stressful events. Regulation implies that adjustments in responses occur to ensure accuracy of operation of multiple organ systems (Porges, 1996). Inherent in that regulation process is the harmonious interaction of multiple areas of the nervous system as the brain strives for balance and organization.

Self-Regulation

Self-regulation is the ability of biological systems to adjust to changing conditions (Ryan, Kuhl, & Deci, 1997). Self-regulation suggests that individual organisms are capable of producing automatic internal adjustments to maintain order (Schore,

self-regulation:
the ability to adjust to changing conditions through internal processes that are coupled with behaviors to maintain a sense of control

1994). However, self-regulation also encompasses behaviors initiated to reduce distress, using internal and external processes to monitor, evaluate, and modify reactions to existing conditions (Thompson, 1994). Self-regulation is an essential element of development and maturation that supports meaningful interactions with the environment not only in infancy but throughout life (Als, 1986; Cicchetti, 1994; Davidson & Sutton, 1995; Fox, 1994; Hofer, 1994; Schore, 1994). For example, thumb-sucking by a tired, fretful infant can soothe and comfort. Participating in leisure occupations such as aerobic exercise, meditation, or yoga can reduce feelings of stress. Listening to loud, fast, upbeat music might keep one alert while working. Engaging in such self-regulating behaviors can mobilize the needed resources to facilitate one's own sense of internal order and control of underlying arousal processes. As such, regulatory abilities encompass a vast range of neural areas and systems and involve an interplay of excitatory and inhibitory mechanisms (Porges, 1996).

Homeostasis

homeostasis:
the maintenance of internal stability through automatic adjustments and coordination of physiologic systems

Homeostasis refers to the maintenance of internal stability through the coordination of organ systems that automatically adjust to environmental changes (Bear, Connors, & Paradiso, 2001). An organism achieves homeostasis through mechanisms of neural regulation involving the rhythmic interaction of multiple physiological systems and encompassing thousands of neuron processes that regulate arousal (Thompson, 1994). Biological systems operate to maintain order and balance.

Modulation

modulation:
the process by which incoming neuronal signals are adjusted in intensity to ensure internal order

Modulation of impulses generated by new and ongoing events is necessary for homeostasis. Modulation adjusts the intensity of incoming neuronal signals to levels that are appropriate to the situation (Bear et al., 2001), which ensures order in internal operations as the organism receives new input and assimilates it with existing reactions. Modulation reflects a process by which the nervous system alters the excitability and responsiveness of neuronal circuits (Noback, Strominger, & Demarest, 1996). Modulation changes the quality and speed of neuron response to stimuli in sensory, motor, and association components so that in any situation, the individual can focus on the most important events that will support function and performance.

Sensory Integration and Regulation

Sensory integration is based upon the adequate receipt and modulation of sensory information that the organism then uses to regulate behavior and emotions. Ayres (1972) recognized the importance of regulation in sensory integration when she suggested that the suppression of input was as vital to the process of neural integration as the activation of input. She described sensory integration as an intricate and complex process performed at all levels of the nervous system. Ayres promoted the idea that sensory input provides nourishment to the brain. An individual whose nervous system does not interpret signals appropriately from the surroundings might be deterred from purposeful interactions with the environment. Learning and maturation are sometimes restricted in persons who are not able to utilize fully the various forms of sensory information inherent in daily life experiences. Self-regulation and sensory integration are interdependent and interrelated processes.

The behavior of the child who seeks massive amounts of sensory input through random, unfocused activity might indicate that the day-to-day routine is not generating enough neural energy to satisfy the brain's need for information from the environment. The child might not be able to readily register the tactile, proprioceptive, and vestibular input typically produced while climbing, running, and jumping and therefore can be deprived of important information needed to develop adequate postural reactions, body awareness, or a sense of position in space. The lack of such information could impede the child's ability to perform self-care, household, or classroom tasks. With disruption in self-regulation, the child seeks needed input through random activity that might be additionally disorganizing. In such cases, sensory integration intervention attempts to increase the variety and richness of the environment by creating opportunities for enhanced sensory input and adaptive behaviors, thereby facilitating neural regulation.

For the child who lacks adequate sensory discrimination, sensory integration intervention aims to increase sensory cues by providing sensory experiences that are more stimulating. For example, playing with foaming soap or digging in the sandbox provides increased tactile input to the hands prior to tasks requiring fine motor coordination (Case-Smith, 1991; Exner, 1995). Such stimulation might increase recognition and awareness of the hands, providing the brain with a sensory foundation for skilled movement. Fast motion on a scooter board activates the vestibular system and helps to facilitate the posture and sitting balance needed for dressing at home or working at a desk in the classroom.

Emotional reactions to sensory stimuli can indicate the underlying state of the nervous system. Emotional reactions must be flexible, responsive to the situation, and enhancing to performance to support adaptation (Thompson, 1994). Excess or flattened emotional responses during sensory play can indicate poor sensory registration and inadequate self-regulation. Children who are hypervigilant to the sensory conditions in the routine of daily life might be unable to engage in appropriate playful or social interactions because they are constantly distracted by irrelevant sensory events. They might withdraw from contact or exhibit strong emotion-charged and negative reactions to new experiences, which suggests hyperresponsiveness to sensory input. Such behaviors can indicate an overexcited and poorly modulated nervous system. In an attempt to reduce neural excitability and augment sensory modulation, therapists use treatment strategies that promote calming, such as slow motion or deep touch-pressure. Such input might assist the brain in its drive to be organized.

Evidence throughout the neuroscience literature supports the use of active sensory experiences to enhance self-regulation as a basis for learning, brain maturation, and neural organization (Davidson, 1994; Derryberry & Reed, 1996; Ryan et al., 1997; Schore, 1996, 1997). However, the passive application of sensory stimulation is rarely justified unless the clinician uses extreme caution and care. Doing and engaging with the environment have greater impact because self-directed activity challenges the nervous system to be self-regulating (Ryan et al., 1997). Rigid external demands intended to control behavior are likely to compromise the internal resources required to carry out purposeful actions (Ryan et al., 1997). Self-generated actions in an environment designed to improve the integration of sensory input and promote self-regulation provide tremendous therapeutic value. Ayres (1972) understood the importance of self-direction and active engagement of the child in the therapeutic process and used this insight to facilitate child-directed activity as a major component of sensory integration therapy.

Neuronal Basis of Regulation

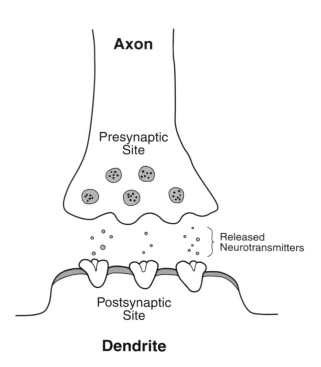

Axon

Presynaptic
Site

}Released
Neurotransmitters

Postsynaptic
Site

Dendrite

Figure 5.1.

Synaptic transmission occurs at chemical synapses
when neurotransmitters are released from the
presynaptic site into the synaptic cleft. Binding of
the neurotransmitter at the postsynaptic surface
can open or close channels to cause excitation or
inhibition of an electrical signal.

habituation:
a decrease in
synaptic firing and
behavioral response
to a repeated non-
threatening stimulus

sensitization:
increased synaptic
firing in response
to a repeated
noxious stimulus

Neuronal Activity and Synaptic Transmission

A series of events occurring within the CNS at the cellular level can have a significant effect on the individual's behavioral responses to environmental stimuli. Synaptic transmission is a means by which neurons influence the excitability of adjacent cells (Shepherd & Koch, 1998). Neurotransmitters released at a synapse can determine whether excitation or inhibition of a neuronal impulse will occur at the postsynaptic site. Neurotransmitters released from presynaptic endings can affect receptors on the postsynaptic surface (Figure 5.1).

Input from adjacent cells constantly barrages each neuron in the CNS. As a result, postsynaptic receptors can receive excitatory and inhibitory inputs simultaneously from numerous sources, then integrate these multiple inputs to determine whether the cell will fire or remain silent (Kandel, Schwartz, & Jessel, 1995).

Habituation and Sensitization: Simple Forms of Learning Based on Neuron Response

Neuroscientists have defined two simple forms of learning, habituation and sensitization, that occur at the neuronal level (Kandel et al., 1995). Changes in neuronal sensitivity occur as a result of the amount and type of stimuli that the neuron receives.

Habituation is a decrease in response at a synapse upon repeated presentation of a nonthreatening stimulus. Simple organisms demonstrate habituation as behavioral disregard of repetitive stimuli (Bear et al., 2001; Kandel et al., 1995). Proposed mechanisms of habituation include an elevated threshold for firing or depletion of neurotransmitters necessary for firing. Habituation has the potential to affect behavior in several ways. It might help an individual ignore nonrelevant events or surrounding distractions and focus on the important features of a situation. Consequently, by reducing unnecessary synaptic action, habituation can reduce distractibility and enhance the ability to attend for appropriate periods. For children with developmental disabilities, distractibility often impedes performance. Failure of the nervous system to habituate might underlie this characteristic, suggesting that the brain finds everything to be novel and interesting. However, this capacity for distraction interferes with the ability to recognize and assimilate the most salient and important features of the task.

Sensitization is an intensified response to a wide variety of stimuli following a strong or noxious stimulus (Bear et al., 2001; Kandel et al., 1995). Sensitization results from heightened neuronal transmission due to a decrease in the firing threshold of individual neurons or an increase in neurotransmitter release. The purpose of sensitization is to assist in potentially dangerous situations by alerting the organism to the surroundings. Sensitization might represent the internal events in persons who exhibit adverse or defensive reactions to one or more types of sensory input because the cells of the nervous system overrespond or fire too easily. This increased response also disrupts the ability to override unimportant stimuli. In contrast to impaired habituation, heightened sensitization creates a feeling that typical stimuli are threatening. For example, most people are not disturbed by a wrinkle in a sock, the rustling of papers by a person sitting nearby, or taking a step off of a curb. The individual who is defensive to sensory signals often perseverates on such stimuli and might go to great lengths to avoid such experiences.

Arousal and Attention: Foundation for Higher-Level Learning

arousal:
increased neuron excitability that mobilizes the internal resources needed to maintain alertness

attention:
the brain's ability to focus on important stimuli for learning

Singly or collectively, inputs from sensory stimuli can affect excitability of the nervous system and influence an individual's level of arousal. Arousal occurs with increased neuronal excitability and cerebral blood flow (Robbins, 1998; Schore, 1997). Heightened electrical activation and excitatory neurotransmitter release mobilize the necessary energy to maintain alertness to surrounding conditions. Adequate neuron action that causes appropriate neurotransmitter release at individual synapses at the right time is an inherent component of arousal. An optimum level of arousal represents the level of neuron excitability needed to remain focused on the task at hand.

Optimum arousal allows individuals to be more aware of incoming stimuli and enhances their attention (Crooks & Stein, 1988). Attention is the brain's ability to focus selectively on the most important stimuli attached to an object or event (Butter, 1987; Porges, 1984) and supports the maintenance of neural regulation (Barkley, 1990; Gillberg & Coleman, 1992; Greenspan, 1992; Ornitz, 1974).

The nervous system balances arousal so as to focus attention for learning. The amount of neuron excitability that maintains an appropriate level of arousal can support and enhance that learning. The synchronous firing of appropriate neurons while the individual is engaged in learning supports the ability to focus and maintain interest in the task. For example, a young infant who has just discovered a new rattle will hold the rattle in front of his or her face while intently examining the features of the toy. This visual examination will often be coupled with mouthing of the object. The child is combining visual, tactile, and proprioceptive senses to gain knowledge of the rattle. Although this might appear to be a very simple example of learning, it is quite complex when considered at the neuronal level. Thousands of neurons fire during each moment of the investigation of the rattle to maintain optimum arousal, providing the brain with the necessary signals to hold the child's interest and form a memory about the object.

Interaction of Multiple Systems

Describing events at the level of the cell only begins to tell the story of regulation. At birth, the human nervous system consists of approximately 100 billion neurons (Whatson & Stirling, 1998). The simultaneous firing of all neurons at once would be devastating and disintegrating. Response regulation requires the integration of neuronal signals from numerous cells at any given moment, but the cells that are selected are specific to the input. This selection process underlies the ability to maintain an optimum level of arousal while inducing the activation of circuits and anatomic areas that support focused attention. Regulation occurs at several levels of the nervous system and results in a coordinated interplay of neuronal activity that supports a behavioral response.

Neuroanatomic Components of Regulation

The maintenance of attention and appropriate arousal is no small accomplishment for the nervous system, with the integration of multiple messages through multiple circuits involving constant coordination between neuroanatomic structures. Interlinking neural systems provide a source for the interplay of excitatory and inhibitory mechanisms that generate a person's responses to the demands of the environment and enhance occupational performance. When even one element fails to operate adequately, the cascading effect can be pervasive. The reticular, limbic, and autonomic systems encompass older structures of the nervous system that are sensitive to changing sensory conditions in the environment and monitor the individual's emotional reactions to change and challenge (Stifter & Jain, 1996). The responses of these older systems, coupled with those of the neocortex, generally lead to maturation and improved performance in several arenas.

Brainstem

Reticular System

In developing the theory of sensory integration, Ayres (1972) emphasized the major role of brainstem structures used in the initial processing and integration of sensory information. In particular, the reticular formation of the brainstem (Figure 5.2) is crucial here. The reticular formation consists of clusters of interconnected neurons with extensive dendritic branches and long axonal projections to higher and lower levels of the nervous system (Gilman & Newman, 1996). The most direct influences on the reticular formation are the sensations produced by pain, light touch, head movement, and sound. Because the first level of synaptic action of the tactile, vestibular, and auditory systems is in the brainstem, responses generated by these sensory systems could be more likely to produce aversive reactions than other types of sensory input. Olfactory, proprioceptive, and visual inputs affect the reticular formation more indirectly through cortical and cerebellar circuits (Gilman & Newman, 1996; Kiernan, 1998).

The reticular formation typically filters out irrelevant stimuli so that only the most important sensory cues pass through to keep the brain informed of events in the environment. Information processed and filtered by the reticular formation contributes to its role in sleep, wakefulness, and arousal. These behaviors are regulated through the ascending pathways of the reticular activating system (Noback et al., 1996). Higher-level structures receiving signals from the reticular formation in turn control the amount of excitability of the reticular formation through reciprocal pathways. The areas involved in this interchange are the hippocampus, hypothalamus, and frontal cortex (Kiernan, 1998).

Sensory input can influence the state of arousal through the reticular system. The excitability of the reticular formation varies depending on the type of sensory information it receives. The tactile system illustrates this point well because some of its distinct anatomical features provide a rationale for using different types of tactile input in therapy. The anterolateral pathways carrying information from the body to the thalamus and somatosensory cortex related to pain and light touch sensations are older and diffuse tracts. As these fibers pass through the brainstem, they extend collateral fibers and terminal branches into the reticular formation. Sensations of pain and light touch warn of danger, facilitating alerting and arousal reactions to enhance survival. Therefore, stimulation of the reticular formation increases brain activity to support vigilance and attention at higher levels.

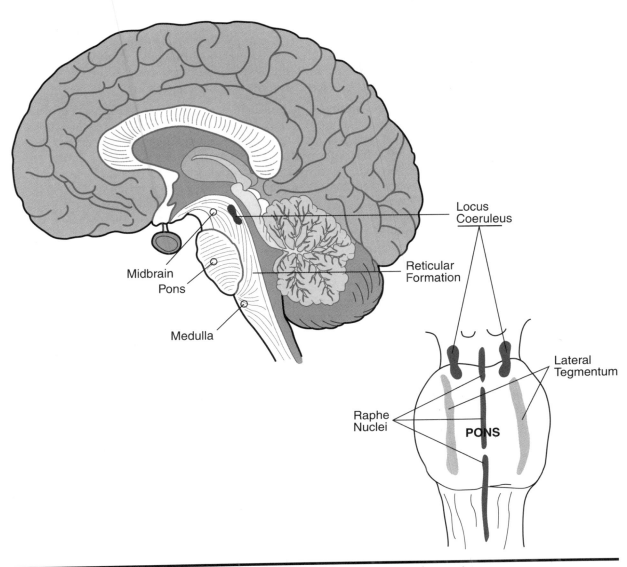

Figure 5.2.   Lateral and frontal view of the brainstem reticular formation

In contrast to the paths for pain and light touch, the newer dorsal pathways for discriminative touch, touch-pressure, and vibration do not extend collateral fibers to the reticular formation as they traverse the brainstem (Martin, 1996). Instead, these signals travel rapidly to the thalamus and somatosensory cortex. As this information spreads through the brain, the cortex acts on the reticular formation in an inhibitory fashion and reduces its excitability. Consequently, applying deep pressure or resistive input to the skin can be a means of reducing aversive reactions in persons who express a dislike of tactile experiences. These treatment strategies attempt to bypass direct activation of the reticular formation that would potentially increase arousal and overreaction to stimuli.

The intensity of a sensory stimulus can also affect the reticular formation. Stronger or more intense stimuli generally have an alerting effect on the reticular system, whereas softer and gentler stimuli can be more soothing and calming and reduce its arousal. Softening the lights, lowering one's voice, or gently rocking the person assists in calming and organizing.

Neurotransmitter Systems of the Brainstem

Distinct groups of cells within the brainstem produce major neurotransmitters called the biogenic amines, including dopamine, norepinephrine, and serotonin. These cell groups form extensive neural connections with widespread areas of the CNS and are significant in their impact on sleep, arousal, attention, and motivation.

Cells in the lateral tegmentum of the pons and medulla and in the locus coeruleus of the pons produce norepinephrine (Figure 5.2). The output branches of the locus coeruleus are more extensive than those of any other nucleus of the nervous system (Noback et al., 1996). Its axons project to the thalamus, hypothalamus, limbic structures, and cerebral cortex. Novel or intense stimuli trigger the release of norepinephrine, which is essential to the modulation of cell firing when released in those target areas throughout the CNS. Norepinephrine produces signals in the main sensory areas of the brain, the parietal, occipital, and temporal lobes, where somatosensory, visual, and auditory stimuli are processed respectively. Such signals might assist in enhancing attention to external events.

Serotonin, produced primarily by a group of reticular formation cells known as the raphe nuclei (Figure 5.2), produces either a modulatory or an augmentative effect at postsynaptic sites. Serotonin supports the learning of avoidance behaviors, influences excitability of lower motor neurons, and affects feeding behavior, sleep states, circadian rhythmicity, and pain responses (Cooper, Bloom, & Roth, 1996). The raphe nuclei distribute signals to the basal ganglia, cerebellum, spinal cord, hypothalamus, and the limbic, frontal, and sensory areas of the cerebral cortex (Gilman & Newman, 1996; Noback et al., 1996). Serotonin is a mood enhancer and is essential to maintaining arousal (Siegel, Agranoff, Albers, Fisher, & Uhler, 1999).

Dopamine's role in attention and arousal is less clear, but it does affect motor function and motivation. Sites of dopamine production include the substantia nigra of the midbrain and cells of the ventral tegmental area medial to the substantia nigra (Figure 5.3). From these midbrain areas, fibers project to the basal ganglia, limbic cortex, and frontal cortex (Kiernan, 1998). Dopamine works through these connections to regulate movement, reduce erratic behavior, and inhibit distracting or irrelevant actions (Siegel et al., 1999).

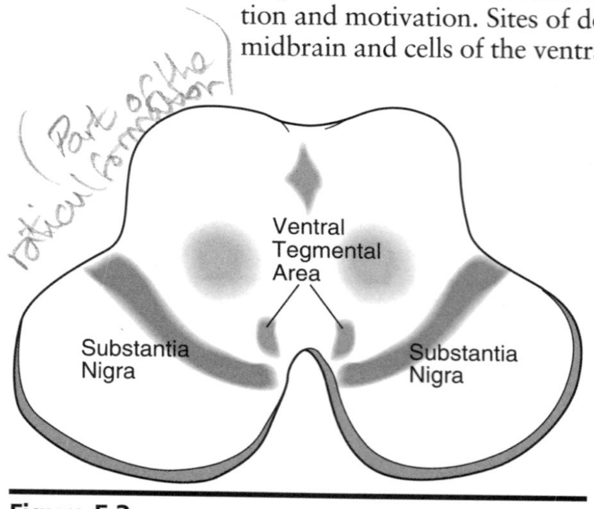

All of these neurotransmitter-producing areas of the brainstem contain nuclear groups of cells that are small in size but have a major effect on multiple CNS areas and therefore on performance. Ayres recognized and emphasized that brainstem-level processes are critical to sensory and neural integration. As the neuroscience literature elucidates in more elaborate ways the functions played by the structures of the brainstem that produce and promote neurochemical responses, researchers and clinicians gain a deeper appreciation for the brainstem's value and the insight that Jean Ayres had in highlighting its significance.

Figure 5.3.

Cross-section of the midbrain, illustrating the location of the substantia nigra and the cells of the ventral tegmental area, which produce dopamine.

A word of caution is in order here in reference to neurotransmitters. Rigorous clinical studies that measure changes in neurotransmitter levels in conjunction with sensorimotor interventions have yet to be done. Such studies could help delineate the effects of sensory integration therapy on neurotransmitter release and synthesis. Such investigations are not simple, however. Researchers must analyze samples of urine, blood, or cerebrospinal fluid for the by-products of neurotransmitter breakdown, known as metabolites. Obviously, this involves medical laboratory analysis and sometimes invasive measures that can limit the feasibility of such studies. Obtaining such information does not necessarily specify which site in the brain or body is metabolizing a particular transmitter substance. Although disorders of regulation are probably disorders of neurotransmitter release and uptake at selected synapses, it is difficult to pinpoint the precise location of the disorder. Clinicians may surmise from observations during treatment that changes in adaptive behavior and performance are a reflection of more adequate biochemical transmission. However, it is important to use caution in making claims about these possible changes without the appropriate data to support those claims. The complexity of the brain's biochemistry is vast, and there is no easy way to simplify it. Speculation might exist about the implications of treatment in this realm, but there is much to be done to validate those ideas.

Hypothalamus

The hypothalamus (Figure 5.4), located at the base of the third ventricle, consists of nuclear groups that affect functions related to species survival. Selected areas of the hypothalamus control eating, drinking, the maintenance of body temperature, the organization of circadian rhythms, hormone regulation, and reproduction (Kiernan, 1998). Projections travel to the peripheral autonomic nervous system, the dorsal motor nucleus of cranial nerve X, the pituitary and adrenal glands, the thalamus, and the prefrontal cerebral cortex, illustrating the widespread effect that the hypothalamus has on neural function. The hypothalamus receives afferents from the retina, prefrontal cortex,

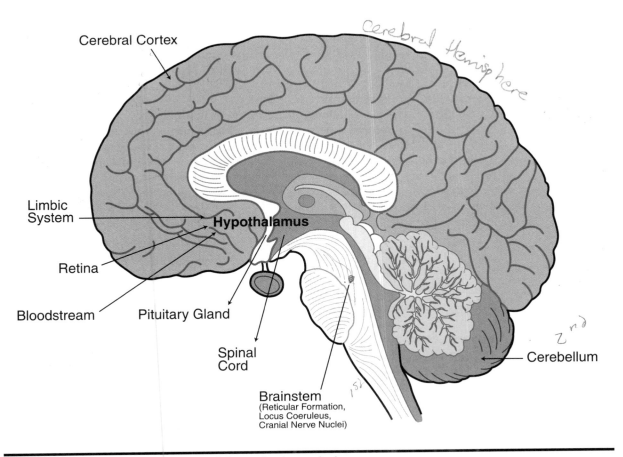

Figure 5.4.   Connections to and from the hypothalamus

thalamus, amygdala, hippocampus, cingulate gyrus, and reticular formation (Kiernan). Projections from the locus coeruleus and raphe nuclei to the hypothalamus produce diffuse modulatory effects on the general excitability of its cells through the release of their respective neurotransmitters (norepinephrine and serotonin). Afferent fibers from taste and visceral sensors also project into the hypothalamus and provide the route by which signals related to feeding can affect the hypothalamus (Brodal, 1992).

The hypothalamus is responsible for control of the autonomic nervous system (ANS), which also plays a significant role in regulatory processes. The ANS (Figure 5.5) innervates glands and cardiac and smooth muscles. Although generally regarded as an efferent system, sensory fibers accompany and are related anatomically and functionally to the motor fibers supplying the viscera (Gilman & Newman, 1996).

The parasympathetic division, operating through cells in the brainstem and sacral spinal cord, regulates the internal organs and maintains reactions for growth, repair, and reproduction. Maturation of the parasympathetic portion of the ANS enhances vagal tone, grading of arousability, and emotional control (Gunnar, 1986; Mangelsdorf, Shapiro, & Marzolf, 1995; Porges, 1996). The vagus nerve, cranial nerve X, is a major component of the parasympathetic system. Its axons travel to the thoracic and abdominal cavities, influencing the actions of the heart, lungs, and digestive and gastrointestinal organs. The vagal system supports digestion, respiration, and the regulation of emotional, motor, and vocal responses through the heart, lung, and oral structures (Porges, Doussard-Roosevelt, & Maiti, 1994). The parasympathetic division of the ANS is a necessary component of self-regulation, promoting homeostasis and coordinated action of body organs and systems.

In contrast, under conditions of perceived threat, the sympathetic subsystem of the ANS activates fight-or-flight reactions for protection and survival. Motor neurons of the sympathetic system reside in the lateral gray matter of the thoracic and upper lumbar levels of the spinal cord in an area known as the intermediolateral cell column (Figure 5.5). The hypothalamus exerts a direct effect on these motor neurons (Kiernan, 1998). From sympathetic cells in the spinal cord, exiting axons traverse the ascending and descending sympathetic chain lying along the vertebral column and travel to visceral organs throughout the head and body. Changes produced in heart rate, blood pressure, sensory conductance, vascular flow, and digestive actions mobilize internal resources to support survival during events that could pose a threat. As a result, activation of the sympathetic nervous system heightens arousal, increases sensitivity to stimuli, and prepares for rapid responses. Stimulation of the sympathetic nervous system produces generalized rather than localized physiological responses, augmented by the release of epinephrine from the adrenal gland into the bloodstream.

Autonomic indicators can guide therapists in their selection of therapeutic interventions and measurement of the impact of those interventions. For example, pupil dilation, irregular respiration, increased heart rate, and blanching or flushing of the skin signal that the sympathetic system is activated. Porges (1996) implicated poor autonomic regulation in high-risk infants who exhibit periods of apnea, bradycardia, poor organization of sucking and swallowing, and high-pitched vocalizations. Such responses deter growth and adaptation and indicate severe distress. Additionally, cues from preterm infants indicative of dysregulation include more time spent in fretful, hyperalert states, averted and fixed gaze, dramatic color changes, gagging, coughing, yawning, sighing, diffuse motor activity, restlessness, and crying (Als, 1986). These behaviors can persist in children with marked developmental delays and are key indicators of the underlying neurobehavioral state of the individual, especially in those who are nonverbal. These behaviors cue therapists to alter treatment strategies by reducing the complexity of the intervention and providing soothing input that decreases overarousal.

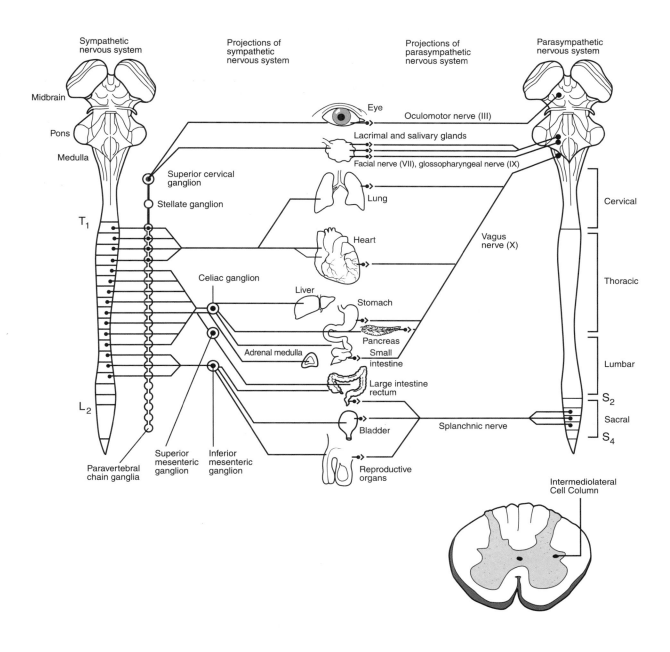

Figure 5.5. The autonomic nervous system viewed from the posterior brainstem and spinal cord

On the right, the parasympathetic portion originates from cell bodies located in cranial nerves III (oculomotor nerve), VII (facial nerve), IX (glossopharyngeal nerve), and X (vagus nerve) and in the sacral cord (S_2 to S_4). The sympathetic portion on the left affects the same glands and organs via splanchnic nerves and the sympathetic chain ganglia that lie alongside the vertebrae. Cell bodies are located in the intermediolateral cell column at the T_1 to L_2 levels of the spinal cord.

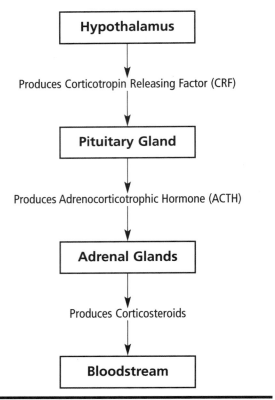

Hypothalamus

Produces Corticotropin Releasing Factor (CRF)

Pituitary Gland

Produces Adrenocorticotrophic Hormone (ACTH)

Adrenal Glands

Produces Corticosteroids

Bloodstream

Figure 5.6. The hypothalamo-pituitary-adrenal axis (HPA)

The regulation of physiologic responses to stress is another responsibility of the hypothalamus. Connections with the pituitary gland provide the hypothalamus with routes to initiate the release of stress hormones. The hypothalamic-pituitary-adrenocortical system (HPA axis) (Figure 5.6) regulates reactions to stress and uncertainty (Thompson, 1994). In a stressful situation, the hypothalamus produces corticotropin releasing factor (CRF) that stimulates the pituitary gland to release adrenocorticotrophic hormone (ACTH). ACTH activates receptors on the adrenal gland to produce stress or steroid hormones, primarily cortisol (Stansbury & Gunnar, 1994). Cortisol, as it circulates in the bloodstream, activates essential body resources needed to sustain physiologic functions during stressful situations (Gilman & Newman, 1996). Cortisol can affect structures of the limbic system involved in emotion, learning, memory, and self-regulation.

Limbic System

The limbic system is the seat of the emotions, linking structures of the temporal lobe with widespread areas of the brain. Connections from the limbic system to the reticular formation and areas of the brain involved in sensory processing moderate emotions in conjunction with incoming information. The hypothalamus is a component of the limbic system and is the route by which autonomic responses are activated to reflect the individual's emotional state. Additional structures of the limbic system (Figure 5.7) include the amygdala, the hippocampus, the parahippocampal gyrus (situated in the temporal lobe adjacent to the hippocampus), the anterior thalamus, the septal area of the basal forebrain, and the cingulate gyrus lying over the corpus callosum (Gilman & Newman, 1996).

Amygdala

For years, researchers have recognized the amygdala as the site where basic emotions are activated. In humans, stimulation of the amygdala produces anxiety (Brodal, 1992; Kiernan, 1998). Stimuli interpreted as dangerous can activate the amygdala (LeDoux, 1996), which receives input from the reticular formation and its neurotransmitters. New or intense stimuli processed via the reticular formation have the potential to alert the amygdala. The amygdala can then act on the hypothalamus and stimulate cortisol production via the HPA axis. The amygdala also communicates with all sensory association areas of the brain as well as the brainstem, thalamus, basal ganglia, hippocampus, and frontal cortex, thereby increasing the potential to excite broader areas of the CNS.

The frontal cortex and the amygdala share reciprocal connections. Through these connections, the frontal cortex can moderate the reactions of the amygdala and inhibit overactivation of emotional responses. The frontal cortex affects "rational" thinking and reflection as an individual considers potential outcomes and solutions to problems during emotional experiences. Using logical thoughts works to the person's benefit, assisting the individual in solving complex problems and reducing anxiety in

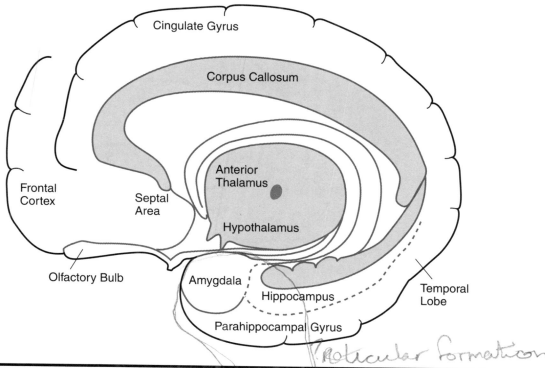

Reticular Formation

Figure 5.7.   Structures of the limbic system

Important structures include the amygdala, hippocampus, hypothalamus, septal area, anterior thalamus, and cingulate gyrus.

new situations. Researchers suspect that the reciprocal connections between the frontal cortex and the amygdala take as long as the first decade of life to myelinate fully. This might explain why children's emotions are sometimes more intense and less easily modulated than those of an adult.

Past experiences, thoughts, and perceptions can exert a strong influence on the excitability of the amygdala. People can literally think themselves into a frenzy or alternatively, into a state of well-being. Persons who are easily overwhelmed by stimuli sometimes elicit a pattern of neuronal activation that impedes the ability of the frontal cortex to regulate the amygdala. Sometimes referred to as a "learned response," this pattern has a potent physiological basis whereby the amygdala is influenced more strongly by inputs from the reticular formation than those of the frontal cortex. Increased reticular activation and heightened arousal reduce cortical inhibition while the amygdala simultaneously receives further stimulation.

In light of these considerations, it is important to recognize the impact of positive emotional experiences during therapy. Engaging children in meaningful play during sensory integration therapy can facilitate positive emotional reactions that promote more productive behaviors and the creation of pleasant memories. Offering opportunities for a child to be invested happily in therapeutic tasks can have a positive effect on the amygdala and increase feelings of security and self-esteem. Ayres (1972) encouraged practitioners to use the child's emotional response as a gauge for measuring the impact of sensory integration therapy. This continues to be one of the most valuable indicators that therapists can use to determine the success of treatment.

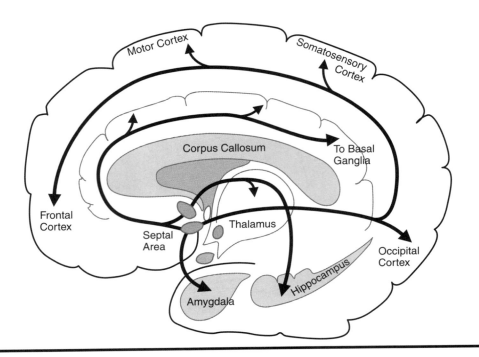

Figure 5.8.

Acetylcholine affects widespread areas of the brain from cells that originate in the septal area of the forebrain. Note the location of the cells and their routes of impact.

Septal Area

Cells in the septal region (Figure 5.8) produce acetylcholine, a neurotransmitter. Nerve fibers originating in the septal region spread widely throughout the cerebral cortex and are the route by which acetylcholine can affect widespread areas of the brain. Acetylcholine has a facilitatory effect on the cells of the cerebrum and contributes significantly to attention (Gilman & Newman, 1996).

Hippocampus

The hippocampus lies under the temporal horn of the lateral ventricle along the medial surface of the temporal lobe and has a role in learning and memory through habituation to non-novel stimuli. The hippocampus inhibits the reticular formation and the amygdala so the individual can focus on an ongoing task. Researchers have also linked the hippocampus to the formation of memories for long-term storage. Although the hippocampus is not the repository of memories, it improves the storage of important information in those locations of the CNS related to the sensory events that occurred at the time the memory was first created (Kandel et al., 1995). For example, a highly visual experience will become anchored primarily in the occipital lobe, whereas auditory stimuli are more likely to engage cells in the temporal cortex. Signals that link the activation of the hippocampus with simultaneous activation of specific sensory areas of the brain provide a basis for memory storage. The more intense the sensory conditions under which information was gathered, the more salience can be attached to the situation and the easier it can be to retrieve those memories when the sensory conditions are again available (Kandel et al., 1995).

Limbic Connections and Memory Formation

The link between the hippocampus and other widely dispersed areas of the brain occurs through the Papez circuit (Papez, 1937). Sensory areas of the cerebral cortex influence the entorhinal cortex of the temporal lobe, which lies lateral and adjacent to the hippocampus (Figure 5.9). The entorhinal cortex sends this sensory information to the hippocampus (Gilman & Newman, 1996; Martin, 1996). From the hippocampus, the fornix provides a link to other brain areas, including the septal area of the forebrain, the thalamus, and the hypothalamus. The hippocampus receives highly processed sensory information about the internal and external worlds (Gilman & Newman). Information transferred to the anterior areas of the CNS can be redistributed to the temporal lobe and the hippocampus via a path known as the cingulum. The cingulum travels through the cingulate gyrus and accesses multiple areas of the cerebral cortex through reciprocal circuits. The cingulum also returns information to the entorhinal cortex and hippocampus. The circuit defined by Papez, linking the hippocampus to other critical sites at the base of the cerebrum, might provide the route by which the appropriate sensory or association areas of the brain receive and store long-term memories for later use.

Emotions play a significant role in memory formation. Whereas the amygdala can trigger the release of CRF from the hypothalamus during a stressful situation, the hippocampus acts as a regulator by inhibiting CRF release. Steroid receptors in the hippocampus are part of a control mechanism regulating the release of cortisol via the hypothalamus. The presence of a highly emotional stimulus persists in activating the

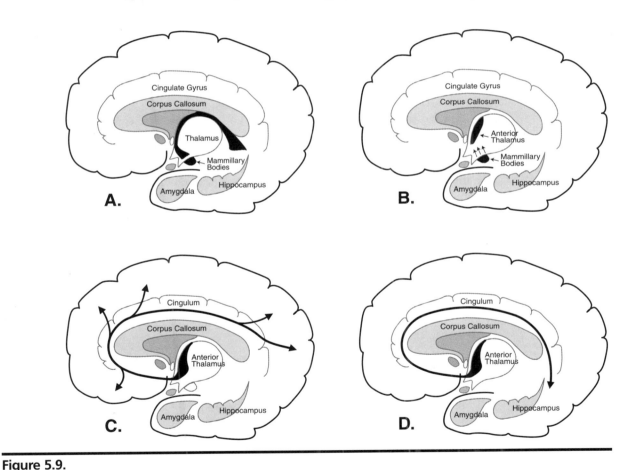

Figure 5.9.

The best-known circuit by which communication is linked between the structures of the limbic system and other areas of the brain is the Papez circuit. Signals from the hippocampus travel via the fornix to the mammillary bodies, then to the anterior thalamus. From there the fibers of the cingulum distribute signals to the cerebral cortex and back to the hippocampus.

amygdala. Such persistence soon impedes the ability of the hippocampus to regulate hypothalamic activation of the HPA axis that would reduce the production of cortisol.

Constant stress interferes with the ability of the hippocampus to lay down new memories (LeDoux, 1996). The hippocampal memory system, through the Papez circuit, provides conscious remembrances that can have multiple meanings not usually equated with fear. Unconscious memories established by fear-provoking circumstances operate through an amygdala-based memory system (LeDoux, 1996). Retrieval of such memories produces bodily responses that invoke preparations for danger. McEwen (1992) demonstrated that prolonged stress results in irreversible depletion of dendrites in the hippocampus. Children who have experienced significant distress (such as abuse) and war veterans with posttraumatic stress disorders have reduced hippocampal volumes (Bremner, Randall, Scott, & Bronen, 1995). Although release of epinephrine and norepinephrine during mild stress can enhance memory, prolonged and intense stress that increases circulating steroid hormones such as cortisol has a serious and detrimental effect on the hippocampus. It is important to reduce stress responses in children who overreact to various sensory events. Distress affects not only the emotional state of the individual but also the potential to learn and remember new information (Graham, Heim, Goodman, Miller, & Nemeroff, 1999). Establishing rapport and a trustful working relationship with clients is critical and apparently has powerful and long-ranging implications.

Cerebrum

Right Hemisphere

The right hemisphere of the cerebrum has a role in the regulation of emotion. Attuned to the environmental panorama, the right hemisphere has an advantage over the left in evaluating the general conditions of the environment. The right hemisphere gives priority to stimuli that are related to survival (Davidson, 1994). The early-developing right hemisphere plays an essential role in processing facial expressions and responding to the melodic features of speech (Schore, 1997). The right hemisphere is central to human bonding and attachment and to the development of reciprocal interactions within the mother-infant regulatory system. Orienting to novel stimuli occurs at a much higher rate in the right hemisphere than in the left and is essential to the regulation of attention. Lesions of the right hemisphere lead more often to attention disorders and distractibility than similar lesions on the left (Heilman, Bowers, Coslett, Whelan, & Watson, 1985). In contrast to the consecutive "linear" analysis of information by the left hemisphere, the processing of the right hemisphere is "nonlinear," based on multiple converging signals that occur in light of incoming sensory information (Schore, 1997).

Prefrontal Cortex

The anterior and lateral portions of the frontal lobe also contribute to the regulation of nervous system activity and emotions (Figure 5.10). These areas support reasoning, judgment, and problem solving (Kiernan, 1998). As the cerebral cortex matures through experience and environmental interaction, the frontal areas assume more prominence in regulating and inhibiting the older systems. Cortical inhibition of arousal emerges gradually throughout infancy (Dawson, Panagiotides, Klinger, & Hill, 1992). For example, from 2 to 4 months, an infant's attention span increases, the sleep-wake cycle follows a pattern of circadian organization, primitive reflexes decline, and more emotional responsiveness is evident. Attention allows an individual to focus on selected information in order to gather meaning from encounters with objects and persons in the environment (Butter, 1987). However, this does not

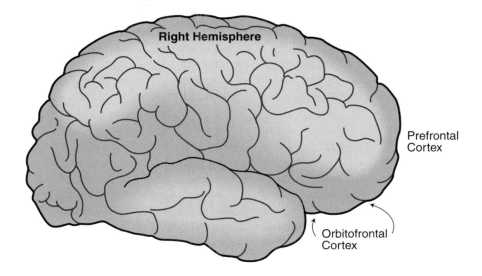

Figure 5.10. The prefrontal and orbitofrontal regions of the anterior lobe of the cerebrum

imply that the mature individual is rigidly fixated on events, but rather that attention can shift easily between events. Attention assumes an important regulatory function in emotional responses very early in life (Thompson, 1994).

Orbitofrontal Cortex

The orbitofrontal cortex (Figure 5.10), located on the medial and ventral surface of the frontal lobes, is involved in reciprocal interactions between the caregiver and the infant (Schore, 1996). The orbitofrontal cortex is larger in the right hemisphere and develops earlier in infancy than the more dorsal and lateral portions of the cerebral cortex. Axons from the visual, olfactory, somatosensory, and auditory cortices converge here. Connections with the brainstem and hypothalamus provide circuits for autonomic regulation, arousal, and attention. These circuits support approach behaviors by which the baby can direct eyes, head, and hands toward objects for investigation. The orbitofrontal system matures during the last half of the second year, which is a critical time for the appearance of many adaptive capacities (Schore, 1997). These advances reflect the role of the frontal lobe in the development of self-regulatory behavior (Dawson, 1994). The orbitofrontal system is a central component by which the forebrain circuits concerned with the recognition and interpretation of life experiences affect regulatory responses (Wolf, 1995).

Conclusion

The neuroanatomic areas identified here represent key areas involved in regulatory behavior. The preceding discussion suggests that regulation is a multifaceted process that occurs at all levels of the nervous system and is affected by a variety of factors. Sensory input can facilitate or impede self-regulating responses and behavior. In assessing and treating children with developmental disabilities who cannot cope with or extract meaning from multiple incoming sensory signals, practitioners must determine ways to facilitate growth-enhancing experiences. Simple solutions to the problems observed might not be readily available. It is probable that the implications of dysregulation in the life of the affected person are extensive and require a prolonged period of management.

Sensory integration therapy can offer important and essential elements that contribute to the positive management of these problems by engaging the child in purposeful actions and by creating the opportunity for self-regulation to develop through these actions. The development of self-regulation does not occur overnight in children who are maturing at typical rates. In the child with a developmental delay, the process takes longer but can be enhanced through interventions that facilitate the child's interest, participation, and achievement of goals.

References

Als, H. (1986). A synactive model of neonatal behavioral organization: Framework for the assessment of neurobehavioral development in the premature infant and support of infants and parents in the neonatal intensive care unit. *Physical and Occupational Therapy in Pediatrics, 6*(1 & 2), 3–55.

Ayres, A.J. (1972). *Sensory integration and learning disorders.* Los Angeles: Western Psychological Services.

Barkley, R. (1990). *Attention deficit hyperactivity disorder: A handbook for diagnosis and treatment.* New York: The Guilford Press.

Bear, M.F., Connors, B.W., & Paradiso, M.A. (2001). *Neuroscience: Exploring the brain* (2nd ed.). Baltimore: Lippincott Williams and Wilkins.

Bremner, J.D., Randall, P., Scott, T.M., & Bronen, R.A. (1995). MRI-based measurement of hippocampal volume in patients with combat-related PTSD. *American Journal of Psychiatry, 152,* 973–981.

Brodal, P. (1992). *The central nervous system: Structure and function.* New York: Oxford University Press.

Butter, C.M. (1987). Varieties of attention and disturbances of attention: A neuropsychological approach. In M. Jeannerod (Ed.), *Neurophysiological and neuropsychological aspects of spatial neglect* (pp. 1–23). New York: Elsevier.

Case-Smith, J. (1991). The effects of tactile defensiveness and tactile discrimination on in-hand manipulation. *The American Journal of Occupational Therapy, 45,* 811–818.

Cicchetti, D. (Ed.). (1994*). Development and psychopathology: Special issue: Neural plasticity, sensitive periods and psychopathology.* New York: Cambridge University Press.

Cooper, J.R., Bloom, F.E., & Roth, R.H. (1996). *The biochemical basis of neuropharmacology.* New York: Oxford University Press.

Crooks, R.L., & Stein, J. (1988). *Psychology: Science, behavior and life.* New York: Holt, Rinehart and Winston.

Davidson, R.J. (1994). Asymmetric brain function, affective style, and psychopathology: The role of early experience and plasticity. *Development and Psychopathology, 6,* 741–758.

Davidson, R.J., & Sutton, S.K. (1995). Affective neuroscience: The emergence of a discipline. *Current Opinion in Neurobiology, 5,* 21–24.

Dawson, G. (1994). Frontal electroencephalographic correlates of individual differences in emotional expression in infants. *The development of emotion regulation: Biological and behavioral considerations. Monographs of the Society for Research in Child Development, 59,* 135–151.

Dawson, G., Panagiotides, H., Klinger, L.G., & Hill, D. (1992). The role of frontal lobe functioning in the development of infant self-regulatory behavior. *Brain and Cognition, 20,* 152–175.

Derryberry, D., & Reed, M.A. (1996). Regulatory processes and the development of cognitive representations. *Development and Psychopathology, 8,* 215–234.

Exner, C. (1995). Remediation of hand skill problems in children. In A. Henderson & C. Pehoski (Eds.), *Hand function in the child: Foundations for remediation* (pp. 197–222). St. Louis: Mosby.

Fox, N. (1994). Dynamic cerebral processes underlying emotion regulation. *Monographs of the Society for Research in Child Development: The Development of Emotion Regulation, 59*, 152–166.

Gillberg, C., & Coleman, M. (1992). *The biology of the autistic syndromes.* New York: Cambridge University Press.

Gilman, S., & Newman, S.W. (1996). *Essential of clinical neuroanatomy and neurophysiology.* Philadelphia: F.A. Davis.

Graham, Y., Heim, C., Goodman, S., Miller, A., & Nemeroff, C. (1999). The effects of neonatal stress on brain development: Implications for psychopathology. *Development and Psychopathology, 8*, 545–565.

Greenspan, S.I. (1992). *Infancy and early childhood: The practice of clinical assessment and intervention with emotional and developmental challenges.* Madison, CT: International Universities Press.

Gunnar, M. (1986). Human developmental psychoneuroendocrinology: A review of research on neuroendocrine responses to challenge and threat in infancy and childhood. In M. Lamb & A.L. Brown (eds.), *Advances in developmental psychology* (pp. 51–103). Hillsdale, NJ: Lawrence Erlbaum.

Heilman, K.M., Bowers, D., Coslett, H.B., Whelan, H., & Watson, R.T. (1985). Directional hypokinesia: Prolonged reaction times for leftward movements in patients with right hemisphere lesions and neglect. *Neurology, 35*, 855–860.

Hofer, M. (1994). Early relationships as regulators of infant physiology and behavior. *Acta Paediatrica. Supplementum, 397*, 9–18.

Kandel, E.R., Schwartz, J.H., & Jessel, T.M. (1995). *Essentials of neural science and behavior.* Norwalk, CT: Appleton and Lange.

Kiernan, J.A. (1998). *Barr's The human nervous system: An anatomical viewpoint.* Philadelphia: Lippincott Williams and Wilkins.

LeDoux, J. (1996). *The emotional brain: The mysterious underpinnings of emotional life.* New York: Simon and Schuster.

Mangelsdorf, S., Shapiro, J. R., & Marzolf, D. (1995). Developmental and temperamental differences in emotion regulation in infancy. *Child Development, 66*, 1817–1828.

Martin, J.H. (1996). *Neuroanatomy: Text and atlas.* Stamford, CT: Appleton and Lange.

McEwen, B.S. (1992). Paradoxical effects of adrenal steroids on the brain: Protection versus degeneration. *Biological Psychiatry, 31*, 177–199.

Noback, C.R., Strominger, N.L., & Demarest, R.J. (1996). *The human nervous system.* Media, PA: Williams and Wilkins.

Ornitz, E.M. (1974). The modulation of sensory input and motor output in autistic children. *Journal of Autism and Childhood Schizophrenia, 4*, 197–215.

Papez, J.W. (1937). A proposed mechanism of emotion. *Archives of Neurology and Psychiatry, 79*, 217–224.

Porges, S.W. (1984). Physiologic correlates of attention: A core process underlying learning disorders. *Pediatric Clinics of North America, 31*, 371–385.

Porges, S.W. (1996). Physiological regulation in high-risk infants: A model for assessment and potential intervention. *Development and Psychopathology, 8*, 43–58.

Porges, S.W., Doussard-Roosevelt, J., & Maiti, A.K. (1994). Vagal tone and the physiological regulation of emotion. *The development of emotion regulation: Biological and behavioral considerations. Monographs of the Society for Research in Child Development, 59*, 167–186.

Robbins, T.W. (1998). Arousal and attention: Psychopharmacological and neurophysiological studies in experimental animals. In R. Parasuraman (Ed.), *The attentive brain* (pp. 189–220). Cambridge, MA: MIT Press.

Ryan, R.M., Kuhl, J., & Deci, E.L. (1997). Nature and autonomy: An organizational view of social and neurobiological aspects of self-regulation in behavior and development. *Development and Psychopathology, 9*, 701–728.

Schore, A.N. (1994). *Affect regulation and the origin of the self: The neurobiology of emotional development.* Hillsdale, NJ: Lawrence Erlbaum Associates.

Schore, A.N. (1996). The experience-dependent maturation of a regulatory system in the orbital prefrontal cortex and the origin of developmental psychopathology. *Development and Psychopathology, 8,* 59–97.

Schore, A.N. (1997). Early organization of the nonlinear right brain and development of a predisposition to psychiatric disorders. *Development and Psychopathology, 9,* 595–631.

Shepherd, G., & Koch, C. (1998). Introduction to synaptic circuits. In G. Shepherd (Ed.), *The synaptic organization of the brain* (pp. 1–36). New York: Oxford University Press.

Siegel, G.J., Agranoff, B.W., Albers, R.W., Fisher, S.K., & Uhler, M.D. (1999). *Basic biochemistry: Molecular, cellular and medical aspects.* Philadelphia: Lippincott, Williams and Wilkins.

Stansbury, K., & Gunnar, M. (1994). Adreno-cortical activity and emotion regulation. *Monographs of the Society for Research in Child Development, 59,* 108–134.

Stifter, C.A., & Jain, A. (1996). Psychophysiologic correlates of infant temperament: Stability of behavior and autonomic patterning from 5 to 18 months. *Developmental Psychobiology, 29,* 321–333.

Thompson, R.A. (1994). Emotion regulation: A theme in search of definition. *The development of emotion regulation: Biological and behavioral considerations. Monographs of the Society for Research in Child Development, 59,* 25–52.

Whatson, T., & Stirling, V. (1998). *Development and flexibility.* New York: Springer-Verlag.

Wolf, S. (1995). Psychosocial forces and neural mechanisms in disease: Defining the question and collecting the evidence. *Integrative Physiological and Behavioral Science, 30,* 85–94.

6

Proprioception:

A Cornerstone of Sensory Integrative Intervention

ERNA IMPERATORE BLANCHE, PH.D., OTR, FAOTA

ROSEANN C. SCHAAF, M.ED., OTR/L, FAOTA

Activities rich in proprioceptive stimuli are an important component of a program using a sensory integrative approach. Recently, there has been an increase in interest in the use of this specific sensory modality for children with a variety of disabilities. The potential benefits and uses of proprioception quickly are becoming part of the mainstream literature (Kranowitz, 1998; Miller, Goldson, & Hanft, 1998). Therapists, teachers, parents, and others frequently discuss proprioception, yet they often misunderstand and misinterpret it. This confusion seems to relate to lack of clarity regarding terminology and definitions as well as to too few controlled studies that investigate the role of proprioceptive stimuli in typical and atypical functioning. This chapter focuses on the use of proprioception in sensory integration theory and practice. Hopefully this information will serve as a foundation for more advanced study and examination of the role of proprioception and how clinicians can use it for children with sensory integrative dysfunction.

When Ayres first discussed proprioception in 1972, she referred to it as "information arising from the body, especially from muscles, joints, ligaments and receptors associated with bones" (Ayres, 1972a, p. 66). She added that proprioceptive information assumed a critical role in sensory integration, influencing motor actions and modulating emotional state (Ayres, 1972a). She viewed proprioceptive flow as exerting excitatory influences on the autonomic nervous system and the cortex that could enhance one's emotional state. In addition, she described sensory impulses arising from the musculoskeletal receptors as "providing an adequate anatomical route for inhibitory influences" (Ayres, 1972a, p. 69). Ayres recognized proprioception as an important component of the sensory integrative process in its contribution to movement, visual form, space perception, and arousal level. Today, the use of proprioception to increase body awareness, improve motor coordination, help modulate arousal level, and aid in the processing of sensation through other sensory systems is a strong and defining feature of the sensory integrative approach.

Seeking to understand the mechanisms that produce the effects observed clinically during activities that increase proprioceptive input raises many questions but provides few answers. The variety of and differences in definitions of proprioception in the literature and the anatomical ambiguity or lack of specific localization of the proprioceptive system create a challenge when trying to determine the effects of proprioception functionally and clinically. The literature examining proprioception often varies in its definitions. Some authors include vestibular elements, others do not; some include joint afferent, kinesthetic, and tactile sensations, and others do not. Authors classify proprioception in different ways, some considering which receptors are triggered or how this sensation is represented and carried in the nervous system (from a neuroanatomical point of view and from a system point of view), and others according to the functions affected by proprioception. Even the sensory integration literature focusing on the effect of sensory experiences on movement and behavior suggests that the differentiation between activities that provide proprioceptive input through self-initiated movement and those that provide vestibular or tactile input needs clarification (Ayres, 1989; Baranek, Foster, & Berkson, 1997; Bowen, Shippa, Tatum, & White, 1999; Fisher, 1991; Ray, King, & Grandin, 1988; Stallings-Sahler, 1998).

This chapter presents a functional view of proprioception as an arousal modulator, a component of motor control, and a major organizer of sensations arising from the body, acknowledging that the anatomic localization (i.e., specific pathways and subcortical and cortical destinations) plays a significant role in dictating function. Proprioceptive activities are a pivotal factor in a therapeutic program of sensory integration because of proprioception's capacity to affect arousal level specifically by calming and organizing an individual who is experiencing overstimulation. It is difficult to separate proprioceptive sensations and consider them in isolation when the various sensory systems work together to provide a significant foundation for moving, interacting, and being. However, focusing specifically on the functions and actions of the proprioceptive system is useful in furthering the understanding of the specific contributions of this sensory system to functional behavior.

The first section of this chapter gives a historical perspective of the pertinent background literature that defines proprioception and its role and functions. A second section presents a typology of proprioceptive dysfunction in an attempt to delineate specific dysfunctions related to the proprioceptive system. The final section discusses the use of proprioception in intervention.

What is Proprioception?

Sir Charles Bell described the sense originating from passive and active movement as the "sixth sense" and defined it as "perceived sensations about the static position or velocity of movement (whether imposed or voluntarily generated) of those parts of the body moved by skeletal muscles, together with perceived sensations about the forces generated during muscular contractions even when such contractions are isometric" (McCloskey, 1988, p. 36). Later authors subsequently referred to these sensations as kinesthetic and proprioceptive senses.

Proprioception Versus Kinesthesia

Sherrington described the proprioceptors as being activated when the organism itself engages in active movement and was careful to differentiate between what he called active movement (i.e., arising from the individual itself) and passive movement (i.e., those resulting from events in the environment) (Evarts, 1981). According to Sherrington (1906), externally produced changes do not affect proprioception in the same way that active movements do. Active movement provides maximal proprioceptive sensation, whereas passive movement provides only minimal use of this sense. This concept of active engagement is important in sensory integration. Active engagement in tasks that provide resistance yields maximal proprioceptive stimulation and has the greatest effect on functional behavior.

Historically, researchers described the proprioceptive system as being subserved by receptors in the muscle spindle and golgi tendon organ, whereas they viewed the receptors in the joint capsule as the source of sensory information leading to conscious awareness or kinesthesia. These early investigators postulated that the muscle spindles were the major contributor to muscle sense and played a role in subconscious motor control (Sherrington, 1906). They viewed kinesthesia as different from unconscious proprioception, believing kinesthetic input to travel via the dorsal column-medial lemniscal system into the somatosensory areas in the cortex. Early research described proprioceptive information, in contrast, as being carried in the spinothalamic system, providing information to the cerebellum. However, some investigators viewed muscle proprioceptive information as subserving kinesthetic sensation and thus generating spatiotemporal maps that are used in the memorization and recognition of motor patterns utilized for coordinated actions (Roll & Gilhodes, 1995; Roll, Gilhodes, Roll, & Velay, 1989). Other literature has suggested that it is impossible to make this clear differentiation because receptors and tracks appear to carry mixed information (Matthews, 1988).

In Ayres' classic text on sensory integration (1972a), the descriptions of proprioception were consistent with the thinking of the time, differentiating proprioception from kinesthesia. She defined kinesthesia as "the conscious awareness of joint position and movement" (Ayres, 1972a, p. 67) contributing to body awareness, visual perception, and praxis: "It is safest to assume that diminished kinesthesis limits the development of visual perception and the body scheme by limiting the amount of information entering the brain during purposeful and manipulative tasks" (Ayres, 1972a, p. 67). In contrast, she saw proprioception as the unconscious sensations arising from muscles, tendons, and bones. She also believed that proprioceptive information arising from the oculomotor muscles contributes to visual perception and fine motor movement (Ayres, 1972a). The tests Ayres developed to evaluate sensory integrative dysfunction laid out her view of proprioception and kinesthesia. In the original *Southern California Sensory Integration Tests* (Ayres, 1972b), as well as the *Sensory Integration and Praxis Tests* (SIPT; Ayres, 1989), Ayres included different subtests that assessed the kinesthetic contributions to movement, motor planning, and the sense of proprioception. Tools for assessing proprioception include the Standing and Walking Balance and Postural Praxis Subtests of the SIPT (Ayres, 1989) and clinical observations.

Since Ayres' time, the literature on proprioception and kinesthesia has suggested that, because the differentiation between these two senses is not functionally accurate, clinicians should consider proprioception and kinesthesia under one sense: proprioception (Fisher, 1991; Fredericks, 1996). Consequently, the term *proprioception* often includes both "active and passive changes in the length and tension of all muscles acting on the moving joint, by distortion of the joint capsule and ligaments, and by deformation of skin. The afferent activity generated by movement comes from all these sources" (Fredericks, p. 102). In this chapter, the word *proprioception* refers to both kinesthesia and proprioception, although the differentiation between conscious and subconscious functions remains.

Proprioceptive Receptors

Different somatosensory receptors contribute differently to the awareness and sense of movement in each joint of the body, depending on the body part required for the action. For example, skin receptors might contribute more significantly to proprioception in small body parts such as the fingers, but the muscle spindle might be the most important proprioceptive receptor in larger body parts such as the knee (Fredericks, 1996). The literature in motor learning and motor control suggests that the efference copy and corollary discharge generated during centrally programmed movements and influenced by central mechanisms contribute to the sense of proprioception (LaRue et al., 1995; Matthews, 1988).

Proprioceptive Integration

Processing of proprioception occurs in at least three different areas in the central nervous system (CNS)—the spinal level, the cerebellum, and the somatosensory cortex—each potentially contributing differently to function. At the spinal level, proprioception detects changes in the length and tension of the muscle and provides a constant stream of information to the cerebellum via the spinocerebellar tracks. At the level of the cerebellum, this information integrates with vestibular information and contributes to postural control and a sense of gravity. Cerebellar-vestibular connections might also be involved in the observed modulating effect of proprioceptive input on vestibular input.

Proprioceptive-Tactile Integration

At the level of the somatosensory cortex, the proprioceptive information is integrated with the tactile system via the dorsal column-medial lemniscal pathway. This pathway carries information to the somatosensory cortex, where it enables primarily discrimination of touch and proprioception. This somatosensory information also might contribute to the planning and execution of refined movements. Wing, Haggard, and Flanagan (1996) have described the regulatory effects of movement and, therefore, proprioception over the tactile system at this level of the CNS.

Because the proprioceptive system often works together with touch and/or movement and gravity, discussions of proprioception often include the tactile and vestibular systems. Although they function together in behavior, it is helpful to clarify their unique contributions. The tactile system provides information about the external environment (exteroception) rather than information about the body per se. Additionally, tactile receptors respond to contact that occurs passively on the external surface of the body (i.e., the skin), whereas proprioceptive receptors respond to a muscle contraction or a joint movement.

Although touch is not truly a proprioceptor, the tactile system does function closely with the proprioceptive system to provide important information about the body. As a result, clinicians often group touch with proprioception and refer to touch, proprioception, and kinesthesia as a somatosense (body sense); however, grouping touch with proprioception has created some confusion in intervention. For example, therapists have used the term *proprioceptive activities* to describe activities that provide deep touch-pressure, such as pretending to make a sandwich by wedging the child between two mattresses, or using a stretchy pressure garment during functional tasks. In reality, these activities provide tactile input in the form of touch pressure to the skin and should be distinguished from proprioceptive-based activities during which the child is *actively resisting* the pillows to move out of a position or pushing against an elastic-fabric swing or tunnel while moving.

Proprioceptive-Vestibular Integration

It is important to distinguish the proprioceptive system from the vestibular system. The vestibular system provides information about movement of the head through space and the body's orientation in reference to gravity. As such, proprioception functions with the vestibular and visual systems in the acquisition of postural control, oculomotor control, and feedforward required to anticipate actions in time and space (Fisher, 1991; Shumway-Cook & Woollacott, 1995). It is important to recognize that there are some activities that produce both vestibular and proprioceptive experiences, and other activities that afford the opportunity for increasing either proprioception or vestibular input. For example, jumping on a trampoline and running produce both types of input; however, swinging in a supported position provides primarily vestibular input, and pushing, biting, and clenching supply primarily proprioceptive input.

Finally, although it is possible to delineate proprioception in terms of its receptors, pathways, and function, it is important not to lose sight of the fact that during daily activity, the individual is receiving, integrating, and utilizing a multitude of sensory inputs from a variety of sources using multiple receptors. It is the ability to integrate and utilize this multisensory information for the purpose of engaging in meaningful occupation that is the central focus of therapy using a sensory integration approach.

An Emerging View of Proprioception: Discriminative and Modulatory Functions

The information presented in the previous section lays a foundation for the proposed functional account of the proprioceptive system. This functional view considers the contribution of the proprioceptive system to movement and behavior, specifically to the overall arousal state and emotional tone, the organization of body awareness, and body scheme, and views proprioception as a basis for the physical sense of self and its interactions with the external world. Similar to other sensory systems, proprioceptive sensations can serve both modulatory and discriminatory functions.

The Modulating Role of Proprioception

In terms of the modulating or regulatory role of proprioception, anecdotal evidence suggests that proprioception exerts a regulatory influence over other sensory systems, including the vestibular and tactile systems, as well as a regulatory influence on arousal level in general. Regarding vestibular sensation, proprioception most likely helps regulate overresponsivity to movement. The modulating effects of proprioception on the tactile system might help to decrease overresponsivity to touch and maintain an optimal level of arousal (Koomar, Szklut, & Cermak, 1998; Kranowitz, 1998). The modulating influence of proprioception over other senses appears to occur at the level of the cerebellum, thalamus, and somatosensory cortex (Wing et al., 1996).

Discriminative Proprioception

The discriminative function of the proprioceptive system manifests itself in the calibration of movement in space and time. For example, a person threading a needle matches discrete proprioceptive, tactile, and visual stimuli to coordinate the necessary movements. The discriminative aspect of proprioception functions with the visual and tactile systems to produce the coordinated movement. Discriminative proprioception works closely with the tactile system as a basis for body scheme and somatopraxis (Ayres, 1972a, 1989). Ayres (1989) addressed the interaction between these systems when she coined the term *somatodyspraxia,* a disorder in which children exhibit decreased scores in two tests assessing aspects of proprioception, the Kinesthesia and Standing and Walking Balance subtests of the SIPT. Because the Kinesthesia subtest assesses tactile and kinesthetic processing, somatodyspraxia is a dysfunction in the discrimination of tactile sensation *and* proprioception. In addition to contributing to praxis, the discriminative aspects of proprioception play an important role in timing motor actions, providing a spatiotemporal frame of reference, and assisting in the perception of weight (Roll & Gilhodes, 1995; Roll et al., 1989; LaRue et al., 1995). Children with coordination disorders as well as those with sensory integrative disorders might have impairments in these discriminative aspects of proprioception (Hoare & Larkin, 1991; Laszlo, 1998).

The ability to discriminate vestibular-proprioceptive information might also contribute to awareness of the person's relationship to gravity, postural control, and the ability to execute projected action sequences (Fisher, 1991). This discriminative aspect of proprioception is the basis for discrete functions required for postural control, motor coordination, and motor planning. In addition, the proprioceptive system also might be responsible for the perception of speed, duration, and direction of movement (Roll et al., 1989) and thereby contribute to the ability to project actions in time and space (Fisher, 1991).

The modulating and discriminatory functions of the proprioceptive-vestibular and proprioceptive-tactile systems function together and provide an important foundation for sensory integration. For example, during performance of a skilled action such as a sports activity, the discriminative aspects of the proprioceptive system work with the regulatory functions to allow for the superimposition of coordinated movement on body awareness, a safe relationship with gravity, and postural control. Although these systems are indistinguishable in the individual with adequate sensory integration, a variety of difficulties can result when these systems are not functioning adequately, which the following section describes.

A New Framework for Understanding Proprioceptive Dysfunction

The existing literature does not provide an adequate description of disorders in the proprioceptive system. Luria (1973), Sacks (1985), Ayres (1972a), and Laszlo (1998; Laszlo, Bairstow, & Bartrip, 1988) are some of the few authors who have addressed these disorders. Luria described "postural apraxias" or "afferent kinesthetic apraxia" as a type of praxis deficit in which the individual loses the afferent basis of movement and cannot perform properly differentiated hand movements. Luria postulated that these disorders result from a lesion of the secondary zones of the postcentral cortex, and such individuals exhibit poor adaptation to the somatosensory characteristics of an object. Sacks described a woman who lost her sense of proprioception and, with that, her body awareness and safe relationship to gravity. Ayres (1972a) proposed that proprioception and kinesthesia influence muscle tone, the excitatory state of the individual, visual perception of space, and motor planning. In addition, she held that proprioception contributes to postural control and the sense of gravity (Ayres, 1972a).

From Ayres' suggestions, then, researchers have surmised that proprioceptive dysfunction might manifest in one or all of these areas. Consequently, clinicians assume that activities rich in proprioception enhance muscle tone, arousal level, visual perception of space, motor planning, postural control, and awareness of gravity. Clinically, children who seek muscle and tendon sensation (proprioception) and deep pressure through resistive active movement probably are demonstrating a specific type of proprioceptive dysfunction called proprioceptive seeking, whereas other children display a lack of awareness of the proprioceptive sense (Dunn, 1997).

Dunn (1997) and Blanche (1999) have expanded this dichotomous classification of proprioceptive dysfunction to include the different patterns of proprioceptive dysfunction that can coexist in one child. These patterns include hyporesponsivity to proprioceptive input, seeking of proprioceptive input, and proprioceptive sensitivity. In addition, researchers have described gravitational insecurity (GI) as a multisensory processing deficit that also includes some aspects of poor proprioceptive processing (Fisher, 1991). This typology provides a framework for assessing the proprioceptive system and the functional limitations that can result, and for making clinical judgments regarding the presence or absence of a dysfunction in the proprioceptive system.

Hyporesponsivity to Proprioceptive Input

Children who are hyporesponsive to proprioceptive stimuli demonstrate poor awareness and discrimination of proprioception and consequently have a poor ability to use proprioceptive input for adaptive behavior (see Table 6.1). These children exhibit some or all of the following signs: break toys easily and appear clumsy, exhibit low (functional) postural tone, and demonstrate tactile discrimination deficits. They enjoy proprioception when it is available, such as engaging in a tug-of-war with the therapist or another child. They also tend to tighten up or "fix" to provide themselves with the necessary input and to increase proximal stability for distal movement.

It is interesting to note that some children might be hyporesponsive not only to proprioceptive stimuli but also to other stimuli as well, showing a partial or total profile of hyporesponsivity to sensory input (Dunn & Westman, 1997; see also chapter 4 of this text, An Ecological Model of Sensory Modulation: Performance of Children With Fragile X Syndrome, Autistic Disorder, Attention-Deficit/Hyperactivity Disorder, and Sensory Modulation Disorder, by Miller, Reisman, McIntosh, & Simon). Typically, poor proprioceptive awareness coexists with poor tactile discrimination and might be

Table 6.1. Typology of deficits associated with the proprioceptive system

---

Hyporesponsivity or poor discrimination of proprioceptive input
- Breaks toys easily
- Exhibits low (functional) muscle tone
- May exhibit hyporesponsivity to touch
- May tighten up or "fix"

Seeks proprioceptive input to modulate state of arousal
- Exhibits sensory modulation deficits in other systems (tactile, vestibular), seeks large amounts of proprioceptive input to help modulate other sensory systems
- Bites, pushes, hits, scratches, bumps, hurls, bangs
- Behaviors can appear or be labeled "aggressive"
- Moves fast, can appear clumsy
- Likes chewy and hard foods
- Can exhibit self-stimulatory (banging head, biting hands, etc.), hyperactive, and/or unsafe behaviors

Gravitational insecurity, vestibular-proprioceptive disorder
- Becomes anxious when the relationship to gravity is challenged
- Moves slowly and carefully
- Becomes anxious when feet are off the ground
- Becomes anxious with objects approaching

Proprioceptive sensitivity
- Cries in weight-bearing positions
- Cries when joints are moved
- Is unable to move or chooses not to move
- Often present in children with greater degrees of physical involvement

---

implicated in somatodyspraxia (Ayres, 1989) as well as the "postural apraxias" or "afferent kinesthetic apraxia" as described by Luria (1973).

It is also important to distinguish proprioceptive hyporesponsivity from proprioceptive seeking. Although both groups of children might seek out and enjoy proprioceptive stimuli behaviorally (Dunn & Westman, 1997), those with hyporesponsivity present with poor praxis and are less physically active in providing themselves with the necessary proprioceptive input. Studies of children with coordination disorders reveal that some of these deficits might relate to proprioceptive or kinesthetic deficits (LaRue et al., 1995; Laszlo, 1998; Laufer & Hocherman, 1998; Lord & Hulme, 1987).

Intervention for children who are hyporesponsive to proprioception should incorporate appropriate organizing activities that are rich in proprioceptive feedback and that generate an adaptive response. Such activities are key to using the proprioceptive system to enhance arousal level, improve body awareness, and facilitate praxis (see Table 6.1).

Proprioceptive Seeking

Children who actively seek proprioception often engage overactively in behaviors that provide significant proprioceptive input. Clinicians have interpreted this behavior as an attempt to gain proprioceptive input to help modulate arousal level and responsiveness to sensory input in other systems, primarily the tactile and vestibular systems (Kranowitz, 1998; Koomar et al., 1998). These disorders are similar to Ayres' (1972a) description of the proprioceptive system as a modulator of the excitatory state. The sensory integration literature has given this aspect of proprioception an increasing amount of emphasis over the last 10 years (Dunn & Westman, 1997; Royeen & Lane, 1991; see also chapter 4 of this text).

Children in this group are very active in their search for proprioceptive input and often appear hyperactive and unsafe. For example, they might run quickly and crash repeatedly into the matted walls of the school gymnasium. Their unsafe actions, however, seem to relate to an active search for input, not poor coordination. Children who are seeking proprioceptive input often seek it in ways that others perceive as inappropriate and sometimes label as "aggressive." For example, these children provide themselves with proprioception by chewing on nonfood or hard food items, biting, pushing, hitting, scratching, bumping, hurling, and banging. They sometimes exhibit behaviors labeled as "self-stimulatory" (banging head, biting hands, etc.). In addition, although they can exhibit adequate control over their movements when they are functioning at their optimal level of arousal, they still appear clumsy in many instances when increasing the speed of their actions due to overstimulation.

Finally, seeking of proprioceptive input can be a manifestation of a larger sensory modulation dysfunction. Such children who seek proprioceptive input often present with sensory modulation deficits in other sensory systems (such as the tactile and vestibular systems) as well (see Table 6.1).

Gravitational Insecurity

The literature describes gravitational insecurity (GI) as a disorder in the vestibular system, specifically inadequate sensory processing of gravity, although studies also have implicated poor processing of proprioception and visual perception of space (Ayres, 1972a; Weisburg, 1984). Behaviorally, the individual with GI becomes anxious when his or her relationship to gravity changes, such as when the feet are not on the ground and the person loses his or her reference point for the relationship of his or her body to gravity.

The child with GI often utilizes the proprioceptive sense to help modulate visual and vestibular information. As a result, the child becomes anxious when not receiving adequate amounts of proprioceptive input through weight bearing, such as when feet are off the ground. The child tends to move carefully, negotiating changes in the supporting surface with difficulty. Activities rich in propriopception can help the child with gravitational insecurity modulate the vestibular system and also reinforce body awareness, thereby increasing the child's comfort with position changes.

Proprioceptive Sensitivity

Children with proprioceptive sensitivity are hyperresponsive to proprioceptive stimuli and often demonstrate anxiety and irritability in response to it (Blanche, 1999). Some of the signs presented by this group of children include anxiety and discomfort when their joints are moved passively, discomfort when placed in weight-bearing positions, and a calming response to vestibular input as long as it is provided by holding the child in a static position. Children who are hypersensitive to proprioceptive input can exhibit postural control problems; however, therapists cannot address the postural control problems because of the anxiety these children experience as a result of imposed movement of body parts.

Clinical experience suggests that children presenting with this type of modulation disorder are often very young and have been found to have seizure disorders or severe forms of developmental disorders. More typically, children with proprioceptive sensitivity become distressed when their limbs are moved passively. Children with GI, in contrast, react when they are high above the ground or when their feet do not touch the ground, but they tolerate passive movement of the extremities and are often able to move actively. A reasonable question is whether these children are hypersensitive to proprioceptive input, or exhibit a form of gravitational insecurity (Blanche, 1999) (see Table 6.1).

Postural Insecurity?

Ayres described gravitational insecurity and postural insecurity as having similar characteristics. She held that GI encompassed a modulation disorder in the vestibular, proprioceptive, and visual systems, whereas postural insecurity was a disorder manifesting in the inability to maintain a stable posture against gravity or insecurity arising from the postural deficits (Ayres, personal communication, 1985). At the time of her death, research had not clearly established this differentiation. Was proprioceptive sensitivity the behavior Ayres was describing when she originally referred to postural insecurity as different from gravitational insecurity?

In children with developmental disabilities who often exhibit additional postural control deficits having a neuromotor base, the differentiation between postural control difficulties (often referred to as postural insecurity) and sensory modulation deficits (such as gravitational insecurity) is pivotal because intervention strategies for each differ greatly. Whereas facilitation is effective in addressing postural control deficits, children with GI respond negatively to this challenge to their center of gravity (Blanche, 1999; Blanche, Botticelli, & Hallway, 1995). In addition, it is important to differentiate postural control deficits and GI from proprioceptive hypersensitivity and hypersensitivity to movement. Therapists can make this distinction by assessing the child's comfort with changes relative to gravity when the child's posture is properly secure.

The Use of Proprioception in Intervention

Activities rich in proprioception are a key element in sensory integration intervention. Although other intervention approaches recommend activities that provide much proprioceptive input, the focus of intervention and the clinical reasoning process the therapist uses are markedly different from those of sensory integration. For example, the neurodevelopmental treatment approach (NDT), myofascial release, and other neuromotor techniques use resistive exercises, weight bearing, approximation, elongation, and traction.

Most of these approaches utilize the sensory input to influence motor performance. In contrast, sensory integration intervention uses proprioceptive input primarily to affect the arousal level, to increase body awareness, to modulate vestibular and tactile input, and to increase the feedback that a child receives from a motor response. With the sensory integration perspective, the child procures proprioception through self-initiated movements whenever possible, rather than through positioning or externally applied forces. For example, the therapist might ask the child to push, carry, or pull heavy loads, thus increasing resistance and maximizing proprioceptive sensation. Intervention strategies not based on sensory integration provide passive proprioceptive input through weight-bearing positions, or by stretching, elongating, or providing traction to the person's body (Bobath, 1984; Boehme, 1988). In sensory integration intervention, a therapist utilizes proprioceptive input to help modulate the level of arousal and to enhance motor planning, whereas traditional neuromotor approaches use proprioceptive input to affect reflexes and automatic postural reactions.

The use of proprioception is a significant component of sensory integration intervention, but in a different way from neuromotor approaches. The following three points summarize proprioception's importance:

- Proprioception functions primarily as an organizer of the person or the self, allowing the child to experience the sensations while maintaining an adequate arousal level.

- Proprioception integrates interoception with exteroception, and this bridge plays a major role in the acquisition of body awareness, praxis or motor planning, and a sense of self (Sacks, 1985).

- Proprioception is an integral component of self-initiated actions, providing a sense of the body upon which movement is superimposed.

Assessing the Child's Specific Needs for Proprioceptive Input

Frequently clinicians are unclear about when, how, and why to use activities rich in proprioception. The following questions can help guide the clinical reasoning process and clarify the use of proprioception in the assessment and intervention process. Keep in mind that the use of proprioception as part of the sensory integrative approach is a complex and multifaceted issue.

- What types of difficulties is the child experiencing in his or her daily occupations, and how do these difficulties relate to poor body awareness, arousal level, and motor planning that might be due to proprioceptive dysfunction?

- If the child is seeking input, what type of input is the child seeking, and why?

- If the child is having difficulty processing information through other sensory channels, what types of proprioception might be useful in helping the child organize actions in the environment?

- Does the child have problems in the modulation or discrimination of proprioceptive input?

Answering these questions will help to identify patterns of dysfunction and aid in choosing the most appropriate intervention.

What types of difficulties is the child experiencing in his or her daily occupations?

Being aware of the reason for referral or the difficulties the child is having in the performance of daily occupations provides important information about how sensory integrative problems might be influencing the child's behavior. Deficits in proprioception might affect the child's motor coordination and/or the child's ability to regulate his or her own behavior. If the child exhibits difficulties in motor coordination affecting such areas as handwriting and sports, the therapist needs to investigate the discriminative aspects of proprioception. If the child is seeking large amounts of input through what might be viewed as maladaptive behaviors (biting, pinching, hitting, or rough play), then it is important to assess the child's ability to modulate input so as to plan intervention accordingly. For example, if the child has difficulty with handwriting because of decreased proprioceptive sensation, then the therapist can gear intervention to increase that input. If the child is having difficulty sleeping because of an inability to modulate the level of arousal, proprioceptive activities might be useful to help the child attain and maintain a more regulated state. Another example is the child who is tactually hypersensitive and, as a result, has difficulty managing a variety of foods orally. In this case, the therapist can use proprioception to help the child modulate tactile input and thereby decrease sensitivity to allow for acceptance of a greater variety of foods.

If the child is seeking input, what type of input is the child seeking, and why?

Children with SI dysfunctions often seek different types of proprioceptive input and for different reasons (Dunn, 1997). Consequently, it is important to consider both the **intensity** and **type** of proprioceptive stimuli the child is seeking. For example, some children seek input to joint receptors through traction, and others seek input to muscle receptors through active coactivation. Likewise, intervention needs to address the child's specific sensory needs in both intensity and type.

Intensity refers to the amount of input the activity offers. For example, crashing provides more intense input than leaning on the caregiver, and jumping on a trampoline produces more intensity of input than standing.

Type of proprioceptive input refers to the specific activities the child is seeking. Behaviors such as crashing, bumping, and leaning suggest a need for a combination of deep pressure (tactile) and proprioception, whereas behaviors such as biting, holding, and pinching suggest that the child has a need for primarily muscle, joint, and tendon input (Koomar et al., 1998; Kranowitz, 1998). Behaviors such as running/crashing and jumping suggest a need for a combination of vestibular and proprioceptive input.

Other types of input include the use of compression and traction. Compression occurs in jumping, weight bearing, and pushing. The child experiences traction when being pulled while holding onto a rope or when hanging on a trapeze. In this latter example, the child is co-contracting the musculature in the hands and fingers and gaining traction of the shoulders and elbows. In this case, the child will most probably have to co-contract to stabilize the trunk.

Finally, although the therapist might interpret the child's behavioral displays as sensation seeking from a sensory integrative perspective, it is equally important to consider other explanations of the child's behavior. From a behavioral perspective, for example, the observed behavior of running and crashing might be a learned attention-seeking behavior, or it might be a symptom of hyperactivity. Although it is tempting to interpret behaviors from only one perspective, the therapist must always consider other potential explanations as well.

If the child is having difficulty processing information through other sensory channels, how might proprioception be useful in helping the child organize actions in the environment?

Understanding how the child processes information through other sensory channels provides a basis for determining how to use proprioception in that child's intervention. If the child does not exhibit modulation deficits in other sensory systems, then the child's searching for proprioceptive input suggests poor registration, a decreased response, or hyperresponsivity to proprioceptive input. It is then important to relate this search for input with the functional deficit and shape intervention accordingly. For example, if the child exhibits poor modulation in other systems, it will be important to pair activities rich in proprioception with an adaptive response that includes maintenance of the optimal level of arousal in spite of the existence of a variety of sensory experiences. On the other hand, if the child's functional disorder includes poor motor planning, the therapist will need to pair the proprioceptive input with an adaptive response that includes activities requiring coordinated actions. In addition, it is important to understand the interaction of proprioception with other sensory systems such as vestibular processing or tactile processing.

Proprioception as an organizer is often the source of confusion in sensory integration intervention. For example, therapists sometimes use a weighted vest to treat children who are in need of deep pressure and/or proprioception. However, rather than use the vest indiscriminately, clinicians must examine the type of input that the weighted vest provides and the type of disorders that respond to the child's wearing it. If the child exhibits a decreased response to proprioceptive input and decreased postural tone, the therapist should carefully examine the implications of vest use because of the impact of the increased weight on postural control. The choice to use a weighted vest depends on each child's functional difficulties, the core sensory processing issues, and the child's individual response to the input provided by the vest. When a therapist prescribes a weighted vest, it is important to consider carefully the ultimate goal of its use (modulation, increased postural tone, increased body awareness) as well as define the expected behavior or goal of its use. In addition, the therapist will need to continually monitor the child's response to wearing the vest and make adjustments as needed.

Does the child have problems in the modulation or discrimination of proprioceptive input?

This question requires thorough investigation of the child's movements and behavior and includes consideration of the issues mentioned in the three preceding questions. This careful analysis yields information about whether there is a modulation deficit, a discrimination deficit, or some combination of both. The need for proprioception as a modulator often accompanies an arousal or regulatory disorder, whereas the need for proprioception to assist with discrimination often but not always accompanies hyporesponsivity in other sensory systems as well. The typology proposed above provides a mechanism for identifying proprioceptive disorders and distinguishing modulation from proprioceptive disorders.

Using This Information to Help the Child Organize Actions in the Environment

When considering why the child is seeking or resisting increased amounts of proprioception and how intervention will address the child's difficulties, it is important to keep in mind the nature of the functional difficulties uncovered in pursuing answers to the first question. For example, the child might be seeking proprioceptive input because of its calming effect. The child might bite, crash, and hit in an attempt to modulate his or her response to sensory input through other systems. In this case, activities rich in proprioception coupled with an adaptive response that includes modulation of the arousal level (which then decreases disruptive behaviors) would be useful (Koomar et al., 1998; Kranowitz, 1998; Linderman & Stewart, 1999; Williams & Shellenberger, 1996). In contrast, the child with poor body awareness and motor planning might require intense proprioceptive stimulation from activities that are alerting and facilitory and that couple with adaptive responses that challenge motor planning, such as jumping on a trampoline while assuming simple body positions and postures. Finally, the child who is overly sensitive to proprioceptive sensation might avoid movement and need to have opportunities for safe activities of limited intensity and duration, such as crawling up an inclined ramp. Refer to Table 6.2 for intervention suggestions. In all cases, safety is of primary importance, as is the need to create opportunities for adaptive responses grounded in meaningful and motivating activities.

Table 6.2. Specific Suggestions for Activities That Offer Opportunities for Enhancing Proprioceptive Input

- Use weights during activities: a weighted jacket, bean bags of different weights.
- When you need to move equipment, use the opportunity and ask the child to help with the pushing, pulling, and lifting.
- Encourage proprioceptive input through co-contraction: wheelbarrow walking, lying quadruped, or participating in activities while prone on elbows. Make sure that the child uses active proximal joint stability.
- Facilitate weight shifts when in weight bearing to activate the muscles.
- Have the child push and pull you or another adult who is sitting on a scooter board or swing.
- Play tug-of-war.
- Play "push-of-war" in which the child, in various weight-bearing positions, pushes a large therapy ball to other children in a game aimed at keeping the ball within the circle of children.
- Use a trapeze or large hoop to pull the child when he or she is on a scooter board. Encourage elbow flexion during the activity to make sure that the child is pulling actively.
- To enhance proprioception in the hands, provide play dough that offers high resistance. Therapy putty can be helpful.
- When the child is riding a moving piece of equipment, provide uneven vestibular stimulation (e.g., jerky, bumpy road) so that the child needs to use proximal joint stability.
- To provide proprioceptive and tactile input, use inner tubes as "bumper cars," or roll the child inside a stack of inner tubes.
- Have climbing equipment that children can use (e.g., steep, soft ramp leaned against the wall; ropes; ladders).

Summary

This chapter has attempted to bring to the literature a topic that professionals have discussed anecdotally in sensory integration theory and intervention principles. The chapter presents four patterns of dysfunction in the proprioceptive system to summarize and categorize the clusters of symptoms that frequently appear together and are related to the proprioceptive system. The proposed typologies provide a foundation for continued exploration of the contributions of proprioception to functional behavior, to behavioral dysfunction related to the proprioceptive system, and to intervention strategies that utilize proprioception and treat proprioceptive dysfunction. The authors intend this chapter to serve only as a beginning of the discussion.

Works Cited

References

Ayres, A.J. (1972a). *Sensory integration and learning disorders*. Los Angeles: Western Psychological Services.

Ayres, A.J. (1972b). *Southern California Sensory Integration Tests*. Los Angeles: Western Psychological Services.

Ayres, A.J. (1989). *Sensory Integration and Praxis Tests*. Los Angeles: Western Psychological Services.

Baranek, G.T., Foster, L.G., & Berkson, G. (1997). Tactile defensiveness and stereotyped behaviors. *American Journal of Occupational Therapy, 51*, 91–95.

Blanche, E.I. (1999). *The somatosensory system*. Western Psychological Services, University of Southern California. Unpublished lecture notes.

Blanche, E.I., Botticelli, T.M., & Hallway, M.K. (1995). *Combining neuro-developmental treatment and sensory integration principles: An approach to pediatric therapy*. Tucson, AZ: Therapy Skill Builders.

Bobath, B. (1984). The neuro-developmental treatment. In D. Scutton (Ed.), *Management of the motor disorders of children with cerebral palsy* (pp. 6–18). London: Spastics International Medical Publications.

Boehme, R. (1988). *Improving upper extremity function: An approach to assessment and treatment of tonal dysfunction*. San Antonio, TX: Therapy Skill Builders.

Bowen, M., Shippa, J., Tatum, L., & White, J. (1999). Weighted vests: School-based occupational therapy practitioners provide insight on utilization. Unpublished study completed at Shenandoah University's Program in Occupational Therapy, May 1999, under the guidance of Barbara Chandler and Yvonne Teske.

Dunn, W. (1997). The impact of sensory processing abilities on the daily lives of young children and their families: A conceptual model. *Infants and Young Children, 9*, 23–35.

Dunn, W., & Westman, K. (1997). The Sensory Profile: The performance of a national sample of children without disabilities. *American Journal of Occupational Therapy, 51*(1), 25–34.

Evarts, E. (1981). Sherrington's concept of proprioception. *Trends in Neuroscience*, 44–46.

Fisher, A. (1991). Vestibular-proprioceptive processing and bilateral integration and sequencing deficits. In A. Fisher, E. Murray, & A. Bundy (Eds.), *Sensory integration: Theory and practice* (pp. 69–104). Philadelphia: F.A. Davis.

Fredericks, C. (1996). Basic sensory mechanisms and the somatosensory system. In C. Fredericks & L. Saladin (Eds.), *Pathophysiology of the motor system* (pp. 78–104). Philadelphia: F.A. Davis Company.

Hoare, D., & Larkin, D. (1991). Kinaesthetic abilities of clumsy children. *Developmental Medicine and Child Neurology, 33,* 671–678.

Koomar, J., Szklut, S., & Cermak, S. (1998). *Making sense of sensory integration* (Cassette Recording No. BCIS2). Boulder, CO: Bell Curve Records, Inc.

Kranowitz, C.A. (1998). The out-of-sync child: Recognizing and coping with sensory integrative dysfunction. New York: The Berkley Publishing Group.

LaRue, J., Bard, C., Fleury, M., Teasdale, N., Paillard, J., Forget, R., & Lamarre, Y. (1995). Is proprioception important for the timing of motor activities? *Canadian Journal of Physiological Pharmacology, 73,* 255–261.

Laszlo, J. (1998). Letter to the editor. *Developmental Medicine and Child Neurology, 40,* 70–71.

Laszlo, J., Bairstow, P.J., & Bartrip, J. (1988). Clumsiness or perceptuo-motor dysfunction? In A.M. Colley & J.R. Beech (Eds), *Cognition and action in skilled behavior* (pp. 293–309). North-Holland: Elsevier Science Publisher.

Laufer, Y., & Hocherman, S. (1998). Visual and kinesthetic control of goal-directed movements to visually and kinesthetically presented targets. *Perceptual and Motor Skills, 86*(3 Pt 2), 1375–1391.

Linderman, T.M., & Stewart, K.B. (1999). Sensory integrative-based occupational therapy and functional outcomes in young children with PDD: A single subject study. *American Journal of Occupational Therapy, 53,* 208–213.

Lord, R., & Hulme, C. (1987). Kinesthetic sensitivity of normal and clumsy children. *Developmental Medicine and Child Neurology, 29,* 720–725.

Luria, A.R. (1973). *The working brain—An introduction to neuropsychology.* London: Penguin Books.

Matthews, P. (1988). Proprioceptors and their contribution to somatosensory mapping: Complex messages require complex processing. *Canadian Journal of Physiological Pharmacology, 66,* 430–438.

McCloskey, D.I. (1988). Kinesthesia, kinesthetic perception (pp. 36–38). In J. Wolfe (Ed.), *Sensory systems II: Senses other than vision.* Boston: Birkhauser.

Miller, L.J., Goldson, E., & Hanft, B. (1998). *SI network: Sensory integration resource center* [On-line]. Littleton, CO: The KID Foundation. Available: http://www.sinetwork.org/

Ray, T., King, L., & Grandin, T. (1988). The effectiveness of self-initiated vestibular stimulation in producing speech sounds in an autistic child. *Occupational Therapy Journal of Research, 8*(3), 186–190.

Roll, J.P., & Gilhodes, J.C. (1995). Proprioceptive sensory codes mediating movement trajectory perception: Human hand vibration-induced drawing illusions. *Canadian Journal of Physiological Pharmacology, 73,* 295–304.

Roll, J.P., Gilhodes, J.C., Roll, R., & Velay, J.L. (1989). Contribution of skeletal and extraocular proprioception to kinaesthetic representation. In M. Jeannerod (Ed.), *Attention and performance* (pp. 549–566). Hillsdale: Lawrence Erlbaum Associates.

Royeen, C.B., & Lane, S.J. (1991). Tactile processing and sensory defensiveness. In A.G. Fisher, E.A. Murray, & A.C. Bundy (Eds.), *Sensory integration: Theory and practice* (pp. 108–136). Philadelphia: F.A. Davis.

Sacks, O. (1985). The disembodied lady. In O. Sacks (Ed.), *The man who mistook his wife for a hat.* New York: Harper Collins.

Sherrington, C.S. (1906). *The integrative action of the nervous system.* New Haven: Yale University Press.

Shumway-Cook, A., & Woollacott, M. (1995). *Motor control: Theory and practical applications.* Baltimore: Williams and Wilkins.

Stallings-Sahler, S. (1998). Sensory integration assessment and intervention with infants. In J. Case-Smith (Ed.), *Pediatric occupational therapy and early intervention* (2nd ed., pp. 223–254). Boston: Butterworth-Heinemann.

Weisburg, M.A. (1984). The role of psychophysiology in defining gravitational insecurity: A pilot study. *Sensory Integration Special Interest Section Newsletter 7,* 1–4.

Williams, M.S., & Shellenberger, S. (1996). *How does your engine run? A leader's guide to the Alert program for self-regulation.* Albuquerque, NM: Therapy Works.

Wing, A., Haggard, P., & Flanagan, J. (1996). Role of primary somatosensory cortex in active and passive touch. In A.M. Wing, P. Haggard, & J.R. Flanagan (Eds.), *Hand and brain: The neurophysiology and psychology of hand movements* (pp. 329–347). San Diego, CA: Academic Press.

Additional Readings

Anderson, E., & Emmys, P. (1996). *Unlocking the mysteries of sensory dysfunction.* Arlington, TX: Future Horizons, Inc.

Ayres, A.J. (1971). Characteristics of types of sensory integrative dysfunction. *American Journal of Occupational Therapy, 7,* 329–334.

Bard, C., Fleury, M., Teasdale, N., Paillard, J., & Nougier, V. (1995). Contribution of proprioception for calibrating and updating the motor space. *Canadian Journal of Physiological Pharmacology, 73,* 246–254.

Case-Smith, J. (1991). The effects of tactile defensiveness and tactile discrimination on in-hand manipulation. *American Journal of Occupational Therapy, 45,* 811–818.

Cordo, P. (1995). Proprioceptive coordination of discrete movement sequences. *Canadian Journal of Physiological Pharmacology, 73,* 305–316.

Edelson, S.M., Edelson, G.M., Kerr, D.C.R., & Grandin, T. (1999). Behavioral and physiological effect of deep pressure on children with autism: A pilot study evaluating the efficacy of Grandin's Hug Machine. *American Journal of Occupational Therapy, 53,* 145–152.

Fleury, M., Bard, C., Teasdale, N., Paillard, J., Bole, J., Lojoie, Y., & Lamarre, Y. (1995). Weight judgment: The discrimination capacity of a deafferented subject. *Brain, 118,* 1149–1156.

Ghez, C., & Sainburg, R. (1995). Proprioceptive control of interjoint coordination. *Canadian Journal of Physiological Pharmacology, 73,* 273–284.

Henderson, A., & Duncombe, L. (1982). Development of kinesthetic judgments of angle and distance. *Occupational Therapy Journal of Research, 2,* 131–144.

Jones, L. (1988). Motor illusions: What do they reveal about proprioception? *Psychological Bulletin, 103,* 72–86.

Matthews, P. (1998). Muscle sense. In J. Wolfe (Ed.), *Sensory systems II: Senses other than vision* (pp. 54–55). Boston: Birkhauser.

McCloskey, D.I., Cross, M.J., Honner, R., & Potter, E.K.. (1983). Sensory effects of pulling or vibrating exposed tendon in man. *Brain, 106,* 21–37.

Minami, T., & Matsui, A. (1998). Interactions: Timing and force control of finger-tapping sequence. *Perceptual and Motor Skills, 86,* 1395–1401.

Sanes, J.N., & Shadmehr, R. (1995). Sense of muscular effort and somesthetic afferent information in humans. *Canadian Journal of Physiological Pharmacology, 73,* 223–233.

Stuart, D. (1988). Muscle receptors, mammalian. In J. Wolfe (Ed.), *Sensory systems II: Senses other than vision* (pp. 51–52). Boston: Birkhauser.

Tracey, D.J. (1985). Joint receptors and the control of movement. In E.V. Evarts, S.P. Wise, & B. Bousfield (Eds.), *The motor system in neurobiology* (pp. 178–182). New York: Raven.

Van der Meulen, J.H.P., van der Gon, J.J.D., Gielen, C.C.A.M., Gooskens, R.H.J.M., & Willemse, J. (1991). Visuomotor performance of normal and clumsy children, I. *Developmental Medicine and Child Neurology, 33,* 40–54.

Van der Meulen, J.H.P., van der Gon, J.J.D., Gielen, C.C.A.M., Gooskens, R.H.J.M., & Willemse, J. (1991). Visuomotor performance of normal and clumsy children, II. *Developmental Medicine and Child Neurology, 33,* 118–129.

Vargas, S., & Camilli, G. (1999). A meta-analysis of research on sensory integration treatment. *American Journal of Occupational Therapy, 52,* 189–198.

Willoughby, C., & Polatajko, H. (1995). Motor problems in children with developmental coordination disorder: Review of the literature. *American Journal of Occupational Therapy, 49,* 787–794.

The Evolution of the Concept of Praxis in Sensory Integration

Erna Imperatore Blanche, Ph.D., OTR, FAOTA

Praxis is a topic that many disciplines—including neuropsychology, neurosciences, movement sciences, speech and language pathology, physical therapy, developmental psychology, and occupational therapy—have studied. Each discipline offers a unique contribution to the understanding of praxis. For example, the neurosciences focus on the neurological sites associated with the various components of praxis; the movement sciences describe the role of praxis during motor skill acquisition; physical therapy describes intervention strategies that focus on motor performance; and speech and language pathology concentrates on oral motor and language components of praxis. Within occupational therapy, sensory integration theory has made a significant contribution not only to the development of intervention strategies addressing praxis disorders but also to the understanding of sensation as an important underpinning of praxis (Ayres, 1966, 1977, 1985, 1989).

The relationship between praxis and the ability to integrate sensory information has developed and expanded throughout the history of the development of sensory integration theory. To understand the association between sensory integration and praxis, it is helpful to retrace historically the trajectory of knowledge development in this area, then update traditional concepts with new data and theories.

Evolution of the Concept of Motor Planning as it Relates to Sensory Integration

Ayres was one of the first researchers to describe a relationship between praxis and sensory processing, specifically a relationship between somatosensory processing and motor planning. Based on factor analysis done with the *Southern California Sensory Integration Tests* (SCSIT, Ayres, 1972b) and later with the *Sensory Integration and Praxis Tests* (SIPT, Ayres, 1989), she described a group of children with decreased tactile discrimination and concurrent difficulty with motor planning simple actions such as imitating nonpurposeful gestures (Ayres, 1965, 1989). Ayres (1969, 1972a) also described another group of children with decreased muscle tone, decreased bilateral motor coordination, and poor postural-ocular abilities. Although at first she did not describe the exact nature of the neurological relationship between these variables, she considered bilateral motor coordination deficits to be a different type of motor coordination disorders, not necessarily dyspraxia (Ayres, 1969, 1971a, 1972a). Ayres (1979) associated poor bilateral motor coordination, poor postural control, and learning disabilities with vestibular functions but did not necessarily consider them the same as dyspraxia. Throughout the 1980s, Ayres continued to focus primarily on the relationship between motor planning and somatosensory processing (1985); however, she did not dismiss a relationship between motor planning and vestibular processing.

During the 1970s, Ayres also described praxis as the equivalent to motor planning and used both terms interchangeably (1979). However, in 1985, she described two other components associated with motor planning/praxis: ideation or conceptualization and execution. In this germinal monograph, she defined praxis as "that neurological process by which cognition directs motor action" (Ayres, 1985, p. 23), ideation as "the concept of possible object-person interaction and some idea of what might take place during that interaction" (p. 20), action planning as "the intermediary process which bridges ideation and motor execution to enable adaptive interaction with the physical world" (p. 23), and execution as the motor expression of ideation and motor planning.

Fisher (1991) expanded on Ayres' conceptualization by using contemporary motor control theories to describe the motor and cognitive components contributing to the individual's interaction with the environment through praxis (see Figure 7.1). To produce a more complete picture of the process of praxis and motor control, Fisher clarified in this model the role of such concepts as neuronal models, feedforward (referred to in the past as efference copy), production feedback, outcome feedback, and motor command in the process of praxis (for a detailed explanation, see Fisher, 1991). Fisher also utilized motor learning theories to define the relationship of the vestibular and proprioceptive systems to praxis. (See the next section in this chapter for an elaboration of the link between praxis and sensory processing.)

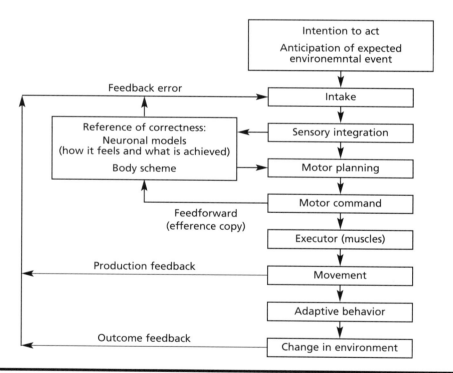

Figure 7.1. Fisher's (1991) schematic model of the process of interaction with the environment

Note. From Vestibular-proprioceptive processing and bilateral integration and sequencing deficits (p. 86), by A. Fisher, 1991, in *Sensory integration: Theory and practice,* edited by A. Fisher, E. Murray, and A. Bundy. Philadelphia: F.A. Davis. Copyright 1991 by F.A. Davis. Reprinted with permission.

With Fisher's (1991) model, it is also possible to clarify how ideation and motor planning might distinguish actions that require praxis from other forms of motor actions such as innate automatic reactions and/or practiced skills. Ayres (1989) clearly differentiated between children with execution deficits due to neuromotor problems and children with dyspraxia whose problems originated in the neural processes preceding the execution. According to Fisher's model, the motor command activates motor plans that the central nervous system (CNS) has already formed, and execution refers to the actual performance of the motor plan carried out by lower levels of the CNS, the muscles, and the joints.

The differentiation between poor skill development because of execution deficits resulting from neuromotor problems and poor skill development due to difficulties in motor planning is important for planning intervention. For example, poor activation of motor commands occurs in children with cerebral palsy who exhibit disorders in the activation of the muscles needed for the execution of a task. Children with neuromotor disorders often lack the components of movement necessary to perform motor acts. For example, they are unable to perform sequential finger touching and are also unable to pick up small objects that require a pincer grasp. These deficits might result from the inability to isolate the movements of the thumb and the index finger from the movements of all other fingers and the wrist, or tonal abnormalities might prevent these children from bringing the finger pads together. In contrast, children with dyspraxia might be able to isolate finger movements and have all other neuromotor components necessary to do a sequential finger-touching task but lack the ability to organize and plan the components into an adaptive interaction with the physical environment. They might be unable to perform new and unfamiliar motor activities such as sequential finger touching but have no difficulty with habitual activities such as picking up small objects requiring the pincer grasp. This observation indicates that the components of the movement (isolated finger movements and ability to bring finger pads together) are present, but the ability to plan the movements in sequence and outside the usual context is not. Two distinct disorders of movement that can coexist are evident here: difficulty with motor execution due to poor ability to activate the necessary muscles, and poor praxis due to an inability to organize the movement components to carry out the task. These difficulties require different intervention strategies.

Praxis and motor skills have some features in common but also exhibit some differences. Praxis and motor skills are both goal-directed, result in finely coordinated and accurate actions (that require feedback), need to be organized sequentially, require cognitive skills to understand knowledge of results, require the ability to accommodate movements to the needs of the situation, are learned, and include an aspect of tool usage (Exner & Henderson, 1995). The differences might stem from the fact that praxis also influences the ability to learn new motor skills and to interact effectively with a continuously changing physical world, whereas skill is the product of that learning. Therefore, it is possible to assess praxis only in a novel task or a task requiring adaptation to moving objects or environments (e.g., playing ball), whereas skill development can be assessed during the performance of novel or habitual tasks.

Support for the Relationship Between Praxis and Sensory Integration

Clinical observations, neurological studies, and motor learning theories all support the relationship between motor planning deficits and tactile and proprioceptive processing deficits. Ayres first described the relationship between tactile discrimination and motor planning in 1964, then further substantiated this relationship with the factor analytic studies published in 1971(b) and 1989. Although Ayres did not describe a clear relationship between motor planning and vestibular processing, Fisher (1991), based on Ayres' work, described a relationship between praxis and vestibular/proprioceptive processing as evidenced in the SIPT factor of Bilateral Integration and Sequencing (BIS). Fisher noted that difficulties with BIS can be accompanied by difficulties in projected action sequences, oculomotor control, and postural control and consequently result in deficits in praxis. Since this 1991 publication, researchers and educators in sensory integration, continuing with Ayres' tradition, have described praxis disorders related to sensory integration as associated with deficits in somatosensory processing (tactile and proprioceptive) or vestibular/proprioceptive processing Cermak, 1991; Fisher, 1991; Mulligan, 1998; Blanche, 1999).

Mulligan's (1998) factor analysis confirmed Ayres' findings about the relationship between low scores in motor planning tests and low scores in the tactile discrimination tests. Mulligan's analysis of 10,961 SIPT scores submitted to Western Psychological Services between 1989 and 1993 demonstrated the existence of four factors (dyspraxia, visual perceptual deficit, somatosensory deficit, and bilateral integration and sequencing deficit) that correlated highly with each other (Mulligan). Researchers in other disciplines also noticed the possible relationship between motor coordination and proprioception (LaRue et al., 1995; Laszlo, 1998; Laszlo, Bairstow, & Bartrip, 1988; Laufer & Hocherman, 1998; Lord & Hulme, 1987).

Studies of the neuroanatomical connections within the brain also support the relationship between motor planning and tactile and proprioceptive processing. The premotor area (area 6) and the motor area (area 4) of the cortex (which are responsible for planning the movement according to the goal and shaping the movement according to specific features in both stationary and moving environments) receive tactile and proprioceptive information from the somatic sensory cortex (Kandel, Schwartz, & Jessell, 1995). Consequently, somatosensory information influences motor planning and motor performance.

Motor control theories also corroborate the relationship of the sensory systems to praxis. As the systems approach to motor control and motor development evolved, so did the appreciation of the role of perception and sensory processing in motor behavior. Shumway-Cook and Woollacott (1995) describe motor control as the interaction between sensation, action, and cognition. As a result, contemporary views of sensation as an important contributor to motor performance now support the relationship that Ayres originally made between sensation and praxis.

Sensory information is necessary in many ways when an individual purposefully interacts with the environment.

- Sensory information from the body and the environment is necessary in the initial intake of information, before the decision to act takes place.

  In making a decision to kick a ball, for example, the individual needs to gather visual information about the position of the ball, somatosensory information about his or her body position relative to the action he or she is planning, and vestibular/proprioceptive information in reference to the individual's position in space.

- Sensory information is necessary in ideation in that previous interactions with the environment contributed to the elaboration of action plans that the individual subsequently utilizes in choosing a goal for the action.

  In the ball-kicking example, the individual's decision to kick the ball rests on previous memories of successful and nonsuccessful interactions with balls.

Ideation or conceptualization is the cognitive ability the individual needs to create the idea or concept to allow purposeful interaction with the environment. Integrating sensory information contributes to ideation because ideation develops from previous interactions with the environment. These interactions become meaningful and the individual remembers them because of the sensory experience the interactions generated. Disorders in ideation can occur because of decreased cognitive abilities or because previous sensory experiences did not register and therefore did not become meaningful. Because the goal of sensory integration intervention is to improve somatosensory awareness and integration as a basis for praxis, intervention for ideation deficits is most useful for individuals who have a sensory integration deficit and less useful for individuals who exhibit cognitive deficits not related to sensory processing.

- Integrating sensory information from the environment and the body is necessary in the construction of motor plans (Ayres, 1984).

- Adequate processing of sensory information is necessary in the collection of feedback from the action and from the effect of one's actions in the environment. Being able to process feedback adequately helps in the construction of motor programs that the individual can utilize for future actions in the environment.

  In the ball-kicking example, the person's memory stores up for future use sensory information about the temporal and spatial parameters needed for successful interactions with the ball.

Finally, as the understanding of the components of praxis expands, so does the understanding of how praxis affects the performance of occupations. To further the theoretical development of praxis in sensory integration, this text includes three chapters that address different aspects of praxis. Using contemporary theories, Giuffrida (chapter 8, Praxis and Motor Planning) and May-Benson (chapter 9, A Theoretical

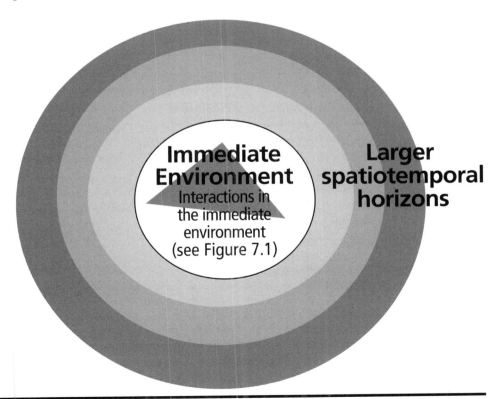

Figure 7.2. Short-term and long-term relationship of praxis to daily life

Model of Ideation in Praxis) expand on the components of praxis, and Blanche and Parham (chapter 10, Praxis and Organization of Behavior in Space and Time) expand on the relationship between praxis and organization of behavior by describing the impact of sensory processing deficits on the perception of time and space. Figure 7.2 illustrates the relationship between sensory integration and praxis or the interaction with the physical world, and expands on this model from an occupational science perspective to illustrate the impact of praxis on organization of behavior and ultimately on the life of the individual. As research accumulates, the construct of praxis develops, and contemporary theories elucidate the interaction between systems, it appears that the relationship first described by Ayres between sensory processing and praxis gains support.

In 1985, Ayres wrote in the foreword of *Developmental Dyspraxia and Adult-Onset Apraxia:*

> While these are *my* final words on the subject, they must not be *the* final words. There is yet much to be learned about developmental dyspraxia.

As others have done before, the writers in this book responded to the challenge.

Works Cited

Quotations on pages 126 and 130 from *Developmental Dyspraxia and Adult-Onset Apraxia* by A.J. Ayres (1985) have been reprinted with permission by Sensory Integration International.

References

Ayres, A.J. (1964). Tactile functions, their relation to hyperactive and perceptual motor behavior. *American Journal of Occupational Therapy, 18,* 6–11.

Ayres, A.J. (1965). Patterns of perceptual-motor dysfunction in children: A factor analytic study. *Perceptual Motor Skills, 20,* 335–368.

Ayres, A.J. (1966). Inter-relationships among perceptual-motor functions in children. *American Journal of Occupational Therapy, 20, 68–71.*

Ayres, A.J. (1969). Deficits in sensory integration in educationally handicapped children. *Journal of Learning Disabilities, 2,* 160–168.

Ayres, A.J. (1971a). Characteristics of types of sensory integrative dysfunction. *American Journal of Occupational Therapy, 25,* 329–334.

Ayres, A.J. (1971b). Deficits in sensory integration in educationally handicapped children. *Journal of Learning Disabilities, 2, 44–52.*

Ayres, A.J. (1972a). *Sensory integration and learning disorders.* Los Angeles: Western Psychological Corporation.

Ayres, A.J. (1972b). *Southern California Sensory Integration Tests.* Los Angeles: Western Psychological Services.

Ayres, A.J. (1977). Cluster analyses of measures of sensory integration. *American Journal of Occupational Therapy, 31,* 362–366.

Ayres, A.J. (1979). *Sensory integration and the child.* Los Angeles: Western Psychological Corporation.

Ayres, A.J. (1984). *Adaptive behavior as a therapeutic process.* Unpublished manuscript.

Ayres, A.J. (1985). *Developmental dyspraxia and adult-onset apraxia.* Torrance, CA: Sensory Integration International.

Ayres, A.J. (1989). *Sensory Integration and Praxis Tests.* Los Angeles: Western Psychological Services.

Blanche, E.I. (1999). *Praxis and dyspraxia handouts.* Unpublished lecture notes presented as part of the Sensory Integration Perspectives Course, University of Southern California, Los Angeles, in conjunction with Western Psychological Services.

Cermak, S. (1991). Somatodyspraxia. In A. Fisher, E. Murray, and A. Bundy (Eds.), *Sensory integration: Theory and practice* (pp. 138–170). Philadelphia: F.A. Davis.

Exner, C., & Henderson, A. (1995). Cognition and motor skill. In A. Henderson & C. Pehoski (Eds.), *Hand function in the child: Foundations for remediation* (pp. 93–110). St. Louis: Mosby.

Fisher, A. (1991). Vestibular-proprioceptive processing and bilateral integration and sequencing deficits. In A. Fisher, E. Murray, and A. Bundy (Eds.), *Sensory integration: Theory and practice* (pp. 71–107). Philadelphia: F.A. Davis.

Kandel, E., Schwartz, J., & Jessell, T. (1995). *Essentials of neural science and behavior.* Norwalk, CT: Appleton and Lange.

Laszlo, J. (1998). Letter to the editor. *Developmental Medicine and Child Neurology, 40,* 70–71.

Laszlo, J., Bairstow, P.J., & Bartrip, J. (1988). Clumsiness or perceptuo-motor dysfunction? In A.M Colley & J.R. Beech (Eds.), *Cognition and action in skilled behavior* (pp. 293–309). North-Holland: Elsevier Science Publisher.

LaRue, J., Bard, C., Fleury, M., Teasdale, N., Paillard, J., Forget, R., & Lamarre, Y. (1995). Is proprioception important for the timing of motor activities? *Canadian Journal of Physiological Pharmacology, 73,* 225–261.

Laufer, Y., & Hocherman, S. (1998). Visual and kinesthetic control of goal-directed movements to visually and kinesthetically presented targets. *Perceptual and Motor Skills, 86*(3), 1375–1391.

Lord, R., & Hulme, C. (1987). Kinesthetic sensitivity of normal and clumsy children. *Developmental Medicine and Child Neurology, 29,* 720–725.

Mulligan, S. (1998). Patterns of sensory integration dysfunction: A confirmatory factor analysis. *American Journal of Occupational Therapy, 52*(10), 819–828

Shumway-Cook, A., & Woollacott, M.H. (1995). *Motor control theory and practical applications.* Baltimore: Williams and Wilkins.

Praxis, Motor Planning, and Motor Learning

Clare Giuffrida, Ph.D., OTR, FAOTA

Sensory integration as a conceptual model has its origins in the neurobiological and neurobehavioral theories of the early 1960s. A.J. Ayres originally developed this model for occupational therapy interventions with children having sensory integration dysfunction, and it has since undergone several revisions by Ayres (1985) and others (Fisher, Bundy, & Murray, 1991). The constructs and organizing principles relevant to this model have changed to reflect current knowledge in occupational therapy, neurobiology, child development, developmental psychology, and motor behavior. Interest and research from other fields concerning children with learning disabilities have also affected the development and understanding of sensory integration disorders, theory, and intervention.

Ayres proposed sensory integration as a method of intervention for children experiencing sensory processing deficits resulting in learning or performance problems (Ayres, 1972). Children with learning and motor planning disorders show characteristic limitations in their role performance in the classroom, at home, or at play. However, the difficulty these children have with performance is not necessarily related to a specific physical impairment (such as cerebral palsy) or a motor control deficit (such as inadequate force production). Rather, their problems stem from their inability to conceptualize, plan, program, remember, or execute the necessary actions supporting performance. However, this inability to plan (dyspraxia) manifests primarily as a developmental movement dysfunction in that the process of thinking about as well as organizing, constructing, and performing motor-based activity expresses itself through action.

Ayres (1985) defined motor planning as a uniquely human skill that is not strictly a neuromotor function but one that uses the neuromotor system for execution. In developmental dyspraxia, the problems lie in the psychological processes and neural activity associated with creating movement ideas and/or with organizing, planning, and using novel movements appropriately and spontaneously. Dyspraxia is a developmental dysfunction. Unlike adult apraxia, developmental dyspraxia is not a disruption of an acquired process but rather the failure of the developmental motor planning process to emerge early in the child's life.

Clinicians now recognize the sensory integration frame of reference for praxis as an effective intervention for children with learning disorders as well as children with developmental disabilities and accompanying motor problems due to sensory integrative dysfunction. Children with a variety of disorders can experience problems with motor planning that are not directly related to the neuromotor condition of their specific disability. It is possible that a child with cerebral palsy could have both a neuromotor condition interfering with movement and difficulty with developing the idea and/or the movement plans needed for an activity such as dressing. Therefore, to treat children with a variety of disorders effectively, it is helpful to understand how both motor control and motor learning contribute to the process of motor planning.

This chapter presents the contemporary concepts and principles that reflect the current knowledge essential to understanding the motor planning processes in the child with developmental disabilities. To familiarize the reader with the different perspectives on motor planning problems, the text discusses the terms currently in use to describe children and adults with motor planning problems. The chapter incorporates an information-processing model as a means for exploring and understanding the typical processes of motor learning and motor planning in the individual. The chapter also reviews information-processing studies relevant to motor planning problems in children. This review emphasizes the research with children with Down syndrome because these investigations lend insight into neurological differences in these children that might be contributing to their motor planning problems. The final section of this chapter suggests intervention strategies and provides direction for future research with children with developmental disabilities and motor planning problems.

Redefining Praxis: From *Clumsiness* to *Developmental Dyspraxia* to *Developmental Coordination Disorder* to *Specific Developmental Disorder of Motor Function*

Praxis

The development and learning of skilled movements and control is a primary means by which a child attains mastery of self and develops competency with toys and tools present in the environment (Morris, 1997). This developmental process is related to praxis, which Ayres defined as the uniquely human skill enabling the brain to conceptualize, organize, and direct purposeful interactions with the world (Ayres, 1985). Praxis, a product of normal motor learning, is fundamental to a child's acting on the environment, necessary for getting dressed, learning to write, or playing. If praxis does not emerge, the result is developmental dyspraxia, a developmental motor planning disorder.

Impaired motor planning and learning abilities in children are relatively common developmental problems (Conrad, Cermak, & Drake, 1983). In adults, apraxia is a disorder of purposeful learned movements not due to a physical impairment such as weakness or paralysis. The literature on adults cites specific abnormalities in the overall process of motor planning, learning, and coordination as apraxia. The literature dealing with children's disorders, however, refers to these problems in children as *clumsiness* (Gubbay, 1975), *developmental dyspraxia* (Ayres, 1972; Cermak, 1985; Denckla, 1984), *Developmental Coordination Disorder* (DCD) (American Psychiatric Association, 1994) and/or *Specific Developmental Disorder of Motor Function* (SDDMF) (World Health Organization, 1992).

Insights From the Adult Apraxia Literature

Rothi and Heilman (1997) defined apraxia as a neurological disorder of learned purposive movement skill that is not due to a deficit in the peripheral sensory or motor systems. Individuals with apraxia commonly have static or progressive central nervous system dysfunction such as occurs in cerebrovascular accidents or Alzheimer's disease. Investigators of adult apraxia originally regarded apraxia as a motor production disorder manifested in multiple ways and closely related to aphasia.

Interest in adult apraxia has shifted through the years to an increased emphasis on understanding the cognitive and symbolic aspects of this disorder. Adult apraxia results in the loss of the ability to formulate, plan, select, or retrieve movement plans already acquired or previously learned. Ideational and ideomotor apraxia refers to specific losses in these aspects of motor planning in adults with apraxia (De Renzi & Lucchelli, 1988; Hecaen & Rondot, 1985; Paillard, 1982; Poeck, 1985; Roy & Square, 1985).

Within the adult apraxia literature, Roy and Square (1985) proposed a dual conceptual and production system as the basis of human action. They explained action as dependent on the interaction of conceptual knowledge about tools, objects, and actions (e.g., knowing what a hammer is) and experiential knowledge about tools, actions, and objects (e.g., knowing how to use a hammer to hit a nail). Information contained in the motor programs or production system for action provides support to the conceptual knowledge about an object or a gesture.

Investigators have occasionally attempted to relate adult apraxia to a sensory basis, but most efforts to do this have occurred in the developmental domain (Ayres, 1972; Gubbay, Ellis, Walton, & Court, 1965). More often, researchers have related adult apraxia to a disturbance in the use of meaningful gestures. This results in an inability to respond appropriately to commands, as might happen when pretending to use a hammer or waving goodbye. The person might be unable to fold a towel on request or imitate or spontaneously produce previously learned skills such as dancing (Rothi & Heilman, 1997). These difficulties suggest that the problem in adult apraxia results from a disconnection or disruption in central nervous system processing that the individual uses to access, translate, recall, and/or execute action plans.

Clumsiness and Developmental Dyspraxia

Gubbay (1975) described the clumsy child as having decreased ability to perform skilled movements despite normal intelligence; exhibiting no primary defects in other sensory, motor, or cognitive functions; and demonstrating normal findings on conventional neurological tests. He proposed a multifaceted etiology for the problem related to structural brain changes resulting in functional differences in children's motor performance.

On the other hand, Ayres (1972, 1985) defined apparent "clumsiness" in children as a possible reflection of the child's inability to plan and execute a nonhabitual motor task such as playing hopscotch. Ayres (1985) attributed these problems to disturbances in central nervous system processing and the inadequate utilization of sensory information for body scheme development and for action planning. She interpreted developmental dyspraxia as a disorder primarily of sensory information integration and planning. In explaining movement planning, Ayres (1985) also described different classes and types of actions as indicating normal or disrupted motor planning or as examples of other forms of motor behaviors. In her lectures, Ayres gave an example of a dog using its hind paw to scratch automatically. She described the dog's scratching not as a motor planning or learned act but one that was innate to the species, hardwired and biologically determined. Ayres emphasized that motor behavior consisted of a repertoire of movements and that children with developmental dyspraxia had problems with learned movements, not necessarily with innate automatic movement patterns. In their explanation of developmental dyspraxia, Fisher et al. (1991) implicated some possible neurological mechanisms associated with the specific movement dysfunction, dyspraxia. They proposed that specific problems in feedforward and feedback motor control mechanisms in children contribute to problems with motor planning.

In 1990, Goodgold-Edwards and Cermak, drawing from the motor learning literature, described and characterized children with developmental dyspraxia as having the following movement-related problems:

1. difficulty organizing and integrating sensory information, especially somatosensory and vestibular input necessary for action. This problem appears as a poor response to environmental cues that influence their actions, such as when a child grasps a bat too tightly or stands stiffly to bat.

2. difficulty learning general rules or strategies concerning classes of movement. This problem is evident when a child is unable to recall having previously thrown a ball and cannot determine in a new situation how far or fast to throw the ball.

3. difficulty taking advantage of perceptual cues (such as the speed and spatial location of an object) to be able to regulate actions. This type of impairment is evident when a child runs too far or to the wrong place to catch a ball, or when a child writes in the wrong place on the page. These children do not develop anticipation or readiness for action easily.

4. difficulty analyzing task demands and problems with effectively using knowledge of performance and feedback from ongoing actions to plan subsequent actions. Such children are unable to improve their performance because they cannot modify their performance by constructing more accurate action plans. These children do not use feedback appropriately to guide or correct their actions and consequently have difficulty learning feedback-dependent actions and serial skills.

5. difficulty solving movement problems and adapting behavior to new or unexpected situational demands. These children have problems transferring what they have learned to new situations or slightly different circumstances.

In general, children with dyspraxia understand the goal for actions but often are not capable of planning their actions effectively. Their movements frequently exhibit poor timing, are not scaled to the task, and/or are inappropriate to the task demands. These children's mental representations of their actions are limited or impoverished, and the inability to match the outcomes of their performance with the feedback from their actions also limits these children. Additionally, the inability of these children to be ready for future actions can hamper performance. Lack of premovement readiness, anticipation, and organization affects their movement behavior adversely so that their responses appear delayed or excessive (Goodgold-Edwards & Cermak, 1990).

Developmental Coordination Disorder (DCD) and Specific Developmental Disorder of Motor Function (SDDMF)

Two terms that have recently come into use in the literature referring to children who are clumsy and children with developmental dyspraxia are *Developmental Coordination Disorder* (DCD) (American Psychiatric Association, 1994) and *Specific Developmental Disorder of Motor Function* (SDDMF) (World Health Organization, 1992). The American Psychiatric Association first introduced DCD into the literature in 1987 and has refined and expanded this term in the fourth edition of the *Diagnostic and Statistical Manual of Mental Disorders* (*DSM-IV*; American Psychiatric Association, 1994). The essential features of this diagnostic category include the same criteria as for the clumsy child syndrome initially defined by Gubbay (1975) while raising the question as to whether developmental dyspraxia is synonymous with or distinct from DCD (Missiuna & Polatajko, 1995). The diagnostic criteria for DCD in *DSM-IV* include late motor milestones and poor motor performances (neither of which are due to a general medical condition) that interfere significantly with the child's academic achievement and activities of daily living. Consequently, this category includes children with motor planning problems who are experiencing problems with planning activities and also children who can plan movements but are delayed or clumsy in their movements. The more recent classification of DCD also allows for "the presence of mental retardation accompanying motor difficulties if the motor problems are in excess of those usually associated with it" (American Psychiatric Association, 1994, p. 53). This classification also allows for the additional presence of attention-deficit and hyperactivity disorders, with both diagnoses given if the criteria for both disorders are present.

According to the criteria for SDDMF, a child must demonstrate inadequate motor skills that adversely affect daily activities in the home and in school. Although the tenth edition of the *International Classification of Diseases (ICD-10)* excludes major neurological diseases from their criteria of SDDMF, both the *DSM-IV* classification and the *ICD-10* claim that children with this disorder can manifest neurodevelopmental immaturities or soft neurological signs such as choreiform movements of the limbs, mirror movements, and bilateral hyper- or hyporeflexia (Miyahara & Mobs, 1995). SDDMF includes children with clumsy child syndrome, DCD, and developmental dyspraxia. This diagnostic category therefore encompasses various motor problems using one term, SDDMF.

Addition of the terms DCD and SDDMF to the literature describing developmental motor problems has created new concerns and discussions about sensory integrative dysfunction, developmental dyspraxia, and clumsy child syndrome (Blanche, 1998; Missiuna & Polatajko, 1995). A recent question is whether these terms are interchangeable or not, and whether they are descriptive of distinct types of motor performance problems. Although different authors use these terms interchangeably, they are not fully synonymous and consequently are confusing in reports of research with children having motor performance problems. For example, the inclusion criteria for DCD allow for delays in motor planning, motor coordination, and/or motor delay interfering with a child's age-appropriate activities. Therefore, a child with DCD can have motor planning problems, but not all children classified as DCD have motor planning problems: some will have delayed motor development or have only clumsiness. For a better understanding of this issue as well as future research needs in this area, refer to the more recent writings of Blanche, Missiuna and Polatajko, Willoughby and Polatajko (1995), and Polatajko, Fox, and Missiuna (1995).

From Idea to Action

This section reviews current concepts in motor learning and planning related to developmental disabilities and presents a synthesis of the ideas important to understanding the motor learning and motor planning process in children who are typical, "clumsy," or have developmental disabilities.

Ayres' early work on sensory integration and praxis focused on explaining the neuroanatomical and neurophysiological underpinnings of developmental dyspraxia. More recent work by Fisher et al. (1991) introduced supplementary knowledge about motor control and learning relevant to praxis. Fisher at al. focused on the role of sensory information and feedback in the processing, learning, and regulation of movements. Contemporary motor behavior research has extended beyond these cognitive-motor and neuroanatomical explanations of movement to encompass the physical dynamics as well as the multiple contextual factors influencing movement planning and learning (Giuffrida, 1998; Haugen & Mathiowetz, 1995). A discussion of these areas and their impact on motor planning is beyond the scope of this chapter; in addition, research in these areas has not yet contributed to the understanding of motor planning in atypical populations. There is, however, substantial research about information processing and motor learning and planning problems in children who are "clumsy" and in children with Down syndrome. Furthermore, through neuroimaging techniques, researchers are increasingly relating cognitive-based activity to function and dysfunction of the central nervous system. These lines of research help to clarify the relationship of neuroscientific findings to cognitively directed motor functioning in children.

Information-Processing Accounts of Skilled Actions

The motor-learning literature offers several information-processing models of motor learning and motor control. These types of models can give insight into the motor planning process in children with developmental disabilities and the research with persons having Down syndrome. These models are a foundation for a clearer grasp of how information-processing capabilities underlie normal performance, how knowledge of ideas and goals guides actions, how understanding and meaning become linked to action, and how the motor planning process can be disrupted or disturbed in children with developmental disabilities such as Down syndrome.

Structure and Nature of Information Processing

In the learning of, planning for, and execution of movements, a subtle interplay of individual, task, and environmental factors occurs as the child's cognitive, sensory, perceptual, motor, and other subsystems interface with task and the environment. To relate movement planning to information processing, it helps to think of persons as processors of information, like computers with hardware and software that interact, using information input to produce output. This information-processing framework provides a way to grasp how an individual processes, stores, and uses incoming information to determine skilled motor activity (Lord & Hulme, 1987a).

In information-processing models of performance, three distinct processing stages mediate the transformation and organization of information, resulting in skilled behavior (Smyth & Glencross, 1986). The information-processing approach assumes that performance results from a finite number of processes. These processes account for the perception and cognitive processing of the sensory information and the programming of the required response. Movement execution therefore depends on sensing and perceiving the environment in order to act effectively. Consequently, most information-processing models of skilled action take into account many movement aspects: the registering and processing of incoming sensory information, important environmental features and movement goals that elicit and/or organize the movement, feedback processes involved in both the learning and the regulation of movements, the role of recall, and the processes necessary for execution of the movement. Models of movement learning and planning describe the process of movement planning from the intake of sensory information through the formation of responses, with different stages of processing, learning, memory, and movement execution co-occurring (Schmidt, 1991).

Schmidt (1991) put forth a simple information-processing model, upon which Light (1991) and Mulder (1991) have elaborated. In this model, the individual registers, attends to, and translates information or sensory input from original input to output. Typically the information-processing stages related to movement output describe the flow of information into and through the system. This flow begins with sensory registration and stimulus identification and proceeds to response selection and response production (Figure 8.1).

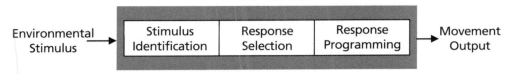

Inside the CNS

Environmental Stimulus → | Stimulus Identification | Response Selection | Response Programming | → Movement Output

Figure 8.1. Light's (1991) model of information processing (CNS = central nervous system).

Note. From Information processing for motor performance in aging adults (p. 69), by K. Light, 1991, in *Movement Science,* Alexandria, VA: American Physical Therapy Association. Copyright 1991 by American Physical Therapy Association. Adapted with permission.

Each stage of processing requires time. To study how individuals process and act on information, researchers have measured how much time individuals spend on processing in each stage and under what conditions the response speeds vary (Light, 1991; Van Dellen & Geuze, 1988). For example, sensing, encoding, and perceiving significant environmental stimuli occur in the information identification stage. Factors affecting this processing stage include the clarity of the information input as well as the intensity and the complexity of the information the individual is processing (Light, 1991). Humans respond most quickly to sharp, intense, and simple environmental cues.

During stimulus identification, the first stage of information processing, the person analyzes information from a variety of sources, such as vision, kinesthesia, or other sensory avenues, while assembling and recognizing the components of information (Sellers, 1995). The person must also determine the significance of the information (Mulder, 1991). In this stage, the individual can detect patterns of movement (such as whether a ball is moving), which results in a representation of the information that is then forwarded to the next stage. In this first stage, attention and memory processes come into play because the person must attend to relevant environmental information and recognize its meaning in order to respond. The knowledge stores around the information representation are dynamic, forming the background for ascribing meaning to patterns. A child riding a scooter attaches meaning to the movement and realizes that he or she is moving through the environment as the scooter comes down the ramp. Once the stimulus identification stage provides information about the nature of the environmental information, response selection can occur (Figure 8.2).

In this stage of response selection, the task is to decide which movement to make in response to

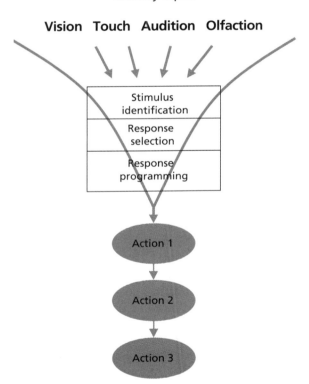

Figure 8.2. Model proposed by Schmidt and Wrisberg (2000) shows the sensory information coming into the system and being processed, and actions resulting.

Note. From *Motor Learning and Performance* (p. 80), by R. Schmidt and C. Wrisberg, 2000, Champaign, IL: Human Kinetics Books. Copyright 2000 by Human Kinetics Books. Reprinted with permission.

the salient information (Light, 1991). In the response selection stage, the sensory information translates to motor output. Response selection involves a central decision process that determines the required response to the environmental information. This processing stage resolves uncertainty about which response to make. A child coming down a ramp on a scooter while holding a beanbag decides to throw the beanbag at a toy bowling pin to the side of the ramp. The child selects a throwing response to knock down the toy bowling pin. The child does not select the option of holding onto the beanbag, hitting the toy bowling pin with the scooter, or any other available response. Reaction time experiments indicate that as compatibility between stimulus (the distance and placement of the toy relative to child on the scooter) and response (the child throwing with the right or left arm) increases or anticipation of events occurs, the child processes information more quickly (Light). This means that, with practice, the child on the scooter will respond and act more quickly. The child also builds up expectations of what to do in future similar contexts. The time required to process information will increase, however, if the child has too many responses from which to choose or if the task becomes more complex and requires multiple actions for the child to select, organize, and plan. A more complex response would be to throw the beanbag at a target, then turn the scooter to avoid an obstacle. According to information-processing accounts of movement, the more complex, two-part action of throwing and turning on the scooter would take longer to plan than the simpler response of throwing.

The final stage of information processing, response programming, begins when the individual decides on or selects a response such as throwing in response to the task demands. In this stage, movement planning, structuring, and response activation occur (Light, 1991). The child organizes and programs the code or instructions for appropriate actions, which travel to the motor apparatus for execution. The motor behavior literature is least clear about this stage and how the individual constructs, learns, and implements planned movements. Schmidt (1991) indicated that in this stage, individuals apply the rules they have learned about movements to specific situations by setting the details or the response parameters of the movement. Mulder (1991) also identified this stage as being rule-dependent and involving both planning and specifying the motor control parameters of the particular action. According to Mulder, the planning aspect involves the sequencing of the action or the ordering of the elements of the plan. In the response programming stage, the person assigns movement parameters to the motor program to order and control the specific movement, such as throwing the beanbag at the toy bowling pin (Figure 8.3).

In the response-programming stage, the motor system gets ready for producing the response and retrieves a general motor program to control and direct the specific movement (Schmidt, 1991). In the example of the child on the scooter, the child has a rule in memory for throwing that is activated by the meaningful information encoded from the environment by the child. Then, as the child rides the scooter, he or she is able to call up and implement a specific action using the appropriate control parameters for the general motor program to achieve success. In this stage, sensory consequences result from the intrinsic and extrinsic feedback from the action, as well as the outcomes of the action. This feedback enters into the development of future action plans as the individual uses the feedback and augmented knowledge of the movement outcome to refine future actions and to develop the ability to detect errors.

In all information-processing stages, attention or the general capacity to process information is critical to performance. In some cases where motor behavior is automatic or already well-learned, attentional demands are minimal. Where attention is necessary to select among movement choices, more controlled processing occurs and attentional demands are even greater. Individuals also use memory for movements to support the movement planning process.

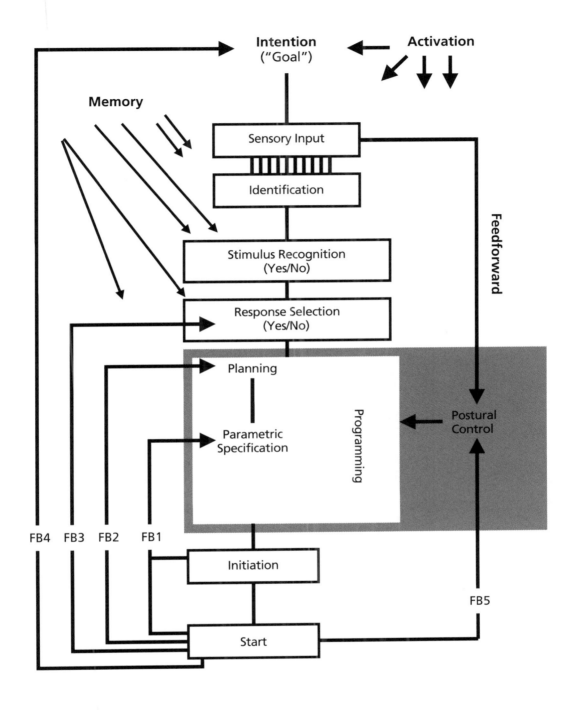

Figure 8.3. Mulder's (1991) model explains planned movements that are feedback-dependent.

Note. From A process-oriented model of human motor behavior: Toward a theory-based rehabilitation approach (p. 199), by T. Mulder, 1991, in *Movement Science,* Alexandria, VA: American Physical Therapy Association. Copyright 1991 by American Physical Therapy Association. Adapted with permission.

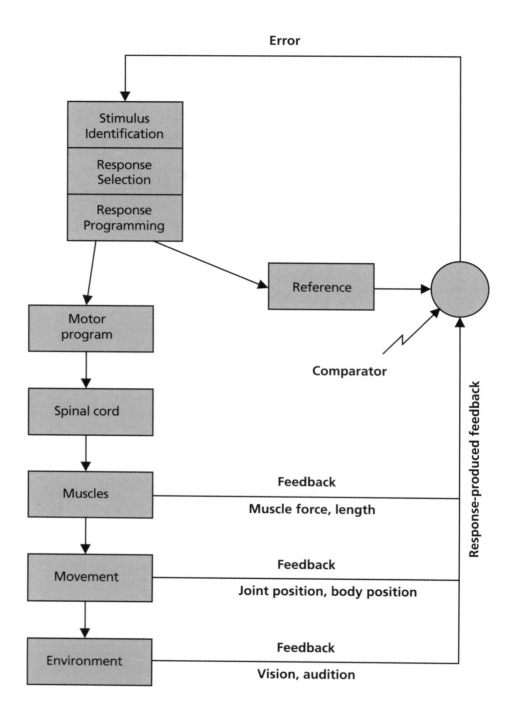

Figure 8.4. Elements of the closed-loop control system integrated with the stages of processing (Schmidt & Wrisberg, 2000).

Note. From *Motor Learning and Performance* (p. 95), by R. Schmidt & C. Wrisberg, 2000, Champaign, IL: Human Kinetics Books. Copyright 2000 by Human Kinetics Books. Reprinted with permission.

Movement Learning

Schmidt (1991) expanded on this basic conceptual model of information processing to hypothesize about how individuals learn and control slow or feedback-dependent movements (closed-loop) and fast, nonfeedback-dependent (open-loop) movements. In the case of closed-loop control, the person has a goal or intends to move. In this model, the person's executive decision-making processes consist of all operations involved in the three information-processing stages. Once these processing stages are complete, the person's commands travel to the effector system. At the same time, a learned reference of correctness of how the movement is to feel is sent to a movement comparator within the system. This reference of correctness represents the expected feedback or feel of the movement, and the person making the movement contrasts the actual feedback from the movement with the expected feel of the movement. Movement errors are the differences that the person senses between the actual movement, the outcome of the movement, and the intended movement. Differences or error signals between the intended movement and the actual movement pass back to the system so that the person can correct or update the movement for the future.

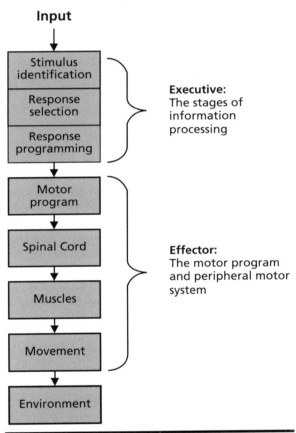

Input

Executive: The stages of information processing

Effector: The motor program and peripheral motor system

Figure 8.5. An expanded open-loop control system for human performance

The executive level contains the stages of information processing (Schmidt, 1991).

Note. From *Motor Learning and Performance: From Principles to Practice* (p. 91), by R. Schmidt, 1991, Champaign, IL: Human Kinetics Books. Copyright 1991 by Human Kinetics Books. Reprinted with permission.

For example, as movement occurs, the person generates a sensory template of the movement. The person's actual movement results in feedback from the movement, which is compared to the sensory template. Mismatches between the sensory template and the movement can lead to corrections in the movement, if time allows. Figure 8.4 displays a hypothetical model of a person's goal-directed movement from this motor control and information-processing perspective.

This model depends on the individual's having an executive or decision-making component, a program for the movement, a comparator or learned reference of correctness, and response feedback from the generated movement. The model helps to account for the learning and control of slow, controlled, or tracking movements, such as when a child maneuvers on a scooter or steers a toy.

If the environment is predictable and stable, open-loop control in the individual can occur. The individual's conscious, executive, decision-making level evaluates the environment, quickly processing information. The person programs and initiates movement in the response-programming stage, with control quickly passing to the movement level (Schmidt, 1991). In this case, it is the person's motor programs, rather than the decision making or feedback from the processing stages, that control the movements. With practice, the individual can build and combine motor programs, which leads to the ability to organize actions in advance that the individual carries out without much modification from sensory feedback. With this style of control, the person's central nervous system mediates the action, rather than the person's using feedback to control the movement or build up the movement plan (Figure 8.5).

The following account proposes how action unfolds according to an individual's intent, goals, and task demands.

Schmidt (1991) proposed that, prior to moving, the mover first analyzes the requirements of the action and the environmental conditions along with his or her intention for action. For example, an individual's actions will vary according to whether the person is planning to throw or catch a beanbag. Precision in information processing becomes critical to movement performance because the information the person processes and attends to helps the mover organize the action to meet the task requirements. The information to which the child attends allows the child to know that he or she has to throw rather than catch the beanbag. The individual's goals, the task requirements, and the environmental conditions affect how the individual attends to, registers, and recognizes the information. All of these factors affect the movement outcome.

For example, there are numerous ways to throw a beanbag. The possibilities depend on the specific environmental context, such as the person's posture (sitting or lying on a scooter); the position of the person relative to the beanbag; the place, shape, and size of the beanbag; and the purpose of the action, such as throwing or catching. The individual's actions form in response to the salient properties of objects (such as a toy's rigidity or pliability), the function of the object, and the individual's intent. With repetition and practice, the person learns specific actions, organizes them, later selects the learned action, and executes the movement. The person's movements also result in establishing an appropriate postural basis from which to perform all subsequent actions requiring motor planning.

Information-processing accounts of movement learning and control therefore depend on the changing relationship between input and output in the system. Using mental operations (such as attention, working memory, and long-term memory for the movement), the individual acts on the information. The person organizes his or her actions by registering, interpreting, and storing meaningful information. With practice, the person develops rules about the relationship of the task's goal, the environmental demands for the movement, the sensation of the movement, the outcomes of the movement, and the feedback from the movement. Schmidt (1991) additionally proposed that feedback from both internal and external sources (such as knowledge about the movement outcome and the pattern of the movement) helps to develop a learned reference of the movement, which assists in movement recognition and recall (Figure 8.6).

Schmidt's (1991) original explanation of movement learning described the movement schema as a set of rules that provides the foundations for a decision or motor act. The process of schema formation includes abstraction and association of the initial movement conditions such as the task requirements, environmental conditions, the movement goal, the sensory consequences (how the movement felt, looked, and sounded), the movement parameters (such as the force, speed, and duration of the movement) and the movement outcome. The schema can take the form of a recall (motor) schema or a recognition (sensory) schema. Schmidt hypothesized that schemas develop from bits of information related to past experiences, which are abstracted and combined into movement rules.

Once the individual learns the movement well, the need for attentional resources and memory becomes minimal. In developing meaningful actions, the person appears to interconnect knowledge structures about movements that developed through practice,

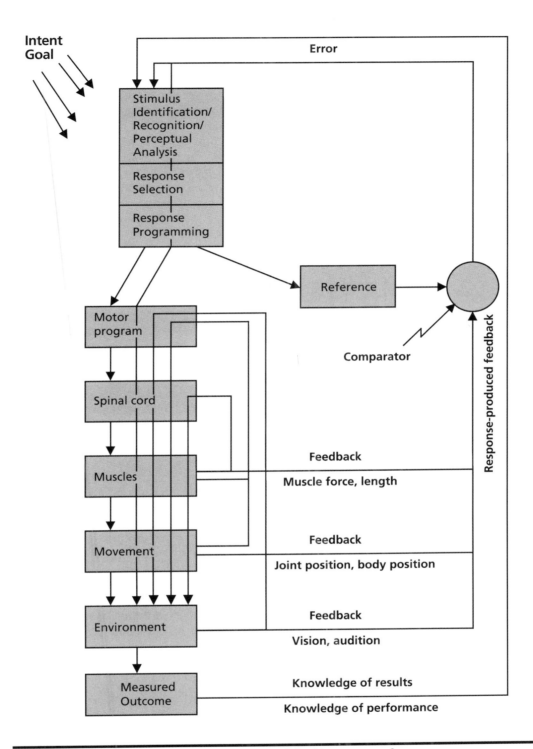

Figure 8.6. An information-processing model of human performance (Schmidt & Wrisberg, 2000).

Note. From *Motor Learning and Performance* (p. 116), by R. Schmidt & C. Wrisberg, 2000, Champaign, IL: Human Kinetics Books. Copyright 2000 by Human Kinetics Books. Reprinted with permission.

making access to motor plans more automatic and less effortful (Schwartz & Buxbaum, 1997). A child can develop problems with motor planning, information processing, or schema formation in many ways, including difficulties with attention, activational resources, and/or memory. Because motor learning is heavily dependent on visual and proprioceptive input, investigators have focused on these specific modalities as the source of difficulty in children who are clumsy (McConnell, 1995). Likewise, persons with learning impairments might not be using feedback appropriately, might rely too heavily on visual guidance to monitor and regulate movements, and/or might have poor error detection abilities and thereby have problems developing a learned reference of correctness. The child with motor planning difficulties might be very slow to develop the rules or action plans and/or might execute poorly formed or inappropriate plans. Children with developmental disabilities who also have specific sensory impairments, motor impairments, attentional problems, or learning problems are probably at greater risk for motor planning problems.

Motor Control

Along with the learning and preparation of movement plans, another element that is helpful in understanding movement is the control of movement. Two major theoretical models, closed-loop and open-loop control systems, introduced in the section on Movement Learning, explain how an individual learns to control movement. Closed-loop control systems use feedback, require a reference of correctness, involve a calculation of error, and allow subsequent corrections to control ongoing movement. Open-loop systems do not use feedback or error correction mechanisms for movement control but send preprogrammed instructions to effector mechanisms (Schmidt, 1991). Open-loop systems are dependent on feedforward control, in which information moves ahead to prepare a part of the system for upcoming sensory feedback or a future motor command. Investigators refer to the central mechanism for open-loop processes as a motor program

The Motor Program

Keele (1968) introduced the concept of the motor program, a set of muscle commands that forms before a movement sequence begins and allows the sequence to be carried out uninfluenced by feedback. However, Keele wrote this definition when the major controversy in motor control research revolved around the extent of influence of sensory feedback on skilled movement. Accordingly, Keele proposed the motor program to account for movements not dependent on sensory feedback. Although the original term has met with criticism on many accounts, a subsequent motor program definition by Rosenbaum (1991) maintained the underlying concept for programmed movements. In current motor control theory, a motor program is a functional state of the system that allows the preparation of particular movements, classes of movements, and sequences of movements to occur. Rosenbaum dismissed the controversiality of the programming concept, suggesting that it was the original explanation of programming, which tied specific muscle commands to movement programs, that was controversial. Rosenbaum likened programming to using the concept of memory in the literature, suggesting that the programming concept acts to invite inquiry into the nature of motor preparation and control, how biomechanical properties of the skeletomuscular system are represented, and how physical interactions with the environment can be taken into account. Accepting this explanation as a contemporary definition of a motor program minimizes the issues surrounding the concept. It is possible, therefore, to retain the idea of an automated, sequenced act supported by the capacity of the central nervous system to respond.

Stages of Learning

In children with movement-planning disorders, the mover's stage of learning influences movement preparation. There are three stages for movement learning: cognitive, associative, and automatic (Schmidt, 1991). All stages utilize cognitive resources, but cognition becomes less important as movement preparation becomes more automatic. These stages describe the different levels of skill development and should not be confused with the information-processing stages. Where the child is in these learning stages, however, can affect how the child processes information and plans.

For example, in the cognitive stage of learning, tasks are new to the learner, and the child must learn what is relevant and significant in the context of the task. In this stage, the learner is beginning to figure out what to do and is beginning to attempt to do it. The child is starting to identify verbally the goals of the task, what to do or not do, when to do it, how to do it, and what to listen to or look at when doing the task. Riding on a scooter for the first time means learning and remembering how to get on the scooter, how to push off, and how to throw a beanbag accurately at a toy while moving on the scooter.

Once the child has solved most of the cognitive problems of doing the task, the child shifts to organizing more effective movement patterns to produce the action in the motor stage. For example, the child now easily gets on and pushes off with the scooter. He or she is able to throw the beanbag at a toy with some accuracy, does not forget to do it, and does not stop the scooter in order to throw. In this stage, performance is improves rapidly, consistency increases, and the child uses feedback to be more consistent. Self-talk is less important, anticipation develops, and the child can monitor his or her own feedback and detect and verbalize errors.

In the final stage of movement learning, the child or learner moves automatically, and the motor program or automated sequences of action do not require attention. In this stage, the action requires decreased attentional demands, and the person is free to perform higher-order cognitive planning activities. The child can develop game strategies and complex elaborations of a skill, such as being able to swing on a trapeze and consistently let go at the right time to maneuver onto other swinging trapezes. In this stage, the child appears very confident, online task analysis can be disruptive, and child can use self-talk for strategy development. In this last stage, the child can easily access and implement movement memories, which frees more cognitive capacity for other aspects of doing. Children with developmental dyspraxia can progress very slowly through these stages, and therapists need to be aware of children's problems in learning to move and plan automatically. These children can also have considerable difficulty in developing automatic play routines for activities such as soccer and basketball.

Research on Information-Processing Accounts of Motor Planning

From a motor-learning perspective, several studies have investigated information-processing capabilities in children with motor learning and/or planning problems. However, these studies are difficult to interpret because the studies classify children with motor planning problems as clumsy, which is not always synonymous with a planning problem. This section reviews these studies, though, because they shed some light on the sensory information processing model of skilled action, the components of movement learning and planning, and possible strategies to use with children who have developmental disabilities and motor planning problems.

Information-Processing Research With Typical Children With Coordination and Planning Disorders

Information-processing research in children who are developing typically except for some coordination problems has focused on whether children with DCD or clumsiness have difficulties with the information processing or executive aspects of movement learning and planning, the learning and memory for action plans, or the sequencing and programming of response specifications for planned movements.

Several studies have investigated stimulus identification and recognition in children with movement problems by comparing these children to children of the same age without movement problems. These studies identified differences primarily in sensory functioning, information processing, and motor control in children with movement problems.

Sensory Deficits

Vision and kinesthesia are two of the most frequently studied sensory systems in motor learning due to their primary role in movement learning and provision of feedback for movement control (Sellers, 1995). Hulme, Biggerstaff, Moran, and McKinley (1982) suggested that the visual and kinesthetic systems, as well as the linkage of these systems, are essential for the learning of motor skills.

In movement learning, the person's use of the visual modality provides information about the depth and distance of objects from the person; the location, shape, and size of objects; guidance of extremities; and potential movement correction (Sellers, 1995). In a series of investigations, Hulme et al. (1982) and Hulme and Lord (1986) examined visual spatial perception in children with clumsiness and in control groups of children developing typically. Hulme et al. noted that children with clumsiness had problems in judging spatial distance, slopes of objects in the environment, and linear length. These investigators focused their research on examining the role of visual perception, kinesthesia, and cross-modal perception in children who were developing typically and in children with clumsiness. The children made successive judgments of the length of straight lines using vision and kinesthesia separately and together. Children with clumsiness were less accurate in their kinesthetic, visual, and cross-modal judgments of length than the children who were developing typically. Correlations between these children's performance in the visual condition of this task and their motor ability were substantial, whereas the correlation between their performance in the cross-modal, kinesthetic, and motor ability conditions was not. Although Hulme et al. have argued that visual perceptual problems could be causally related to motor problems in children with clumsiness, further research in this area has not defined a causal relationship between visual perception deficits and motor ability. Hulme and Lord (1986) suggested that memory performance and poor ocular motor control could not explain deficient performance on visual judgment of length. These studies suggest that problems with visual spatial processing interfere with motor performance but do not fully explain the role of perceptual processing of visual spatial information in children who are clumsy.

In another series of investigations, O'Brien, Cermak, and Murray (1988) and Murray, Cermak, and O'Brien (1989) studied perceptual motor abilities and motor skill performance in children with clumsiness and learning disabilities and in children who were developing typically. In these studies, investigators tested children on visual perceptual, visual motor, and motor proficiency tests. The study by O'Brien et al. found that the degree of clumsiness in these children correlated significantly with the degree of visual perceptual and visual motor impairments the children exhibited. The later study by Murray et al. found that the children's degree of clumsiness as measured by the *Test of Motor Impairment* (Stott, Moyes, & Henderson, 1984) correlated significantly with the children's performance on the *Sensory Integration and Praxis Tests'* Space Visualization, Motor Accuracy, and Design Copy subtests (Ayres, 1989). These investigators concluded that clumsiness appears to relate to some aspects of visual perceptual ability, but they cautioned against assuming that all children with clumsiness have visual perceptual problems.

A later study (van der Meulen, Denier van der Gon, Gielen, Gooskens, & Willemse, 1991) investigated the role of visual feedback in goal-directed movements in children who were developing typically and children with clumsiness. Investigators found that for fast, goal-directed movements, children with clumsiness differed significantly from the children who were developing typically. The children with clumsiness had markedly slower movement times and more inconsistency in their movements during the early, fast phase of the movement than did the children who were developing typically. The children with clumsiness appeared to use visual feedback, instead of open-loop motor control, as a strategy to improve accuracy of performance. Open-loop control was not an effective movement strategy for children with clumsiness. These children seemed to rely more heavily on visual guidance to control movement than the children who were developing typically.

Along with the studies of vision and kinesthesia by Hulme and Lord (1986) and Lord and Hulme (1987a, 1987b, 1988), other studies have investigated the role of kinesthesia and the sensory linkage of vision, kinesthesia, or proprioception in children with clumsiness. Kinesthesia is the sensory information obtained through the different sensory receptors indicating body and limb position and movement speed, direction, and force. Kinesthesia is necessary for skill development (Jarus & Gol, 1995), although its role might be important but not crucial.

Bairstow and Laszlo's (1981) studies of the role of kinesthesia indicated that kinesthetic sensitivity correlated with motor function, and impaired sensitivity contributed to clumsiness. The investigators tested children with clumsiness and determined that they had problems with kinesthetic sensitivity, spatial-temporal programming, and temporal programming. The children subsequently received different kinds of training, including specific kinesthetic training, training in all processes specific to their problems, training only in spatial and temporal programming, and general fine or gross motor skill training. The researchers found that training in all processes and kinesthetic training alone significantly improved the children's performance on a test of motor proficiency.

Other investigators have heavily criticized these studies, disagreeing over the methods that Bairstow and Laszlo (1981) used to determine and treat kinesthesia impairment. Lord and Hulme (1987b) examined the claims made by Laszlo and colleagues for the Kinesthesia Sensitivity Test (KST; Bairstow & Laszlo) by using performance on the KST and measures of motor performance to compare children who were developing typically and children who were clumsy. Lord and Hulme found that, although the children with clumsiness did poorly on the motor tests, their performance on the KST did not differ significantly from the children who were developing typically. Lord and Hulme concluded that the KST is not a satisfactory instrument with which to measure kinesthetic ability in children who are clumsy.

Others (Doyle, Elliott & Connolly, 1986; Hoare & Larkin, 1991) also questioned the reliability of the KST and whether a single test is sufficient to assess kinesthesia, or whether clinicians need to assess kinesthesia across conditions. Because kinesthesia, like visual perception, is a multimodal construct and task specific, future evaluations should look at these children across a wide range of tasks to determine the problems as well as the advantages, if any, of kinesthetic training (Sellers, 1995).

More recent studies of visual perception and proprioceptive processing in children who are clumsy have investigated whether intrasensory processing is more adequate than intersensory processing and whether deficits in these areas stem from a developmental delay or a deficit. Sigmundsson, Ingvaldsen, and Whiting (1997) investigated intersensory and intrasensory processing of the visual and proprioceptive modalities in a group of 8-year-old children whose difficulties had been identified as "clumsy with hand-eye coordination problems." The investigators compared this group's performance on a pointing task using vision, proprioception, or vision and proprioception to the performance of a group of 5-year-olds and a group of 8-year-olds on the same task under the same sensory conditions. The children identified as clumsy performed less well than both groups of children for the visual and visual-proprioceptive condition. The results suggested that problems with clumsiness result more from a deficit than a delay. However, when the children had to locate the targets proprioceptively, the performances of the children with clumsiness were similar to the 5-year-old children but inferior to the performance of the 8-year-old children, seeming to support a developmental lag for proprioception. In further analysis of the performance of the preferred and nonpreferred hand under the visual and visual-proprioceptive conditions, the investigators also found a significant discrepancy in hand performance of the children with clumsiness relative to children who were developing typically. The investigators suggested that this difference in hand performance could have pathological significance and might relate to delayed maturation of the corpus callosum, resulting in impairment of hemispheric transfer of information. They stated that further study would be necessary to obtain evidence for or against that proposition.

In summary, several studies from the visual perceptual, kinesthetic, and proprioceptive processing perspectives have identified a relationship between clumsiness and problems with intersensory and intrasensory processing. Findings in this area are inconclusive and emphasize the need for further studies to examine the relationship between sensory processing and coordination and the relationship among processing delays, deficits, and clumsiness.

Information-Processing Deficits

Many studies have found evidence that children with clumsiness experience difficulty with the speed and accuracy of processing information. Most of these studies examined children with clumsiness and children with typical development, comparing their responses to processing information and organizing and executing a response under different task conditions. These investigations sought to determine whether the children with clumsiness had problems with response selection and motor programming. Three different studies of simple and choice reaction time (Schellekens, Scholten, & Kalverboer, 1983; Smyth & Glencross, 1986; Van Dellen & Geuze, 1988) found that children with clumsiness had longer reaction and movement times than children who were developing typically. These studies suggest that clumsy children might search longer for the appropriate response or experience delays with the cognitive decision-making process of response selection.

Using a simple reaction-time task and a coincident timing task, Henderson, Rose, and Henderson (1992) had children anticipate when to intercept a target in order to be accurate. Children with *Developmental Coordination Disorder* had longer movement and reaction times than children who were developing typically. Henderson et al. attributed these delays to the children's requiring longer times to search for and retrieve the response or the appropriate stimulus-response mappings from working memory. Taking present and previous findings in information processing into account, they further proposed that the difficulty for these children is not low stimulus-response incompatibility, but rather that this delay serves as an indicator of general resource depletion in the planning and execution of movements. They also predicted that children with DCD would experience more difficulties during tasks with low stimulus-response compatibility and demanding and complex responses.

To determine how response selection and response programming contribute to slow or inaccurate performance, Van Dellen and Geuze (1988) tested these processes in children with clumsiness. In measurements of both reaction and movement times, children who were clumsy responded differently from typically developing children. The investigators concluded that the cognitive decision process of response selection contributed to the slow responses of these children but not to their inaccuracy. Furthermore, these children seemed to have problems adapting their movements to changes in the environment and task demands. Their difficulty with stimulus-response compatibility might explain why these children have more problems with learning new tasks.

Geuze and Kalverboer (1987), investigating timing and tapping, found that children with clumsiness were not able to alter their tapping tempo on demand but tended to tap at a set, regular pace. If these children receive inaccurate or inconsistent feedback from their movements, their motor programs will be less efficient. They will more than likely need more time to plan their movements and be less consistent or have more variable movements. Furthermore, if these children are having problems with response selection, as noted in some studies, these children might also be having difficulty with mapping the environmental conditions to the appropriate response selection.

Using a rotary pursuit task, Lord and Hulme (1988) investigated motor program development in children with clumsiness. This study matched children with clumsiness and children who were developing typically for age and sex, then examined each group's performance on learning the rotary pursuit task. The children with clumsiness varied in their performance on this task as measured by time on target, hit rate, and mean hit length. One subgroup seemed to develop motor programs, but another subgroup deteriorated in performance and did not seem to be able to develop motor programs. The overall poor performance of these children on this task seemed to relate more to their inability to use visual feedback than their inability to develop motor programs. In a similar study, Smythe (1991) investigated motor programming and the use of feedback for movement control in children with clumsiness. He demonstrated that these children had substantial difficulty with motor programming, leading to a greater dependence on feedback for movement control.

In summary, investigators using a motor programming perspective to investigate response selection and motor programming capability have found that children with clumsiness are slower to initiate and execute complex movements due to motor programming deficits and difficulties in the response selection stage. Children with clumsiness might be unable to make use of feedback and to build up preprogramming capabilities. Based on these studies, however, it is difficult to determine whether these are the sole motor programming problems for these children.

Motor Control Deficits

Once the individual organizes a movement to meet task and environmental demands, the person needs to set the specifications for the control of displacement, movement, amplitude, and speed. Recent motor control studies have found that children with clumsiness fixate posturally more than children who are developing typically. They appear to freeze the movement, similar to young children first learning to move (Damiano, 1993; Vereijken, Whiting, Newell, & von Emerick, 1992). Larkin and Hoare (1992) found that children with clumsiness used reciprocal activation instead of coactivation as a stability strategy for balance control. The children also corrected postural sway inconsistently, using both proximal-distal and distal-proximal activation.

In summary, studies of motor control in children with clumsiness found that these children demonstrated different patterns of sequencing and poor anticipation and had difficulty controlling movement speed and force of the movement (Larkin & Hoare, 1992). The researchers often interpreted these motor control differences as deficits because their patterns were different from those demonstrated by children who are developing typically.

Studies of Children With Down Syndrome

Several theories have attempted to account for the praxic disorders in individuals with mental retardation because these individuals display movement problems similar to those occurring in children with dyspraxia (Elliott, Edwards, Weeks, Lindley, & Carnahan, 1987; Elliott, Gray, & Weeks, 1991; Elliott & Weeks, 1990, 1993a, 1993b; Elliott, Weeks, & Elliott, 1987; Elliott, Weeks, & Gray, 1990; Elliott, Weeks, & Jones, 1986). Consequently, many studies have examined movement learning, information processing, and cerebral organization in children with Down syndrome as a way to understand movement planning and the possible role of cerebral functioning in movement for children who are typical and those who are atypical.

There is considerable research interest in children with Down syndrome because these children have known problems with motor performance, and they have specific deficits related to their condition. Other children with retardation can also have extensive central nervous system impairments affecting motor performance. In forms of retardation not associated with Down syndrome, the nature and extent of brain damage can be unknown but might overlap with that of children with Down syndrome. Increasingly, studies are comparing children with movement problems to children with retardation of unknown etiology and to children with Down syndrome to investigate the similarities and differences of their problems and to examine the possible pathology contributing to dysfunction.

In Luria's (1961) early work, he proposed that individuals with mental retardation do not develop verbal control over their motor behaviors, including the planning and execution of the behavior. Verbal regulation or reminders about the movement are not helpful in effecting learning for individuals with mental retardation, as they are for individuals with typical motor learning. In 1981, Anwar specifically proposed that individuals with Down syndrome are unable to use motor programs due to their deficits in visual motor integration. This is similar to the finding for children with clumsiness (Smythe, 1991). Similarly, Henderson, Morris, and Frith (1981) proposed that children with Down syndrome have impairments in the timing component of movements but not the spatial aspect. These problems contribute to the children's difficulty in matching their movements to the task, such as knowing when to extend one's arms to catch a ball successfully. In a study of tracking in children with Down syndrome, children with mental retardation etiology unknown, and children with typical development, Henderson et al. concluded that children with Down syndrome have limited ability to use predictability in timing. The investigators interpreted this as difficulties with learning to preplan the timing of their movements or deficits in the temporal aspect of motor programming. The children with Down syndrome, however, showed no greater impairment in their ability to use spatial predictability (e.g., where to orient one's hands to catch a ball) than other children with retardation or the children who were developing typically.

Several investigations over the years have proposed that within the population of retarded individuals, the children with Down syndrome are less well coordinated than their peers of similar mental age without Down syndrome. Therefore, investigators have studied children with Down syndrome more extensively in regard to their motor planning, information-processing capabilities, and cerebral organization and specialization.

To gain more insight into speech perception, production, and movement organization in individuals with Down syndrome, Elliott and his colleagues (Elliott, 1985; Elliott, Edwards, et al., 1987; Elliott et al., 1986, 1990, 1991; Elliott & Weeks, 1990, 1993a, 1993b; Elliott, Weeks, et al., 1987) conducted a series of investigations of cerebral organization and specialization. These investigators proposed that individuals with Down syndrome have speech perception lateralized in the right hemisphere, which differs from individuals with typical development. In contrast, both populations have movement organization and sequencing lateralized in the left hemisphere. In dichotic listening tests, individuals with Down syndrome exhibited a left ear/right hemisphere advantage, compared with a group of typical adults who demonstrated a right ear/left hemisphere advantage. Other studies by Elliott and colleagues investigated lateral manual asymmetries and transfer of training in individuals with Down syndrome and individuals who were developing typically. They found similar patterns of performance, suggesting that speech production and movement organization were localized in the left hemisphere for right-dominant individuals with and without Down syndrome.

These investigators concluded that typically developing right-dominant individuals experience ease of translation from speech perception to movement sequencing to speech production because all of these mechanisms are lateralized in the same (left) hemisphere. In individuals with Down syndrome, the speech perception mechanism is lateralized in the right hemisphere, whereas motor sequencing and speech production are lateralized in the left hemisphere. Elliott and associates proposed that this specific atypical cerebral organization and right-hemisphere specialization for speech perception in individuals with Down syndrome is the basis for this group's specific deficit in planning and production of speech and complex motor acts based on verbal cues and commands.

Other studies of information processing and brain behavior relationships in individuals with Down syndrome indicate that these individuals differ in specific information-processing capabilities from individuals matched with them for mental and chronological age. These differences, however, are not a function of cerebral organization but cerebral responsiveness.

Several studies have suggested that evoked related potentials (ERP) obtained from individuals with Down syndrome differ in several respects from those of subjects without retardation. Using components of auditory-event-related potentials, Lincoln, Courchesne, Kilman, and Galambos (1985) investigated information-processing capabilities in children with Down syndrome and children who were developing typically. By comparing the children with Down syndrome to control groups matched by chronological and mental age, the investigators hoped to distinguish whether ERP patterns reflect abnormal processing structure and capacity or maturationally delayed processing structure and capacity. In a previous study, Squires, Galbraith, and Aine (1979) had indicated that children with Down syndrome had visually evoked potentials (VEP) that were different from what is typical, suggesting that these children process incoming visual stimuli more slowly. In that study, it was unclear whether the differences in VEP were due to maturational delay or true differences. The study by Lincoln et al., which used auditory information, found that children with Down syndrome had deficits related to sensory and cognitive information processing for which immature mental development could account. Based on this study and other evidence in the literature, these investigators concluded that these children had significant impairments in (a) speed of orienting and categorizing auditory information, (b) organizing a motor response necessary for motor planning acts, and (c) processes necessary for effectively utilizing immediate auditory memory. In addition, this study indicated that some of these differences might be associated with brain pathology likely to be involved in the development of memory. Lincoln et al. further suggested the possibility of hippocampal disorders in children with Down syndrome because the hippocampus plays an important role in memory, assessing whether information is meaningful and how it should be classified (Luria, 1973).

In summary, the studies on information processing and cerebral organization in individuals with Down syndrome indicate that there are neuroanatomical, stimulus identification, and perceptual analysis differences in these children that contribute to motor planning deficits. Likewise, research has demonstrated that these children have problems with programming temporal aspects of movement that influence movement execution. Further studies of cerebral organization and specialization in children with developmental disabilities might shed additional light on the processes supporting motor planning and programming in these children.

Motor Learning Based Intervention Strategies

Children can experience problems of a sensory, perceptual, and/or cognitive nature that contribute to dyspraxia. Intervention programs for these children need to consider the causes of their problems as well as an understanding of the movement process. For example, if the child's movement problems stem from perceptual difficulties, intervention can encompass verbal mediation and cuing. Conversely, if the problem results from poor motor learning and use of feedback, the child might need more practice opportunities using different forms and amounts of feedback necessary for learning. Teaching these children new skills or teaching them to perform activities of daily living can be a challenge, but practitioners should approach the task systematically, with a clear grasp of how motor learning and information processing co-occur.

The following suggestions for teaching children with motor planning problems come from the motor learning literature with an emphasis on use of cognitive processes, sensory integration or polysensory and multimodal approaches, and learning and memory strategies (see also Figure 8.7).

1. Use visually directed strategies and verbal mediation (Goodgold-Edwards, & Cermak, 1990). Ask the child to look at what he or she is doing and where he or she is going. Demonstrate the action to the child so the child has a visual model of performance to imitate. Imitation is usually easier than generating the action independently. For verbal mediation and monitoring, have the child verbally indicate what he or she is to do, then have the child talk about what he or she has done. This supports the child's thinking about future actions as well as recalling those actions once completed.

2. Use visual and tactile cues or multimodal stimulation to enhance the development of feedforward (open-loop) and feedback (closed-loop) actions. The use of multimodal information with verbal and visual mediation can augment the feedback in the learning process and facilitate planning.

3. Once the child can respond independently to visual or verbal cuing and appears to have a stable goal and idea of different actions and goals, increase task complexity. Having the child plan multistep procedures can increase task demands.

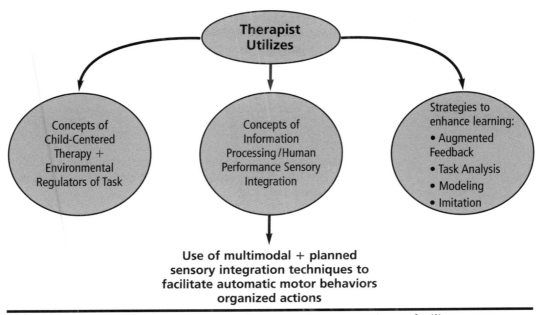

Figure 8.7. Overview of interaction of intervention strategies to facilitate movement planning in children (adapted from Croce, 1993).

Note. From A review of the neural basis of apractic disorders with implications for remediation by R. Croce, 1993, in *Adapted Physical Activity Quarterly, 10,* p. 206. Copyright 1993 by Human Kinetics Books. Adapted with permission.

4. The following approaches focus on incorporating tactile, proprioceptive, and sequential motor planning variables and developing a visual and verbal reference for the action plan (Hagen, 1987). Croce (1993) has elaborated on these strategies with specific recommendations for enhancing learning according to a motor learning approach. For example,

To increase conscious awareness of sensorimotor planning and execution, have the child:

- cognitively analyze sensorimotor task components. Provide sensory motor experiences and tasks from which the child can benefit, and involve the child in determining the movement experiences that could be beneficial to him or her. Such activities might include having the child think through and talk about the experiences in which he or she will engage for the specific session.

- predict the sensorimotor elements necessary to produce the intended action. For example, you might have the child tell you how far or fast he or she will ride on a scooter to accomplish a certain movement goal.

- monitor tactile, proprioceptive, and visual feedback as the child attempts the motor response. Provide augmented feedback about the goal and/or specify the feedback in the specific situation. Have the child give feedback about his or her performance. Ask the child, for example, "Did it feel right? Did you see what you did? Was that what you planned to do?"

- analyze feedback in relation to the predicted sensorimotor response. Have the child elaborate on the feedback from the planned action and whether it matched the expected consequences. For example, "Did the beanbag hit the target? If not, why not?"

- make adjustments to the response on the basis of feedback. In this case, have the child think about and verbalize the changes that he or she will make in the next attempt at the goal in order to be successful.

To establish the learned sensory reference of correctness for the motor behavior, have the child:

- establish a visual-verbal referent for the target behavior. Demonstrate or verbalize to the child about the expected action so that the child has the goal in mind.

- establish the ability to assume a position on the basis of the visual-verbal reference pattern. Have the child practice the expected action sequence while you give feedback.

- increase his or her ability to use the visual-verbal reference pattern cognitively to initiate and control the behavior. For example, have the child visualize the expected action sequence, then mentally practice or verbalize it prior to initiating the action.

- facilitate the ability to produce the target behavior volitionally. Give the child multiple opportunities in different situations to produce the target behavior.

To establish and increase the individual's ability to assume a targeted position or goal-directed motor behavior based on a visual-verbal reference pattern, have the child:

- increase the ability to identify a visual representation of the target on the basis of verbal referents. In this case, give the child visual opportunities to select the behavior based on verbal descriptions. Use picture cards of action sequences matched to verbal descriptions.

- develop a cognitive basis from which to attempt to facilitate purposeful gestural movements. Provide the child with ample opportunities to use gestures to describe meaningful situations or to mime.

- increase his or her cognitive ability to use a visual and verbal reference. Give the child opportunities to imitate or describe how to act, and also to recall these experiences.

- initiate and control movement by focusing on child-centered therapy. Allow the child to direct his or her session as much as possible, and structure the environment to elicit adaptive responses from the child.

To form relationships among the goal, the initial condition, the outcome, and the response specification (schema development), have the child practice under variable conditions and demands, and use appropriate feedback and physical guidance. This will help skill learning, retention, and transfer.

- Incorporate the child's goals as essential to intervention. It is important to practice and learn what is most important to the child for a successful therapy outcome.

- To help a child learn rules and use of contextual cues, point out rules and similarities, and help the child think through the situation and problem solve his or her movements in space (Goodgold-Edwards & Cermak, 1990).

- Provide feedback about the consequences of the child's actions as well as the success of the actions.

- Use attention-reducing or -enhancing environments so the child can attend more effectively to the learning process as well as filter and abstract the necessary information to motor plan.

- Provide increasing environmental demands on memory for actions, because all forms of memory functions are important to motor planning. Encourage the child to rehearse verbally what he or she is to do, and have the child recall how the action felt.

- In skill building, provide a model at first, but then allow the child to recall the action plan in the same and different contexts.

- Always center the intervention on purposeful, meaningful, and child-centered activity that maximizes the use of the environment, the task, and the child's goal-directed movements.

- Establish specific goals with the child, and use these to gauge successful intervention outcomes.

Most of these recommendations encourage the child to participate more actively in the session and encourage therapists to structure sessions so those children with motor planning difficulties can use different strategies to maximize the learning experience. The emphasis here is on variety of movement experiences, as well as more conscious awareness from the therapist and the child about movement planning. Movement learning is a process that entails more than integration of sensory information. These more conscious aspects of movement learning can compliment a sensory integrative approach during the intervention process. With children who have other disabilities, it is also important to remember that their specific pathology might limit optimal performance and that compensatory strategies might also be helpful to maximize functioning.

Summary

Developmental dyspraxia is the inability to execute nonhabitual movements. A.J. Ayres defined this disorder in the 1960s and devised occupational therapy interventions based on a sensory integration approach. This chapter presented current knowledge on this topic in the motor learning area to elaborate on this movement dysfunction and to shed some light on this problem in children with developmental disabilities.

This chapter also presented an information-processing account of skilled action and reviewed research pertinent to this model in children with clumsiness and children with Down syndrome. Research suggests that differences in cerebral organization and cerebral responsiveness contribute more to the specific motor planning difficulties in children with Down syndrome than in children with comparable mental delays. The information-processing model takes into account the role of sensory information in both the learning and the planning of goal-directed movements. Application of this model, along with understanding of how sensory integration is important to movement, can support more effective interventions with children who have motor planning problems.

The chapter reviewed possible interventions for children with dyspraxia based on prevailing theoretical accounts and current research. Because minimal information exists on this problem in children with developmental disabilities, investigation in this area is important. Further research with children with developmental disabilities and motor planning problems can increase the knowledge about the different disorders and enhance understanding of dyspraxia, as in the research with children who have Down syndrome. It is more than likely that continuing research into a variety of disorders (such as attention-deficit disorders, Autistic Disorder, cerebral palsy, and spina bifida) will expand the knowledge of movement and planning disorders in atypical populations as well as children who are developing typically.

References

American Psychiatric Association. (1994). Category 315.40. Developmental Coordination Disorder. *Diagnostic and statistical manual of mental disorders* (4th ed. Revised), 53–55. Washington, DC: Author.

Anwar, F. (1981). Motor function in Down's syndrome. In N.R. Ellis (Ed.), *International review of research in mental retardation: Vol. 10*. New York: Academic Press.

Ayres, A.J. (1972). *Sensory integration and learning disorders*. Los Angeles: Western Psychological Services.

Ayres, A.J. (1985). *Developmental dyspraxia and adult-onset apraxia*. Torrance, CA: Sensory Integration International.

Ayres, A.J. (1989). *Sensory Integration and Praxis Tests*. Los Angeles: Western Psychological Services.

Bairstow, P.J., & Laszlo, J.I. (1981). Kinaesthetic sensitivity to passive movements and its relationship to motor development and motor control. *Developmental Medicine and Child Neurology, 23*, 606–616.

Blanche, E.I. (1998). Intervention for motor control and movement organization disorders. In J. Case-Smith (Ed.), *Pediatric occupational therapy and early intervention* (pp. 255–276). Boston: Butterworth-Heinemann.

Cermak, S. (1985). Developmental dyspraxia. In E.A. Roy (Ed.), *Neuropsychological studies of apraxia and related disorders* (pp. 225–248). Amsterdam: North Holland.

Conrad, K.E., Cermak, S.A., & Drake, C. (1983). Differentiation of praxis among children. *American Journal of Occupational Therapy, 37*, 466–474.

Croce, R. (1993). A review of the neural basis of apractic disorders with implications for remediation. *Adapted Physical Activity Quarterly, 10*, 173–215.

Damiano, D. (1993). Reviewing muscle contraction: Is it a developmental, pathological or a motor control issue? *Physical and Occupational Therapy in Pediatrics, 12*(4), 3–20.

Denckla, M.B. (1984). Developmental dyspraxia: The clumsy child. In M.D. Levine & P. Saltz (Eds.), *Middle childhood: Development and dysfunction* (pp. 729–741). Baltimore: University Park Press.

De Renzi, E., & Lucchelli, F. (1988). Ideational apraxia. *Brain, 111*, 1173–1185.

Doyle, A.J.R., Elliott, J.M., & Connolly, K.J. (1986). Measurement of kinaesthetic sensitivity. *Developmental Medicine and Child Neurology, 28*, 188–193.

Elliott, D. (1985). Manual asymmetries in the performance of sequential movement by adolescents and adults with Down's syndrome. *American Journal of Mental Deficiency, 90*(1), 90–97.

Elliott, D., Edwards, J.M., Weeks, D.J., Lindley, S., & Carnahan, H. (1987). Cerebral specialization in young adults with Down's syndrome. *American Journal of Mental Deficiency, 91*(5), 480–485.

Elliott, D., Gray, S., & Weeks, D.J. (1991). Verbal cuing and motor skill acquisition for adults with Down's syndrome. *Adapted Physical Activity Quarterly, 8*, 210–220.

Elliott, D., & Weeks, D.J. (1990). Cerebral specialization and the control of oral and limb movements for individuals with Down's syndrome. *Journal of Motor Behavior, 22*(1), 6–18.

Elliott, D., & Weeks, D.J. (1993a). Cerebral specialization for speech perception and movement organization in adults with Down's syndrome. *Cortex, 29*, 103–113.

Elliott, D., & Weeks, D.J. (1993b). A functional systems approach to movement pathology. *Adapted Physical Activity Quarterly, 10*, 312–323.

Elliott, D., Weeks, D.J., & Elliott, C.L. (1987). Cerebral specialization in individuals with Down's syndrome. *American Journal of Mental Retardation, 92*(3), 263–271.

Elliott, D., Weeks, D.J., & Gray, S. (1990). Manual and oral praxis in adults with Down's syndrome. *Neuropsychologia, 28*(12), 1307–1315.

Elliott, D., Weeks, D.J., & Jones, R. (1986). Lateral asymmetries in finger-tapping by adolescents and young adults with Down syndrome. *American Journal of Mental Deficiency, 90*(4), 472–475.

Fisher, A., Bundy, A., & Murray. E. (1991). *Sensory integration: Theory and practice.* Philadelphia: F.A. Davis

Geuze, R.H., & Kalverboer, A.F. (1987). Inconsistency and adaptation in timing of clumsy children. *Journal of Human Movement Studies, 13,* 421–432.

Giuffrida, C. (1998). Motor learning: An emerging frame of reference for occupational performance. In M.E. Neistadt & E.B. Crepeau (Eds.), *Willard & Spackman's occupational therapy* (9th ed., pp. 560–565). Philadelphia: Lippincott-Raven.

Goodgold-Edwards S., & Cermak, S. (1990). Integrating motor control and motor learning concepts with neuropsychological perspectives on apraxia and developmental dyspraxia. *American Journal of Occupational Therapy, 55*(5), 431–439.

Gubbay, S.S. (1975). *The clumsy child: A study of developmental apraxic and agnosic ataxia.* London: W. B. Saunders.

Gubbay, S.S., Ellis, E., Walton, J.N., & Court, S.D.M. (1965). Clumsy children: A study of apraxic and agnosic deficits in 21 children. *Brain, 88,* 295–312.

Hagen, C. (1987). An approach to the treatment of mild to moderately severe apraxia. *Topics in Language Disorders, 8,* 35–40.

Haugen, J.B., & Mathiowetz, V. (1995). Contemporary task-oriented approach. In C.A. Trombly (Ed.), *Occupational therapy for physical dysfunction* (pp. 510–527). Baltimore: Williams and Wilkins.

Hecaen, H., & Rondot, P. (1985). Apraxia as a disorder of a system of signs. In E.A. Roy (Ed.), *Studies of apraxia and related disorders* (pp. 75–97). Amsterdam: North-Holland Elsevier.

Henderson, S.E., Morris, J., & Frith, U. (1981). The motor deficit in Down's syndrome children: A problem of timing? *Journal of Child Psychology and Psychiatry, 22*(3), 233–245.

Henderson, L., Rose, P., & Henderson, S. (1992). Reaction time and movement time in children with a developmental coordination disorder. *Journal of Child Psychology and Psychiatry, 33*(5), 895–905.

Hoare, D., & Larkin, D. (1991). Kinaesthetic abilities of clumsy children. *Developmental Medicine and Child Neurology, 33,* 671–678.

Hulme, C., Biggerstaff, A., Moran, G., & McKinley, I. (1982) Visual, kinaesthetic and cross-modal judgments of length by normal and clumsy children. *Developmental Medicine and Child Neurology, 24,* 461–467.

Hulme, C., & Lord, R. (1986). Clumsy children—A review of recent research. *Child: Care, Health and Development, 12,* 257–269.

Jarus, T., & Gol, K. (1995). The effect of kinesthetic stimulation on the acquisition and retention of a gross motor skill by children with and without sensory integration disorders. *Physical and Occupational Therapy in Pediatrics, 14*(3/4), 59–73.

Keele, S.W. (1968). Movement control in skilled motor performance. *Psychological Bulletin, 70,* 387–403.

Larkin, D., & Hoare, D. (1992). The movement approach: A window to understanding the clumsy child. In J. J. Summers (Ed.), *Approaches to the study of motor control and learning* (pp. 413–419). Amsterdam: Elsevier Science Publishers.

Light, K. (1991). Information processing for motor performance in aging adults. In J. Rothstein (Ed.), *Movement Science* (pp. 68–75). Alexandria, VA: American Physical Therapy Association.

Lincoln, A.J., Courchesne, E., Kilman, B.A., & Galambos, R. (1985). Neuropsychological correlates of information-processing by children with Down syndrome. *American Journal of Mental Deficiency, 89*(4), 403–414.

Lord, R., & Hulme, C. (1987a). Kinaesthetic sensitivity of normal and clumsy children. *Developmental Medicine and Child Neurology, 29,* 720–725.

Lord, R., & Hulme, C. (1987b). Perceptual judgments of normal and clumsy children. *Developmental Medicine and Child Neurology, 29,* 250–257.

Lord, R., & Hulme, C. (1988). Patterns of rotary pursuit performance in clumsy and normal children. *Journal of Child Psychology and Psychiatry, 29*(5), 691–701.

Luria, A.R. (1961). *The role of speech in the regulation of normal and abnormal behavior.* London: Pergamon Press.

Luria, A.R. (1973). *The working brain.* New York: Basic Books.

McConnell, D. (1995). Processes underlying clumsiness: A review of perspectives. *Physical and Occupational Therapy in Pediatrics, 15*(3), 33–52.

Missiuna, C., & Polatajko, H. (1995). Developmental dyspraxia by any other name: Are they just clumsy children? *The American Journal of Occupational Therapy, 49,* 619–627.

Miyahara, M., & Mobs, I. (1995). Developmental dyspraxia and developmental coordination disorder. *Neuropsychology Review, 5*(4), 245–268.

Morris, M. K. (1997). Developmental dyspraxia. In L.J.G. Rothi & K.M. Heilman (Eds.), *Apraxia: The neuropsychology of action* (pp. 245–269). East Sussex, UK: Psychology Press.

Mulder, T. (1991). A process-oriented model of human motor behavior: Toward a theory-based rehabilitation approach. In J. Rothstein (Ed.), *Movement Science* (pp. 198–207). Alexandria, VA: American Physical Therapy Association.

Murray, E., Cermak, S., & O'Brien, V. (1989). The relationship between form and space perception, constructional abilities and clumsiness in children. *American Journal of Occupational therapy, 44,* 623–627.

O'Brien V., Cermak, S., & Murray, E. (1988). The relationship between visual perception motor abilities and clumsiness in children with and without learning disabilities. *American Journal of Occupational Therapy, 42,* 359–363.

Paillard, J. (1982). Apraxia and the neurophysiology of motor control. *Philosophical Transactions of the Royal Society, B298,* 111–134.

Poeck, K. (1985). Clues to the nature of disruptions to limb praxis. In E.A. Roy (Ed.), *Neuropsychological studies of apraxia and related disorders* (pp. 99–109). Amsterdam: North-Holland.

Polatajko, H., Fox, A.M., & Missiuna, C. (1995). An international consensus on children with developmental coordination disorder. *Canadian Journal of Occupational Therapy, 62*(1), 3–6.

Rosenbaum, D. (1991). *Human motor control.* San Diego, CA: Academic Press Limited.

Rothi, G.L., & Heilman, K. (Eds.). (1997). *Apraxia: The neuropsychology of action.* United Kingdom: Psychology Press.

Roy, E.A., & Square, P.A. (1985). Common consideration in the study of limb, verbal and oral apraxia. In E.A. Roy (Ed.), *Neuropsychological studies of apraxia and related disorders* (pp. 111–161). Amsterdam: North-Holland.

Schellekens, J.M.H., Scholten, C.A., & Kalverboer, A.F. (1983). Visually guided hand movements in children with minor neurological dysfunction: Response time and movement organization. *Journal of Child Psychology and Psychiatry, 24*(1), 89–102.

Schmidt, R. (1991). *Motor learning and performance.* Champaign, IL: Human Kinetics Books.

Schmidt, R., & Wrisberg, C. (2000). *Motor learning and performance* (2nd ed.). Champaign, IL: Human Kinetics Books.

Schwartz, M., & Buxbaum, L.J. (1997). Naturalistic action. In L.J.G. Rothi & K.M. Heilman (Eds.), *Apraxia: The neuropsychology of action* (pp. 269–287). East Sussex, UK: Psychology Press.

Sellers, J.H. (1995). Clumsiness: Review of causes, treatments, and outlook. *Physical and Occupational Therapy in Pediatrics, 15*(4), 39–55.

Sigmundsson, H., Ingvaldsen, R.P., & Whiting, H.T.A. (1997). Inter- and intrasensory modality matching in children with hand-eye coordination problems: Exploring the developmental lag hypothesis. *Developmental Medicine and Child Neurology, 39,* 790–796.

Smyth, R.R., & Glencross, D.J. (1986). Information processing deficits in clumsy children. *Australian Journal of Psychology, 38*(1), 13–22.

Smythe, T.R. (1991). Abnormal clumsiness in children: A defect of motor programming? *Child: Care, Health and Development, 17,* 283–294.

Squires, N.K., Galbraith, G.C., & Aine, C.J. (1979). Event-related potential assessment of sensory and cognitive defects in the mentally retarded. In D.H. Lehmann & E. Callaway (Eds.), *Human evoked potentials* (pp. 397–413). New York: Plenum

Stott, D.H., Moyes, F.A., & Henderson, S.F. (1984). *The Henderson Revision of the Test of Motor Impairment.* San Antonio, TX: The Psychological Corporation.

Van Dellen, T., & Geuze, R.H. (1988). Motor response processing in clumsy children. *Journal of Child Psychology and Psychiatry, 29*(4), 489–500.

Van der Meulen, J.H.P., Denier van der Gon, J.J., Gielen, C.C.A.M., Gooskens, R.H.J.M., & Willemse, J. (1991). Visuomotor performance of normal and clumsy children in fast goal-directed arm-movements with and without visual feedback. *Developmental Medicine and Child Neurology, 33,* 40–54.

Vereijken B., Whiting, H.T.A., Newell, K.M., & von Emerick, R.E.A. (1982). Free(z)ing degrees of freedom in skill acquisition. *Journal of Motor Behavior, 24,* 133–142.

Willoughby, C., & Polatajko, H. (1995). Motor problems in children with developmental coordination disorder. *American Journal of Occupational Therapy, 49*(8), 787–793.

World Health Organization. (1992). *The ICD-10 classification of mental and behavioural disorders. Clinical descriptions and diagnostic guidelines.* Geneva, Switzerland: Author.

A Theoretical Model of Ideation in Praxis

Teresa A. May-Benson, M.S., OTR/L

Therapists working in the area of sensory integration routinely work with children who have motor planning or praxis problems. Within this population, therapists often identify a subgroup of children who appear to have particular difficulties with knowing what to do or how to conceptualize what to do with objects in their environment. Ayres (1985) referred to this difficulty in knowing "what to do" as a problem with ideation. These children often stand out from other children with motor planning problems in their inability to come up with play ideas or to determine goals for motor activities. These children often stand and watch others, sometimes refuse to participate in play, and tend to be followers. They often are "bored" and unable to play alone without an adult directing their interactions with objects. There is a marked lack of variation in their play, because they tend to use all toys in similar ways. When asked, "What do you want to do today?" or "What can you do with this toy?" they typically respond, "I don't know!" Ayres believed these children to be especially impulsive, distracted, and overactive. They also tend to be disorganized, lack persistence with tasks, and become easily upset by failure. In contrast, a child with motor planning problems but adequate ideation is able to identify ideas and goals for play but is unable to organize a motor plan to achieve that goal. In summary, the child with ideational problems has difficulty identifying new or unfamiliar goals for object interactions.

Clinicians typically face many obstacles in identifying, assessing, and treating these children with ideation problems because of the difficulties in separating problems in ideation from problems in motor planning. Ayres stated, "the lack of a firmly established, clear definition of praxis with unanimity of opinion indicates that this human function is not well understood and that its disturbance has not attracted much attention from the health professions" (1985, p. 8). This lack of a well-defined theoretical basis to understanding praxis in general and the ideational aspect of praxis in particular makes assessment and treatment of ideation problems, as distinct from motor planning problems, particularly difficult. To date, investigators have not been able to define adequately or research extensively the concept of ideation as a separate process from motor planning. Therefore, the purpose of this chapter is to explore the concept of ideation as a specific component of praxis, develop a working definition of ideation, examine the neurological and neurophysiological contributions to ideation, and provide a model of the construct of ideation within the praxis framework.

Researchers traditionally have examined difficulties in action performance in children and adults from different perspectives, including motor control theories, dynamic systems theory, and neuropsychological models of praxis. Although all of these perspectives contribute to the larger picture, this chapter focuses on action performance from neuropsychological perspectives and models of praxis because this is the framework that pediatric occupational therapists use most often. Ayres described praxis within this framework as the process or "ability of the brain to conceive of, organize, and carry out a sequence of unfamiliar actions" (1979, p. 183) and further specified that "when a motor pattern . . . becomes habitual, it no longer requires motor planning nor does it reflect skill in praxis" (1973, p. 170). This description specified that praxis is a process that occurs when action performance involves conceptualization of an act, organization of the motor components, and execution of a sequence of nonhabitual or nonlearned actions. Further, Paillard (1982) identified praxis as "the operations that intervene between the mental representation that a subject has of his body and the physical world that surrounds it, and the intentional triggering of an appropriate act as directed within the framework of that reality" (p. 112). Consequently, praxis is the framework one uses when examining action performance as a process involving person-environment interaction that includes the conceptualization of a mental representation of both the person and the physical world, identification of goals for that interaction, organization of a plan to attain the goal, and the actual motor execution of the actions (see Figure 9.1). To date, the praxis literature in occupational therapy has focused primarily on the motor planning and execution aspects of action performance, and although occupational therapists routinely state the importance of ideation as a part of the praxis process (Ayres, 1985; Cermak, 1991; Kimball, 1993), the ideational or conceptualization aspect of performing intentional actions as a part of praxis has received minimal attention.

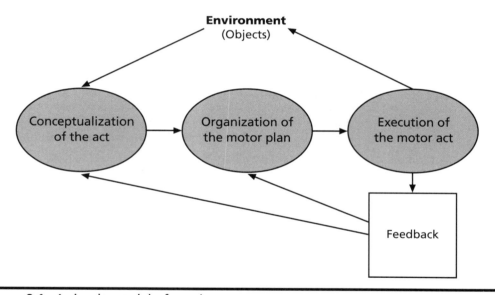

Figure 9.1. A simple model of praxis

Defining Ideation

The lack of a concise definition of ideation limits the occupational therapist's understanding of this process in children. No clear definition of ideation is presently available in the dyspraxia literature. *Webster's College Dictionary* (Random House, 1995, p. 667) broadly defines an *idea* as "any conception existing in the mind as a result of mental understanding, awareness or activity; a thought, conception or notion; a plan of action, intention; a concept developed by the mind; a mental image." *Ideation* and *ideate* refer to the formation of the idea or conception. The psychological and neuropsychological literature examines these specific concepts of mental image, conceptualization, intention, and so forth, as different constructs, making it difficult to obtain a clear understanding of ideation. However, there is clearly a relationship between these terms and the conceptualization of ideation as a part of praxis. This definition suggests that an idea involves selection of a goal for action but is a more complex representation of that action than just identification of the final static end-point of the action.

Within the occupational therapy literature, Ayres (1985) described ideation and emphasized its dynamic nature, stating that

> [I]deation or conceptualization is central to the theory of dyspraxia. . . . [It] is a cognitive or thinking process. Before one can engage purposefully or adaptively with a physical object, large or small, one must first have the concept of possible person-object interaction and some idea as to what might take place during that interaction. . . . Ideational praxis is an essential skill underlying all use of objects to obtain a goal that may or may not be independent of the objects. It includes all tool use. . . . (p. 20)

Although Ayres did not provide a clear definition of ideational praxis, she specified ideation as being a process particularly linked to interaction with the environment and specifically identified the relationship of this process to object or tool use and goal attainment.

The occupational therapy literature often describes children with ideational difficulties (Ayres, 1985; Cermak, 1985, 1991), but except for one study by physicians Deuel and Doar (1992), no formal study has examined the possibility of ideational deficits in children. Clinically, occupational therapists have described children with ideational deficits as not recognizing play opportunities with objects. Such children tend to use equipment in simplified ways and often do not participate until they watch others interact with the objects in the environment. These children also break toys often through inappropriate use (Ayres, 1985; Cermak, 1985, 1991). Ayres (1985) subsequently hypothesized that children with ideational deficits have difficulty identifying possible appropriate interactions with objects in their environment.

Ideation in Adult-Onset Apraxia and its Relation to Dyspraxia in Children

In contrast to the lack of information on ideation in the dyspraxia literature, clinicians have recognized ideational deficits in adult populations with brain injury since the early part of this century. Hugo Liepmann specifically discussed deficits in ideation in his original works on apraxia in adults. He proposed that voluntary actions were the direct result of mental ideas of the movement and the motor response those ideas evoked. He believed that environmental stimuli evoked visual and kinesthetic "engrams" or "memory images" to be used in the formation of these motor ideas. He also proposed that the *idea* consisted of the purpose (or goal) of the action and of possible ways of performing the action (cited in Luria, 1966). Therefore, he viewed an *idea* as a gestalt image of a desired action that encompassed a global purpose as well as an undefined sense of various possibilities for achieving that goal. The *motor plan* involved the selection and ordering of one specific set of actions ultimately identified for the completion of the desired idea. *Motor execution* then entailed the selection and ordering of specific muscle and joint movements necessary to carry out the identified motor plan.

Based on this viewpoint, Liepmann identified three forms of apraxic disturbance in adults: *limb-kinetic, ideomotor,* and *ideational apraxias.* Investigators have generally accepted these three classifications over the years, with various modifications and specifications proposed by various researchers. *Limb-kinetic apraxia* refers to a deficit in the ability to program the individual joint and muscle movements within a motor plan and represents a deficit in motor execution. *Ideomotor apraxia* refers to a deficit in the ordering or planning of the movements within an action and, although rarely referred to as such in the adult literature, likely represents a deficit in motor planning. *Ideational apraxia* is a deficit in the ability to conceptualize the idea of a gestalt action involving objects, evidenced in activities that involve the visualization of the interactions among multiple actions and objects to achieve a goal (see Table 9.1). For example, ideational apraxia in the activity of mailing a letter could appear as an inability to fold the paper, put it in an envelope, seal the envelope, and stamp the letter in the correct order, using the objects correctly (e.g., putting the letter, not the stamp, in the envelope). The individual is unable to conceptualize the activity of mailing the letter as a whole. The person can motor plan individual components, such as placing the paper in the envelope, but might not fold it first. This individual has lost the gestalt idea of actions necessary to reach a goal. As a result, congruent with Ayres' (1985) description of ideational problems in children, clinicians viewed ideational apraxia in adults to be a deficit in the ability to identify possible appropriate interactions with objects and possible appropriate means of achieving the desired goal.

Poeck (1982, 1983, 1985, 1986) particularly supported the view of ideational apraxia as a deficit in the ability to conceptualize the interactions of multiple objects in adults. He stated that ideational apraxia is a disturbance in the conceptual organization of a movement, characterized by an impairment in carrying out sequences of actions requiring the use of multiple objects in the correct order necessary to achieve an intended purpose. He identified the ability to conceptualize appropriate interactions and use among *multiple* objects as an important part of ideation. In contrast to Poeck, De Renzi and colleagues (De Renzi, 1985; De Renzi, Pieczuro, & Vignolo, 1968) identified ideational apraxia as a fundamental "agnosia of object use" or lack of knowledge of object use that was evident in the use of either *single* or *multiple* objects.

Roy and colleagues (Roy, 1978, 1982, 1983; Roy, Elliot, Dewey, & Square-Storer, 1990; Roy & Square, 1985) further identified the role of object use in ideation and conceptualization of actions. In contrast to Liepmann's traditional view of apraxia (cited in Luria, 1966), Roy and colleagues proposed that apraxia consists of deficits in *production* of actions and deficits in *conceptualization* of actions (with two distinct types of conceptual deficits). Production apraxia includes deficits in the execution of the motor act. Conceptual apraxia, however, is a deficit in the abstract knowledge of aspects of object/tool and action interactions. The first type of conceptual apraxia is a primary planning apraxia involving specific deficits in the spatial understanding of actions. The second type of conceptual apraxia is a secondary planning apraxia with deficits in sequencing the components of the gestalt plan. The researchers believed that conceptual apraxias require knowledge of objects'/tools' properties or affordances and the potential actions that could be used on the object as well as the knowledge of various actions that might utilize specific object properties. For example, knowledge of object properties that could be acted upon manifests in the recognition of the solid property of a wooden stool to stand upon versus the unstable property of a rocking chair. Knowledge of actions that could be used on various object properties evidences itself in a child's play when the child encounters an empty box. The child might climb in the box, turn it around, sit in it, throw it, or climb on it. In addition, conceptualization requires knowledge of the serial order of actions needed to interact with objects appropriately. For example, one must hold a hammer by the handle (not the head) and move it up and down with precision to drive a nail into a board.

In recent years, Heilman and colleagues (Heilman, Maher, Greenwald, & Rothi, 1997; Ochipa, Rothi, & Heilman, 1997) have expanded and modified Roy's typology. In this model, deficits in the production system include problems integrating and interpreting

Table 9.1. Comparison of Terminology in Adult Apraxia and Dyspraxia

Apraxia	Dyspraxia
Ideational Apraxia	**Ideation**
A disorder in conceptualization of a motor act in relationship to interactions with objects. (Involves the ability to conceptualize a goal and the action necessary to achieve that goal.)	The ability to conceptualize interactions with objects. (Involves the ability to identify a goal and some sense of how to achieve that goal.)
Example of Function: "I want to mail a letter. I need to fold the paper, put it into the envelope, seal it, and stamp it in order to mail the letter."	*Example of Function:* "I want to throw the ball into the basketball hoop."
Example of Dysfunction: Told to mail the letter, the adult does not know how to organize that process although the person knows all the components.	*Example of Dysfunction:* The child does not know what to do with the ball. Does not know that the ball can be thrown in the hoop.
Ideomotor Apraxia	**Motor Planning**
A disorder in the ability to sequentially order the motor elements of an act. (Involves the ability to sequence the motor action necessary to complete an action.)	The ability to plan or sequence a motor act. (Involves the ability to plan and order the actions necessary to achieve a goal.)
Example of Function: "To fold the paper, I need to reach out and grasp the bottom of the paper and bring it to the top."	*Example of Function:* "I will do a lay-up shot. I need to run to the right of the basket, jump up on one foot, raise my arm, and drop the ball in the basket."
Example of Dysfunction: The adult does not know how to sequence body movements to complete the action. The person reaches into the air before grasping the paper to fold it over.	*Example of Dysfunction:* The child does not know how to approach the basket or what position the body should be in to make the shot.
Limb-Kinetic Apraxia	**Motor Execution**
A disorder in the motor programming of motor movements. (Involves the programming of joint angles, muscle tension, force needed, and limb positions to complete the motor plan.)	The ability to execute a motor plan. (Involves the programming of joint angles, muscle tension, force needed, and limb positions to complete the motor plan.)
Example of Function: "I need to reach out with my arm extended so far with my fingers held just so to grasp the paper for folding."	*Example of Function:* "I need to raise my arm so high, jump up with so much force in exactly this spot, and hold the ball just so."
Example of Dysfunction: The adult overshoots the edge of the paper and crumples the paper in the hand while trying to grasp the edge.	*Example of Dysfunction:* The child lifts arms only to shoulder height and slams the ball on the floor very hard.

spatial and temporal information for task performance. These investigators viewed deficits in the conceptual system as problems in knowledge of the mechanical function of tools and objects and proposed that conceptual apraxias occur in two areas, associative and mechanical. These researchers identified associative problems as relational deficits in tool-action or tool-object knowledge, similar to Roy's model described previously. However, mechanical problems involve demonstrating deficits in understanding the mechanical nature of problems and the nature of affordances that tools

Table 9.2. Views of Ideation in Adult-Onset Apraxia and Dyspraxia

Author	Contribution to Praxis Theory	Definition of Ideational Apraxia
Liepmann (cited in Luria, 1966)	Identified two types of deficits in apraxia: 1. Ideomotor: primary problem with gestures and imitation 2. Ideational: deficit in object use	Held that ideas included a purpose/goal and possible ways of performing the action to achieve goal Defined ideational apraxia as a deficit in the sequential use of an object
Poeck (1982, 1983, 1985, 1986)	Identified: 1. Ideomotor apraxia: Impaired selection of the elements which constitute a movement 2. Ideational apraxia: impaired sequencing of actions	Defined ideational apraxia as an impairment in carrying out sequences of actions requiring the use of various objects in the correct order necessary to achieve an intended purpose as a consequence of a disturbance in the conceptual organization (sequencing) of movements
De Renzi (1985); De Renzi et al. (1968)	Identified ideomotor and ideational apraxia	Defined ideational apraxia as the inability to demonstrate the use of actual single or multiple objects, fundamentally an "agnosia of use"

Roy & Square (1985)	Identified:
	1. Production apraxia
	2. Two types of conceptual apraxia:
	  a. Primary planning apraxia
	  b. Secondary planning apraxia
		Used the term conceptual apraxia to refer to a deficit in tool use including aspects of knowledge of objects, knowledge of actions and objects, and knowledge of serial order of actions

Heilman & Rothi (1993); Heilman, Maher, Greenwald, & Rothi (1997); Ochipa, Rothi, & Heilman (1989, 1992)	Identified conceptual and production aspects of praxis as described by Roy	Used the term ideational apraxia to refer to patients who could not sequence acts; used conceptual apraxia to describe a deficit in content errors in the actual use of objects
Cermak (1985)	Applied Roy's model of apraxia to children	Likened primary planning apraxia to ideational deficits

provide. This type of problem involves more associative and relational difficulties between recognizing object or tool properties as well as recognizing what type of interaction is necessary to solve a problem (e.g., knowledge that a screwdriver is the most appropriate tool for tightening a screw). This typology places a heavy emphasis on the ability to associate object qualities with actions appropriate for their use (see Table 9.2).

Cermak (1985) applied Roy's model of adult apraxia to children with dyspraxia. She likened developmental dyspraxia as defined by Ayres (1973, 1979) to the planning apraxia in Roy's model. She equated the dyspraxic child who is generally disorganized with Roy's primary planning apraxia. She compared the child with clumsiness related to poor perceptual skills and decreased body awareness to the secondary planning apraxia. Finally, she linked the incoordinated child who has no problems identifying or approaching a task to the executive apraxia. However, investigators have not researched this conceptualization of dyspraxia in children empirically. In addition, Cermak did not specify any problems with ideation, although the overall disorganization associated with the primary planning apraxia most fits the child with ideational difficulties.

Other research on dyspraxia has also recognized different types of praxis problems in children (Ayres, Mailloux, & Wendler, 1989; Cermak, Coster, & Drake, 1980; Conrad, Cermak, & Drake, 1983; Dewey & Kaplan, 1994); however, these studies have examined different subtypes of motor planning problems only and have not addressed ideational problems in the child with dyspraxia. To date, only one study (Deuel & Doar, 1992) has examined the possibility of ideational problems in children. This study utilized Liepmann's (cited in Luria, 1966) adult apraxia model of ideational and ideomotor apraxias with a population of children to identify problems in ideation and motor planning.

In summary, the adult-onset apraxia literature recognizes a dichotomy between conceptual or ideational deficits and motor production deficits, suggesting that deficits in ideation might be different from motor production problems. Investigators have also applied this conceptualization to children with dyspraxia. In adults with apraxia, ideational deficits typically appear as the inability to know how to achieve an identified goal in either novel or familiar tasks. These adults have difficulty completing familiar, everyday tasks such as preparing a cup of coffee or setting a table. In contrast, ideational problems in children most often appear as the inability to identify the goals for novel object interactions or action performance. These children are often able to perform familiar and routine activities adequately but are unable to find new ways of using toys or engaging in novel activities.

A Proposed Model of Ideation in Praxis

As mentioned previously, researchers have not examined ideation in children thoroughly, nor have they developed a codified/unified model of ideation within a praxis framework. The proposed model of ideation in praxis, represented pictorially in Figure 9.2, may serve as a framework for understanding the processes involved in the formation of ideas prior to performance of actions as well as the various internal and external influences on ideation. This model views ideation as a dynamic process that includes the function of determining an intentional global goal for action and the potential means for attaining that goal. In this model, an idea reflects the conceptualization of potential interactions of a person with objects or the environment. For a child, an idea might be, "I want to throw this ball into that hoop." The idea involves the goal of getting the ball in the hoop and a general sense of throwing the ball to achieve that goal. Motor planning requires selection of the specific means of throwing the ball accurately into the hoop.

Within the ideation process, the initiation of goal determination begins with an intentional process in response to internal or external stimuli. An idea results from a cognitive conscious awareness of the need for a goal-directed action. Intentional goals build from previous knowledge of actions and object functions. These two components form the basis for knowing which objects are appropriate for specific actions. In the basketball example, the child sees a basketball hoop, a basketball, and a baseball bat in the back yard. The hoop, ball, and bat provide external, environmental stimuli for action. There are internal stimuli in the form of a desire to play. The child uses previous knowledge to know that the ball, and not the bat, is for going through the hoop. This information then contributes to the idea of "I want to throw this ball into that hoop."

On a physiological level, determination of an intentional goal immediately and simultaneously generates a motor image of the desired goal. Production of the motor image of the specific goal leads to a simultaneous preparation of the postural sets and motor actions needed to achieve the intended goal. Generation of the motor image and

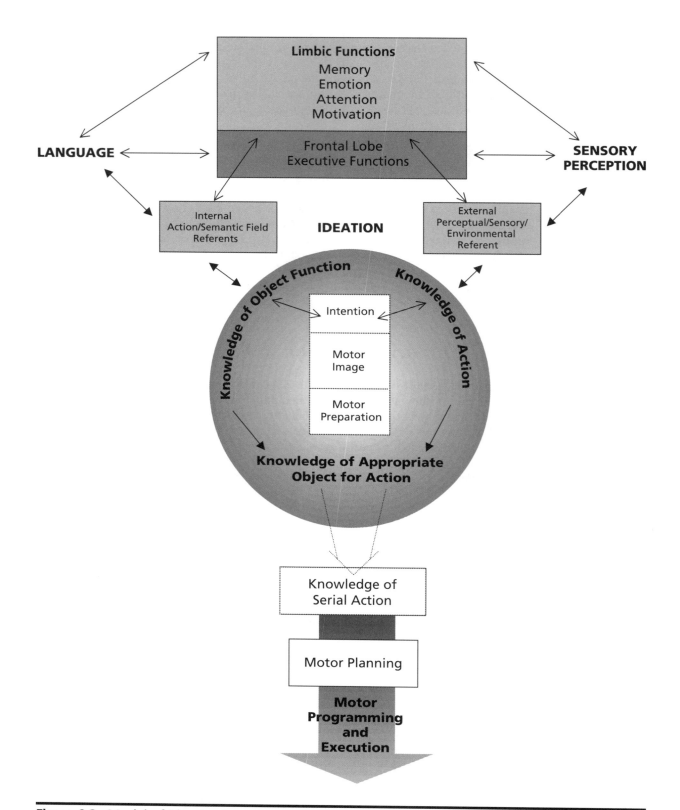

Figure 9.2. Model of ideation in action performance

preparatory motor sets feed into a general knowledge of possible action sequences that can lead to the desired goal. The process of ideation then moves into the process of motor planning, which selects and organizes a specific sequence of actions that are necessary to accomplish the intended goal. The process of motor programming of the specific limb movements then occurs for the execution of the action. As the individual executes the action, feedforward and feedback information contributes to changes in the immediate motor plan and can influence a change in the overall idea. In throwing a ball into a hoop, the child generates a motor image of him- or herself as a basketball star performing a flawless lay-up. The child motor plans a lay-up shot, but the execution is less graceful than that of the initial image. The child changes the motor plans to be more accurate, and the motor image of the idea of throwing the ball into the hoop becomes more realistic.

Ideation, particularly the development of intention, originates from external and internal influences or referents. External referents are perceptual, sensory, or environmental in nature and can influence and are influenced by cognitive executive functions, limbic functions, memories, attention, motivation, emotions, and so forth. Internal referents typically are language-based semantic inputs influenced by cognitive, executive, or limbic functions. This model, therefore, allows for two circuits for initiation of intentional actions, one driven by external environmental inputs such as object qualities, perceptions, and so forth, and the other by language and internal motivations and drives.

This is an integrated model that supports the concept of ideation as a process separate from motor planning and motor execution. This model views ideation as a process composed of intentions, motor images of goals, and preliminary motor preparations. Cognitive knowledge of object functions, actions, and appropriate objects for actions is necessary to form intentions and plans to achieve desired goals. External sensory perceptions are one foundational means of forming ideas for action plans. The environmental attributes or object affordances can provide a primary referent for ideation of actions. Internal language, thoughts, motivations, and so forth are another foundational means of forming ideas. The following sections examine and review the literature supporting the various components of this model.

Neuropsychological Basis of Ideation

Review of the research in adult apraxia, neuropsychology, and neurophysiology is useful in examining the role and manifestation of ideational problems in adults with apraxia and children with dyspraxia. The literature suggests that ideation of a motor action involves the development of an intention and a motor image of a desired goal or action. Bruner (1973) examined "intention" in relation to the organization of early skilled actions in children. He stated that early motor performance serves two basic purposes: interactions with others and mastery over tools and objects. According to Bruner, infants develop motor competence through intention, feedback, and various patterns of action that occur between these processes. Regarding the role of intention in motor development, he stated that intention begins as an initial internal physiological arousal state in infants, although he did not expand on the "origin" of intention. He proposed that, behaviorally, intention has a number of observable components, comprised of an anticipation of the outcome (or goal) of an act, a selection (or plan) of appropriate means to achieve the goal, a sustained "direction of behavior" during the act, a "stop order" occurring at the end of the act, and a means of adaptation of the act based on feedback during the act. This description is similar to the concept of praxis.

Bruner (1973) described the capacity for intention as being present at birth, although not fully developed. He stated that the constituent parts of a given act are initially ordered only loosely and do not develop into the appropriate temporal order without practice and feedback. Once well developed, these skills can then become the basis for more complex actions. Bruner added that certain "preadapted patterns of manipulatory activity" exist that can be evoked by vision alone, such as groping in response to a previously unmanipulated object. Bruner's model of action performance in infants involves the identification of an initial intentional "arousal state" that can arise from a variety of unknown internal mechanisms and possibly by some external stimuli such as vision. This "intentional" state in infants might be analogous to the "ideation" state in older children and adults.

In more recent years, Jeannerod (1994) proposed a model of action planning that stressed the role of motor intention and motor imagery in the representation of action goals in adults. According to Jeannerod, motor behavior consists of a representational part and an overt part, components that investigators can observe and describe separately. Jeannerod considered generation (or ideation) of motor actions to be driven by internal goal representations (or ideas) built from knowledge of and input from the environment. Object attributes can provide stimuli for internal representations when the objects are the goal of an action. For example, 3-year-old Harry has received a small package with a new toy inside. Struggling to remove the plastic wrapping, he looks around and immediately grabs a toy screwdriver lying among the other toys scattered about the floor. He then uses the screwdriver to open the package successfully. He is able to determine that the screwdriver has properties that will open the package, in contrast to the properties of the toy car or stuffed animal lying nearby. Action generation depends on a "pragmatic" or "practical" form of mental imagery or representation that varies from "semantic," consciously accessible forms of mental imaging. In other words, given a specific object or tool, the child will have greater ideation if he or she is able to imagine, "How might I use this object in this situation?" versus adhering strictly to "What is this object supposed to be used for?" In addition, according to Jeannerod, motor images are functionally inseparable from automatic motor preparations that occur when one intends to perform an action. For example, Kecia stands at the top of a platform looking at a large pile of pillows below her. "I'm going to jump," she shouts as she simultaneously and automatically crouches down, leans forward, flexes her arms, and tightens her muscles in preparation for jumping into the pile below her. The motor readiness to jump occurs instantaneously with the idea of jumping.

The work of Bruner (1973) and Jeannerod (1994) emphasized the need for an initial "intention" (or idea) prior to producing a motor action. Bruner proposed that intention in children is accompanied by an increased arousal state, and that formation of a global goal and plan of action is necessary for the execution of motor acts. Jeannerod in particular stressed the formation of a motor image of the gestalt action, contending that this image is functionally inseparable from physiological motor state preparations that occur upon construction of the motor image. According to these two authors, intention and motor image are integral to the concept of ideation.

The Role and Function of the Environment in Ideation

Many investigators have emphasized the role of the environment in ideation. Bruner (1973) and Jeannerod (1994) proposed that the qualities of objects in the environment can provide the external referents for motor images or intentions to act. Ayres (1985) stressed the role of the environment in her claim that "praxis is expressed in a manner which is dependent upon the environment invitation and demand. Praxis is context dependent and the physical environment elicits and determines the idea and the motor plan" (p. 6).

The Gibsons (J.J. Gibson, 1977; E.J. Gibson, 1970, 1982, 1988) advocated the role of the environment in ideation most clearly in their ecological model of motor performance. In the Gibsonian framework, objects possess particular attributes that, within the context of a given environment, invite or elicit interaction. Within this model, the environment drives ideation and the perceptual attributes of the environment provide the stimulus for action. As in Bruner's (1973) model, the ability to recognize and act on the affordances of the environment is present to some extent at a very early age and develops in complexity over time. The Gibsons considered this ability to be essential for the development of exploratory behaviors, perception, and acquisition of knowledge of the environment. Consequently, external referents or sensory inputs can drive or generate ideas for action performance. The qualities of objects or affordances themselves provide one means of generating ideation. In a sensory integration frame of reference, the ability to present environmental affordances at an appropriate level is a primary means of developing praxis. Accordingly, the clinician may use a bottom-up approach to treatment of ideational problems by structuring the environment and the objects within it to elicit desired actions from the child. For instance, setting up a "mountain" of large foam blocks with a desired toy at the top would facilitate the idea of climbing when the child entered the room. Using the inherent affordances of objects in the environment can contribute to the child's store of "pragmatic" uses of objects and contribute to the child's understanding of possible object-action interactions.

The Role and Function of Language in Ideation

The Gibsons (J.J. Gibson, 1977; E.J. Gibson, 1970, 1982, 1988) supported the role of external referents in the generation of ideas and motor actions; however, other researchers such as Luria (1966) and Ojemann (1982) have advocated for the importance of the roles of language and cognitive functions in the development of motor actions. Luria (1966) highlighted the importance of environmental stimuli but also emphasized the role of internal referents, particularly speech, as a primary, integral part of the production of voluntary motor actions. He described language as necessary for independent, goal-directed motor actions.

Ojemann (1982) and Ayres (1985) also stressed the close relationship of language functions and motor actions. Ojemann proposed that language and motor functions share many cortical brain structures and that damage to these sites results in deficits in language and action performance. He described common structures located not only in the cortex but also at the subcortical thalamic level. Ayres (1985) further supported this relationship between language and action, hypothesizing that ideation in praxis is associated closely with language functions. Like Luria, she questioned whether ideation is a general neurophysiological function that could subserve praxis as well as general behavioral organization. Clinically, she identified children with language problems as having the greatest difficulties with ideation. Therefore, language appears to have a connection with ideational processes, although the nature of this relationship is not clear at this time.

MacKay (1983, 1985) proposed a different theory of how actions are planned, represented in the brain, and produced as action sequences that might further the understanding of ideation in motor actions. He emphasized the relationship between cognitive knowledge of actions and motor knowledge (which involves the timing, force, and motor programming aspects of actions) in the development of motor actions. Like Luria and Ayres, he particularly stressed the role of language in the development of motor organization. He put forth a node model of cognitive and motor organization to address the cognitive aspects of motor performance. He posited that brain neurons are organized in functional units that he referred to as nodes. The nodes are organized hierarchically into various levels with interconnections between and within levels. Priming and linking nodes at the various levels activate motor actions as a result of internal and external inputs.

This model emphasized the top-down activation of motor nodes, with higher-level "mental" processes initiating the motor activation process. The mental nodes activate muscle movement nodes that in turn activate sensory analysis nodes; these then provide feedback to the mental nodes. These various node levels are organized into several systems that control action. The most relevant system to ideation in praxis is the pragmatic system that MacKay (1983, 1985) proposed to link language and action. MacKay suggested that this system is responsible for the function of integration of perception, speech, action, goal setting, rate setting, evaluative functions, and the determination of output mode. Within this system, "ideas" originate with global goals based on information from language and attitudinal processes and generate general action plans. MacKay postulated that ideational apraxia in adults could be the result of a disconnection of the action and speech systems or a disruption in the interactions of the sequencing nodes.

In conclusion, Luria, Ojemann, and Ayres supported the role and importance of language as a primary referent for ideation. MacKay also emphasized the role of language and proposed a functional model for this relationship. Although his model is a highly functionally oriented theory that does not attempt structural explanations, it does give some insight into the influence of cognitive and language processes on the development of goal-directed actions. Accordingly, the clinician may also use a top-down approach to facilitating ideation by using language to emphasize actions or object properties to encourage ideation. For instance, the clinician might help the child analyze a swing: "Sam, this swing is on stretchy cord. It goes up and down. What could we do with it?" or "Molly, look at the bolster swing. How many ways could we ride it?" Using a conscious, language-driven approach to expand and generalize the child's semantic knowledge of possible object-action interactions provides an additional avenue for ideation.

Neuroanatomical Basis of Ideation

Examination of the neuroanatomical and physiological information available regarding ideation, intention, and motor planning is helpful in identifying why, how, and what aspects of the praxis process are involved in ideation. The literature suggests that the brain structures receiving, organizing, and integrating information related to ideation fall within three primary categories: the sensorimotor areas, the frontal lobe, and the limbic system.

Sensorimotor Areas

The sensorimotor areas involve the primary sensory and motor strips just anterior and posterior to the central gyrus of the cerebral cortex. Luria (1966, 1973) identified this area, along with the parietal lobe and the frontal lobe of the brain, as being of primary importance in the organization, planning, and execution of actions. Within the parietal lobe, primary sensory areas 3, 2, and 1 receive direct sensory inputs from the environment and the periphery of the body. Association areas 5 and 7 integrate this sensory information and relate it to other information, previous actions, and so forth. The association areas, along with areas 39 and 40 (the angular gyrus and supramarginal gyrus) identify targets, select limb positions, and prepare the spatial orientation needed for actions based on the incoming sensory information. This information from the posterior parietal areas of 5, 7, 39, and 40 is vital in providing preplanning, target, and tactile/visual/spatial information necessary for goal-directed actions and the development of ideas.

The preprocessed and integrated information from the posterior parietal areas goes directly to a variety of prefrontal lobe structures, including the primary motor area for direct motor responses and the supplemental motor area (SMA) for further integration and motor planning. Corollary copies of the information travel to the basal ganglia and cerebellum for additional levels of motor processing. The SMA (the medial portion of area 6) is the primary area for the organization of motor actions. It is in the SMA that the gestalt motor image of an idea and the component movements for the motor plan develop. The arcuate premotor area, which forms the lateral portion of area 6, serves primarily a motor programming function, in contrast to the ideational and motor planning functions performed by the SMA. Accordingly, the SMA appears to be the primary structure responsible for the development and conceptualization of specific motor plans to achieve a goal (Ghez, 1991). From these findings, it is possible to hypothesize that much of what is called ideation (i.e., goal recognition and motor imaging of gestalt actions) occurs within the SMA.

The SMA, however, is also influenced by and receives inputs from many brain structures, including the prefrontal brain areas controlling executive functions such as regulation of behavior, long-term planning, and goal-directed behavior. Language processing areas 21 and 22 and sensory areas 3, 2, and 1 also project directly to this area, providing internal language and external sensory referents as well as feedforward and feedback information. Finally, there are indirect connections from the limbic system, particularly the anterior cingulate cortex, hippocampus, basal ganglia, and cerebellum that project through area 4 to this area and provide internal referents from memories, emotions, motivation, and so forth. In praxis, the SMA appears to serve as a center for the imaging of ideas and development of motor plans.

Classic studies by Roland, Larson, Lassen, and Skinhof (1980) corroborated these functional and structural divisions. Using cerebral blood flow studies, these investigators showed that when subjects performed simple motor acts not requiring motor planning (such as flexing and extending a finger), the primary sensory and primary motor areas were the only brain areas activated. Completing a simple novel sequential motor task, such as sequentially touching the thumb to fingers, activated the SMA and the primary motor areas, indicating that the SMA was necessary to plan the sequential motor task but not the simple motor act. Simply imagining or internally rehearsing the same task without motor execution activated only the SMA, pointing to the importance of the SMA in motor imaging. Asking subjects to complete a continuous motor task motorically, such as tracing a spiral pattern in the air with their index finger, activated both the SMA and premotor areas along with primary sensory and motor areas. This interaction suggests that the premotor area is necessary for executing continuous control of the movement based on external sensory feedback and feedforward mechanisms but that it is not necessary for discrete sequential movements, as in the previous task. Asking subjects to complete a complex maze task by moving their finger in specific directions to verbal commands required numerous brain areas, including the SMA, premotor area, language areas, frontal association areas, and primary sensory, primary motor, and posterior parietal association areas. This study and others like it (Sirigu et al., 1996) support the role of the SMA in the planning of novel motor actions. Simple, learned actions do not require the involvement of this brain structure. In addition, the activation of the SMA when subjects only imagined but did not perform motor actions substantiates the specific role of the SMA in ideation as a cognitive process.

It is therefore possible to conclude that the sensorimotor areas provide the primary neuroanatomical connections for the use of a bottom-up external referent approach to ideation.

Frontal Lobe

In addition to sensorimotor information, the SMA receives information from frontal lobe structures that influence the development and formation of ideas. Luria (1966, 1973) advocated the role of the executive functions of the frontal lobe in influencing conceptualization, proposing that the frontal lobe system is responsible for the organization and preservation of goal-directed action. According to Luria (1966), complex actions require a defined overall goal. The frontal lobe performs the functions of selecting movements related to the overall goal, allows verbal or conscious mediation of the act, and compares the results of the action with the original intention. Luria postulated that the intention for motor action develops in the frontal system with the aid of internal speech mechanisms and other incoming sensory inputs. He noted deficits in initiation and maintenance of goal-directed actions, often seen in children with ideation problems, in his patients with frontal lobe damage (1973), supporting the role of frontal lobe functions in ideation.

From Luria's perspective, the frontal lobe serves a largely regulatory function in initiating and sustaining the goal-directed action. It contributes to the identification of a goal but does not appear to have a role in the formation of motor images or the actual formation of specific action-related ideas. The functions of the frontal lobe are also connected intimately to the limbic system, which also contributes to initiation and goal identification. As a result, through frontal lobe connections, the clinician can facilitate ideation with conscious, cognitively-oriented approaches, especially those that are language-oriented.

Limbic System

Goldberg (1985) proposed a connection between the frontal lobe, motor actions, and the limbic system. His Premotor Concept Model hypothesized mechanisms for limbic influences on motor processes, suggesting that there is a dual structural and functional division in the premotor area of the prefrontal cortex that occurs during the formation of brain structures. He proposed that the SMA and the arcuate premotor area originate phylogenetically from different brain structures. This difference in origin allows for two pathways of influence for motor functions. According to this model, the arcuate premotor area originates from the insular lobe, specifically the piriform area, and deals with perception, recognition, and association of external stimuli, particularly responsive actions in relation to environmental feedback. Conversely, the model proposed that the SMA develops ontogenetically from the paralimbic cortex, specifically the anterior cingulate cortex and the hippocampus, and deals with generation of actions initiated by internal referents and inputs. This origination of the SMA from the paralimbic cortex affords a cortical connection with current limbic structures that might provide a means for limbic-controlled memory and emotions to influence ideation. This dual structural division of the premotor area supports the influence of both external and internal stimuli in ideation.

About the same time as Goldberg (1985), Brooks (1986) proposed a model of motor learning that further hypothesized limbic structural and functional connections in action performance. However, Brooks discussed issues of "insight" and motivation in relation to learning novel motor tasks that Goldberg did not address. Brooks proposed that the limbic system, particularly the amygdala and anterior cingulate gyrus, was vital in developing insight and motivation to purposive, intentional, skilled activity. In examining motor learning in monkeys, Brooks determined that monkeys became skillful at given motor tasks only after they had gained "insight" into the nature of the task. He stated that "learning to perform a task well requires an understanding of its nature. In other words, knowing *what* to do must precede learning *how* to do it. . ." (p. 30). This "knowing what to do" might be analogous to ideation or being able to conceptualize a given goal for an action. The learning "how to do it" corresponds to motor planning.

Brooks (1986) identified four components necessary for motor learning: motivation, insight into appropriate behavior, motor skill, and attention. The limbic and sensorimotor systems interact through direct and indirect circuits to determine what to do (insightful behavior) and how to do it best (motor skill). Like Goldberg (1985), Brooks proposed that the cortical premotor areas, particularly the supplementary motor area, receive various modulating inputs from a variety of limbic structures. The hippocampus and amygdala in the limbic system provide memory formations and attach affective meaning to the memories, with the amygdala playing an important role in providing relevance to the environmental context of actions. Influences from the hypothalamus, amygdala, and cingulate cortex drive motivation to action, especially related to searching for satisfaction of internal drives. "Creation of motivation" occurs possibly through convergence of limbic and nonlimbic inputs on the cerebral association areas, including the supplementary motor area (Brooks, 1986). The "insight" or "knowing" proposed by Brooks might be part of the ideational aspect of developing "ideas" of what to do in novel motor activities. Consequently, building memory stores of appropriate object-action interactions through experience, especially "affective" or presumably pleasurable experiences, can facilitate future "insight" and ideation.

In summary, numerous structures, processes, and functions participate in the generation of ideas (see Table 9.3). Neuroanatomical evidence corroborates the influence of sensory, language, executive, and limbic inputs on the supplemental motor area that might contribute to the development of global action ideas or conceptualizations. Accordingly, ideas and plans originating in the SMA are highly dependent on inputs from internal referents and structures as well as external inputs (Ghez, 1991). It is possible, then, that the foundations of ideation originate in executive, language, or limbic functions, However, it appears that a gestalt integration of these influences

Table 9.3. Summary of Neuroanatomical Correlates of Ideation

Brain Area	Function Related to Ideation
Parietal Lobe Primary Sensory Areas 3, 2, 1	Receives direct sensory inputs from the body and the environment
Sensory Association Areas 5, 7	Integrates multiple sensory inputs and serves as relay to other parts of the brain
Areas 39 and 40 (Angular Gyrus and Supra-Marginal Gyrus)	Identifies targets in the environment, selects limb positions, and prepares spatial orientations needed for actions
Premotor Area Area 6—medial portion (Supplemental Motor Area [SMA]) Area 6—lateral portion (Arcuate Premotor Area)	Receives feedforward inputs for execution of continuous motor movements Primary area for organization and motor planning of actions, especially complex tasks Proposed area for formation of motor images and ideas Performs motor programming functions for limb positions, trajectories, force, etc.
Frontal Lobe	Performs executive functions of identifying goals and initiating and maintaining task performance and attention
Limbic System Hypothalamus, Amygdala, and Cingulate Cortex Hippocampus and Amygdala	Provides insight and motivational influences to SMA and frontal areas Attaches emotional tone to memories and actions Provides relevance to environmental context of actions

with external inputs into an "idea" does not occur until all the various inputs reach the SMA. Therefore, this chapter proposes that an "idea" as a gestalt goal-directed motor image does not occur until the SMA, although language, prefrontal, limbic, and sensorimotor structures influence the formation of this image.

Figure 9.3 presents a model of the interrelationship of the functions and brain areas involved during the praxis processes of ideation, motor planning, and execution. Ideation as a process involves the functions of goal identification and development of global motor images that provide the basis for motor planning. The frontal and limbic lobes of the brain, along with language, provide internal referents to the SMA that contribute to the formation of concepts and plans. The actual planning and execution processes of praxis involve the functions of programming actions and ordering the motor elements necessary to complete actions. Motor planning of specific actions entails primarily the premotor area, with posterior parietal and SMA areas being more involved with increasingly complex tasks. This planning process then forms the foundation for motor production of the intended act. Motor production occurs mainly in the primary sensory and motor areas. This model might help clinicians better separate the individual components of the praxis process.

Conclusions and Clinical Applications

Given that the literature on praxis has paid little attention to the concept of ideation, this chapter has attempted to organize the information on ideation into a unified model. The model set forth in this chapter proposes that ideation, as a part of praxis and action performance, is a dynamic process that involves the identification of a motor goal, a gestalt motor image of possible means of achieving the desired action, and the concurrent physiological preparatory motor sets. This view of ideation requires the contributions of object-action and action-object knowledge in the formation of this process and includes language as an internal referent and the environment as an external referent through perception of object affordances.

Understanding the contributions of these various components to ideation can assist clinicians in better identifying and treating children with ideational difficulties. Using Figure 9.2 as a guide, clinicians have multiple avenues for facilitating ideation in their

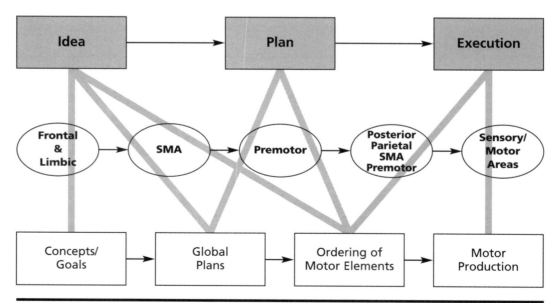

Figure 9.3.   Model of the relationship between praxis processes, functions, and structures.

clients. The therapist may use a bottom-up approach emphasizing external referents and affordances from the environment, utilizing such cues as, "Look, this ball is round. It's soft and it rolls. Is that a good thing to stand on? This stool is hard and it's stable. Is it a good thing to stand on?" The therapist may also use a more top-down, language-based approach to emphasize object-action interactions with cues such as, "Here is a ball, a stool, and a tire. What could you use to climb up on top of this clubhouse?" Or the therapist could emphasize possible actions for use with objects, such as, "Here is a hoop to play with. What are all the different things you could do with it? You could spin it like a top, swing it on your arm, put it over your head, or throw it like a flying saucer." Building a child's knowledge of potential uses for objects or functions of objects, possible actions that the child can use on a variety of objects, and how to combine various objects and actions through actual experience is vital to developing the memory stores necessary for ideational skills. Helping the child to recognize possible person-object-environment interactions is central to developing ideation. Facilitating generalization of specific object-action interactions is also particularly important in promoting ideation in novel situations.

Works Cited

Quotations on pages 163, 165, and 172 from *Developmental Dyspraxia and Adult-Onset Apraxia* by A.J. Ayres (1985) have been reprinted with permission by Sensory Integration International.

References

Ayres, A. (1973). *Sensory integration and learning disorders*. Los Angeles: Western Psychological Corporation.

Ayres, A. (1979). *Sensory integration and the child*. Los Angeles: Western Psychological Corporation.

Ayres, A. (1985). *Developmental dyspraxia and adult-onset apraxia*. Torrance, CA: Sensory Integration International.

Ayres, A., Mailloux, Z., & Wendler, C. (1989). Developmental dyspraxia: Is it a unitary function? *Occupational Therapy Journal of Research, 7*, 93–110.

Brooks, V. (1986). How does the limbic system assist motor learning? A limbic comparator hypothesis. *Brain Behavior Evolution, 29*, 29–53.

Bruner, J. (1973). Organization of early skilled action. *Child Development, 44*, 1–11.

Cermak, S. (1985). Developmental dyspraxia. In E. Roy (Ed.), *Advances in psychology: Vol. 23. Neuropsychological studies of apraxia* (pp. 225–248). New York: North-Holland.

Cermak, S. (1991). Somatodyspraxia. In A. Fisher, E. Murray, & A. Bundy, (Eds.), *Sensory integration: Theory and practice* (pp. 137–165). Philadelphia: F.A. Davis.

Cermak, S., Coster, W., & Drake, C. (1980). Representational and nonrepresentational gestures in boys with learning disabilities. *American Journal of Occupational Therapy, 34*, 19–26.

Conrad, K., Cermak, S., & Drake, C. (1983). Differentiation of praxis among children. *American Journal of Occupational Therapy, 37*, 466–473.

De Renzi, E. (1985). Methods of limb apraxia examination and their bearing on the interpretation of the disorder. In E.A. Roy (Ed.), *Neuropsychological studies of apraxia and related disorders* (pp. 45–64). New York: North-Holland.

De Renzi, E., Pieczuro, A., & Vignolo, L. (1968). Ideational apraxia: A quantitative study. *Neuropsychologia, 6*, 41–52.

Deuel, R., & Doar, B. (1992). Developmental manual dyspraxia: A lesson in mind and brain. *Journal of Child Neurology, 7*, 99–103.

Dewey, D., & Kaplan, B. (1994). Subtyping of developmental motor deficits. *Developmental Neuropsychology, 10*(3), 265–284.

Ghez, C. (1991). Voluntary movement. In E. Kandel, J. Schwartz, & T. Jessell (Eds.), *Principles of neural science* (pp. 609–625). Norwalk, CT: Appleton & Lange.

Gibson, E.J. (1970). The development of perception as an adaptive process. *American Scientist, 58,* 98–107.

Gibson, E.J. (1982). The concept of affordance in development: The renascence of functionalism. In W. Andrew Collins (Ed.), *The concept of development: The Minnesota symposia on child psychology: Vol. 15* (pp. 51–81). Hillsdale, NJ: Erlbaum.

Gibson, E.J. (1988). Exploratory behavior in the development of perceiving, acting and the acquiring of knowledge. *Annual Review of Psychology, 39,* 1–41.

Gibson, J.J. (1977). The theory of affordances. In R. Shaw & J. Bransford (Eds.), *Perceiving, acting, and knowing* (pp. 67–82). Hillsdale, NJ: Erlbaum.

Goldberg, G. (1985). Response and projection: A reinterpretation of the premotor concept. In E. Roy, (Ed.), *Advances in psychology: Vol. 23. Neuropsychological studies of apraxia* (pp. 251–266). New York: North-Holland.

Heilman, K., Maher, L., Greenwald, M., & Rothi, L. (1997). Conceptual apraxia from lateralized lesions. *Neurology, 49,* 457–464.

Heilman, K., & Rothi, L. (1993). Apraxia. In K. Heilman & E. Valenstein (Eds.), *Clinical neuropsychology* (pp. 141–163). New York: Oxford University Press.

Jeannerod, M. (1994). The representing brain: Neural correlates of motor intention and imagery. *Behavioral and Brain Sciences, 17,* 185–245.

Kimball, J.G. (1993). Sensory integrative frame of reference. In P. Kramer & J. Hinojosa (Eds.), *Frames of reference for pediatric occupational therapy* (pp. 87–167). Baltimore: Williams & Wilkins.

Luria, A. (1966). *Higher cortical functions in man.* New York: Basic Books.

Luria, A. (1973). *The working brain.* New York: Basic Books.

MacKay, D. (1983). A theory of the representation and enactment of intentions. In R. Magill, (Ed.), *Advances in psychology: Vol. 12. Memory and control of action* (pp. 217–229). New York: North-Holland.

MacKay, D. (1985). A theory of the representation, organization and timing of action with implications for sequencing disorders. In E. Roy, (Ed.), *Advances in psychology: Vol. 23. Neuropsychological studies of apraxia* (pp. 267–308). New York: North-Holland.

Ochipa, C., Rothi, L., & Heilman, K. (1989). Ideational apraxia: A deficit in tool selection and use. *Annals of Neurology, 25,* 190–193.

Ochipa, C., Rothi, L., & Heilman, K. (1992). Conceptual apraxia in Alzheimer's disease. *Brain, 115,* 1061–1071.

Ojemann, G. (1982). Interrelationships in the localization of language, memory, and motor mechanisms in human cortex and thalamus. In R. A. Thompson & J. R. Green (Eds.), *New perspectives in cerebral localization* (pp. 157–175). New York: Raven Press.

Paillard, J. (1982). Apraxia and the neurophysiology of motor control. *Philosophical Transactions of the Royal Society of London, Series B: Biological Sciences, B298,* 111–134.

Poeck, K. (1982). The two types of motor apraxia. *Archives of Italiennes de Biologie, 120,* 361–369.

Poeck, K. (1983). Ideational apraxia. *Journal of Neurology, 230,* 1–5.

Poeck, K. (1985). Clues to the nature of limb praxis. In E. Roy, (Ed.), *Advances in psychology: Vol. 23. Neuropsychological studies of apraxia* (pp. 99–110). New York: North-Holland.

Poeck, K. (1986). The clinical examination for motor apraxia. *Neuropsychologia, 24,* 129–134.

Random House. (1995). *Random House Webster's College Dictionary.* New York: Author.

Roland, P., Larsen, B., Lassen, N., & Skinhof, E. (1980). Supplementary motor area and other cortical areas in organization of voluntary movements in man. *Journal of Neurophysiology, 43,* 118–136.

Roy, E. (1978). Apraxia: A new look at an old syndrome. *Journal of Human Movement Studies, 4,* 191–210.

Roy, E. (1982). Action and performance. In A. Ellis (Ed*.), Normality and pathology in cognitive function* (pp. 265–298). London: Academic Press.

Roy, E. (1983). Neuropsychological perspectives on apraxia and related action disorders. In R. A. Magill (Ed.), *Advances in psychology: Vol. 12. Memory and control of action* (pp. 293–321). New York: North-Holland.

Roy, E., Elliot, D., Dewey, D., & Square-Storer, P. (1990). Impairments to praxis and sequencing in adult and developmental disorders. In C. Bard, M. Fleury, & L. Hay (Eds.), *Development of eye-hand coordination across the life span* (pp. 358–384). Columbia, SC: University of South Carolina Press.

Roy, E., & Square, P. (1985). Common considerations in the study of limb, verbal and oral apraxia. In E. Roy (Ed.), *Advances in psychology: Vol. 23. Neuropsychological studies of apraxia and related disorders* (pp. 111–161). New York: North-Holland.

Sirigu, A., Duhamel, J., Cohen, L., Pillon, B., Dubois, B., & Agid, Y. (1996). The mental representation of hand movements after parietal cortex damage. *Science, 273,* 1564–1568.

Praxis and Organization
of Behavior in Time and Space

Erna Imperatore Blanche, Ph.D., OTR, FAOTA

L. Diane Parham, Ph.D., OTR, FAOTA

Praxis is an organizational process that manifests itself in motor control as well as in general organization of behavior. This organizational process requires adequate perception and integration of spatial and temporal constraints. Difficulties in processing information about space and time, therefore, can result in inefficient movement as well as more generally disorganized behavior. Children with dyspraxia, who often exhibit motor planning deficits as well as difficulties with organization of behavior, might have a dysfunction in the perception and organization of spatial and temporal cues received from the environment. A dysfunction in this basic spatio-temporal organizational mechanism manifests itself throughout the life span as difficulty in organizing activities and occupations in increasingly more complex spatiotemporal environments.

The toddler who builds a tower, the child who runs to catch the ball, the adolescent who prioritizes school obligations upon returning home, and the person who moves to another country to work are examples of individuals engaging in daily activities that require organization of actions in time and space. Whereas a baby takes only a few seconds to put one block on top of another and moves the hand within the immediate reach space, an adult who chooses to move overseas organizes behavior in a much more expansive spatial and temporal context. The ability to organize space and time is a developmental process that is often impaired in individuals with developmental disabilities. This impairment can affect a person's ability to participate fully in culturally and personally meaningful occupations related to work, play, and self-maintenance.

Organization of behavior in time and space is a recurrent topic in occupational therapy, often described in relation to deficits in praxis (Roy, 1978; Ayres, 1985; Cermak, 1985). Although children with developmental dyspraxia typically exhibit organizational problems, investigators have not clarified the relationship between praxis and organization of behavior. The orchestration of daily occupations requires organization of behavior. Clark, Wood, and Larson (1998) coined the term *orchestration of daily occupations* to mean the "ideation, composition, execution, ordering, and other qualitative aspects of occupations" to create a daily routine (p. 17). The orchestration of daily occupations is central to the practice of occupational therapy, particularly in treating individuals who have developmental disabilities or disorders in praxis.

This chapter focuses on the relationship between the ability to organize motor actions and the ability to organize daily occupations. The chapter begins with a review of the literature linking praxis to organization of behavior and concepts of time and space, followed by the description of a model integrating the concepts of organization of time and space in different contexts. The final section describes the model's applicability to clinical practice.

Basic Concepts of Praxis and Organization of Behavior

Praxis: Ayres Revisited

The organization of performance components into occupations, and occupations into daily routines, has been a central theme in occupational therapy and occupational science (Ayres, 1989; Clark et al., 1998; Parham, 1998). However, the literature has not fully described the process by which an individual organizes movement into occupations, and occupations into daily rounds of activities.

Ayres (1972, 1979, 1985, 1989) is one of the few writers who has linked organization of movement to the organization of daily occupations. Ayres described praxis and organization of behavior as closely related because dysfunction in praxis often accompanies disorders in organization of behavior (1985). She defined praxis as an "aptitude that underlies conceptualization, planning, and execution of skilled adaptive interaction with the physical world" (Ayres, 1989, p. 11). In treatment, clinicians often focus on the motor planning aspect of dyspraxia when addressing handwriting, dressing, and participation in adaptive physical education. Motor planning involves timing and sequencing actions in space to produce a goal-oriented action. Practitioners seldom address ideation (the ability to conceptualize a new action) and organization of behavior in broad time-space contexts, due to priorities of the funding sources or because of the lack of knowledge to address these concepts efficiently. However, praxis and organization of behavior are related because dysfunctions in praxis affect organized behavior (Ayres, 1985, 1989). Ayres believed that the link between praxis and organization of behavior lay in ideation, conceptualization, or some other central organization process; however, she had not fully clarified this relationship at the time of her death (Ayres, 1985, 1989).

Ayres' thoughts about praxis and ideation over the last few years of her life provide some insight into her ideas about the relationship of praxis to organized behavior. In her published lecture entitled *Developmental Dyspraxia and Adult Onset Apraxia*, she defined praxis as a "uniquely human skill that enables us to interact effectively with the physical world" (Ayres, 1985, p. 1). Here she discussed praxis as a cognitive process encompassing ideation and motor planning. She wrote, "Perhaps ideation is the very first step in the development of the ability to organize behaviors relative to the physical environment" (Ayres, 1985, p. 21). She wondered, "Could ideation or conceptualization, as a generalized neurophysiological function, serve both praxis as well as a more extensive organization of behavior?" (Ayres, 1985, p. 22). In this lecture, she speculated that ideation, as a fundamental aspect of praxis, might lay the foundation for organization of behavior (Ayres, 1985).

In Ayres' last publication, the manual of the *Sensory Integration and Praxis Tests* (1989), she continued to define praxis as "a uniquely human aptitude that underlies conceptualization, planning, and execution of skilled adaptive interaction with the physical world" (p. 11). However, she expanded on this idea to emphasize the relationship between praxis and the doing of everyday occupations:

> Praxis is the ability by which an individual figures out how to use his or her hands and body in skilled tasks such as playing with toys, using tools (including a pencil and a fork), building a structure (whether a toy block tower or a house), straightening up a room, or engaging in many occupations.

> Praxis is more "behavior" than it is "motor coordination." Although smoothness of motor output is needed to accomplish skilled, goal-directed tasks in the environment, practical ideation and planning are required

to govern these actions. . . . Together, sensory integration and praxis provide one of the most critical links between the environment and human behavior. They enable the informational transactions to occur between the organism and the rest of the world which are basic to the organization of behavior. (Ayres, 1989, p. 11)

Ayres identified praxis as a fundamental organizational process that involves ideation, motor planning, and execution of purposeful actions. According to this viewpoint, praxis is a process in which one mentally generates an idea of what to do and organizes a temporal sequence of actions within the spatial contexts of the physical world to participate in real-world occupations. Further, Ayres noted that "conceiving, planning, and executing adaptive action is a major means by which sensation is made meaningful and translated into a body percept" (1989, p. 11). This assertion implies that praxis contributes to the construction of some aspects of the self. Praxis (including ideation) involves the organization of actions into meaningful occupations (organization of behavior) and influences the construction of the self. Building on this conceptual framework, the authors of this chapter propose that praxis is a critical ability in the organization of occupations into a daily round of activities (orchestration of daily occupations). One may ask, then, How does dyspraxia affect the individual's organization of behavior and orchestration of occupations in a broad sense, beyond the execution of simple motor actions? The section in this chapter on Applications to Occupational Therapy addresses this important question.

Organization of Behavior

Part-Whole Relationship

Organization of behavior requires that the individual has a concept of the whole (the purpose) in relation to the parts, which necessitates that spatial maps contribute to the concept of the whole and sequencing abilities that allow the temporal ordering of the parts to the whole. Recast into a sensory integration framework, organization of behavior involves praxis because sequencing of actions in time is necessary. Furthermore, this sequencing of action is organized in relation to spatial maps generated by sensory integrative processes.

Sequencing

Many authors have described the relationship between praxis and sequencing (Ayres, 1985; MacKay, 1985; Roy & Square, 1985; Fisher, 1991). Ayres defined sequencing of actions as "making transitions from one limb position to another" (1985, p. 70). However, sequencing also functions to organize actions mentally into occupations and to orchestrate occupations into a daily round of activities in the larger spatiotemporal horizon. As a result, sequencing is a process utilized not only in planning motor actions but also in organizing occupations and planning daily events.

MacKay (1985) explored the concept of an underlying organization process responsible for coordinated movements and purposeful organized environmental interactions. For MacKay, the underlying process required sequencing and timing. He proposed four levels of organization of movement and behavior: the muscle movement system, the movement concept system, the action plan system, and the pragmatic system. Each of these systems represented an increasingly more complex organization of time and space.

The muscle movement system controls the organization of muscle movements, determining strength, speed, and direction of specific movements. Movement occurs when a muscle sequence node activates specific sets of muscle fibers. This node provides content, sequence, and timing of the action.

The movement concept system involves general categories of movement and simple movements that require coordination of more than one muscle, such as pressing a key or shifting gears while driving. This system specifies the selection of the movement and the sequence of movements.

The action plan system concerns intentional, purposeful actions an individual can achieve through different movements, such as going to the bakery or driving to work (MacKay, 1985). In contrast to movement concept systems, action plan systems involve movement of the entire body in space, deal with a novel rather than an automated action, and require the use of feedback (MacKay). The action plan accounts for organizing and sequencing movements into intentional purposeful actions. Motor planning, which enables actions to be organized into occupations, fits in this catagory.

The pragmatic system integrates all forms of behaviors. It provides strategies and evaluations, including attitudes and values, of the social, psychological, and physical representations of the world. The pragmatic system sets the purpose and the spatial parameters for the action and determines the mode of output (i.e., language, motor) (MacKay, 1985). The pragmatic system ties into sequential rules when prioritizing occupations in terms of importance for the person. Therefore, the pragmatic system contributes to the organization of occupations into a meaningful daily routine.

MacKay (1985) described three basic components responsible for organizing actions, which he called nodes. Nodes have general properties that have neural representation and are relevant to the organization and execution of behavior. MacKay identified the three types of nodes according to their function: content nodes, sequence nodes, and timing nodes. Content nodes are "theoretical units representing the form or component of an action" (p. 273), sequence nodes are mechanisms that activate and organize content nodes into sequential order, and timing nodes determine the rate of a behavior and are closely associated with sequencing nodes. Activation of these nodes occurs within the systems noted in the preceding paragraphs. The mechanism described by MacKay offers a possible explanation for the organizing process that takes place at different levels of functioning. The organizing process occurs when muscle contractions organize into movements, movements become action plans and occupations, and the pragmatic system prioritizes action plans and orchestrates occupations.

The literature alludes to praxis as an organizational process that affects coordinated movements as well as behavior in a larger spatiotemporal context. The three critical processes that underlie this organizational process are ideation, understanding part-whole relationships, and sequencing. The organization of spatial and temporal information plays an important role in these processes. The next section discusses in greater depth the concepts of time and space as they relate to organization of behavior.

Temporal and Spatial Aspects of Organization of Behavior

Locational and Experiential Dimensions

The organization of one's behavior requires perceiving, conceptualizing, and integrating multiple dimensions of time and space. For example, an individual occupies a physical space in the perceived present while projecting into the future by taking into account experiences from the past. Only the perceived present and the physical space a person occupies in the present are real (Fraisse, 1963) and therefore could be considered objective reality. The past, the future, and the space from which the person comes or to which the person goes are subjective experiences existing exclusively in each individual. Transforming these subjective experiences into real actions and behaviors requires organization of a broad spectrum of spatial and temporal constraints.

Time and space have two dimensions: locational space or time and experiential space or time (Parkes & Thrift, 1980). Locational space or time is "space or time that is objectively surveyable, typically geographical territory and calendar or clock time of the physical universe" (Parkes & Thrift, p. 9). Experiential or existential space is "lived space; the inner structure of space as it appears to us in concrete experiences of the world as members of a culture group socialized according to a common set of experiences, signs, and symbols" (Parkes & Thrift, p. 24). Experiential time and space refer to the subjective experience of time and space, including the sociocultural, emotional, and symbolic experience. An example of experiential time is sensing the appropriate time to do something, which is mediated by social circumstances (Parkes & Thrift).

An individual perceives locational time or space through the senses, and experiential time or space is dependent on the person's prior experiences. Therefore, because experiential space and time rest on prior perceptions of locational space and time, altered perceptions of space and time affect the person's experience and memory of a situation.

Perception of Space

Kolb and Whishaw (1990) divided the locational space around an individual into three subspaces, each of which has a distinct neural representation. These three subspaces are body space, which represents the body surface and the body percept (Wapner et al., 1965); grasping space, the space within the person's immediate reach; and distal space, the space that extends beyond grasping. Distal space includes past and present space and the sequence in which events occur in space.

Kolb and Whishaw (1990) also described cognitive space or the representation of space in the brain. Cognitive spaces are representations of all spaces described in the preceding paragraph, as well as space that is not visually available. Cognitive space also requires consideration of the temporal dimension.

Experiential space is a type of cognitive space that is dependent on prior experiences and can change depending on new experiences. Experiential space adds the dimension of meaning to cognitive space. Buttimer (1976) described *experiential space* as the phenomenological view of space in which the "experiencer lives and moves and searches for meaning" (p. 282).

It is possible to differentiate space into body space, grasping space, distal space, cognitive space, and experiential space. Perceptions of space may play a role in establishing a gestalt or a part-whole relationship of the environment. By organizing space, the individual can build a mental map of where the actions occur that are part of a movement synergy, or where the movement synergies, occupations, and daily routines occur. Organizing time plays a role in relating the parts of the action to the whole (the occupation or routine) in a sequential pattern.

The perception of space depends on information that individuals obtain through their senses (Ayres, 1972). Therefore, sensory integrative functions are critical in spatial perception. Perception of space relies on adequate processing of visual (Ayres, 1972; Kolb & Whishaw, 1990), somatosensory, and vestibular input (Ayres, 1972; Hall, 1966). The visual system contributes information about form, shape, depth, size, permeability, position, and distance of objects and environmental features in relation to each other and to the observer. The auditory system supplies information about the spatial location of the person relative to environmental sounds. The tactile and proprioceptive systems provide information about near space, specifically the impinging of objects and people on the body; the weight, texture, and shape of held objects; and the position of body parts in relation to each other. The vestibular and proprioceptive systems provide information about the body's position relative to gravity, orientation and movement of the head through space, and position of body parts in relation to each other (Ayres, 1972). All of these aspects of sensory information work together to provide a cognitive spatial map of the environment and one's location within it. (For further, in-depth description of perception of space, see chapter 15 in this volume, Sensory Integration and Visual Deficits, Including Blindness, by Roley & Schneck.)

Perception of Time

The occupational therapy literature has extensively discussed the issues surrounding visual perception of space (Ayres, 1972; Henderson, 1992, 1992/1993); however, the literature has neglected the importance of the perception of time. Investigators frequently take into account the temporal dimension of sequencing and timing only in relation to specific movement patterns, rather than the molar patterns of orchestrated occupations.

Individuals perceive time by sensing change. According to Fraisse (1963), successive stimuli are integrated in such a way that they can be perceived temporally and sequentially, which characterizes the perception of time. The relative simultaneity is the perceived present. Actions in this ever-changing world depend on the situation in which the person finds him- or herself at a particular instance, as well as on what the person has experienced in the past and what he or she expects in future. Fraisse described the perspective derived from the perceived present, as it connects to the past and the future, as a temporal horizon. Actions take place within a temporal horizon. Temporal horizons are successive temporal perspectives that allow individuals to connect events to each other in the past, present, and future. As the person grows and learns to take into account a progressively larger time frame, the temporal horizons expand. Accordingly, as with space, temporal horizons expand with age.

An individual's notion of time depends on his or her perception of succession and duration (Fraisse, 1963, 1984). The perception of succession and duration occurs through the senses. According to Fraser (1987), the individual has several systems of time: biological time, which represents biologically based or species-specific realities of time such as circadian rhythms; notice time or mature time, characterized by a clear distinction between past, present, and future and by the mental awareness of present and the ability to change attention to different temporal horizons; and sociotemporal time, which represents the collective evaluation of time, socialization of time, and shared time within a social system. Individuals need to integrate these aspects of time to function in the world.

As with the experience of space, the experience of time requires processing sensory cues that when integrated, contribute to the perception of time. To adapt to temporal constraints, one needs to perceive succession, simultaneity, and duration within each sensory system; integrate these perceptual patterns; organize this information to give a clear sense of present in relation to past and future; and organize these aspects of time within the sociocultural milieu. A breakdown at any point within this complex process can interfere with temporal adaptation. For example, dyspraxic patients who exhibit disorganized behaviors have difficulty budgeting time for daily tasks and often are unpunctual and forgetful. Inadequate organization of temporal cues can affect organization of behavior in several temporal horizons.

As noted earlier, perceiving time is dependent on the perception of change, and individuals perceive change through sensing succession and duration (Fraisse, 1963). As a result, the sensory systems that are more sensitive to change play an important role in the perception of time. Fraisse considered hearing as the "main organ through which we perceive change: it is considered as the 'time sense' just as sight is that of space" (1963, p. 83). Hearing plays a critical role in the perception of time through succession of stimuli; however, individuals process the perception of time, as they do the perception of space, through a combination of sensory channels. For example, the vestibular sense also plays an important role in acquiring a sense of time; however, investigators have not fully explained the contribution of the vestibular system (Fraisse, 1963). The relationship between the perception of time and the vestibular system might lie in the way the semicircular canals operate. These canals are sensitive to change because they are stimulated when there is change in velocity of head motion, and they return to resting discharge when velocity is constant (Kandel & Schwartz, 1981). Another sense that could play a role in detecting temporal (and spatial) patterns is the proprioceptive system, primarily because it signals sequential changes in muscle tension during active movements. Interestingly, researchers have found a link between vestibular-proprioceptive difficulties and sequencing disorders (Fisher, 1991).

Most of the other sensory receptors in the body also react to change and constancy. Poppel (1988) explained perception of time with a hierarchical system in which "elementary temporal experiences (ETE) are incorporated at different levels" (p. 134). There are at least four elementary temporal experiences:

- ETE of simultaneity or nonsimultaneity
- ETE of temporal order or succession
- ETE of the subjective present
- ETE of duration

According to Poppel (1988), the most basic ETE is the ability to discriminate between simultaneity or nonsimultaneity of stimuli. This ability is dependent upon the receptor's threshold for nonsimultaneity. The auditory system exhibits the lowest threshold, followed by the somatosensory system. The visual system has the highest threshold. The sensation of simultaneity and nonsimultaneity is mediated at the level of the receptor. In contrast, Poppel proposed that the perception of temporal order or succession is mediated centrally because the perception of temporal order registered by the auditory, visual, and somatosensory systems is the same even though the threshold for simultaneity or nonsimultaneity is different for all three.

The next level of perception of time is the perception of the subjective present, which is dependent upon the integration of successive events into a unit. The present or "perceived present" lasts "only for the duration of the organization which we perceive as one unit" (Fraisse, 1963, p. 84). The time interval for these events to be integrated into a unit perceived as the present is 2 to 3 seconds. According to Poppel (1988), this perception is dependent on the sensory system's ability to hold information for only 2 to 3 seconds.

Poppel (1988) proposed that perception of duration, the highest level of the hierarchical taxonomy of time perception, cannot be accounted for by a physiological process. Traditionally, investigators thought that duration depends on how much information an individual has processed in a given interval. If the informational content is low, then the duration appears to be short; if informational content is high, then the duration appears to be long. However, this pattern contradicts the subjective experience of the passage of time. If one is in a situation with low informational content, then time appears to slow down, and if one is in a situation of high content, then time appears to fly. Poppel (1988) described this contradiction as the time paradox.

If individuals process perception of simultaneity, succession, and perceived present through the senses, then children with sensory processing disorders are likely to have impairments in time perception. Consequently, children with sensory processing disorders sometimes exhibit poor organization of behavior because of inadequate sensory processing involved in the perception of time and space, rather than exclusively because of deficits in higher-level processing skills such as ideation and cognition.

Integrating Space and Time to Organize Behavior

Spatiotemporal Units

As noted previously, the senses contribute in different ways to the perception of space and time. Organization of spatial and temporal qualities of incoming sensory information allows individuals to perceive the present. The present, in turn, provides a reference point for the future and a frame for the conceptualization and planning of future actions. Therefore, organization of space and time is essential in the development of praxis and the organization of occupations into coherent daily routines. Spatial and temporal cues must be packaged so that the processes of ideation and motor planning can allow the person to construct and engage in occupations.

The locational and experiential dimensions of both space and time integrate into spatiotemporal units that assist in the organization of behavior. One term that refers to the integration of locational and experiential time and space is *place*.

Parkes and Thrift (1980), writing from a chronogeographic perspective, discussed the experience of place as a familiar mental and social environment, which includes the outer and inner experiences of the individual.

Another concept that describes the experiential qualities of time-space is *lifeworld*, a term used in the phenomenological literature to describe the "culturally defined spatiotemporal setting or horizon of everyday life" (Buttimer, 1976, p. 277). This concept takes into account the sociocultural milieu. Buttimer proposed that individuals perceive everyday activities in a holistic manner without prereflection or within a taken-for-granted experience and described the lifeworld experience as an "orchestration of various time-space rhythms" (p. 289). The individual needs to synchronize physiological rhythms, cultural rhythms, work style rhythms, and physical functional rhythms to establish rhythmic patterns of activities (Shapcott & Steadman, 1978).

Spatiotemporal Horizons

Individuals integrate space and time into a sense of place at different horizons of interaction. These spatiotemporal horizons expand along a continuum, from the near horizon of here and now to the farthest, most expansive horizon that includes experiential space of the past and the imagined future. The individual's life trajectory involves an expansion of these horizons of space-time organization (Fraisse, 1984) so that over time, one becomes capable of orchestrating actions in increasingly broader space and time perspectives. For example, the very young infant organizes the immediate locational time-space horizon and begins to organize behavior using experiential space and time. As the person develops and matures, the time-space horizons expand to longer time frames and broader life-spaces that are highly experiential, with strong cultural patterning. A competent adult is able to organize actions in multiple spatiotemporal horizons in order to participate fully in complex human interactions. Disability or chronic health problems can constrict or distort the horizons as the individual becomes less able to negotiate his or her lifeworld freely.

Individuals with praxis difficulties typically experience problems related to proximal space and time. The motor control literature extensively describes these problems in relation to coordination of movement. However, the difficulties experienced by individuals with praxis problems are not always confined to motor coordination but can also involve problems related to time management and interpersonal skills, and it is not uncommon to find that disruptions extend into more distal horizons of time and space, including experiential dimensions in the sociocultural milieu.

Successful organization of behavior requires simultaneous organization of multiple spatiotemporal horizons and the ability to shift back and forth fluidly from one horizon to another. It is useful to consider five spatiotemporal horizons upon which occupations take place. These horizons are tentative concepts that future study very likely will modify. The selection of these horizons is somewhat arbitrary, because there are an infinite number of them. The five spatiotemporal horizons discussed here are Body Space in the Present, Reach Space in Proximal Time, Available Space in Proximal Time, Cognitive Space in Extended Time, and Imagined Space in Distant Time.

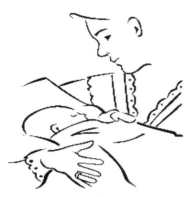

The infant organizes the spatial constraints of the body in the present.

Body Space in the Present

The nearest horizon that the individual needs to organize is the space occupied by one's own body within the perceived present. Organization of this information enables the individual to generate a sense of physical self in the here and now. This spatiotemporal horizon begins to be constructed at birth and continues throughout the lifespan. Biotemporal rhythms, which in infancy include heartbeat, respiratory, and sleep-wake patterns (Pierce, 1997), contribute to the organization of this spatiotemporal horizon.

As the infant organizes space and time within this horizon, he or she begins to develop a sense of physical self that comes into play when moving and interacting with objects and people. This sense of self establishes what Hall (1966) describes as intimate distance. Intimate distance defines the boundaries of the immediate space. Intimate social interactions that include close contact impinge upon these boundaries.

The primary senses that convey information at this distance are the tactile, proprioceptive, and smell receptors. Vision and audition play a minor role (Hall, 1966). Touch, as the most personally experienced sensation, conveys information not only about location and spatial properties of objects, including people, but also about changes in heat and texture in the immediate environment (Hall, 1966).

Body scheme is a product of the organization that occurs within this horizon, arising from two experiences: a spatial gestalt experience based on sensory information and an ever-changing dynamic of possible actions superimposed on it (Wapner et al., 1965).

For a newborn infant, occupations that occur within this spatiotemporal horizon include such activities as breastfeeding and cuddling with the caregiver. For an adult, occupations in the Body Space in the Present horizon include hatha yoga, receiving a massage, and cuddling with a loved one.

Reach Space in Proximal Time

The horizon of Reach Space in Proximal Time integrates reaching space (Kolb & Whishaw, 1990), or what Hall (1966) described as personal space or distance, within a locational time frame of minutes to hours. Interactions within this horizon rely on visual and auditory information in addition to the sensory information of the Body Space in the Present horizon. Object exploration (through manipulation, mouthing, and interaction with toys that offer simple responses to simple actions) helps develop the perception of space within the immediate reach (Pierce, 1997). A later stage within this horizon requires a combination of object use, as in nesting and disassembling puzzles (Pierce).

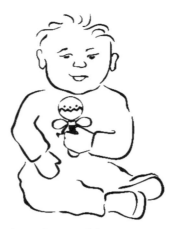

The baby organizes the reaching space and the immediate past and future.

The organization of time and space within this horizon of interaction enables coordinated limb movements without displacing the entire body. Coordination, at its most basic level, is the "co-ordering of muscle activity" (Sugden & Keogh, 1990, p. 2). The individual uses feedforward, anticipation of future temporal and spatial location, to guide the extremities (Fisher, 1991). Occupations that individuals can perform within this horizon (such as sewing, writing, or playing the piano) involve maintenance of a stable base. Children with praxis difficulty might be able to learn to organize their actions within this horizon (e.g., writing) but can have great difficulty organizing actions in broader horizons that involve moving the entire body through space and time.

Hall (1966) termed the experiential space organized at this horizon as personal distance. One's culture dictates what is the appropriate personal distance, For example, Americans tend to maintain more space between people than individuals from some other cultures. Children with learning disorders and developmental disabilities often have difficulties managing the culturally appropriate distance of interaction. They approach strangers, situating themselves closely to initiate an interaction.

Moving Through Proximal Space and Time

At the horizon of Moving Through Proximal Space and Time, the individual performs movements that require organization of space occupied by displacements of the entire body while taking into account prior as well as near future sequences of events (Kolb & Whishaw, 1990). The space organized in this horizon is the visually perceived space, regardless of size. Interactions within this horizon do not require the person to infer or conceptualize space beyond what he or she immediately perceives. Occupations that take place within this horizon include playing soccer, dancing, and cooking.

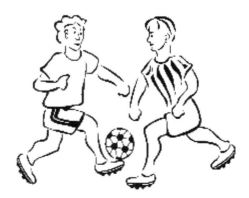

The child organizes the visually available space in the immediate past and future.

Organization of space and time in this horizon requires complex motor planning. In addition to feedback from previous actions, feedforward is critical in projecting actions into the future. For example, when playing soccer, the individual first must perceive the spatial location of all players and the ball, then anticipate their changing positions during the next few seconds so that when the ball moves, the player knows where and how to reposition his or her body. The individual uses his or her repertoire of past experiences to plan future actions in the immediate space and time frame.

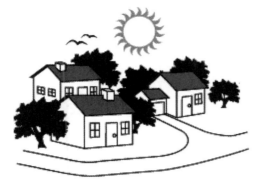

The person organizes the familiar spaces in the extended time.

Moving Through Cognitive Space in Extended Time

Within the horizon of Moving Through Cognitive Space in Extended Time, one orchestrates streams of occupations into the daily round of activities. The space that the person organizes encompasses the neighborhood or the town; the time extends to hours, days, and even weeks. The organized space no longer includes only the visually perceived space but also a cognitive representation of the space the individual does not perceive immediately. Kolb and Whishaw (1990) referred to this cognitively represented space as cognitive space.

Henderson (1992) defined cognitive space as "our internal representation of real space, our spatial memory, spatial concepts and spatial thinking" (p. 3). She described cognitive space as including mental images of objects and spaces that the individual can manipulate mentally, cognitive maps of the environment that can be real or inferred through previously sequentially perceived stimuli, and a "spatial memory by which we select our actions" (p. 3). The capacity to move through cognitive space opens up vast potentials for interactions with the environment.

In this spatiotemporal horizon, the person organizes streams of occupations into a daily routine, utilizing extended spans of space and time to group occupations into meaningful blocks such as "time at the park," "time at school," "housework," "work," and "errands." Within each block are strings of occupations that the person has organized at more proximal spatiotemporal horizons. For example, the individual might sequentially do paper work, attend a meeting, and have lunch with co-workers, organizing these occupations in his or her mind as a block of space-time called "work."

Temporal rhythm plays an important role at this level of spatiotemporal organization. Not only must the individual group occupations into blocks of space-time, but he or she must also synchronize these blocks with the occupations of other people.

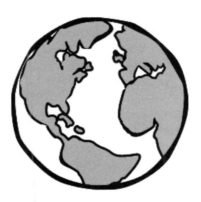

The person builds on previous skills and organizes the cognitive or imaginary in the extended time.

In westernized cultures, the use of clocks is imperative in synchronizing these patterns with other individuals. Patients with poor organization of behavior are often late and can seem disoriented in time.

Imagining Action in Distant Time

Organization within the spatiotemporal horizon of Imagining Action in Distant Time requires taking into account long-term goals and values, ambitions, and interests. Examples of actions at this level include planning a vacation for the following month or planning to go to school in the coming fall. Past experiences and the present situation shape people's perception of the future

(Fraisse, 1984). Taking into account the distant future also requires conceptualization of that future in potential spaces that could be as large as cities, countries, and continents.

People organize this time in different ways. Some do not plan more than a few weeks ahead, and others carefully establish goals and plan their path for the next few years. Most people, when asked about their future, have certain plans about where they are going or where they would like to be in the future. Research in this area with individuals who have disabilities is extremely limited.

A Conceptual Model of Praxis and Organization of Behavior

Analysis of the literature on praxis and organization of behavior gives new insights to the understanding of how to strategize intervention for individuals with developmental disabilities. This section presents a conceptual model or cognitive map that represents the authors' current synthesis of this literature.

In this model, praxis and organization of behavior require integrating sensory information and conceptualization of potential actions in space and time. Integrating sensory input is necessary for the organization of spatiotemporal patterns. Conceptualization refers to the ideational skill of projecting imagined actions from the present into future temporal horizons. These basic elements of praxis are prerequisite for complex organization of behavior. In this model, organization of behavior is a complex outcome of praxis that involves integration and sequencing of locational and experiential space and time into the five spatiotemporal horizons discussed in the preceding section of this chapter.

Case Study: Pete

Pete is an attractive 20-year-old who presently attends an Ivy League school. He is a bright young man with excellent writing skills, whom his family and friends describe as charming but disorganized. An examination of his developmental history shows that the disorganization started early. Pete's mother's pregnancy was uneventful, as was Pete's delivery. Although he attained motor milestones on time during his first year, the family observed that the quality of his movements was slightly atypical. His mother, an occupational therapist, noticed that he exhibited decreased extensor muscle tone, his scapulae were held in abduction with shoulders protracted, and proximal joint stability was poor, suggesting poor organization of body space in the present.

When presented with novel tasks such as feeding himself a cracker, Pete tended to revert to earlier patterns of interaction, such as trying to grab the food with his mouth rather than with his hands. Pete also exhibited poor oral motor control: lip closure around the spoon was not automatic, and muscle tone around the oral area was so low that his mouth was open much of the time. Although his parents were concerned, they could not find a professional who would address Pete's needs when he was an infant. During the first years of life, Pete's difficulties were evident in his organization of reach space in proximal time.

Pete enjoyed being read to and playing with puzzles and cars. When he was 3 years old, his delays became more evident: although he appeared to understand language, his verbal skills were significantly below age. His pediatrician referred him to a speech pathologist and an occupational therapist. The occupational therapist identified a vestibular processing deficit, affecting postural control and motor planning skills.

At 5 years of age, after 2 years of intervention, Pete entered the primary grades, where he was considered an intelligent child; however, he had difficulties with handwriting, organization of material, and physical education. Motor planning skills were poor, primarily in activities requiring anticipation of actions in time and space, such as playing ball. His organizational deficits were evident in his movements through proximal space and time.

As the school years progressed, Pete's difficulties in motor planning were no longer important in his life. He made friends with ease and, at his parents' encouragement, he participated in one sport activity per week. Pete's poor organization of cognitive space and extended time was evident in his forgetfulness, messiness, and untidiness. For example, when he had a science project that required constructional skills, Pete easily chose the topic and developed it, but he skillfully managed to engage his parents and siblings in the actual construction. During the primary-grade years, Pete often forgot his backpack at school or in the park, had to be awakened many times every morning, and sometimes forgot to wear socks or underwear when going to school.

Because he was an excellent student, Pete entered a highly academic high school. During the high school years, Pete no longer played team sports. To stay in shape, he participated in track. He developed his writing abilities and received many awards, but he still had difficulties managing distant time to meet deadlines and often stayed up all night to finish projects. Pete's disorganization became his main shortcoming. He had difficulty organizing himself temporally to get a driver's license, even after some of his friends made appointments for him to take the driving test. He also continued having difficulty organizing himself in space. When his room needed cleaning so he could go out, his friends came to help. The process of applying to college required his parents' intervention in rewriting the application and monitoring the due dates.

In college, Pete continues to show signs of disorganization. As his world expands, his poor organization of time and space has a greater impact on his environment. However, he continues to use social strategies to help him cope with the tasks that require organization of distant time and cognitive space. These include organizing his friends the day before classes start so they show him the way around campus, following his classmates' lead when it is time to meet the deadlines to sign up for courses every semester, relying on his roommate to wake him up in the morning, and enlisting his friends when it is time to move his belongings from the dorm to storage during the summer.

Pete is majoring in English and art. Both fields will require that he organize cognitive imaginative worlds that do not rely heavily on the management of space and time. His difficulties most likely will be evident in daily tasks, such as getting an apartment, paying the bills on time, and meeting deadlines. If he is successful, he probably will benefit from hiring a personal assistant.

Applications to Occupational Therapy

The conceptual model described in this chapter is a helpful cognitive tool for identifying praxis problems at the different levels of complexity represented by the five spatiotemporal horizons. It can also be a useful heuristic for designing interventions that provide support for praxic development at these different horizons. It is possible to analyze disorders in the organization of space and time by considering the child's behavior within the frame of one spatiotemporal horizon as well as across several of the horizons. The model suggests that problems in praxis initially appearing in the most proximal horizons are later evident in more expansive spatial and temporal units. Some of the key propositions of sensory integration theory already contain this assumption embedded within them. For example, sensory integration theory proposes that poor body scheme (a function of the spatiotemporal horizon of Body Space in the Present) leads to motor planning difficulties (involving the horizons of Reach Space in Proximal Time and Moving Through Proximal Space and Time). The model put forth in this chapter would elaborate on this proposition by predicting that the praxic difficulties interfering with body scheme and motor planning early in life will affect the child's interactions with more distant and abstract dimensions of space and time as the child matures.

One line of reasoning in intervention planning is to focus intervention efforts on the most proximal horizon involved, because it is the dimension in which the praxis problems initially emerge. For most children with praxis difficulties, this approach would implicate body scheme as the target for remediation. However, the authors' clinical experience suggests that, although this approach might be useful in the initial stages, intervention will be more effective if therapy directly addresses increasingly broader and more abstract space-time dimensions. As with sensory integration intervention in general, practitioners must exercise clinical judgment in gauging when, how, and how much to increase challenges, taking into consideration the child's age and developmental status, the nature of the child's problems, the family's concerns and priorities, and the child's aspirations. With these caveats in mind, the following paragraphs suggest some of the kinds of therapeutic activities that might be useful in addressing development within each spatiotemporal horizon.

Table 10.1 presents a summary of the spatiotemporal horizons considered in this chapter, along with related disorders and suggested intervention techniques.

Within the spatiotemporal horizon of Body Space in the Present, the most proximal level of this conceptual model, lie sensory processing problems affecting body scheme and the ability to act on one's own body. In general, intervention at this level aims to help the child experience intimate space in the present time through exploration of touch and proprioceptive sensations. Treatment approaches that address body scheme difficulties within this spatiotemporal horizon include exploration of deep touch pressure, vibration, and other tactile inputs and activities that augment proprioception, such as pushing and pulling against resistance. Informal games involving imitation of simple facial or whole-body movements place greater demands on organization of

Table 10.1. Summary of Spatiotemporal Horizons

Spatiotemporal Horizon	Spatial Constraints Organized	Temporal Constraints Organized	Possible Disorders	Intervention
Body Space in the Present	The body and its boundaries	Present	Poor body scheme, use of feedback	Have child explore body through touch, proprioception
Reach Space in Proximal Time	Space available through reach	Immediate past and future	Poor fine motor coordination, graphomotor skills, motor planning	Use tools, handwriting, arts and crafts, tabletop games and activities
Moving Through Proximal Space and Time	Visually available space	Immediate past and future	Problems using feedforward to plan whole-body movements	Control the size of the visually available space
Moving Through Cognitive Space in Extended Time	Cognitive space, generally familiar or known places	Extended time (e.g., a day)	Problems in sequencing tasks, organizing events mentally	Have child visualize the familiar. Use maps of familiar space. Organize daily routine
Imagining Action in Distant Time	Cognitive space; may be distant or imaginary place	Very distant or extended time (e.g., a year)	Same as above but evidenced in larger horizons	Create stories and plans that take place in distant time and space. Use maps of unfamiliar time/space

body scheme. For older children and adults, helpful intervention approaches include those that focus attention on body sensations, such as Feldenkrais methods, and occupations such as hatha yoga.

At the spatiotemporal horizon of Reach Space in Proximal Time, the child might exhibit inefficiencies in the ability to utilize sensory feedback as well as feedforward to perform occupations that require reach, grasp, transfer, and organization of the immediate space-time matrix from a relatively stationary position. Encouraging the child to manipulate, mouth, and reach for toys helps the child integrate peripersonal space and time extending from the immediate present to the immediate future. Playing simple cause-and-effect games also encourages temporal awareness of immediate future (Pierce, 1997). Treatment approaches that address more complex actions within this spatiotemporal horizon include activities that focus on fine motor coordination and challenge postural control in prone, seated, or standing positions. Examples of such activities are drawing and painting, many crafts, handwriting, keyboarding and computer work, and seated games such as cards, checkers, and board games.

At the spatiotemporal horizon of Moving Through Proximal Space and Time, the difficulties children exhibit involve problems with organizing action plans to perform occupations within the visually available environment. Therapists working from a sensory integration perspective often deal with organization of behavior within this horizon. In intervention at this horizon level, clinicians can use objects to assist the child in organizing space (Pierce, 1997). For example, the therapist might encourage the child to transport objects from one spatial location to another, or to use a heavy push-toy that slows motor activity and increases awareness of movement in distal space (Pierce). Therapists can also address awareness of distal space and future time by having the child move through space independently to reach a pre-chosen destination in the room. It is possible to manipulate spatial parameters so that the demands on spatial organization grow as the child's skills develop, such as limiting the visually available space to a dollhouse or a large box, or expanding it to the size of a small room or a large gym. It might be effective to constrain the child's movement through space by having the child move on a piece of suspended equipment, or to unconstrain movement by allowing the child to move freely in space. If difficulty anticipating the trajectory of whole-body movements in time and space is apparent, intervention can involve grading of projected action sequences, as described by Fisher (1991).

To function effectively within the spatiotemporal horizons of Moving Through Cognitive Space in Extended Time and Imagining Actions in Distant Time, the individual needs to have well-developed ideation and the ability to visualize space, sequentially organize actions, and orchestrate occupations into coherent routines. Clinicians can design treatment approaches to support the development of these abilities. For a relatively simple treatment activity, the therapist makes a map of a room, marking places where he or she has hidden toys. The child then uses the map to finds the objects.

To address the horizon of cognitive space and the daily unit, therapists can have the child consciously plan the daily routine and describe his or her activities, including when and where the child performed them, for the past day. These challenges often reveal poor conceptualization of daily routines. For example, Mary, a 13-year-old girl with hemiplegia and praxis difficulties who attended a regular school, reportedly had difficulty getting her chores done at home. When asked to describe the sequence of activities that she performed during the day, Mary's response was quite limited. She named simple actions, such as putting on socks, and forgot large streams of activities, such as having lunch with her friends. Mary seemed to describe the events that were difficult for her and therefore might have been salient in her memory, but she seemed to struggle with conceptualizing her activities as falling into patterns of coherent, meaningful routines.

More abstract challenges within the most distant spatiotemporal horizons might include asking a child to make up stories and plans involving actions taking place in a distant time (in 30 minutes, tomorrow, next week, or next year) and/or in a distant location (the next room, the house next door, the local shopping center, or another town). Therapists can grade these challenges from proximal to distal, moderating challenges to time conceptualization with challenges to space conceptualization (i.e., moderating high challenge to time concept with low challenge to space concept, and vice versa). Diagrams or "maps" of temporal sequences, as well as maps of unfamiliar places, are useful in expanding the child's competencies in the most distant spatiotemporal horizon.

In summary, this continuum of space-time interactions helps explain why individuals with inadequate praxis can experience difficulties in organizing their actions at different horizons of interaction. Treatment aimed at organization of behavior requires careful consideration of the spatiotemporal horizons that might affect the child's ability to reach treatment goals. Occupational therapists can address organization of behavior by helping the child develop the ability to perceive and organize space and time across increasingly more abstract and complex spatiotemporal horizons.

Acknowledgment

The authors are grateful to Ruth Zemke for influencing the ideas presented in this paper.

Works Cited

Quotation on page 184 from *Developmental Dyspraxia and Adult-Onset Apraxia* by A.J. Ayres (1985) have been reprinted with permission by Sensory Integration International.

Excerpts on pages 184 and 185 from *Sensory Integration and Praxis Tests* by A.J. Ayres, copyright © 1989 by Western Psychological Services. Reprinted by permission of the publisher, Western Psychological Services, 12031 Wilshire Boulevard, Los Angeles, California, 90025, U.S.A. Not to be reprinted in whole or in part for any additional purpose without the expressed, written permission of the publisher. All rights reserved.

Quotation on page 187 from *Times, Spaces, and Places—A Chronogeographic Perspective* by D. Parkes and N. Thrift (1980) have been reprinted with permission from John Wiley and Sons.

References

Ayres, A.J. (1972). *Sensory integration and learning disabilities*. Los Angeles: Western Psychological Services.

Ayres, A.J. (1979). *Sensory integration and the child*. Los Angeles: Western Psychological Corporation.

Ayres, A.J. (1985). *Developmental dyspraxia and adult-onset apraxia*. Torrance, CA: Sensory Integration International.

Ayres, A.J. (1989). *Sensory Integration and Praxis Tests*. Los Angeles: Western Psychological Services.

Buttimer, A. (1976). Grasping the dynamism of lifeworld. *Annals of the Association of American Geographers, 66*(2), 277-292.

Cermak, S. (1985). Developmental dyspraxia. In E. Roy (Ed.), *Neuropsychological studies of apraxia and related disorders* (pp. 225–248). Amsterdam: Elsevier Science Publishers.

Clark, F., Wood, W., & Larson, E. (1998). Occupational science: Occupational therapy's legacy for the 21st century. In M. Neistadt & E. Crepeau (Eds.), *Willard and Spackman's occupational therapy* (9th ed., pp. 13–21). Philadelphia: J.B. Lippincott.

Fisher, A. (1991) Vestibular-proprioceptive processing and bilateral integration and sequencing deficits. In A. Fisher, E. Murray, & A. Bundy (Eds.), *Sensory integration: Theory and practice* (pp. 71–107). Philadelphia: F.A. Davis.

Fraisse, P. (1963). *The psychology of time*. New York: Harper and Row.

Fraisse, P. (1984). Perception and estimation of time. *Annual Reviews Psychology, 35,* 1–36.

Fraser, J.T. (1987). *Time—The familiar stranger*. Amherst, MA: The University of Massachusetts Press.

Hall, E. (1966) *The hidden dimension*. New York: Anchor, Doubleday.

Henderson, A. (1992). A functional typology of spatial abilities and disabilities—Part I. *Sensory Integration Quarterly, 20*(3), 1–6

Henderson, A. (1992/1993). A functional typology of spatial abilities and disabilities—Part II. *Sensory Integration Quarterly, 20*(4), 1–5

Kandel, R., & Schwartz, J. (1981). *Principles of neural science*. New York: Elsevier North Holland, Inc.

Kolb, B., & Whishaw, I. Q. (1990). *Fundamentals of human neuropsychology* (3rd ed.). New York: W. H. Freeman.

MacKay, D. (1985). A theory of the representation, organization and timing of action with implications for sequencing disorders. In E.A. Roy (Ed.), *Neuropsychological studies of apraxia* (pp. 267–302). Amsterdam: North Holland.

Parham, L.D. (1998). What is the proper domain of occupational therapy research? *American Journal of Occupational Therapy, 52,* 485–489.

Parkes, D., & Thrift, N. (1980). *Times, spaces, and places—A chronogeographic perspective*. Chichester, Great Britain: John Wiley & Sons.

Pierce, D. (1997). The power of object play for infants and toddlers at risk for developmental delays. In D. Parham and L. Fazio (Eds.), *Play in occupational therapy for children* (pp. 86–111). St. Louis: Mosby-Year Book, Inc.

Poppel, E. (1988). Time perception. In J.M. Wolfe (Ed.), *Readings from the Encyclopedia of Neuroscience: Sensory systems II—Senses other than vision* (pp. 134–135). Boston: Birkhauser.

Roy, E.A. (1978). Apraxia: A new look at an old syndrome. *Journal of Human Movement Studies, 4,* 191–210.

Roy, E., & Square, P. (1985). Common considerations in the study of limb, verbal, and oral apraxia. In E. Roy (Ed.), *Neuropsychological studies of apraxia* (pp. 111–161). Amsterdam: North Holland.

Shapcott, M., & Steadman, P. (1978). Rhythms of urban activity. In T. Carlstein, D. Parkes, & N. Thrift (Eds.), *Timing space and spacing time* (pp. 49–74). London: John Wiley & Sons.

Sugden, D., & Keogh, J. (1990). *Problems in movement skill development.* In H.G. Williams (Series Ed.), *Growth, motor development, and physical activity across the life span.* Columbia, SC: University of South Carolina Press.

Wapner, S., Werner, H., de Ajuriaguerra, J., Cleveland, S., Critchley, M., Fisher, S., & Witkin, H. (1965). *The body percept.* New York: Random House.

Werner, H. (1965). Introduction. In S. Wapner, H. Werner, J. de Ajuriaguerra, S. Cleveland, M. Critchley, S. Fisher, & H. Witkin (Eds.), *The body percept* (pp. 3–8). New York: Random House.

Additional Readings

Geschwindt, N. (1975). The apraxias: Neuronal mechanisms of disorders of learned movement. *American Scientist, 63,* 188–195.

Goodgold-Edwards, S., & Cermak, S. (1990). Integrating motor control and motor learning concepts with neuropsychological perspectives on apraxia and developmental dyspraxia. *American Journal of Occupational Therapy, 44*(5), 431–439.

Hall, E. (1983). *The dance of life—The other dimension of time.* New York: Anchor Books Doubleday.

Kelly, J. (1981). Vestibular system. In E. Kandal & J. Schwartz (Eds.), *Principles of neural science* (pp. 406–418). New York: Elsevier.

Miller, N. (1986). *Dyspraxia and its management.* Rockville, MD: Aspen.

Zerubavel, E. (1981). *1*Berkeley, CA: University of California Press.

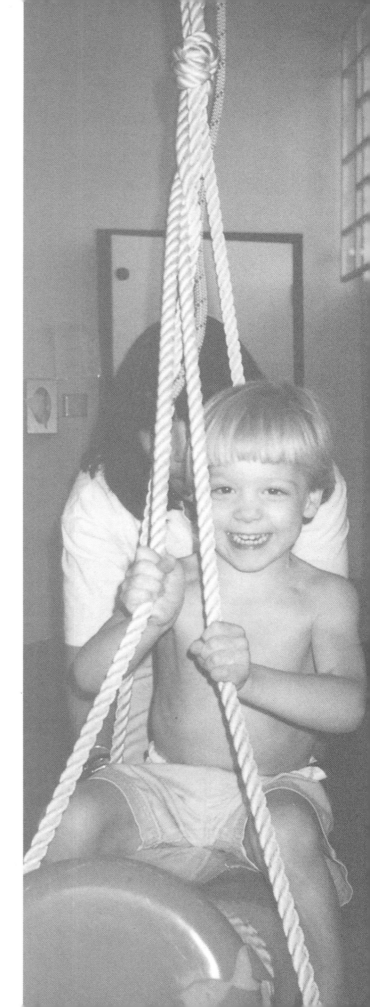

Clinical Reasoning and the Use of Narrative in Sensory Integration Assessment and Intervention

Janice Posatery Burke, Ph.D., OTR/L, FAOTA

Introduction

The term *clinical reasoning* describes both the conscious and unconscious or tacit knowledge and problem solving used by practitioners when they provide occupational therapy. Like many professionals such as architects, psychologists, and physicians, the therapist draws on the facts that are present in the situation as well as the subtle, soft details in order to make the best decision for intervention. A therapist using clinical reasoning is collecting, analyzing, and interpreting both objective and subjective information about the person's needs to create an accurate profile of the individual. In addition to this specific data, the therapist also is using his or her store of knowledge about the kinds of problems that occupational therapy can address, his or her own clinical experience, and clinical intuition to develop an idea of what needs to be done and how it should unfold.

To be effective, practitioners begin by applying the rules and information they have learned from course work in the social sciences (including cultural anthropology, psychology, and social psychology) and the hard sciences (including biology, anatomy, and physiology), combined with their clinical experience. For example, in a given case a therapist might apply knowledge of human motivation and socialization with what he or she knows from working with people of similar cultural and age groups. In addition, the therapist will use his or her understanding of body mechanics, physical functions of the various body systems, and disease and wellness concepts. Because the focus of occupational therapy transcends the mechanical functions of the body to the broader view of the whole person, practitioners must go beyond simply applying their knowledge of body mechanics and focus their attention on the particulars of the person. An interactive approach combined with clinical reasoning can facilitate the therapist's ability to tailor his or her absolute knowledge to each person's specific complexities.

Technical fields such as manufacturing and production depend on reasoning that is linear. The path to solving a problem or to achieving a goal is straight and direct, with clear and specific barriers and constraints to consider and either confront and resolve or avoid. Health and human service professions such as occupational therapy are quite different in the reasoning required to solve problems. In these professions, the path to problem solution lies in the pattern that reflects the specific concerns and factors accompanying a person's profile. Factors a therapist must consider in the clinical reasoning process include:

- Physical and psychosocial status of the individual in relation to his or her age
- Severity of the presenting problem and other associated physical and psychosocial issues

- Personality and temperament of the person
- Ethnic and cultural background
- Socioeconomic status
- Everyday living, school/work life of the person
- Educational background
- Special skills and interests
- Family obligations, values, and needs
- Multiple roles the person holds (e.g., family member, student)

The profile of information is not easy to predict and will vary from one person to the next, reflecting a person's identity and history. Similarly, the path to solving the problem often changes and shifts as intervention unfolds and the person responds in his or her own way. To generate a reasonable and effective approach for each client, the occupational therapist must consider multiple pieces of information, details, and insights, defining the specific problem at hand and developing ideas about the needs for intervention as well as the best strategies and techniques to support success. This information drives an intervention plan that the therapist implements and evaluates, refines and re-evaluates in an ongoing cycle of reasoning.

A therapist frequently develops a working hypothesis or idea about a problem, its causes, and possible solutions. This hypothesis will go through repeated revisions and iterations as the therapist tries different solutions and evaluates their effectiveness. Because each individual has a unique background and past experiences, there often are surprises and unpredictable reactions to intervention that become evident only during and after intervention rather than before. The therapist must be focused on the *expected* outcome, the progress the client is making toward it, and the unexpected or unpredicted outcomes that develop.

This flexibility is especially critical in the application of sensory integration principles and practices. Each child exhibiting a sensory integration dysfunction brings a unique profile of strengths and needs as well as a specific personality, a distinctive background and history, and a particular family, home, school, and neighborhood. The child's response to therapy will vary because of the state of the central nervous system on any given day but also because of the child's unique characteristics as a person and the supports and constraints that are present in daily life. This requires the therapist to be alert to the child's reactions and to modify and revise the intervention plan accordingly. The capacity to create improvisations during intervention and the ability to evaluate the child in an ongoing process are hallmarks of clinical reasoning and are skills that develop in therapists as they become more experienced and proficient in their craft.

This chapter explores the clinical reasoning literature outside of occupational therapy as well as within the field in order to identify key concepts that provide insight into the clinical reasoning process. A case example illustrates how therapists who provide sensory integrative interventions use clinical reasoning.

Clinical Reasoning as it Looks in Action

How practitioners think in action has been the focus of researchers and professionals in fields such as nursing, physical therapy, psychotherapy, social work, urban planning, and architecture. Their findings underscore the importance of the practitioner's thinking and reasoning in problems that involve people. For example, Dreyfus and Dreyfus (1980, 1986) worked with chess players and airline pilots to develop an explanation of the process of skill acquisition. They described this ontogeny of skillfulness as a continuum from novice to expert, a developmental progression based on increasing skills in reasoning and reflection as a result of experience. According to Dreyfus and Dreyfus, the progression in skill is contingent upon the skill learner developing more and more sophisticated strategies for identifying and making sense of the information presented in any given situation. The researchers termed this process *situation appraisal*.

Benner (1984) applied the Dreyfus model to clinical nursing practice in a study that combined interviews and participant observation with novice to expert nurses. Benner found that specific clinical skills and reasoning behaviors correlated to development and experience. In addition, Benner described a wide range of nursing practice behaviors (the helping role, the teaching-coaching relationship, diagnosis and monitoring, medication and therapy) and the concomitant reasoning processes that accompanied them.

In a later study, Benner and Tanner (1987) identified what they came to call the *intuitive quality of clinical judgment* in nurses. Their work underscored the legitimacy of the kind of knowledge that develops from experienced kinds of knowing. Based on accounts from nurses, these authors described specific intuitive-based behaviors that nurses use in their everyday practices, further supporting the belief that intuition is an essential part of clinical judgment.

Donald Schon, a philosopher, scholar, and urban planner, has written in depth on the process by which an individual develops and uses professional knowledge. Among the behaviors he identified and analyzed were reflection-in-action, the improvisational quality of reasoning, and naming and framing the problem. Schon (1983) described reflection-in-action:

> Both ordinary people and professional practitioners often think about what they are doing, sometimes even while doing it. Stimulated by surprise, they turn thought back on action and on the knowing which is implicit in action. They may ask themselves, for example, "What features do I notice when I recognize this thing? What are the criteria by which I make this judgment? What procedures am I enacting when I perform this skill? How am I framing the problem that I am trying to solve?" Usually reflection on knowing-in-action goes together with reflection on the stuff at hand. There is some puzzling, or troubling, or interesting phenomenon with which the individual is trying to deal. As he tries to make sense of it, he also reflects on the understandings that have been implicit in his action, understandings that he surfaces, criticizes, restructures, and embodies in further action. (p. 50)

Schon's description included a consideration of the professional's dual activities of doing and thinking, an interplay that occurs simultaneously, informing the actions and decisions that one makes while "in the midst of the performance" when you are "thinking on your feet" (1983 p. 54).

In a further exploration of the reflection-in-action process, Schon used the notion of improvisation to capture the sequence of recognizing "how well it has been working, and on the basis of these thoughts and observations, changing the way you have been doing it" (1983, p. 55). These abilities to make refinements, switch course, and modify and adapt an activity as it is unfolding are characteristic of a therapeutic approach such as sensory integration intervention. A therapist helps a child select an activity and, based on the child's performance, creates improvisations in order to produce conditions that will elicit a therapeutically desirable adaptive response. The original plan shifts according to what occurs, what the therapist observes, how the child reacts and responds, and how the therapist modifies the activity.

Donald Schon (1983) identified problem setting and the notion of naming and framing as critical in the work of a professional.

> When we set the problem, we select what we will treat as the "things" of the situation, we set the boundaries of our attention to it, and we impose upon it a coherence which allows us to say what is wrong and in what directions the situation needs to be changed. Problem setting is a process in which, interactively, we *name* the things to which we will attend and *frame* the context in which we will attend to them. (p. 40)

This approach to problem solving allows the practitioner to organize information in order to make sense of it and provide a start point or entry for intervention. The framing that occurs will vary based on clinicians' professional training, experience in different practice arenas, work history with patients, the theories they use to organize and guide their thinking, and their own personal philosophies.

In an article entitled "Conceptual Models in Psychiatry," Lazare (1973) illustrated the concept that clinicians name and frame the problem according to a specific theoretical point of view. Using one case, the author presented four contrasting theoretical interpretations (medical, psychological, behavioral, and social) of the same data. Clearly, each perspective directs the practitioner to select information that is most relevant given the particular set of lenses through which the practitioner is viewing the case. For example, the medical model focuses on "etiology, pathogeneses, signs and symptoms, differential diagnosis, intervention and prognosis" (p. 346). In contrast, the social model looks at "ways in which the individual functions in [the] social system" (p. 347) and how a "socially disruptive event" such as a death of a partner, a long-distance move, or similar significant social event affects the person.

Clinical Reasoning in Occupational Therapy

Occupational therapists also have investigated ideas about clinical reasoning in a broad range of practice concerns such as evaluation, intervention, and the educational process that prepares future therapists. From the very beginnings of occupational therapy education and formalized development of the profession, the training of future therapists has emphasized careful matching of the therapeutic task to the person while being watchful of the individual's reaction, carefully appraising and revising the intervention plans. The in-depth clinical fieldwork period that is part of the training in occupational therapy underscores the belief that a clinician cannot develop clinical reasoning from book or classroom learning alone. An understanding of the practice develops and undergoes refinement in "real-life" training situations where the student can learn from an experienced mentor how to frame problems, think intuitively, make clinical judgments, reflect-in-action, and develop a repertoire of skills on which to rely in any given situation.

In her explanation of the "thinking that guides practice," Rogers (1983, p. 601) took a broad view of clinical reasoning, describing the phenomenon as a synthesis of skills that includes ethics, art and, science. Rogers set out a series of reasoned questions and considerations that are embedded in the process of assessment and intervention. This explication of the reasoning process mirrored the work of Benner (1984), Benner and Tanner (1987), and Schon (1983, 1987). Others, such as Rogers and Masagatani (1982) and Barris (1987), described the process of clinical reasoning in the evaluation process. Fondiller, Rosage, and Neuhaus (1990) and Neuhaus (1988) discussed what clinical reasoning looks like when operating uniquely in occupational therapy with a specific set of the professional values and ethical concerns. Looking more specifically at professionalism, Parham (1987) presented the importance of autonomy, reflection, and the use of theory to guide practice as the essential components of a professional.

Mattingly and Fleming each contributed significantly to occupational therapists' understanding of the clinical reasoning process, studying in-depth a group of practitioners in a large urban rehabilitation hospital. Their numerous publications have described in detail the nuances of occupational therapy practice. They included a definition of the process of clinical reasoning (Mattingly, 1991b), the notion of the therapist as a problem solver with a three-track mind (with different reasoning strategies to match the distinct types of problems to be solved; Fleming, 1991), the narrative nature of clinical reasoning (Mattingly, 1991b), and the conflicts inherent in a view of the body as a machine and the body as a seat of human experience (Mattingly & Fleming, 1994). With the increased recognition of the importance of clinical reasoning stimulated by the work of Mattingly and Fleming, other occupational therapists such as Burke and DePoy (1991), Crepeau (1991), Slater and Cohn (1991), Neistadt (1992), and Cohn (1989, 1991) addressed clinical reasoning in specific groups of practitioners (therapists, leaders, managers, and administrators) and in the classroom and fieldwork experience.

Applying Principles to Sensory Integration

The case study in this section illustrates how therapists use specific clinical reasoning concepts when applying sensory integration theory in their practice of occupational therapy. The selection of the five specific clinical reasoning concepts presented here does not imply that other clinical reasoning concepts are not operating also.

Case Study: Finding Ways for Josh to "Fit In"

Josh was a kindergarten student whose teacher, Ms. R., referred him for an occupational therapy evaluation. Her primary concerns included Josh's difficulty playing and sharing with other children, his refusal to accept changes in classroom routines, and his need to be away from other children during table activities. She also sought help for his significant delays in language and fine motor skills. Josh had a limited vocabulary of about 12 spoken words and six signs. He was able to hold the pencil using a gross grasp, could not use scissors, and had limited manipulation skills. Ms. R. felt overwhelmed by Josh's difficult behavior, such as kicking and screaming when he did not get his way. She discussed her concerns with Josh's mother, who was a strong advocate for her son's inclusion in the typical kindergarten room. Ms. R. felt she had little insight into the nature of Josh's difficulties, did not believe she had established a way to communicate with him, did not understand his behavior, and did not know how to draw him into classroom activities.

Josh was new to his suburban school. He and his family had moved recently from a city 300 miles away to a suburban area outside a large city. He lived with his parents and his older sister, who was in the fourth grade. Both of Josh's parents worked full time outside of the home. Josh spent after school and some weekend time with a sitter who interacted with him and took him to activities such as swimming and park outings. Josh's family was interested in providing activities and interactions for Josh that allowed him to be happy and "a typical kid."

In addition to her concerns about her son's adjustment to his new school setting, Mrs. W. was troubled about problematic behaviors including wrist banging, tearing paper, and hitting his leg with his fist. She also was concerned that Josh was tasting and mouthing dirt as well as other objects in his environment, which posed a serious health and safety risk.

During an occupational therapy assessment, Josh's therapist observed him in a sensory integrative setting. Initially he was reluctant and fearful to get onto and stay on the platform swing without continuous verbal encouragement and close physical contact. Mrs. W. interpreted her son's reluctance on the swing as having to do with "feeling unbalanced and being afraid of falling." As the evaluation session continued, Josh tolerated and, with time, appeared to enjoy the platform and other swings as they moved in horizontal and circular patterns. He enjoyed sitting on, bouncing on, and laying prone over large therapy balls and was able to play a beanbag toss game while prone over a ball, supporting a portion of his weight on his hands and arms and demonstrating fair prone extension postures.

Josh required assistance for proprioceptive activities, including bearing weight on arms, holding and tossing a medicine ball, hitting a hanging tether ball using a weighted bat, throwing beanbags, pulling a heavy bag up into the air using a rope on a pulley, and using a massager. He engaged in all of these activities with obvious pleasure as evidenced by sounds he made, his visual attention to the activity, and his continued involvement. His mother also interpreted his responses as pleasurable.

Josh demonstrated no tactile hypersensitivity in his hands, arms, or legs. However, he was sensitive on his face and mouth, not allowing the therapist to put a whistle to his lips (he turned away on each offering).

Clinical Reasoning Using a Sensory Integration Perspective

The Role of Theory in Clinical Reasoning

The foundation of a practitioner's clinical reasoning rests on the conceptual framework by which the therapist organizes the way he or she thinks. Using a sensory integration conceptual framework, the therapist has a distinct set of information (such as concepts about sensory registration, modulation, and vestibular and proprioceptive input) to apply to a case situation.

Theories, models, and conceptual frameworks all carry with them a set of information that outlines the domain of their concern. This includes an understanding of the problems the therapist must address, the kinds of information the therapist needs to collect as well as the assessment tools and strategies to use, the goals to achieve, and the type of interventions the therapist will decide to implement. Theory also guides the kind of research that can inform an understanding of the problem(s) and the kinds of research methods a researcher can apply to understand the problem(s) further.

Theory is critically important in the process of clinical reasoning. When theory guides practice, the therapist is able to collect and interpret information using an organized and meaningful scheme that contributes to an understanding of what needs to be done. Sensory integration theory has defined concepts and supporting principles, and the relationships among the principles. These components strengthen the therapist's ability to understand what he or she is observing and recording about a child's behavior. Theory also supports the therapist's ability to predict the effects of the intervention he or she will provide. The following description outlines the importance of theory in Josh's case.

> The occupational therapist observed Josh and began to interact with him. Her sensory integration framework led her to ask, "How does Josh take in and process sensory information? What kinds of sensory information does he like? What kinds of sensory information have an organizing effect on him? Disorganizing? Is there a relationship between the kind of sensory information he is receiving, his ability to process it, and his behavior? Is this child over- or underresponsive to certain kinds of sensory information?" Further, she began to construct clinical observation opportunities guided by a sensory integration perspective so that she could construct an understanding of Josh's sensory registration and processing.

A sensory integrative perspective clearly defines the kinds of issues and concerns that a therapist will address. Additionally, in this case example, sensory integration theory played a critical role in developing the therapist's understanding of the problem and guiding the specific interpretation of what was interfering with this child's ability to interact successfully in his environment. Theory is especially interesting to consider in the practice of sensory integration because therapists are in a nearly continuous dialog with themselves about what they can expect to happen, given their theoretical perspective, and what actually does happen, given the individual receiving the intervention.

Narrative

Narrative is a strategy that enables the therapist to understand an individual within the context of the person's everyday life. Using a narrative approach, a therapist can form a collective understanding of the person, the family, his or her culture, and social life in order to focus interventions and outcomes that will be the most meaningful and important to the person and family. Narrative is particularly appropriate for work that focuses on the human experience, because telling stories:

- is a uniquely human characteristic
- is a way that humans make sense of the world
- is a process that allows humans to select and use information about their past to form a vision of the future
- allows the therapist to consider fully any special influences (such as one's culture, social class, ethnicity, and race)

Narrative offers clinicians the opportunity to think beyond the child today and into the future. This prospective storytelling technique is the vehicle for a vision of what might be.

> Therapists are often concerned not simply with reaching a set of objectives, but are concerned that the whole process of therapy should unfold in such a way that patients are given powerful experiences of successfully

met challenges, successes which can give patients the confidence to actively create a maximally independent life for themselves. (Mattingly, 1994, pp. 244–245)

The following narrative questions are useful in framing a child's story.

The present

- What is this child's life like now?

- What are this child's primary roles?

- Who is/are the primary caretaker(s)?

- What is this child able to do within his or her roles? What does the family think about this?

- What is the child unable to do? What does the family think about this?

- What is the child's sensory integrative status?

- How is it affecting role performance?

- How is it affecting interactions and relationships in the family? In the daycare/school setting? In the neighborhood?

- What are the family's priorities for what needs to happen to enhance this child's role functioning?

- Where is the best place for this to happen? In individual occupational therapy? With activities at home? At school?

- Where does this family wish for this child to fit in the community, and what kind of intervention or supports are necessary?

The future

- What will this child be like next year? In 3 years? In 5 years?

- What kinds of roles will this child be able to enact?

- Who will be the primary caretaker(s)?

- What will the child be able to do?

- How will the child's sensory integrative status have changed?

Josh's narrative developed from information about the enactment of his roles as a kindergartner, brother, son, and young member of a community. His teacher had a story for him that spoke of him not fitting into the classroom and not clicking with his teacher or his classmates. In contrast, his mother had a story of Josh as an active "member" of his family, school, and community. His mother's story grew out of a value of finding ways to include Josh, ways to help him meet his needs and fit into his social world. Mrs. W.'s story for her son was very much the story any mother would tell about her child, one that spoke to helping him find his place in a new school and begin to explore the outside world by developing interests (swimming, playing).

Josh's occupational therapist entered Josh's story and asked, "How are Josh's sensory needs interfering with and/or facilitating his story?" The therapist also considered the kinds of activities that would help to provide the sensory input he was seeking in order to increase his ability to interact and participate in school, home, and community. Josh's banging and hitting might well have been signals of his need for proprioceptive input that was more readily accessible, easily registered, and enjoyed. His fearfulness when initially placed on a swing could have been a sign of a hyperresponsive vestibular system combined with limited experiences and postural instability. Josh was a little boy who was having difficulty fitting in at a new school because of his developmental delays and his limited communication skills as well as his sensory integrative problems. He also was in a new environment with a teacher who had not yet learned how to read his signals, communicate with him, or provide the kinds of sensory experiences that would feed his central nervous system.

For the therapist to assist in realizing Josh's story, the clinician needed to help find ways to address his sensory needs within his everyday life with an eye to tomorrow as well as his early elementary school years.

The Three-Track Mind

Fleming (1994) described the therapist's reasoning as three converging sets of strategies that include procedural, interactive, and conditional thinking. Each strategy contains a distinct set of concerns and, in a sense, aims at different components of the person and problem.

Clinical Reasoning Using Three Tracks (Burke, 1997)

- **Procedural Track**

    Purpose: to treat the disability and reduce symptoms

    Point of View: the intervention process has specific powers to influence the disability

    Foci: the medical problem, the treatment procedure or method to remediate it

- **Interactive Track**

    Purpose: therapy with the person

    Point of View: it is important to understand the person

    Foci: "this person" as a social being

- **Conditional Track**

    Purpose: the therapeutic intervention with the person with the disability

    Point of View: various biological, environmental, and social factors influence people differently

    Foci: the person, problems, and potentials within an occupation orientation

In Josh's case example, the therapist was thinking procedurally when considering the kinds of sensory integrative techniques, equipment, and materials needed to help normalize Josh's sensory processing. Similarly, as the therapist developed a menu of ideas for selecting and using sensory materials throughout the day to address Josh's sensory needs, procedural reasoning was the mode. On an interactive level, the therapist was concerned with finding ways to connect with Josh so that he would recognize, respond to, and interact with the therapist; use social skills; and develop a way to be with people. Conditionally the therapist was asking, "How can I be thinking about creating successful experiences within his school, home, and community so that people see Josh, get to know him, understand his needs, and enjoy interacting with him and including him in the everyday world?"

Naming and Framing

Building on the work of Schon (1983), Parham (1987) imported clinical reasoning directly into occupational therapy in her article, "The Reflective Therapist." In describing the occupational therapist as an autonomous professional, Parham outlined the importance of naming and framing in the work of a professional occupational therapist: "Problem setting is as important as problem solving. Applying technical procedures lies within the realm of problem solving. Problem setting refers to identifying the appropriate problem to solve" (p. 556). Parham described problem setting as "a conceptual rather than a technical process. In problem setting, the therapist names what will be attended to in practice, and frames the context for intervention" (p. 557). It is in the naming of the problem and framing of the context that the therapist's clinical reasoning skills come forth.

> Therapists experience these processes most intensely during evaluation and diagnostic sessions. In thinking about Josh, the therapist initially needed to determine whether he was hypo- or hyperresponsive to sensory stimuli. Next, the therapist had to develop an understanding of the type and duration of stimuli that elicited particular responses, and interpret the responses when she manipulated the stimuli (proprioceptive input *during* vestibular activities rather than after or before). Observations of the child's ability to organize behavior, modulate, motor plan, and make adaptive responses under specific conditions further inform the naming and framing.

Reflection in Action

Clinical reasoning propels a therapist into putting together a plan of action, then implementing, evaluating, and modifying that plan. In an ongoing fashion, the therapist thinks about and uses the information learned each time he or she works with the client, both during the interaction and following the session. The therapist asks, "Is this working? Is this what I expected to happen? How shall I change this to be more effective? Shall I continue with this?" This ability to consider and reconsider the client's problems continuously as they evolve in intervention provides further input for the interventions that take place in the immediate moment as well as those that will take place in the future.

> In working with Josh, the therapist was continuously asking herself questions about Josh and his response to movement, touch, and proprioceptive input. Reports of Josh's sensory seeking at home (banging wrists, hitting leg with fist) encouraged the therapist to think about proprioceptive input as a source of pleasure and meaning. Successful trials with bouncing on the therapy ball and bearing weight on hands and arms led to experimenting with the massager and other types of proprioceptive input. Following the session, the therapist reflected on her reflection-in-action and thought about Josh's changing responses over the course of the session, becoming more involved and interactive. This led her to think about how important proprioceptive input was to Josh and how she could devise ways to provide opportunities for such sensory input over the course of the school day to increase interaction.

Summary

Examining the clinical reasoning that informs a therapist's practice brings insight into the multidimensional quality of the therapist's thinking. Judgments and decisions made during therapy depend on complementary as well as competing ideas embedded in the theoretical perspective the therapist is using. The complexity of this phenomenon of reasoning becomes more sophisticated as a practitioner matures from novice to expert. This maturation is grounded in experience and increasingly complex thinking and reasoning skills.

Sensory integration theory provides a rich backdrop for clinical reasoning. Therapists who use sensory integration in practice are privy to a set of concepts and principles to guide their thinking as well as their practice and research considerations. The conscious recognition of the role of clinical reasoning in sensory integration evaluation, intervention, and research allows therapists (novice to expert) to understand, appreciate, and use specific reasoning techniques and skills more effectively as they work with people who have sensory integrative dysfunction.

Works Cited

Quotation on pages 209 and 210 from Mattingly, C., and Fleming, M.H., *Clinical Reasoning: Forms of Inquiry in Therapeutic Practice,* F.A. Davis, Philadelphia, 1994, with permission.

Acknowledgment is made of the source of the material: from "Toward Professionalism: The Reflective Therapist" by D. Parham, (1987). The American Occupational Therapy Association, Inc. Reprinted with permission.

Quotations on page 206 from *The Reflective Practitioner* by D. Schon (1983) have been reprinted with permission by Basic Books, Inc.

References

Barris, R. (1987). Clinical reasoning in psychosocial occupational therapy: The evaluation process. *Occupational Therapy Journal of Research, 7,* 147–162.

Benner, P. (1984). *From novice to expert. Excellence and power in clinical nursing practice.* Menlo Park, CA: Addison-Wesley Publishing Company.

Benner, P., & Tanner, C. (1987). Clinical judgment: How expert nurses use intuition. *American Journal of Nursing, 87,* 23–31.

Burke, J.P. (1997). *Frames of meaning: An analysis of occupational therapy evaluations of young children.* Unpublished doctoral dissertation, University of Pennsylvania, Philadelphia.

Burke, J.P., & DePoy, E. (1991). An emerging view of mastery, excellence, and leadership in occupational therapy practice. *American Journal of Occupational Therapy, 45,* 1027–1032.

Cohn, E.S. (1989). Fieldwork education: Shaping a foundation for clinical reasoning. *American Journal of Occupational Therapy, 43,* 240–244.

Cohn, E.S. (1991). Nationally speaking— Clinical reasoning: Explicating complexity. *American Journal of Occupational Therapy, 45,* 969–971.

Crepeau, E. (1991). Achieving intersubjective understanding: Examples from an occupational therapy treatment session. *American Journal of Occupational Therapy, 45,* 1016–1026.

Dreyfus, H.L., & Dreyfus, S.E. (1980). *A five-stage model of the mental activities involved in directed skill acquisition.* Unpublished report supported by the Air Force Office of Scientific Research (AFSC), USAF (Contract F49620-79-C-0063). University of California at Berkeley.

Dreyfus, H.L., & Dreyfus, S.E. (1986). *Mind over machine.* New York: The Free Press, Macmillan.

Fleming, M. (1991). The therapist with the three-track mind. *American Journal of Occupational Therapy, 45,* 1007–1014.

Fleming, M. (1994). The therapist with the three-track mind. In C. Mattingly & M. Fleming (Eds.), *Clinical reasoning. Forms of inquiry in a therapeutic practice* (pp. 119–136). Philadelphia: F.A. Davis.

Fondiller, E.D., Rosage, L.J., & Neuhaus, B. (1990). Values influencing clinical reasoning in occupational therapy: An exploratory study. *Occupational Therapy Journal of Research, 10,* 41–55.

Lazare, A. (1973). Hidden conceptual models in clinical psychiatry. *The New England Journal of Medicine, 288*(7), 345–351.

Mattingly, C. (1991a). What is clinical reasoning? *American Journal of Occupational Therapy, 45,* 979–986.

Mattingly, C. (1991b). The narrative nature of clinical reasoning. *American Journal of Occupational Therapy, 45,* 998–1005.

Mattingly, C. (1994). The narrative nature of clinical reasoning. In C. Mattingly & M. Fleming (Eds.), *Clinical reasoning. Forms and Inquiry in a therapeutic practice* (pp. 239–269). Philadelphia: F.A. Davis.

Mattingly, C., & Fleming, M. (Eds.). (1994). *Clinical reasoning. Forms of inquiry in a therapeutic practice.* Philadelphia: F.A. Davis.

Neistadt, M. (1992). The classroom as clinic: Applications for a method of teaching clinical reasoning. *American Journal of Occupational Therapy, 46,* 814–819.

Neuhaus, B. (1988). Ethical consideration in clinical reasoning: The impact of technology and cost containment. *American Journal of Occupational Therapy, 42,* 288–294.

Parham, D. (1987). Toward professionalism: The reflective therapist. *American Journal of Occupational Therapy, 41,* 555–561.

Rogers, J. (1983). Eleanor Clarke Slagle Lectureship—1983: Clinical reasoning: The ethics, science, and art. *American Journal of Occupational Therapy, 37,* 601–616.

Rogers, J., & Masagatani, G. (1982). Clinical reasoning of occupational therapists during the initial assessment of physically disabled patients. *Occupational Therapy Journal of Research, 2,* 195–219.

Schon, D. (1983). *The reflective practitioner.* New York: Basic Books, Inc.

Schon, D. (1987). *Educating the reflective practitioner.* San Francisco: Jossey-Bass.

Slater, D., & Cohn, E. (1991). Staff development through analysis of practice. *American Journal of Occupational Therapy, 45,* 1038–1044.

Assessment of
Sensory Integration and Praxis

Mary-Margaret Windsor, Sc.D., OTR/L

Susanne Smith Roley, M.S., OTR

Stacey Szklut, M.S., OT/L

This chapter describes the rationale and procedures for assessment of sensory integration and praxis within an occupational therapy practice framework. The assessment process measures and examines specific components of sensory integration related to the child's engagement in occupation. Formal and informal observations of behavioral symptoms of sensory integrative dysfunction will help the therapist discern underlying deficits that interfere with performance. The interpretation of these findings guides the intervention process to improve performance (Ayres, 1972a). The *International Classification of Disability and Health, Prefinal Draft* (ICIDH-2; World Health Organization, 2000) model of function provides an overarching framework for evaluating the components of sensory integration and praxis relative to a larger scope of issues that support or inhibit the child's performance in context. The assessment process is dynamic and ongoing throughout the therapeutic interaction with the client. Dynamic assessment supports clinical reasoning that associates sensory integration and praxis with levels of function, especially socially relevant outcomes.

Defining Assessment and Evaluation

Historically, occupational therapy literature has used the terms *assessment* and *evaluation* separately and interchangeably but never consistently (McGourty, Foto, Smith, Smith, & Kronsnoble, 1989). Hinojosa and Kramer (1998) provided definitions for occupational therapy that the American Occupational Therapy Association Commission on Practice adopted: *Evaluation* is a general process (gathering, interpreting data); *assessment* refers to a specific tool and is a component of evaluation.

It is important to be aware, however, that other fields (education, psychology, government [IDEA]) often use the terms *assessment* and *evaluation* more loosely than do occupational therapists. Also note that in test development theory, *evaluation* pertains to the process of measuring change of behavior, in contrast to diagnosis or discrimination, the process of identifying behaviors for the purpose of placement within a group. Appendix 12-A provides expanded information about the purposes and uses of quantitative tests.

Evaluating Sensory Integration and Praxis Within the Context of Occupational Therapy

A comprehensive evaluation is a systematic inquiry and investigation. Blanche (2000) proposed that the assessment process is similar to a research project: the clinician formulates the question, gathers the data, and forms a hypothesis. These evolving hypotheses guide the investigation, and the clinician examines the conclusions by gathering additional data. The evaluation process accomplishes three major purposes:

- *identification* of sensory integrative deficits and their impact on activity and participation
- *documentation* of current level of function
- *appraisal/reappraisal* of change based on expected outcomes

The assessment process outlined in Table 12.1. follows the logic of the Occupational Therapy Practice Framework (American Occupational Therapy Association, 2000), which delineates the therapeutic process used in occupational therapy. Within this framework, assessment is an ongoing process throughout the interaction with the client. The evaluation consists of two parts, the occupational profile and the analysis

Table 12.1. Occupational Therapy Assessment Procedure Focusing on Sensory Integration and Praxis

Referral Statement	Issues and Concerns
Define and describe current concerns.	Record reports of actual behaviors that led to request for the assessment. Inquire about the sensory motor components of the child's interactions.
Obtain occupational history.	Inquire regarding the past, existing, and preferred type and pattern of engagement of the individual and family.
Observe.	Observe individual's capabilities with and without assistance in multiple settings as appropriate.
Conduct formal or informal assessment.	Collect data on sensory integration and praxis and related functions.
Synthesize data and its relationship to client concerns and occupational engagement patterns.	Review factor and cluster analyses to determine patterns of dysfunction in sensory integration. Consider use of sensory integration frame of reference in conjunction with other appropriate frames of reference for intervention.
Verify impression with family and child.	Create and record goals and objectives related to functional outcomes based on impressions and client concerns.
Create plan of action.	Recommend duration, length of time, and context in which intervention using a sensory integration frame of reference will occur if appropriate.
Plan for transition.	Determine long-range projected action plan that includes eventual discharge from therapeutic services and involvement in community activities.
Conduct dynamic, iterative assessment.	Conduct ongoing assessment during intervention and modification of intervention plan.
Conduct informal evaluation of outcomes and strategize to enhance outcomes.	Communicate regularly with significant individuals to evaluate and update intervention plan.
Reevaluate, evaluate change.	Compare current data to baseline data.
Revise intervention plan.	Continue, alter, adapt, or end intervention.

of occupational performance. Clinicians monitor intervention through dynamic assessment and measure outcomes through a variety of ongoing evaluations.

Identification

The sensory integrative frame of reference highlights the effects of hidden neurobiological processes on performance (Ayres, 1972a). As such, the evaluation of sensory integration and praxis relies specifically on data from which clinicians hypothesize about the child's neurobiological processing of sensation and its impact on performance. Both formal and informal assessments are effective for this purpose.

Informal Assessments

A variety of frameworks exist for gathering and interpreting information from others about a specific behavior or performance deficit. One behavior can have many different explanations, depending on which theoretical framework the evaluator uses for interpretation. Theoretical frameworks affect expectations of what to assess and analysis of performance components that then determine the intervention approach (Keshner, 1991). Utilizing a sensory integrative approach, the therapist reframes the problems during the analysis by seeing motor performance and behavior and thinking about sensory processing (Ayres, 1979; Blanche, Botticelli, & Hallway, 1995).

The first step in any assessment process is to define and describe clearly the reasons that cause the child, family, or school to seek consultation, evaluation, or intervention (Coster, 1998). The venue for this discussion is typically the intake interview. An occupational history supplies information regarding patterns of real and expected engagement in activities and includes questions about what is important to the child or family, such as taking a family vacation or having friends over for dinner. This background information also examines how the child organizes behavior for accomplishing tasks and activities as well as for planning events within abstract time and space. The therapist then uses information about the child's and family's typical and desired engagement patterns to guide the goals and objectives of the intervention.

A developmental, sensory, or family history furnishes important background information for understanding the child's reactions to sensation. The parents, caretakers, and other professionals who work with the child provide insights into the child's ability to process various types of sensory experiences within different environments and with different levels of support and challenge. Two sensory histories developed specifically for sensory integrative evaluation are the *Sensory Profile* (Dunn, 1999) and the *Evaluation of Sensory Processing* (Parham & Ecker, 2000).

The therapist's direct observations of the child can take place in a variety of settings. Observations within "natural" contexts or environments can provide significant clues to a child's functional capabilities and limitations and are extremely useful. Therapists usually consider "natural" contexts to be typical environments in which the child spends time, such as at home and in school. There is some debate as to whether or not, in a more primitive sense, typical environments are in fact "natural." From a sensory integrative perspective, a sensory integrative-type clinic is possibly a more primitively natural setting in which to assess and treat sensory and motor functions. This argument aside, each context provides information that yields a richer picture of the child.

The client and the therapist together decide the contexts that will provide the most useful evaluation data. Therapists often find it easier to evaluate a younger child in a setting that is familiar to the child. Especially for very young children, novel settings can inhibit otherwise spontaneous exploration and ease of interacting with the environment. On the other hand, the clinic setting that is controlled for quantity and types of activities and sensory demands sometimes provides a better environment in which to assess a child than a busy classroom or household. In some instances, the competing sensory stimuli of the natural environment can hinder the expression of a child's sensory and motor capabilities.

Skilled unstructured observations are often the only means by which to gather information about a child. The therapist makes the observations during child-directed activities rather than during therapist-directed activities. As previously stated, the evaluator makes inferences about the child's ability to organize sensation for use from observations of the child's behavioral responses and adaptations to changing physical and social environmental conditions. The therapist carefully analyzes the child's physical, social-emotional, and cognitive performance and capacity for making adaptive responses. The worksheet in Appendix 12-B (Koomar, Szklut, Ingolia, & OTA-Watertown Staff, 1995) describes specific observations and tasks in which to observe the effects of sensory integration on performance.

Clinical observations of neuromotor functions can be either structured or unstructured (Blanche, 2000). Depending on the examiner, such observations can encompass a broad spectrum of abilities. A clinician must have extensive knowledge of typical and atypical development for accurate interpretation of the observations. Appendix 12-C lists clinical observations of soft neurological signs that contribute to understanding sensory integration dysfunction.

Formal Assessments

The *Sensory Integration and Praxis Tests* (SIPT; Ayres, 1989) are the "gold standard" for evaluating sensory integration and praxis functions. The SIPT is a standardized assessment tool with normative data for a limited age range (ages 4-0 to 8-11), With the exception of postrotary nystagmus (a measure of a reflexive ocular-motor function), the SIPT subtests identify performance-based components that are important to the functions of sensory integration and praxis. This tool measures various aspects of sensory perception and praxis (Ayres, 1989). The SIPT includes 17 subtests belonging to four overlapping categories: (1) motor-free visual perception, (2) somatosensory, (3) praxis, and (4) sensorimotor. The SIPT considers these separate functions not only in isolation of each other but also relative to patterns that investigators have identified through over 30 years of research (Ayres, 1989; Mulligan, 1998a, 1998b).

Generally, the SIPT has limited direct application to many individuals with identified disabilities. This is particularly true for persons who have difficulty in situations requiring performance on request (i.e., comprehension of instruction, attention, manipulation of test items, sensitivity to context, or demonstration of capabilities outside the natural environment). Additionally, because diagnosis using the SIPT is dependent upon comparison to a like-age group with similar experiences, it is hard to determine whether the differences in test scores are attributable to the presence of sensory integration dysfunction or to pathology resulting in delayed neuromaturation.

Although Ayres (1989) stated that the SIPT is not appropriate for children with significant cognitive or motor impairments, children with diagnoses of mild neuromotor deficits or cognitive delays might benefit from the information the SIPT can provide. The SIPT is useful with high-functioning children with Asperger's disorder (Parham, Mailloux, & Smith Roley, 2000). Additionally, investigators have used the SIPT clinically with people who are older than the normative age ranges. In these cases, the SIPT serves as a nonstandardized evaluation of sensory integration and praxis functions. Clinicians must use caution in interpreting information collected outside of the age range for which this test is standardized. When a testing situation does not allow use of the SIPT in a standardized fashion, the examiner can evaluate the areas that the

SIPT covers by observing the child in similar activities. For example, when evaluating a child who is unable to comply with structured requests, then during a more playful period, the examiner can ask the child to follow unfamiliar two- and three-step verbal commands, which are similar to the Praxis on Verbal Command test demands; or invite the child to play Simon Says, which is similar to the Postural Praxis test demands. From the child's responses to these requests, an experienced examiner can make inferences about sensory integration and praxis.

Other than the SIPT, few standardized tools exclusively identify specific neurobiological behaviors related to sensory integration dysfunction. Appendix 12-D describes additional formal assessments such as the Sensory Profile (Dunn, 1999) and the Test of Sensory Functions in Infants (DeGangi & Greenspan, 1989), as well as some current tests that contain behavioral measures associated with sensory integration.

Interpreting Deficits in Sensory Integration

Interpretation of the child's sensory integration and praxis function relative to all the other factors that contribute to development is highly complex. The therapist's knowledge and expertise are critical when evaluating the magnitude of influence of the sensory integrative deficits on performance, especially in light of a preexisting diagnosis. The clinical chapters that follow in this text highlight some of these complexities. Interpretation of the test findings from an individual child is dependent upon several bodies of knowledge: the theoretical foundation of sensory integration; knowledge of the instruments used in evaluation; understanding of typical and atypical development; and clinical reasoning. Ayres' flow chart entitled "The Senses, Integration of Their Inputs, and Their End Products" (1979, pg. 60) provides a model for synthesizing the relationships between sensory systems, functional activities, and end products. Ayres identified the spectrum of sensory integrative deficits through a series of factor and cluster analyses, first with the *Southern California Sensory Integration Tests* (1972b) and subsequently with its revision, the SIPT (1989). (See Parham & Mailloux, 1996, for a summary of these studies.) Fisher, Murray, and Bundy (1991) proposed a model for interpretation of SIPT data and related clinical observations.

Table 12.2 is a worksheet that provides a structure for interpreting a child's evaluation data from the SIPT and other relevant evaluations such as clinical observations. The data are organized into three levels: sensory systems (specifically visual, vestibular, proprioceptive, and tactile), motor and praxis functions, and higher cortical functions. The worksheet provides a structure for analyzing the interrelationships among these variables. Within each box on the worksheet, the clinician identifies the child's performance for that system by listing the scores on the SIPT subtests or noting related observations. The list of items in each box is not inclusive; a clinician may add any relevant data. The worksheet lists the SIPT subtests in order of their importance as indicated by their loading on the cluster and factor analyses (Ayres, 1989). The worksheet takes into account not only single systems but also the relationships among the variables in the different boxes. The proximity of the boxes implies relationships among constructs that Ayres (1989) identified through factor and cluster analyses.

The worksheet leads the therapist to consider sensory processing first. The visual system is the most complex and has multi-layered contributions to function (see chapter 15 by Smith Roley & Schneck). Evaluation of the vestibular system occurs primarily through structured clinical observations (see Appendix 12-B). The somatosensory system consists of two systems, the proprioceptive system and the tactile system. The clinician can best evaluate the proprioceptive system through structured and unstructured observations of movement and body scheme (see chapter 6 by Blanche & Schaaf). The structured subtests of the SIPT are the best tools for assessing the tactile system. Clinicians can most effectively evaluate sensory modulation, which is often

Table 12.2. Diagnostic Worksheet Using the Sensory Integration and Praxis Tests (SIPT; Ayres, 1989) and Related Data*

Visual	Score	Vestibular	Score	Somatosensory	Score	Modulation	Score
Visual spatial SV FG Visual motor DC MAC Visual construction DC CPr Visual praxis CPr MAC DC Clinical observations		Postural SWB Clinical observations Prone Stability Righting Equilibrium Ocular motor PRN Ocular motor control Movement Stabilization		Proprioception KIN SWB OPr Tactile GRA FI LTS MFP Haptic form & space MFP GRA Clinical observations		Response to sensation Overreactive Underreactive Fluctuating Activity level Attention LTS Clinical observations	

Bilateral integration & sequencing	Score	Praxis	Score
BMC SPr OPr GRA MFP Part II (PPr) Clinical observations (i.e., jumping jacks)		PPr OPr PrVC (SPr) (BMC) Play	

Right hemisphere	Score	Laterality	Score	Praxis on verbal command	Score	Left hemisphere	Score
IQ Low performance High verbal Poor visual spatial SV, FG, FI, DC Low frustration Tolerance		SVCU PHU R/L differences Clinical observations		PrVC (low) PRN (high) Poor sequencing OPr, SPr, BMC, SWB, DC		IQ High performance Low verbal Poor sequencing	

Irregular Neurological (*circle if present*): diadochokinesia, thumb/finger, choreoathetosis, finger/nose, associated movements, clonus, increased PRN, tremors, tics, hypersensitivity to movement, seizures, other (*specify*):

Abbreviations of the SIPT

BMC	bilateral motor coordination	FG	figure ground	KIN	kinesthesia	MFP manual form perception
CPr	constructional praxis	FI	finger identification	LTS	localization of tactile stimuli	OPr oral praxis
DC	design copying	GRA	graphesthesia	MAC	motor accuracy	PHU preferred hand use

PPr postural praxis PrVC praxis on verbal command SVCU contralateral hand use
PRN postrotary nystagmus SPr sequencing praxis SWB standing and walking balance
PHU preferred hand use SV space visualization

*Note. From Course manual: From interpretation to intervention: Course 3 of the Comprehensive Program in Sensory Integration, by S. Smith Roley, 1999, Los Angeles: Western Psychological Services. Copyright 1999 by S. Smith Roley. Reprinted with permission.

linked to reactions to somatosensory processing, through sensory history question-naires and parent report (see chapter 4 by Miller, Reisman, MacIntosh, & Simon). Ayres (1972a, 1989) identified relationships among these sensory systems as they affect function. Often the function of one sensory system will affect the others (see chapter 1 by Spitzer & Smith Roley).

The second level of the worksheet examines bilateral integration and praxis. Motor performance is the vehicle through which to measure these constructs. Neuromotor deficits will affect performance on these tests and must be considered as a critical vari-able. During the analysis, the therapist considers the relative contribution of neuro-motor deficits, postural control deficits, and dyspraxia to poor motor performance. Discriminative analysis is necessary to distinguish a vestibular-based bilateral integra-tion and sequencing deficit from a neuromotor or praxis deficit. Often a bilateral inte-gration and sequencing deficit shows a laterality pattern of either equally poor use of both hands or slow development of the non-preferred hand (Smith, 1981). Low test scores in this domain, along with deficient tactile discrimination test scores, indicate developmental dyspraxia (see chapter 8 by Giuffrida). Play scales such as the Knox Preschool Play Scale (Knox, 1997) and observations of unstructured play are extreme-ly valuable in identifying developmental dyspraxia (Parham & Fazio, 1997).

The third level of analysis examines higher-level functions. In the absence of sensory-based deficits, deficits in processing information occur possibly at a cognitive level rather than or in addition to the level of the brainstem (Ayres, 1972a). Cognitive eval-uations such as IQ measures, rather than the SIPT or related instruments, are the appropriate vehicle with which to evaluate these higher-level functions. Dyspraxia on verbal command can indicate a language-based dyspraxia that the examiner can pin-point through the presence of a normal or high postrotary nystagmus score and adequate tactile discrimination test scores (Ayres, 1989). A speech and language or psycho-logical evaluation will often substantiate this impression.

During the evaluation process, it is impossible to evaluate only sensory integration and praxis. Cognitive, emotional, social, and physical processes all affect a child's abil-ities. Children who are referred for an assessment sometimes demonstrate irregulari-ties that stem from neurological deficits such as seizures or tremors. The clinician considers these deficits when interpreting any of the test data. Presence of irregular neurological functions does not necessarily rule out a sensory modulation or sensory processing deficit or dyspraxia. However, neurological irregularities do make it much more difficult to be certain about the extent of predicted benefits from intervention.

Intervention planning is a natural outcome of the identification process. Having identified deficits in certain systems, the examiner begins to hypothesize about the cascade of resulting difficulties. For example, a child who demonstrates deficits in somatosensory processing and praxis is likely to have difficulty learning new tasks and performing skilled tasks with ease in a fast-moving environment and will appear disorganized, especially in novel environments. Intervention will focus on remediat-ing the somatosensory and praxis deficits while enhancing the reported and predict-ed functional deficits. Discrete interpretation of test findings guides and facilitates targeted interventions.

Documentation: Relationship of the Model of Function to Sensory Integration

Documentation of the child's current level of function includes not only a description of sensory perception and planning strengths and weaknesses but also an appraisal of the impact of these strengths and weaknesses on the person's interactions within the context of daily occupation. The ultimate concern of occupational therapists using this frame of reference is not the structure or function of the body or its ability to process sensation but the ability of the child and his or her family to participate in meaningful occupations (Parham & Mailloux, 1996).

The updated ICIDH-2 Beta 2 and Prefinal Drafts (World Health Organization, 1999, 2000) emphasize function and challenge previous assumptions regarding an individual's expected capabilities with regard to the extent and nature of his or her impairment. Function results from the interaction between an individual's health condition, a given context relative to his or her capability during activity, and the individual's ability to participate in that context (see Table 12.3). This model is progressive in its acknowledgment of the role of activity and participation in health and therefore resonates well with occupational therapy (Coster, 1999) and sensory integration theory (Ayres, 1979).

Table 12.3. Model of Function (ICIDH-2 Prefinal Draft)*

Levels of Function	Characteristics	Contextual Factors
Body Structure/Function (Body)	Structural parts, components of movement	Physical, social and attitudinal worlds that influence all levels of function
Activity (Person)	Simple and complex activities and tasks	
Participation (Societal)	Involvement in life situations	

*Note. From ICIDH-2: International classification of disability and health. Prefinal draft, by the World Health Organization, 2000, Geneva, Switzerland: Author. Copyright 2000 by the World Health Organization. Adapted with permission.

Ayres (1979) defined sensory integration as "the organization of sensation for use" (p. 5). Although occupational therapists have traditionally focused their evaluations primarily on sensory integrative and praxis function at the body and clinical activity levels, it is becoming increasingly obvious that the outcomes might be most salient at the activity and participation levels. The dynamic process of sensory integration often has nonlinear results. Likewise, the relationship among the three levels of function (body structure/function, activity, and participation) is interactive but not causal or hierarchical. Change at the body level or the activity level does not automatically result in change at the participation level. Therefore, during current assessment procedures, the outcomes of sensory integrative intervention should include not only changes in sensory perception and planning but also the interaction of the person within the context of daily occupation. In addition, this comprehensive model controls for the inherent problems of an evaluation process limited to either physical impairments that might be difficult or impossible to change or performance of activities without regard to performance in context (Campbell, 1995; Haley, Coster, & Binda-Sundberg, 1994; Haley, Coster, & Ludlow, 1991; World Health Organization, 1980).

The World Health Organization model of function (1999, 2000) promotes the following perspectives:

1. The parts of the model (body structure/function, activities, and participation) are neither hierarchical nor causal to each other.

2. Presence of impairment does not automatically mean that an individual cannot participate in a full, meaningful life; nor does absence of impairment guarantee a full, meaningful life.

3. What brings the child to therapy is a problem in activity performance or participation, not necessarily a diagnostic label or a physical impairment.

4. When working with a chronic disability, therapists have a greater chance of changing functional performance and level of participation than of changing the diagnosis or impairment.

5. The task and context for performance are as important to function as the skills of the person participating.

Application of ICIDH-2 to Occupational Therapy Practice

Body Structure and Body Function (Body Level) assessments include medical characteristics or components such as strength, range of movement, muscle tone, reflexes, and soft neurologic signs. Historically, therapists have used many of the tests to evaluate clients at this level (e.g., portions of the SIPT, Ayres, 1989; *Bayley Scales of Infant Development-II,* Bayley, 1993; *Clinical Observations,* Wilson, Pollock, Kaplan, & Law, 1994). This information is quite useful diagnostically. Results of these assessments do not necessarily predict function, because these assessments examine the person in isolation of his or her social and physical contextual supports.

Activity (Individual Level) describes discrete actions (e.g., walking, sitting, reaching, or in-hand manipulation) and activities (e.g., daily living activities, hygiene, meal preparation, dressing, school performance, leisure, and work) that the client is capable of performing in the environment. Performance can be dependent upon body structure and function for quality and movements. The *Peabody Developmental Motor Scales* (Folio & Fewell, 2000) and some SIPT subtests (e.g., Design Copying and Walking and Standing Balance, Ayres, 1989) assess activities at the individual level. This form of assessment evaluates the child's ability to perform activities but does not answer questions about the child's successful adaptive engagement in natural contexts and environments.

Participation (Societal Level) encompasses performance and engagement in daily life within the context of the opportunities that life provides. Therefore, the participation level refers to desired and expected outcomes (e.g., attendance of a child with cerebral palsy in kindergarten) as well as to factors that support (e.g., wheelchair ramps, personal assistants) or constrain (e.g., poor funding, refusal to accept children with disabilities into a program) achievement of those outcomes. Sensory histories and questionnaires measure functional performance at the participation level. The *Child Behavior Checklist* (6 to 16 years; Achenbach & Edelbrock, 1991) and parts of the *School Function Assessment* (Coster, Deeney, Haltiwanger, & Haley, 1998) assess social participation. Such instruments measure the extent of participation and typically do not yield information regarding restrictions on participation.

Contextual Factors (Personal and Environmental) provide the background features of an individual's life and circumstances, features of his or her physical, social, and attitudinal world. Contextual factors are important because their interactions with the three levels of function (Body, Person, Society) can affect the individual's functional outcome.

The following case study demonstrates application of the ICIDH-2 model to the assessment process. Philosophically, assessment is an interaction in which the client invites the therapist to share his or her professional knowledge and insights about the child. In the midst of analyzing various levels of abilities and limitations, the therapist first and foremost, and without reservation, honors the uniqueness of the child or client.

Bryan

Bryan is a delightful 6-year-old boy with Down syndrome who lives with his mother, his father, and an 8-year-old sister. In the past, he had received early intervention services in his home one time per week and in a center-based group experience every other week. Because he had no physical limitations, his primary service provider was a speech and language pathologist. Bryan's family has had previous assistance in identifying and accommodating to his "special temperament and needs." Home has been a happy, safe place. Upon transition out of early intervention, the local school system assumed responsibility for provision of service.

During the previous academic year, Bryan had a successful preschool experience in a special classroom at the local rehabilitation center. He has recently begun to attend an inclusive kindergarten in his neighborhood school and
is experiencing difficulties. He sometimes will not keep his shirt on in school because it tickles him. He limits his play materials and time because he doesn't like the feel of certain objects, and he has negative behaviors during art projects when his hands get dirty. Sometimes he hits other students on the playground or when working with small groups. His nonacademic and social interactive skills are different from those expected for children in his classroom.

Most of the boys in the class spend much time building cities and roads in the sand table. Bryan does not join them because he likes to keep his hands clean. Some of the children have asked why Bryan tries to take his shirt off in school. Bryan has told them that it tickles and scratches and is uncomfortable, but they don't understand. When the children made cotton snow people to put on their home refrigerators, Bryan refused to participate. After using the bathroom, Bryan often has trouble tucking in his shirt and zipping his pants. His teacher is concerned that he will have difficulty with his winter jacket and boots. At school recently, Bryan has become angry and has pushed or hit other students while standing in line after recess. Bryan does not use the playground equipment and spends recess time chasing other children. They run away from him on the playground because they are afraid he will hit them. Some of his classmates have stated they "don't like him." A neighborhood child and schoolmate had a birthday party but did not invite Bryan. In the past, Bryan had enjoyed "play dates" with former preschool classmates. However, he has not made friends with anyone in his kindergarten class. Initially Bryan liked his new school, but now he has begun to ask to stay home and often cries in the morning.

Bryan's parents and teacher recognize that Bryan is not adapting to school. They are concerned that he is not acquiring the learning and social skills that he will need for a successful academic experience. There is not a goodness-of-fit between Bryan's current fine and gross motor performance, play and social interactions, and the expectations and demands in an inclusive educational setting. The classroom teacher has observed that Bryan has many motor skills and enough cognitive and social abilities to participate in most school tasks, but he does not seem able to use them.

The problem for this child is not simply Down syndrome or sensory integrative dysfunction, although these factors influence his functional abilities. His problem, as described by his teacher and his parents, is that he is not able to participate in classroom learning and social activities. Bryan's parents and teacher have requested an occupational therapy assessment. When Bryan's therapist can state the problem clearly, then she can generate hypotheses to understand, explain, and/or change his behavior. Sensory integration strategies can help Bryan organize and plan better in school; they can also help him to be more comfortable in his sensory world. Bryan will still have Down syndrome with capabilities different from his schoolmates, but he can develop skills to improve the quality and level of participation in his physical, social, and cognitive worlds. Following the introduction of various intervention techniques, observing and recording changed behaviors in Bryan's daily life will quickly verify the hypothesis of sensory integration dysfunction. Besides confirming the presence of sensory integration dysfunction, the therapist and the teacher can use dynamic assessment of Bryan's sensory status and behavioral responses to maximize his potential for purposeful and positive performances and occupation.

The following is an example of the format Bryan's therapist used to organize Bryan's occupational therapy assessment.

1. **Referral or problem statement**

   Statement of client concerns. Typically, this statement includes concerns regarding the child's participation in daily life activities. In Bryan's case, his therapist wrote, "Bryan has difficulty participating with other children his age in a positive fashion during the learning, performance, and social parts of his school day."

2. **Initial intake information**

   Review of school and medical records in order to understand implications of impairment on development, cognition, motor, language, and social interaction. For Bryan, this review drew upon all interpretations of additional data relative to Bryan's diagnosis of Down syndrome.

3. **Occupational inquiry**

   Interview of the child or client, asking questions such as:

   What is Bryan doing or not doing at home and at school?

   What does Bryan enjoy doing at home and at school?

   What is similar to or different from the past at home?

   How does this influence what the family is doing or not doing?

   How does this influence activity in other environments, particularly school?

   What are the desired changes in Bryan's and his family's life?

   What are the desired changes in Bryan's school life?

4. Observation through formal and informal assessment

The therapist conducts observations through structured and unstructured activities in a variety of settings, both in clinical and natural contexts (e.g., school and at home), recording behaviors without interpretation.

Observations at the body structure/function level include:

- Medical diagnosis

- Structural or physical conditions that appear to constrain outcomes (e.g., heart functions or an unstable atlanto-axial joint)

- Strength, endurance, range of motion

- Status and response of the sensory systems (tactile, vestibular, proprioceptive, gustatory, auditory, visual, olfactory) (Ayres, 1972a; Hanft; Miller, & Lane, 2000; Lane, Miller, & Hanft, 2000; Miller & Lane, 2000)

- Sensory registration: sensory detection; recording, noticing, and responding to salient environmental information

- Sensory modulation: neural process of adjusting the intensity, frequency, duration, complexity, and novelty of sensory stimuli leading to strategies for self-regulation

- Sensory discrimination: distinguishing among various aspects and qualities of sensory stimuli

- Use of sensory information to guide behavior

- Praxis: ability to create, plan, and carry out unfamiliar actions and sequences

- Motor skills: postural tone; movement patterns and reactions; gross, fine, and visual-perceptual motor skills; hand use, particularly thumb opposition, grasp pattern, and in-hand manipulation

Selected body structure/function evaluations: The SIPT is not appropriate for this child.

- Note tests in Appendix 12-D. Select a tool such as the *Sensory Profile* (Dunn, 1999) or the *Touch Inventory for Elementary School-aged Children* (Royeen, 1986), or use the *Peabody Developmental Motor Scales* (Folio & Fewell, 2000) with qualitative observation during performance.

- Careful use of structured clinical observations, keeping in mind developmental delay/age

- Sensory motor history or profile

Observations at the activity level include:

- Daily living skills (particularly independence in bathroom skills and dressing)

- Play activities

- Fine motor activities

- Gross motor activities

- Educational activities

- Cognitive activities

Selected activity level evaluations:

- Qualitative observations related to the sensory systems during performance on the *Gross Motor Function Measure* (Russell et al., 1993) and the *Movement ABC* (Henderson & Sugden, 1992)

- Qualitative impressions during completion of the *Wee-Functional Independence Measure* (University of Buffalo, 1998) or the *Vineland Adaptive Behavior Scales* (Sparrow, Balla, & Cicchetti, 1984)

Observations at the participation level include:

- Modification of context and provision of supports that promote Bryan's participation

- Amount of assistance necessary

- Level of acceptance

- Physical barriers or assists

- Social barriers or assists

- Spontaneous participation

Selected participation level evaluations:

- Qualitative impressions related to the sensory motor systems during completion of evaluations such as the *School Function Assessment* (Coster et al., 1998), *Child Behavior Checklist* (Achenbach & Edelbrock, 1991), or the *Parenting Stress Index* (Abidin, 1990)

5. **Compile data and verify impressions**

   Use clinical reasoning (see Chapter 11 by Burke) and knowledge of sensory integration and praxis (see Table 12.2) to interpret the data. The therapist and the client validate the impressions and plan and implement intervention strategies.

6. **Evaluation of change**

   During intervention: Use the dynamic assessment model, informal behavior or performance checklists, and observations (written or video) during therapy and within the natural environment.

   Following intervention: Readminister measures that assess end products and client concerns.

Appraisal/Reappraisal: The Dynamic Assessment of Sensory Integration

Dynamic assessment expands the concept of assessment beyond identification, intervention planning, and intervention effectiveness to include ongoing assessment within the context of intervention. Dynamic assessment is more holistic than the type of assessment typically available through traditional performance-based measures. When it works properly, dynamic assessment is a reciprocal process that links assessment to intervention, supporting the clinical reasoning process discussed by Burke in chapter 11 of this text and converting "opportunistic observation" (Meisels, 1996, p. 43) into a transaction that improves function. Using this type of evaluation on an ongoing basis throughout intervention, therapists can test the hypotheses they generated in the initial assessment process. Practitioners sometimes refer to this type of assessment as *interactive assessment*. The assessment process is not exclusive to the child; instead, assessment includes all significant individuals that constitute the client and caregivers. The early childhood literature notes the importance of inclusive inter-action, that is, observing the effects on a child's performance and interaction when the parents/caregivers participate within the assessment-intervention session(s) (Johnson, 2000; Ahern & Grandison, 2000).

Dynamic assessment has gained recognition in the field of occupational therapy because of its emphasis on functional outcomes and learning in context (Missiuna & Samuels, 1989; Toglia, 1992). Toglia identified three underlying precepts of the dynamic assessment approach: (a) the therapist bases assessment of the child's responsivity to the interaction or reciprocity within the interaction during intervention; (b) the therapist does not view test scores as the sole predictors of client performance; and (c) intervention is neither rigid nor bound to specific order. Dynamic assessment has been successful with children who have neuromotor problems (Easley, 1996) and is similar to Vygotsky's concepts of zone of proximal development and guided participation (Rogoff, 1990). This model of assessment differs from informal and formal or standardized assessments because it takes into account not only the task under examination but also the individual and his or her environment. (May-Benson, 1997).

Evaluation that includes dynamic assessment is not limited to the use of standardized instruments but, in addition to judicious use of criterion-referenced instruments, incorporates activities not normally considered to be assessment instruments. Judgment-based procedures and questionnaires allow the clinician to include information about typical performances and capabilities of the client related to his or her life at home, school, or in the community. Evaluation driven by dynamic assessment is not restricted to program entry and discharge. Rather, practitioners are able to refine and improve intervention procedures continuously in response to the results of the ongoing assessment process intrinsic to those procedures. The development and refinement of dynamic assessment allow the therapist to use performance in context to link assessment and intervention concurrently within the intervention session (Easley, 1996; Haley, Baryza, & Blanchard, 1993; Toglia, 1992). Dynamic assessment therefore provides a structure for moving from performance-based assessment to more ecologically relevant and context-rich assessment that includes observations of activities of daily living, performance during meaningful activities, and participation in more typical settings. Because dynamic assessment captures the process of "best therapy" so well and potentially encompasses the broader view of function and disability within a context, dynamic assessment is an excellent framework for the ongoing assessment/evaluation-intervention process that occurs when utilizing a sensory integrative frame of reference (see Table 12.4).

Table 12.4. Elements of Dynamic Assessment

Primary Elements	Characteristics
Individual	Multifaceted (e.g., social-behavioral skills, motor skills, body type/characteristics, cognitive ability, temperament, sensory acuity)
Task	Novelty, physical attributes, psychological attributes, complexity, actions required, etc.
Environment	Comfortable, supportive, familiar (a spectrum of properties consisting of people, animals, plants, physical entities)
Context	The interaction of the above elements that surrounds the client and provides meaning

As the word *dynamic* indicates, the assessment focuses on the ongoing process of acquiring new skills, with emphasis on investigating the child's ability to modify and improve performance when given adult guidance (Lidz, 1990, 1991, 1995). By identifying cues or environmental components that facilitate or hinder the child's performance, the therapist can provide intervention via formal and structured cues to elicit the child's best performance. The therapist identifies factors that limit the child's response and shares these insights with those who work with the child. The therapeutic focus is on the child's potential to learn new skills rather than on current levels of function. This capacity to facilitate the child's ability to modify performance and benefit from instruction is one of the most important outcomes of the dynamic assessment (Feuerstein, 1979) and is central to the therapeutic relationship and the ongoing process of intervention.

Appropriate use of assessment coexisting with intervention has always been an integral part of sensory integration practice. The therapist's search for the "just-right challenge" during intervention involves this process (Fisher et al., 1991). Using the dynamic-systems framework, a therapist observes a client's eating capabilities during lunch, for example, rather than specific isolated evaluations of oral motor reflexes, grasp/reach patterns, response to textures/smells, and so forth. The evaluator grades the task and gives structured cueing. This process utilizes the foundation skills of activity analysis to adapt the demands in component areas. The evaluator might decrease the number of items presented or reduce the postural, bilateral motor, or planning demands of the activity. Cueing can vary from general "hints" ("Is there another way you might sit on that swing to make it go?") to specific directions ("Turn around on the swing so you can hold the ropes with both hands"). The therapist then investigates the strategies the individual is using and attempts to analyze why the individual made that specific response. This phase of task analysis can utilize interventions such as cognitive or sensory strategies. The evaluator will again have to rely on careful observation and information from parents and other caretakers regarding the individual's best learning modalities and typical strategies. The therapist can also assess these modalities and strategies through careful task adaptation, such as changing specific sensory and motor variables each time the child moves through an activity. Dynamic assessment has many similarities to the intervention process in sensory integration that controls variables to facilitate an adaptive response. During classic sensory integrative intervention, the therapist is vigilant, constantly viewing the child's adaptive responses and modifying the interventions accordingly. The tenets of dynamic assessment fit well with sensory integration intervention that is in fact a dynamic process (see chapter 1 by Spitzer & Smith Roley).

Summary

Sensory integration is one of many processes that influence the life and function of a child, particularly a child with a disability. Identification of specific aspects of the spectrum of disorders related to an individual's sensory integration and praxis allows specificity in intervention planning and outcomes evaluation. Evaluators examine sensory integration and praxis within a broader occupational therapy assessment that emphasizes occupation and participation. A knowledge of test development theory and psychometrics enables the therapist to make informed choices concerning the purpose for testing, the level of function to be measured, and the instruments that best match the purpose and level of assessment. The process of assessment outlined in this chapter guides the therapist in acquiring knowledge and strategies for using clinical or informal instruments in a reliable, unbiased manner. Most often, a single instrument and a single setting will not provide all the information necessary for the evaluation of a single child.

Clinicians must view assessment of sensory integration and praxis relative to the child's overall function across multiple domains and consider sensory integration and praxis in light of the model of function that has evolved from the World Health Organization (1980, 1999, 2000), National Center for Medical Rehabilitation Research (National Advisory Board, 1993), and other sources. This model provides a structure for understanding levels of function and encourages assessment at all three levels—body, person, society. This is particularly important for evaluating sensory integration and praxis in children with disabilities who often are not candidates for direct, standardized measures such as the SIPT

This chapter presented dynamic or interactive assessment as a model that links assessment to intervention and as an effective means for evaluating change during intervention. Dynamic assessment supports the clinical reasoning process, thereby improving effectiveness and reliability in assessment, providing a context with meaning during performance, and allowing "fine tuning" and change during intervention. Such a process of interactive assessment permits timely, appropriate change and modification of the task, the individual, and the environment. Dynamic assessment can also connect assessment and intervention to the everyday life and occupations in the child's natural world.

Outcomes related to sensory integration have been hard to measure because their scope is difficult to define clearly (Dunkerley, Tickle-Degnen, & Coster, 1997). Ayres (1979) included improvements in self-esteem, personal-social skills, and school performance as expected results from sensory integration treatment. However, using these end-product behaviors as outcomes has been problematic due to lack of direct cause-and-effect relationships resulting from sensory integrative intervention. Although sensory integrative and praxis functions of components at the body structure or function level can improve as a result of specific intervention, practitioners are becoming more refined in understanding the effects of enhanced sensory integration and praxis on meaningful and purposeful participation in occupation. The most striking changes that result from sensory integrative intervention in populations with other diagnoses relate to improved participation by the child and improved quality of life for the family (Cohn & Cermak, 1998).

Acknowledgments

The authors extend sincere appreciation to Anthony B. Gerard, Ph.D., and Richard Furbush, M.S., OTR/L, for their editorial review of this chapter.

References

Abidin, R.R. (1990). *Parenting Stress Index* (3rd ed.). Charlottesville, VA: Pediatric Psychology Press.

Achenbach, T.M., & Edelbrock, C. (1991). *Manual for the Child Behavior Checklist and Revised Child Behavior Profile.* Burlington, VT: University of Vermont, Department of Psychiatry.

Ahern, C.A., & Grandison, C.M. (2000). Inclusivity in developmental neuropsychological assessment. *Zero to Three, 20* (4), 23–27.

American Occupational Therapy Association. (2000). *The occupational therapy practice framework: Draft V.* Bethesda, MD: Author.

Aylward, G.P. (1997). Conceptual issues in developmental screening and assessment. *Developmental and Behavioral Pediatrics, 18,* 340–349.

Ayres, A.J. (1972a). *Sensory integration and learning disorders.* Los Angeles: Western Psychological Services.

Ayres, A.J. (1972b). *Southern California Sensory Integration Tests.* Los Angeles: Western Psychological Services.

Ayres, A.J. (1979). *Sensory integration and the child.* Los Angeles: Western Psychological Services.

Ayres, A.J. (1989). *Sensory Integration and Praxis Tests.* Los Angeles: Western Psychological Services.

Ayres, A.J., & Tickle, L.S. (1980). Hyperresponsivity to touch and vestibular stimuli as a predictor of positive response to sensory integration procedures by autistic children. *American Journal of Occupational Therapy, 34,* 375–381.

Bailey, D.G., Jr., & Wolery, M. (1989). *Assessing infants and preschoolers with handicaps.* Columbus, OH: Merrill Publishing Company.

Bayley, N. (1993). *The Bayley Scales of Infant Development* (2nd ed.). San Antonio, TX: The Psychological Corporation.

Berk, R.A., & DeGangi, G.A. (1983). *DeGangi-Berk Test of Sensory Integration.* Los Angeles: Western Psychological Services.

Blanche, E.I. (2000). *Utilizing clinical reasoning in the assessment of children with SI dysfunction.* Videotape in preparation. Torrance, CA: Pediatric Therapy Network.

Blanche, E.I. (2001). The role of observations in the clinical reasoning process. Manuscript in preparation.

Blanche, E.I., Botticelli, T.M., & Hallway, M.K. (1995). *Combining neuro-developmental treatment and sensory integration principles: An approach to pediatric therapy.* Tucson, AZ: Therapy Skill Builders.

Campbell, S.K. (1995). *Physical therapy for children.* Philadelphia: W.B. Saunders.

Carrasco, R.C., & Lee, C.E. (1993, September). Development of a teacher questionnaire on sensorimotor behavior. *Sensory Integration Special Interest Section Newsletter, 16,* 5–6.

Cohn, E.S., & Cermak, S.A. (1998). Including the family perspective in sensory integration outcomes research. *American Journal of Occupational Therapy, 52,* 540–545.

Cook, D.G. (1991). The assessment process. In W. Dunn (Ed.), *Pediatric occupational therapy: Facilitating effective service provision* (pp. 35–72). Thorofare, NJ: Slack.

Coster, W. (1998). Occupation-centered assessment of children. *American Journal of Occupational Therapy, 52,* 337–344.

Coster, W., Deeney, T., Haltiwanger, J., & Haley, S. (1998). *School Function Assessment.* San Antonio, TX: Therapy Skill Builders.

DeGangi, G.A., & Greenspan, S.I. (1989). *Test of Sensory Functions in Infants.* Los Angeles: Western Psychological Services.

Dunkerley, E., Tickle-Degnen, L., & Coster, W.J. (1997). Therapist-child interaction in the middle minutes of sensory integration treatment. *American Journal of Occupational Therapy, 51,* 799–805.

Dunn, W. (1994). Performance of typical children on the Sensory Profile: An item analysis. *American Journal of Occupational Therapy, 48,* 967–974.

Dunn, W. (1999). *Sensory Profile.* San Antonio, TX: Therapy Skill Builders.

Easley, A.M. (1996). Dynamic assessment for infants and toddlers: The relationship between assessment and the environment. *Pediatric Physical Therapy, 8,* 62–69.

Feuerstein, R. (1979). *The dynamic assessment of retarded performers.* Baltimore, MD: University Park Press.

Fisher, A.G., Murray, E.A., & Bundy, A.C. (1991). *Sensory integration: Theory to practice.* Philadelphia: F. A. Davis Company.

Folio, M.R., & Fewell, R.R. (2000). *Peabody Developmental Motor Scales.* Austin, TX: Pro-Ed.

Gillette, N. (1991). The issue is: Research directions for occupational therapy. *American Journal of Occupational Therapy, 45,* 563–566.

Guyatt, G. H., Kirshner, B., & Jaeschke, R. (1992). Measuring health status: What are the necessary measurement properties? *Journal of Clinical Epidemiology, 45,* 1341–1345.

Haley, S.M., Baryza, M.J., & Blanchard, Y. (1993). Functional and naturalistic frameworks in assessing physical and motor disablement. In I.J. Wilhelm (Ed.), *Physical therapy evaluation in early infancy (Clinics in Physical Therapy)* (pp. 225–256). New York: Churchill Livingstone.

Haley, S.M., Coster, W.J., & Binda-Sundberg, K. (1994). Measuring physical disablement: The contextual challenge. *Physical Therapy, 74,* 74/443–82/451.

Haley, S.M., Coster, W.J., & Ludlow, L.H. (1991). Pediatric functional outcome measures. In G.H. Kraft & K.M. Jaffe (Eds.), *Physical medicine and rehabilitation clinics of North America* (pp. 689–723). Philadelphia: W.B. Saunders.

Haley, S.M., Coster, W.J., Ludlow, L.H., Haltiwanger, J.T., & Andrellos, P.J. (1992). *Pediatric evaluation of disability inventory.* Boston: Boston University.

Hanft, B.E., Miller, L.J., & Lane, S.J. (2000). Toward a consensus in terminology in sensory integration theory and practice: Part 3: Observable behaviors: Sensory integration dysfunction. *Sensory Integration Special Interest Section Newsletter, 23*(3), 1–4.

Henderson, S.E., & Sugden, D.A. (1992). *Movement Assessment Battery for Children.* London: Psychological Corporation, Ltd.

Hinojosa, J., & Kramer, P. (1998). *Evaluation obtaining and interpreting data.* Rockville, MD: American Occupational Therapy Association.

Johnson, K. (2000). Inclusive interaction in mental health consultation to the childcare community. *Zero to Three, 20* (4), 15–18.

Jones, C., & Monkhouse-Kleuser, M.A. (1981). *Balcones Sensory Integration Screening* (Rev. ed.). Austin, TX: Occupational Therapy Association, Inc

Jongbloed, L.E., Collins, J.B., & Jones, W. (1986). Sensorimotor Integration Test Battery. *Occupational Therapy Journal of Research, 6,* 131–150.

Keshner, E.A. (1991). How theoretical framework biases evaluation and treatment. In *Contemporary management of motor problems* (pp. 37–47). Alexandria, VA: Foundation for Physical Therapy.

Knox, S. (1997). Development and current use of the Knox preschool play scale. In L.D. Parham & Fazio, L. (Eds.). *Play in Occupational Therapy for Children.* St. Louis: Mosby-Times, Inc.

Koomar, J., Szklut, S.E., Ingolia, P., & OTA-Watertown Staff. (1995). *Sensory modulation and discrimination evaluation.* Unpublished manuscript.

Lane, S.J., Miller, L.J., & Hanft, B.E. (2000). Toward a consensus in terminology in sensory integration theory and practice: Part 2: Sensory integration patterns of function and dysfunction. *Sensory Integration Special Interest Section Newsletter, 23*(2), 1–3.

Lidz, C.S. (1990). The preschool learning assessment device: An approach to the dynamic assessment of young children. *European Journal of Psychology of Education, 2,* 167–175.

Lidz, C.S. (1991). *Practitioner's guide to dynamic assessment.* New York: Guilford Press.

Lidz, C.S. (1995). Dynamic assessment and the legacy of L.S. Vygotsky. *School Psychology, 16,* 143–153.

May-Benson, T. (1997*). Introduction to dynamic assessment: A curriculum guide for occupational therapists.* Unpublished manuscript, Boston University Sargent College, Boston.

McGourty, L., Foto, M., Smith, N., Smith, R., & Kronsnoble, S. (1989). *Uniform terminology for occupational therapy* (2nd ed.). Rockville, MD: American Occupational Therapy Association.

Meisels, S.J. (1996). Charting the continuum of assessment and intervention. In S.J. Meisels & E. Fenichel (Eds.), *New visions for the developmental assessment of infants and young children* (pp. 27–52). Washington, DC: Zero to Three.

Miller, L.J., & Lane, S.J. (2000). Toward a consensus in terminology in sensory integration theory and practice: Part 1: Taxonomy of neurophysiological processes. *Sensory Integration Special Interest Section Newsletter, 23*(1), 1–4.

Miller, L., & Roid, G.H. (1995). *T.I.M.E.— Toddler and Infant Motor Evaluation.* Tucson, AZ: Therapy Skill Builders.

Missiuna, C., & Samuels, M.T. (1989). Dynamic assessment of preschool children with special needs: Comparison of mediation and instruction. *Remedial and Special Education, 10,* 53–62.

Morton, K., & Wolford, S. (1984). *Analysis of Sensory Behavior Inventory* (Rev. ed.). Arcadia, CA: Skills with Occupational Therapy.

Mulligan, S. (1998a). Patterns of sensory integration dysfunction: a confirmatory factor analysis. *American Journal of Occupational Therapy, 52,* 819–828.

Mulligan, S. (1998b). Application of structural equation modeling in occupational therapy research. *American Occupational Journal of Occupational Therapy, 52,* 829–834.

Mulligan, S. (2000a). Evaluating the evidence for occupational therapy using a sensory integration framework. (Submitted for review for publication in AJOT).

Mulligan, S. (2000b). Cluster analysis of scores of children on the Sensory Integration and Praxis Tests, *Occupational Therapy Journal of Research, 20*(4), 256–262.

National Advisory Board. (1993). *Research plan for the National Center for Medical Rehabilitation Research* (NIH Publication No. 93-3509). Washington, DC: U.S. Dept. of Health and Human Services.

Parham, L.D. (1998). The relationship of sensory integrative development to achievement in elementary students: Four-year longitudinal patterns. *Occupational Therapy Journal of Research, 18*(3), 105–127.

Parham, L. D., & Ecker, C. (2000). *Evaluation of sensory processing.* Manuscript in preparation, University of Southern California, Los Angeles.

Parham, L.D., & Fazio, L. (1997). *Play in occupational therapy for children.* St. Louis: Mosby-Times, Inc.

Parham, L.D., & Mailloux, Z. (1996). Sensory integration. In J. Case-Smith, A.S. Allen, & P.N. Nuse (Eds.), *Occupational therapy for children* (3rd ed., pp. 307–356). St. Louis: Mosby.

Parham, D., Mailloux, Z., & Smith Roley, S. (2000). Sensory processing and praxis in high-functioning children with autism. Paper presented at Research 2000, February 4–5, 2000, Redondo Beach, CA.

Provost, B., & Oetter, P. (1993). The Sensory Rating Scale for Infants and Young Children: Development and reliability. *Physical and Occupational Therapy in Pediatrics, 13*(4), 15–35.

Reisman, J.E., & Hanschu, B. (1992). *Sensory Integration Inventory* (Rev. ed.). Hugo, MN: PDP Products.

Rogoff, B. (1990). *Apprenticeship in thinking: Cognitive development in social context.* New York: Oxford University Press.

Royeen, C.B. (1986). The development of a touch scale for measuring tactile defensiveness in children. *American Journal of Occupational Therapy, 40,* 414–419.

Royeen, C.G. (1987). TIP—Touch Inventory for Preschoolers: A pilot study. *Physical and Occupational Therapy in Pediatrics, 7*(1), 29–40.

Russell, D., Rosenbaum, P., Gowland, C., Hardy, S., Lane, M., Plews, N., McGavin, H., Cadman, D., & Jarvis, S. (1993). *Gross motor function measure manual* (2nd ed.). Hamilton, Canada: McMaster University.

Schroeder, C.V., Block, M.P., Campbell, E.T., & Stowell, M. (1979). *SBC Adult Psychiatric Sensory Integration Evaluation.* San Diego, CA: Research Associates, California.

Shumway-Cook, A., & Woollacott, M. (1995). *Motor control: Theory and practical applications.* Baltimore: Williams and Wilkins.

Smith, S. (1981, Winter). Speculations on crossing the midline, dyspraxia, and future perspectives: Synopsis of a seminar in the clinic of A.J. Ayres, Ph.D., August 25, 1981. *Center for the Study of Sensory Integrative Dysfunction Quarterly Newsletter, 2–3.*

Smith Roley, S. (1999). *Course manual: From interpretation to intervention: Course 3 of the Comprehensive Program in Sensory Integration.* Los Angeles: Western Psychological Services.

Sparrow, S.S., Balla, D.A., & Cicchetti, D.V. (1984). *Vineland Adaptive Behavioral Scales.* Circle Pines, MN: American Guidance Service.

Spitzer, S., Smith Roley, S., Clark, F., & Parham, D. (1997). Sensory integration: Current trends in the United States. *Scandinavian Journal of Occupational Therapy, 4:0000-0,* 1–16.

Toglia, J. (1992). A dynamic interactional approach to cognitive rehabilitation. In N. Katz (Ed.), *Cognitive rehabilitation models for intervention in occupational therapy* (pp. 104–143). Boston: Andover Medical Publishers.

University of Buffalo. (1998). *Wee-Functional Independence Measure System SM Clinical Guide* (Version 5.01). Buffalo, NY: Author.

Wilson, B.N., Pollock, N., Kaplan, B.J., & Law, M. (1994). *Clinical Observations of Motor and Postural Skills.* Tucson, AZ: Therapy Skill Builders.

World Health Organization. (1980). *International classification of impairments, disabilities, and handicaps.* Geneva, Switzerland: Author.

World Health Organization. (1999). *ICIDH-2: International classification of functioning and disability. Beta-2 draft, full version.* Geneva, Switzerland: Author.

World Health Organization. (2000). *ICIDH-2: International classification of disability and health. Prefinal draft.* Geneva, Switzerland: Author.

Additional Readings

Anastasi, A., & Urbina, S. (1997). *Psychological testing* (7th ed.). Upper Saddle River, NJ: Prentice Hall.

Arendt, R.E., Maclean, W.E., Jr., & Baumeister, A.A. (1988). Critique of sensory integration therapy and its application in mental retardation. *American Journal on Mental Retardation, 92,* 401–411.

Clark, F.A., Parham, D., Carlson, M.E., Frank, G., Jackson, J., Pierce, D., Wolfe, R., & Zemke, R. (1991). Occupational science: Academic innovation in the service of occupational therapy's future. *American Journal of Occupational Therapy, 45,* 300–319.

Coster, W. (1999). School function assessment: Administration and interpretation. Workshop sponsored by Therapro and OTA Wakefield, March 28, Boston University Sargent College, Boston.

Coster, W.J., & Haley, S.M. (1992). Conceptualization and measurement of disablement in infants and young children. *Infants and Young Children, 4,* 11–22.

Deusen, J. van, & Brunt, D. (1997). *Assessment in occupational therapy and physical therapy.* Philadelphia: W. B. Saunders.

Dunn, W. (1981). *A guide to testing clinical observations.* Rockville MD: American Occupational Therapy Association.

Greenspan, S.I. (1996). Assessing the emotional and social functioning of infants and young children. In S.J. Meisels & E. Fenichel (Eds.), *New visions for the developmental assessment of infants and young children* (pp. 231–266). Washington, DC: Zero to Three.

Greenspan, S.I., & Meisels, S.J. (1996). Toward a new vision for the developmental assessment of infants and young children. In S. J. Meisels & E. Fenichel (Eds.), *New visions for the developmental assessment of infants and young children* (pp. 11–26). USA: Zero to Three: National Center for Infants, Toddlers, and Families.

Greenspan, S.I., & Wieder, S. (1997). An integrated developmental approach to interventions for young children with severe difficulties in relating and communication. *Zero to Three, 17,* 5–18.

Haley, S.M. (1994). Perspective: Our measures reflect our practices and beliefs: A perspective on clinical measurement in pediatric physical therapy. *Pediatric Physical Therapy, 6,* 142–143.

Hertzig, M.E., & Shapiro, T. (1987). The assessment of nonfocal neurological signs in school-aged children. In D. Tupper (Ed.), *Soft neurological signs* (pp.71–93). Orlando, FL: Grune & Stratton.

Hoehn, T.P., & Baumeister, A.A. (1994). A critique of the application of sensory integration therapy to children with learning disabilities. *Journal of Learning Disabilities, 27,* 338–350.

Kaplan, B.J., Polatajko, H.J., Wilson, B.N., & Faris, P.D. (1993). Reexamination of sensory integration treatment: A combination of two efficacy studies. *Journal of Learning Disabilities, 26,* 342–347.

Landman, G.B., Levine, M.D., Fenton, T., & Soloman, B. (1986). Minor neurological indicators and developmental function in preschool children. *Developmental and Behavioral Pediatrics, 7,* 97–101.

Law, M. (1987). Measurement in occupational therapy: Scientific criteria for evaluation. *Canadian Journal of Occupational Therapy, 54,* 133–138.

Lollar, D.J. (1999, May). *ICIDH-2 presentation.* Information presented at the Neurobehavioral Rehabilitation Center Seventh Annual Research Colloquium: Unifying disability, Boston University Sargent College, Boston.

Meisels, S.J., & Fenichel, E. (Eds.). (1996). *New visions for the developmental assessment of infants and young children.* Washington, DC: Zero to Three.

Miller, L.J. (Ed.). (1989). *Developing norm-referenced standardized tests.* Binghamton, NY: Haworth Press.

Trombly, C.A. (1993). The issue is: Anticipating the future: Assessment of occupational function. *American Journal of Occupational Therapy, 47,* 253–257.

Trombly, C.A. (1995). Elenor Clark Slagle Lectureship. *American Journal of Occupational Therapy, 49,* 960–972.

Tupper, D.E. (Ed.). (1987). *Soft neurological signs.* Orlando, FL: Grune & Stratton.

Williamson, G.G. (1996). Assessment of adaptive competence. In S.J. Meisels & E. Fenichel (Eds.), *New visions for the developmental assessment of infants and young children* (pp. 193–206). Washington, DC: Zero to Three.

Yule, W., & Taylor, E. (1987). Classification of clinical soft signs. In D.E. Tupper (Ed.), *Soft neurological signs* (pp.19–43). Orlando, FL: Grune & Stratton.

A Few Words About Formal Evaluations

Purposes and Uses of Quantitative Assessment Tools

The three primary uses for measurement are discrimination (classification), evaluation (change in a construct or function), and prediction (Guyatt, Kirshner, & Jaeschke, 1992; Russell et al., 1993). Particular test types best serve specific purposes (Meisels, 1996).

Discrimination

A discriminative instrument is useful for identifying or classifying an individual based on actions or presence of a characteristic(s). Standardized, norm-referenced tests compare the score of the individual with scores of a specified reference group (norm-referenced testing). The *Sensory Integration and Praxis Tests* (Ayres, 1989) belong to this category: they identify children with sensory integration dysfunction by comparing their test performances to those of a typical age group. In standardized normative testing, sensitivity refers to the ability of the measure to categorize or identify individuals correctly (Aylward, 1997).

Screening Versus Evaluation

In education and psychology (Bailey & Wolery, 1989), screening refers to the process of measuring large groups to identify individuals who are at high risk or exhibit symptoms of a particular condition; additional follow-up with further evaluation is necessary to make the diagnosis. A good screening is usually quick and inexpensive and results in a percentage of false positives (people initially identified as having the condition but, as determined by further assessment, do not have the condition). Evaluation is a more lengthy and complex measurement that results in a diagnosis.

Evaluation

An evaluative measure establishes a baseline of function and allows measurement of change over time, such as during or after intervention. Responsiveness is the feature in a standardized assessment that describes how well that assessment is able to measure change in function. Responsiveness is statistically determined based on subjects' scores and identification of minimal change that the tool's authors considered to be clinically important (Russell et al., 1993). Practitioners may use this type of test to demonstrate efficacy or functional change.

Presently, occupational therapists develop and use tests primarily for discrimination, not evaluation (Gillette, 1991; Haley, Coster, Ludlow, Haltiwanger, & Andrellos, 1992). Such instruments are not responsive to the subtle but meaningful changes within a special population that clearly affect function but are never of a magnitude that would change categorization from the special group to the typical group. Understanding this concept is central to understanding why it has been so difficult to demonstrate efficacy of intervention.

Complex tasks, roles, and participation are essential for tracking change in functional performance (e.g., ability to comb hair or to perform daily living activities more easily are better indexes of change than increased range of motion). Criterion-referenced tests, curriculum-based evaluations, and continuous performance assessments, which deal with mastery of levels of performance that lead to more inclusion, are possible selections for evaluating improved performance (Meisels, 1996). The purpose of such instruments is to measure changes within a targeted behavior, not to measure changes in an individual that would lead to change in group membership (e.g., from a neuro-motor group to a typical group). Children with disabilities can have functional and performance changes but still remain classified as developmentally disabled. Criterion-referenced tests or curriculum-based evaluations allow observation of a greater spectrum of process, often within an ecological context, as well as the actual performance. They are not bound by the artificial confines often necessary in standardized performance-based testing (e.g., a limited number of task presentations while the child sits at a table).

At a less formal level, the practitioner can embed the process of assessment within the process of intervention. Conducting assessment concurrently with intervention allows for subtle changes and tweaking of strategies when providing direct service. Continuous performance or dynamic assessment emphasizing sensory integration (described in depth in the section of this chapter entitled Appraisal/Reappraisal: The Dynamic Assessment of Sensory Integration) comprises a helpful means of ongoing evaluation of the client's performance for therapists.

Prediction

A predictive measure provides an estimate of prognosis (if and when functional status change will occur) and means for developing critical pathways. There is some evidence that, when administered to young children, the SIPT can predict later math and reading difficulties (Parham, 1998). However, more studies are necessary to validate this data. Improving discrimination and evaluation and identifying critical components of function would increase prediction and intervention. The emphasis on causal pathways and evidence-based practice in current medicine demands such undertakings.

Structured Clinical Observations:

*Application to Diverse Populations**

*Note. From "The Role of Observations in the Clinical Reasoning Process," by E.I. Blanche. Copyright 2001 by E.I. Blanche. Reprinted with permission.

Description	Relationship to Sensory Integration Theory	Application to a Diverse Population
Automatic postural control and anti-gravity movements: the ability to regulate the body's position in space for the dual purposes of stability and orientation (Shumway-Cook & Woollacott, 1995). Equilibrium reactions can occur in response to an externally imposed force or tilt in the supporting surface (reactive) or in response to a self-initiated movement (anticipatory).	Hyporesponsivity to vestibular/ proprioceptive input often results in poor development of postural control.	Children with neuromuscular and tonal abnormalities (e.g., cerebral palsy, Down syndrome) often exhibit difficulties with postural control. Children with Autistic Disorder or modulation deficits do not seem to have difficulty with postural control.
Antigravity extension: the ability to extend the trunk against gravity. Often evaluated in the prone extension posture.	Hyporesponsivity to vestibular input often results in poor development of antigravity extension.	Assess in unstructured manner. Children with tonal abnormalities often have problems with antigravity extension.
Antigravity flexion: the ability to flex the head, trunk, and extremities against gravity.	Difficulties with antigravity flexion often occur in children with tactile processing and motor planning deficits.	Assess in unstructured manner. Children with tonal abnormalities often exhibit difficulties with antigravity flexion.
Bilateral motor coordination: the ability to coordinate both sides of the body during symmetrical, alternating, or asymmetrical tasks.	Poor bilateral motor coordination can relate to vestibular/proprioceptive deficits. Sometimes occurs with difficulty with laterality for preferred use of one body side.	Poor bilateral motor coordination is often affected in children with neuromotor deficits and can be affected in children with genetic disorders. Weakness or pathology of one body side will affect both laterality and bilateral motor coordination.
Automatic eye movements: the ability to move the eyes in a coordinated manner. Includes the ability to have smooth eye movements and maintain a stable visual field while moving.	Assess automatic eye movements in their relationship to vestibular/proprioceptive functions.	Children with a variety of diagnoses exhibit difficulty with eye movements not only because of factors related to sensory processing but also because of other motor or neurological issues.
Motor planning: involves bilateral, reciprocal, alternating, or symmetrical limb movements. Ask the client to perform the actions (e.g., jumping jacks) in imitation of the examiner.	Assess motor planning to gauge sequencing, bilateral motor coordination, and the ability to project actions in time and space.	Children with neurological impairments due to a variety of diagnoses often perform poorly on assessment of motor planning because of cognitive limitations, neuromotor difficulties, or poor comprehension.
Neurological tests of cerebellar integrity: Shilder's Arm Extension Test, slow ramp movements, finger to nose, diadochokinesia.	Within the SI frame of reference, clinicians utilize these tools to assess proprioceptive functions.	Children with neurological impairments due to a variety of diagnoses often perform poorly on these tests.
Proximal joint stability: the ability to stabilize proximal joints so precise movement can occur in distal joints. It is a dynamic process that requires contraction of agonists and antagonists around a joint.	Within the SI frame of reference, clinicians interpret deficiencies in proximal joint stability as deficits in proprioceptive functions.	Assess in an unstructured manner. Children with tonal abnormalities often exhibit problems with proximal joint stability.
Response to movement: the ability to process vestibular information. The examiner observes registration and organization of the sensory input.	The child's response to movement experiences relates to muscle tone, postural control, arousal level, ocular motor control, and bilateral motor coordination. Aversive response to movement is related to other functional deficits such as resistance to typical movement activities (e.g., riding in a car, going on fast rides at the fair, riding on a boat).	Observing the response to movement is the best indicator of vestibular/ proprioceptive processing disorders. Children with Autistic Disorder, some types of genetic disorders, and learning disorders can have problems in this area. Children with cerebral palsy can also exhibit deficits in this area.

Overview of Selected Sensory Integration Assessment Instruments*

Test	Purpose	Intended Population	Time Requirement	Amount/Type of Psychometric Testing
Analysis of Sensory Behavior Inventory (Rev. ed.) (Morton & Wolford, 1984)	Screens for SI dysfunction	3 to 22 years with serious behavior problems	—**	No psychometric testing
Balcones Sensory Integration Screening (Rev. ed.) (Jones & Monkhouse-Kleuser, 1981)	Screens for SI dysfunction	Children	—	Interrater reliability
Clinical Observations of Motor and Postural Skills (Wilson, Pollock, Kaplan, & Law, 1994)	Screens for SI dysfunction with a focus on vestibular processing	5 to 9 years	20 min	—
DeGangi-Berk Test of Sensory Integration (Berk & DeGangi, 1983)	Screens for SI dysfunction with a focus on vestibular processing	3 to 5 years	30 min	Domain and construct validity; inter-observer reliability; retest stability; standardized on limited sample
Functional Assessment for Children with Sensory Integration Dysfunction (Cook, 1991)	Assesses the impact of dysfunction on specific functional life tasks	Children with SI dysfunction	—	No psychometric testing; for use as an informal assessment too.
SBC Adult Psychiatric Sensory Integration Evaluation (Schroeder, Block, Campbell, & Stowell, 1979)	Evaluates SI dysfunction	Adults with psychiatric disabilities	75 min	Interrater reliability; internal consistency, concurrent, and clinical validity
Sensorimotor Integration Test Battery (Jongbloed, Collins, & Jones, 1986)	Assesses sensorimotor integration	Adults with a CVA	90 min	Internal consistency; construct, discriminant, and clinical validity
Sensory Integration Inventory (Rev. ed.) (Reisman & Hanschu, 1992)	Screens for SI dysfunction	Individuals with developmental disabilities	30 min	—
Sensory Integration and Praxis Tests (Ayres, 1989)	Test for sensory integration and praxis	4 to 8 years	2.5 hr	Standardized on sample of 1197 children in US and Canada; extensive psychometric testing
Sensory Profile (Dunn, 1994, 1999)	Screens for SI dysfunction by assessing sensory responsiveness	3 to 10 years	—	Normed on national sample
Sensory Rating Scale for Infants and Young Children (Provost & Oetter, 1993)	Screens for SI dysfunction by assessing sensory responsiveness	Birth to 3 years	—	Internal consistency; intrarater and interrater reliability
Sensory Sensitivity Checklist (Ayres & Tickle, 1980)	Screens for SI dysfunction by assessing sensory responsiveness	Children	—	No psychometric testing
Teacher Questionnaire on Sensorimotor Behavior (Carrasco & Lee, 1993)	Screens for SI dysfunction	Children	—	Internal consistency
Test of Sensory Functions in Infants (DeGangi & Greenspan, 1989)	Screens for SI dysfunction by measuring processing and reactivity	4 to 18 months with regulatory disorders or developmental delay	20 min	Interobserver and test-retest reliability
T. I. M. E.—Toddler and Infant Motor Evaluation (Miller & Roid, 1995)	Assesses motor abilities including praxis (motor organization)	4 months to 3.5 years	15–45 min	Standardized
Touch Inventory for Elementary School-Aged Children (Royeen, 1986)	Screens for tactile defensiveness	6 to 10 years	15 min	Interrater and test-retest reliability; internal consistency; criterion-related validity; norms available
Touch Inventory for Preschoolers (Royeen, 1987)	Measures tactile defensiveness	2.5 to 4.5 years	—	Pilot test

**Dashes indicate information was not available.

13

Clinical Applications in Sensory Modulation Dysfunction:

Assessment and Intervention Considerations

Lucy Jane Miller, Ph.D., OTR

Clare Summers, M.A., OTR

Sensory modulation dysfunction (SMD) is "a problem in the capacity to regulate and organize the degree, intensity and nature of response to sensory input in a graded and adaptive manner . . . [that] disrupts an individual's ability to achieve and maintain an optimal range of performance necessary to adapt to challenges in life" (Lane, Miller, & Hanft, 2000, p. 1). Behaviorally, children with SMD can exhibit overresponsivity as they actively seek or avoid sensory input in the environment, or hyporesponsivity and passivity as they fail to orient and respond to typical levels of sensory input in the environment (Miller & Lane, 2000; Dunn, 1997). In addition, *emotional problems* (e.g., anxiety, aggression, tearful and/or tantrum-like symptoms), and *attentional problems* behaviors (e.g., distractibility, impulsivity, disorganization, hyperactivity) frequently occur. SMD can severely impair daily occupations, routines, and roles, and occurs in mild to severe forms (Hanft, Miller, & Lane, 2000; Parham & Mailloux, 1996). Although the core deficit in SMD might be sensory (see chapter 4 of this text), functional problems (i.e., difficulties with social participation, self-regulation, perceived self-competence, and/or performance of home, school, or community tasks) are the usual basis for referrals for occupational therapy (Cohn, Miller, & Tickle-Degnen, 2000).

Responsivity refers to the behavioral response to sensation.

Reactivity refers to the physiological response.

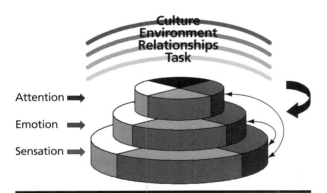

Figure 13.1. The Ecological Model of Sensory Modulation

light shading = underresponsivity
medium shading = normal responsivity
        (a match between the external
        and internal dimensions)
dark shading = overresponsivity
      black = lability, severe overresponsivity
        alternating with severe under-
        responsivity

The Ecological Model of Sensory Modulation

Chapter 4 of this text, An Ecological Model of Sensory Modulation: Performance of Children with Fragile X Syndrome, Autistic Disorder, Attention-Deficit/Hyperactivity Disorder, and Sensory Modulation Dysfunction, details a conceptual model of sensory modulation. This model highlights four *external dimensions* (*culture, environment, relationships* and *task*) and three *internal dimensions* (*sensory processing, emotions,* and *attention*) that affect children with SMD (Figure 13.1). To frame the strengths and limitations of each child, clinicians consider each of these seven dimensions during assessment and intervention planning.

The two case studies in this chapter demonstrate how therapists used this model as a framework to guide assessment, evaluate results of assessment, and plan intervention, considering the supports and demands provided by the *external dimensions,* the types of sensory stimulation that caused the referral symptoms, and how the *sensory processing* problems might have been affecting the children's *emotion* and *attention* processes.

The Assessment and Intervention Process in SMD

The Assessment Process

Parham and Mailloux (1996) summarized the limitations and disabilities in SMD as:

1. decreased social skills and participation in play

2. poor self-confidence and self-esteem

3. difficulties with daily life skills and at school

4. anxiety, poor attention, and poor ability to regulate reactions to others

5. poor skill development in fine, gross, or sensorimotor domains

The assessment process includes a variety of scales that assess the internal and external dimensions that affect a child behavior and functional abilities, including both behavioral and physiological measures. (See Appendix 13-A for more detail about the assessments used in the Sensory Integration Dysfunction Treatment And Research [STAR] Center at The Children's Hospital in Denver, CO.)

At the STAR Center, the assessment process for children with SMD generally follows the sequence listed below.

1. Upon referral, parents receive by mail a detailed medical and developmental questionnaire, which they return prior to evaluation.

2. Clinicians use either the *Sensory Integration and Praxis Tests* (SIPT; Ayres, 1989) or the *Miller Assessment of Preschoolers* (MAP; Miller, 1982, 1988), and *First STEP* (*Screening Test for Evaluating Preschoolers;* Miller, 1993) to test the child.

3. Parents complete the *Short Sensory Profile* (SSP; McIntosh, Miller, Shyu, & Dunn, 1999), the *Parent Rating Scale of the Leiter International Performance Scale–Revised* (Leiter-P; Roid & Miller, 1997), and the *Child Behavior Checklist–Parent Rating Scale* (CBCL; Achenbach, 1991).

4. The parents receive a copy of the *Leiter–R Teacher Rating Scale* (Roid & Miller, 1997) to give to the child's teacher and return at the next visit.

5. The occupational therapist completes the *SMD Behavior During Testing Checklist* (see Appendix 13-B) and *Leiter–R Examiner Rating Scale* (Roid & Miller, 1997).

6. Investigators administer the Sensory Challenge Protocol, a controlled laboratory paradigm that gauges an individual's responsivity to 50 sensory stimuli, with 10 trials in five sensory domains, by continuously sampling the individual's electrodermal reactivity (EDR) after sensation (Miller et al., 1999). (See Appendix 4-B in chapter 4 for details of the Sensory Challenge Protocol.)

7. The therapist conducts and videotapes a parent interview (see Appendix 13-C).

8. The occupational therapist and the psychologist administer other scales (e.g., *Wechsler Intelligence Scale for Children—Third Edition,* Wechsler, 1991; *Multidimensional Anxiety Scale for Children,* March, 1997; March, Parker, Sullivan, Stallings, & Conners, 1997; *Vineland Adaptive Scales,* Sparrow, Balla, & Cicchetti, 1984).

9. The treating therapist reviews the parent interview tape and drafts the Goal Attainment Scale (GAS) (see sample GAS in Appendix 13-D). The therapist reviews the GAS with the parent during a joint session before initiating the intervention.

As a final step in the assessment process, and in preparation for creating the intervention plan, the therapist reflects on the case by posing a series of self-reflective questions such as:

- How does the child perceive vestibular/proprioceptive information? Is the child a "movement seeker" or a "movement avoider"?

- How does the child perceive other sensory stimuli? Does the child seek or avoid tactile, auditory, visual, and olfactory information?

- What is child's emotional reaction in stressful situations? Does child withdraw, show aggression, or become tearful?

- What are the child's motor responses? Does child shut down, stop moving, become hyperactive?

- What affects the child's attention? Does child perseverate or become distractible, inattentive, and impulsive?

The process is iterative with constant questions about how the *external dimensions* affect the *internal dimensions* and how the child might be manifesting underlying neurological or physiological reactions in observable behaviors.

The clinician takes into consideration the family's priorities for intervention. The intervention plan *always* reflects the family's priorities. To ensure that this reflective process includes the family's concerns and goals, the therapist asks her- or himself a series of questions such as: What inputs (sensory and/or compensatory) can we use to help the child master his or her life demands? What can we teach parents, teachers, or others to assist the child in achieving a regulated, "just-right" state, where he or she can learn, play, and relate? Having generated a diagnostic hypothesis related to the seven external and internal dimensions (see the Ecological Model of Sensory Modulation in Figure 13.1), the therapist then designs the first therapy session.

The Intervention Process With SMD

Therapists provide occupational therapy for children with SMD using a sensory integrative frame of reference that is guided by clinical reasoning (Miller, Wilbarger, Stackhouse, & Trunnell, in press; also see chapter 11 in this text, Clinical Reasoning and the Use of Narrative in Sensory Integration Assessment and Intervention, by Burke). The factors guiding intervention are a detailed analysis of the child's *internal dimensions* (sensation, emotion, and attention), an understanding of how the child's *sensory processing* problems might be related to difficulties with other internal dimensions, and insight into how the specific *external dimensions* (*culture, environment, relationships* and *task*) affect the child. In the authors' program, intervention begins in a direct service setting, providing individualized occupational therapy with a sensory integration frame of reference. Each session includes intensive parent education. When ready, the therapist, child, and parent design additional sessions that occur at home, at school, or in the community as dictated by the circumstances.

The STEP-SI clinical reasoning framework (Miller et al., in press) provides structure to the therapist's ongoing thinking process when constructing the direct intervention plan and making observations and decisions during intervention sessions. Each STEP-SI element represents a question clinicians ask before, during, and after each activity in therapy.

Each element can be either a support or a challenge to successful completion of an activity. The therapist uses clinical reasoning (Mattingly & Fleming, 1994; Mattingly, 1991) to analyze the child's responses and to interpret the child's action-reaction, which leads directly to the next activity.

Typically, occupational therapists are the professionals involved in treating SMD (Ayres, 1972, 1989). The objective of intervention is to afford the child sensory or compensatory methods of self-modulating his or her own reactions, first in the clinic and then in daily life situations. Best results seem to occur when children receive individual direct therapy combined with consultation in natural environments (i.e., home, school, and community). For example, in Figure 13.2 Erin and Eric, who are both in direct therapy for SMD, have gone on an outing with their therapist to the pumpkin patch. This activity provides excellent tactile and proprioceptive input within a natural context. Erin's and Eric's parents have accompanied them so that the therapist can use the pumpkin patch activity to show the parents how to use sensory techniques to assist the children in self-regulation.

Intervention is actually an ongoing diagnostic evaluation process in which the clinician considers the contributing factors to poor behavior regulation and explores the supports the child needs to maintain a modulated state in a variety of environments. The clinical reasoning involved in this type of intervention is an iterative process involving rehearsal, careful observation, and ongoing interpretation of responses. Each child is the clinician's "professor," teaching the professionals about him- or herself over the course of the intervention.

In direct intervention, the therapist and the parents work together to assess, support, and challenge the child's ability to modulate sensory information from his or her body and environment. The therapist might start with external

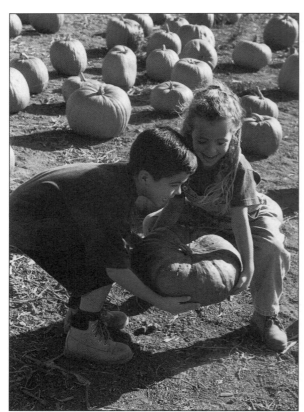

Photo by Shay McAtee.

Figure 13.2. Erin and Eric receive proprioceptive input during activities at the pumpkin patch.

dimensions that are supportive for the child, incrementally adding elements from external dimensions that serve to challenge the child. Then, with the assistance of the therapist, the child is guided to use his or her internal dimensions to regulate activities and be successful. Ultimately the child generalizes this ability so that he or she can maintain a modulated state of arousal without the therapist's support.

The activities often include gross and fine motor activities; however, the goal of therapy is not to improve motor skills (as it might be for children who have developmental motor disorders such as dyspraxia; see Cermak, 1991). For children with SMD, therapists consider intervention a "success" when the child can generalize the type of self-regulation he or she maintained in a clinic setting to the home, school, or community environments. For example, Jeremy came to therapy with severe symptoms of gravitational insecurity. During his direct therapy that occurred once a week for a year, he received intervention to help him integrate the vestibular overreactivity in an appropriate manner. His underlying neural processing might have been altered by direct therapy, and in addition he learned self-regulatory techniques that he could use in natural settings to maintain a modulated state of arousal. In Figure 13.3, Jeremy has gone outside the direct therapy setting to the park and is playing on the merry-go-round. He is able to maintain an appropriate arousal state using the sensory techniques he learned during therapy.

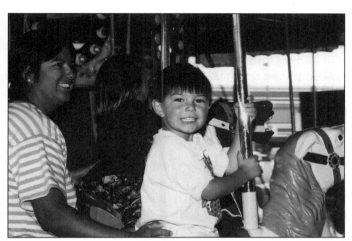

Figure 13.3. Jeremy begins to tolerate slow vestibular stimulation at the park with his therapist.

The children at the STAR Center are also enrolled in an occupational therapy effectiveness research study, consequently each receives occupational therapy for the same amount of time before outcomes are measured. Currently the effectiveness study protocol begins with 5 weeks of individual occupational therapy twice a week in a clinic equipped with suspended equipment, mats, balls, and a variety of swings and other typical sensory integrative toys and objects (Parham & Mailloux, 1996). Parents are present and active during intervention. Typically, after the first 5 weeks of intervention (10 sessions), the therapist/parent team has developed excellent hypotheses about which activities and modalities best promote adaptive, regulated reactions in the child. Then the therapist and parents address larger quality-of-life goals in natural contexts either in the direct service setting or in natural settings. Some parent/therapist teams elect to use all 20 sessions in direct service in the clinic setting.

The therapist and the parents collaboratively plan the remaining 10 sessions to include at least one home and one school visit. During sessions outside the clinic, the questions broaden from the effect of guided and controlled sensation, environment, relationships, and so forth, on activities in the clinic, to the impact of the child's internal dimensions on his or her ability to function well in natural environments. The remaining sessions can be allocated to additional direct service sessions in the clinic; work with parents, teachers, and/or other individuals in natural settings (i.e. babysitter, piano teacher, dance teacher, grandparents etc.); or to other community activities, such as going swimming, buying shoes, or going to a neighborhood playground. The exact nature of the second half of the sessions depends on the needs of the child and family. All children are retested for the effectiveness study at the end of 20 sessions using the initial assessment tools, with the exception of the SIPT. Children whose therapists and parents feel that they need further intervention either extend the treatment time or take a break and return for more intervention at a later time.

Case Study: Kamon

Referral Issues and Assessments

Kamon was an endearing 3-year, 6-month-old boy referred by his family counselor because of extreme oppositional behaviors when dressing. It sometimes took Kamon several hours to dress, and he frequently refused entirely. The family counselor was working on parenting issues and behavior modification, but no improvement had occurred in the dressing problem. Kamon's parents also were concerned because he refused to try most fine motor tasks.

The following sections give the results from MAP, First STEP, SSP, Leiter–P Rating Scales, CBCL, Goal Attainment Scale, and parent interview (all scores transformed to z-scores). Because Kamon refused to finish most fine motor activities on pretest and thereby completed only two MAP subtests, his therapist was unable to obtain final scores on pretest. The discussion below demonstrates how the Ecological Model of SMD served as a framework to synthesize assessment results.

External Dimensions Affecting Function

According to the Ecological Model of SMD, all four external dimensions created significant challenges for Kamon related to his presenting problems. In direct therapy sessions, Kamon's therapist explored each dimension and suggested methods of modifying external dimensions so that the dimensions could become supports rather than demands.

Culture

Kamon was limited by his sensitivity to sensation and withdrew if the sensory demands of his culture became too great. He had a large extended family (more than 40 people) who gathered for holidays and birthdays. At a recent event, Kamon hid under a bed as people arrived, and the family had to instigate an all-out search to find him.

He demonstrated most of his problems at home, despite the fact that both his mother and father were gentle, understanding, and well educated. Because home was "safe" for Kamon, he allowed himself to fall apart and express his feelings there. For example, frequently upon arriving home after school, Kamon would exhibit tantrums, crying, and screaming in response to simple requests by his parents.

Environment

Kamon was extremely sensitive to auditory and visual stimuli, and many family activities (e.g., TV) were troublesome. If the stimulus was too active, bright, or loud, Kamon would dissolve in tears. Leaving the house to shop, eat out, or go to church was stressful because Kamon frequently became overwhelmed and aggressive. Kamon spent most of his time at home playing alone.

Relationships

Kamon "refused" to interact with certain children because of his olfactory sensitivities. For example, he said that the hair of the girl in front of him at school "smelled," his personal rug at circle time was "too rough," and he felt "smothered" by other children. His low Aggressive score (CBCL, -3 SD) reflected his tendency to act out his problems at school. However, the support provided by Kamon's warm, caring teacher allowed him to flourish in school, so far. His parents were concerned that as demands for relationships increased, he might not adapt. A significant discrepancy existed between relationships at home, at school, and in the clinic. During the occupational therapy evaluation, Kamon was shy and withdrawn, rarely interacted with the examiner, and sat in his mother's lap. Low scores on Vineland Socialization domain (−2 SD), Leiter–P Social Abilities (−2.7 SD) and CBCL Social Problems (−2.4 SD) reflected these difficulties.

Task

Most fine motor activities (e.g., puzzles, coloring, building) resulted in tears and refusals. Kamon's parents were concerned that Kamon's refusal to participate in many activities would affect his kindergarten success. They were concerned about how his refusal to play with toys would affect his sense of competence and his friendships.

Internal Dimensions Affecting Function

Sensory Processing

Kamon's extreme hyperresponsivity to sensation showed in his SSP scores (total SSP −4.15 SD; Taste/Smell Sensitivity −5.5 SD; Tactile Sensitivity −4.33 SD; Visual/Auditory Sensitivity −3.0 SD) (see Figure 13.4). The parent interview highlighted the impact of Kamon's heightened reactions to sensations. The therapist hypothesized that Kamon's strong resistance to dressing might have a tactile basis. He was remarkably resistant to certain textures (e.g., fuzzy socks), to tags in clothing, to seams in socks. He would wear only loose-fitting pants, preferring shorts and short-sleeved shirts even in winter. His sensory hyperreactivity interfered with bathing, and he refused to have his hair brushed. Although Kamon enjoyed movement activities at home, he became disorganized and hyperactive when engaged in highly active tasks. His low Vineland score on the Daily Living Skills subtest (−1.9 SD) reflected these problems.

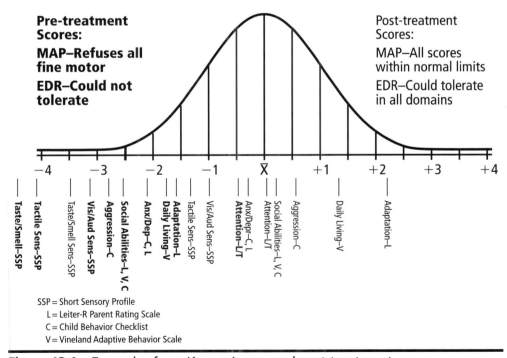

Figure 13.4. Examples from Kamon's pre- and post-treatment scores.

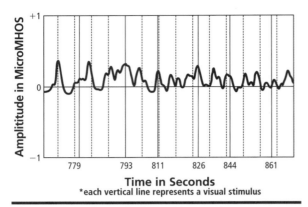

Figure 13.5. Sample from Kamon's electrodermal reactivity recording.

Kamon's sensitivities had an enormous impact on his diet, which was limited to mostly breads and cereals. He refused to be in the kitchen when his mother made dinner because of "bad smells" and refused to sit at the dinner table when it "smelled yucky." His visual and auditory sensitivities made it difficult for the family to spend time together on most activities. He cried upon hearing a hairdryer or shower. Clearly, Kamon's extreme sensory defensiveness was dramatically affecting daily living abilities.

Kamon's electrodermal reactions on the Sensory Challenge Protocol confirmed his physiological sensory reactivity (see Figure 13.5). His hyperreactivity is evident in the high amplitudes, many peaks after each stimulus, and no habituation. His behavior in the "space lab" was hyperactive, and he could barely tolerate the electrodes on his palms.

Emotions

Kamon had significant emotional problems, confirmed by scores on Leiter–P and CBCL. Parent interview and results from the *SMD Behavior During Testing Checklist* reinforced these findings. Parents and the examiner rated Kamon's Adaptation as significantly impaired (< -2 SD); his low Leiter–P score (-1.7 SD) on Moods and Confidence and Energy and Feelings confirmed his Anxious/Depressed score (CBCL, -2.5 SD) (see Figure 13.4).

Attention

Kamon's attention was normal during his occupational therapy assessment and at school ($+.5$ SD). He sat quietly and attended to stories or games at school and in the occupational therapy evaluation, although he refused to do tasks at which he might "fail." His scores from behavior and performance at home indicated difficulties, reflected in his inability to attend to board games, books, drawing, and so forth. Kamon's parents' rating of Attention on Leiter–P was -2 SD (see Figure 13.4).

Kamon's Intervention

Kamon's Goal Attainment Scale Objectives

1. to dress independently and in a timely manner

2. to demonstrate a typical number of tantrums for a child his age

3. to tolerate everyday noises without becoming upset

4. to have his hair brushed on a regular basis

5. to perform age-appropriate fine motor tasks

Parent Education

An important step in Kamon's intervention was parent education related to sensory modulation dysfunction. When Kamon's parents understood the sensory basis of Kamon's difficulties, they began to empathize with how life "felt" to Kamon. They were able to identify, avoid, or prepare better for situations that were threatening to Kamon. Kamon's parents began to understand that because home was "safe," Kamon was secure enough in this place to express his distress. Instead of viewing his home behaviors as his fault or as parenting problems, they realized that his good behavior at school was due to the care and shelter that they provided at home.

Direct Therapy With Sensory Integration Framework

The first step in direct service was to explore the effects of touch pressure/proprioceptive activities to establish whether Kamon would respond positively with calming and decreased sensitivity. His therapists focused on activities that he and his parents could do at home, providing a daily "sensory diet" (Frick et al., in press; Wilbarger & Wilbarger, 1991). Developing home activities was challenging because Kamon continued to "act out" at home.

Kamon attended individual occupational therapy twice a week for 5 weeks where he began to feel safe and try new activities, accepting small challenges. His strong *relationship* with his therapist was a tool that his therapist used to help him try novel games. The therapist provided touch pressure and proprioceptive input as well as vestibular games before novel activities, which helped to regulate Kamon's *sensory* reactivity. Kamon sought *predictability* and responded enthusiastically to pretend play. He did best when therapy followed a set routine. Each session started with massage and joint compression in a playful manner that he called "checking for and fixing broken bones" (massage, joint compression, and traction), a routine that Kamon's parents gradually transferred to his home routines.

Consultation at Home

For the second set of 10 sessions, Kamon's therapist and his parents decided to continue direct clinic-based therapy once a week, to have one school consultation, and to use the remaining four therapy sessions at home. In direct therapy, the therapist tried out games for home and then implemented them during the home visits. Kamon played the "broken-bones" game daily and told his parents, "That broken-bones game helps me get dressed." Kamon began to be aware of how much the games helped him, and he began to prepare himself for situations. Other play activities that provided deep pressure and proprioceptive input included beating up a tent filled with pillows, tug-of-war with a large piece of stretchy fabric, and being a "hotdog in a bun" (under a therapy ball).

During the therapist's home visit, Kamon, his parents, and the therapist visited the nearby park (Figure 13.6). The therapist helped the parents to understand how they could use many of the opportunities at the park to help regulate Kamon's tendency to become dysregulated. In this way, Kamon's parents could continue many of the therapeutic activities begun during his direct therapy sessions through home-based follow-up on their own.

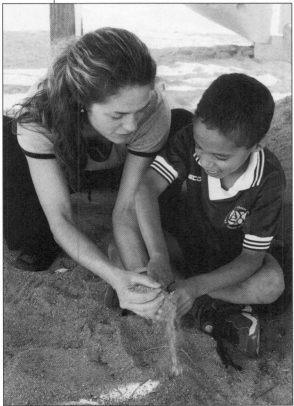

Photo by Shay McAtee.

Figure 13.6. Kamon receives deep pressure and proprioceptive input while playing with his therapist in the sandbox at a nearby park.

Consultation at School

Kamon's therapist observed him at school and provided his teacher with general information related to Kamon's underlying strengths and sensitivities and activities that would fit within a typical classroom. His parents suggested, and the therapist agreed, that Kamon should be allowed to enjoy his successes at school. The team felt that providing additional challenges in the school environment might lead to anxiety at school, so together with the teacher, they set up a routine that would not provide challenges at school.

Outcomes of Intervention for Kamon

Kamon made both qualitative and quantitative changes on testing after 20 occupational therapy sessions (see Figure 13.4, which displays both his pre- and postintervention scores on assessments).

External Dimensions

Kamon's therapist discussed the qualitative changes in the parent exit interview where his parents expressed delight and joy over the changes Kamon had made. However, they noted, "There is still a long way to go." They were thrilled that Kamon could join the family at most dinners and for family activities such as watching TV. After therapy, he could dress himself "most" days and allow his hair to be combed. His tolerance of new or frustrating situations had improved markedly. A significant difference after therapy was the consistent support and understanding that both parents were able to offer him. They no longer felt that something "bad" about their parenting had "caused" his difficulties, and they could help him self-regulate in public places.

Sensory Processing

Kamon's posttreatment lab results indicated a lingering physiological hyper-reactivity (measured by electrodermal reactivity in the laboratory paradigm); however, his behavior in the "space lab" was remarkably different on post-testing. He tolerated all 5 sensory stimuli and allowed the examiner to administer all 10 stimuli in each sensory domain. Quantitatively, Kamon's scores on the SSP showed sensory improvements on all six subtests that had abnormal scores in the pretest condition (average improvement of .80 SD). After therapy, Kamon was able to self-regulate enough to complete the MAP evaluation, with all scores within normal limits. This was a marked improvement over his pretreatment status.

Emotion

At home, his behavior fluctuated. Certain weeks, he was emotionally labile with numerous tantrums; other weeks, he was a delight. However, his parents were optimistic because 5 out of the 6 preceding weeks he had shown "mostly positive behaviors."

Kamon's family decided to "take a vacation" from occupational therapy after the 20 sessions; however, they planned on returning a couple of months before he began kindergarten. They continued to follow through with Kamon's sensory diet and other occupational therapy adaptations at home and when they went as a family to community events and activities.

Case Study: Stevie

Referral Issues and Assessments

Stevie was an outgoing, attractive 5-year, 8-month-old boy with presenting problems of frequent angry outbursts with peers and siblings, extreme hyperactivity in quiet settings, and fear of new activities. He had significant school difficulties because of extremely disruptive and aggressive behaviors. His peers were afraid of him, and his kindergarten was considering expulsion. Stevie was assessed in the laboratory to measure his electrodermal reactivity during the Sensory Challenge Protocol, and the evaluating occupational therapist administered the SIPT, CBCL, SSP, Leiter–R Parent Rating, and Vineland scales. Qualitative measures included Goal Attainment Scaling and parent interview.

External Dimensions Affecting Function

Culture

Stevie's family had many demands for quiet, good behavior. For example, his family belonged to a church that met three times a week, during which there was "quiet worship time." His family stopped participating in church as a family, although both parents still went separately. Family gatherings presented the expectation that "children were to be seen and not heard." Stevie's family, unable to control his hyperactivity, coped by not attending most family events.

Environment

Stevie was upset by new and crowded environments. Stevie's family avoided taking him out of familiar environments. His family had not viewed the environment as an active element that they could manipulate to support Stevie.

Relationships

Stevie was aggressive with peers, siblings, and parents. Interpersonal relations were *always* challenging for Stevie, although he adored his parents, who spent immense energy structuring Stevie when he was near other children or adults.

Task

Stevie was an intelligent, talented little boy. He loved to play with toys that had moving parts and lights or sounds. Tasks were helpful in organizing Stevie's unregulated behavior if an adult could "catch" the disintegration in time.

Internal Dimensions Affecting Function

Sensory Processing

Stevie showed extreme hyporeactive vestibular and proprioceptive processing, manifested by continual sensation seeking. At his occupational therapy evaluation, Stevie was in constant motion, continually chewing on his shirt and other objects. His SIPT scores reflected his poor perception of vestibular and proprioceptive sensations (low scores in Standing and Walking Balance -1.5 SD, Postrotary Nystagmus -2.35 SD), as did his SSP score on Under-Responsive/Seeks Sensation (-4.33 SD). Figure 13.7 gives Stevie's assessment results before his therapy was initiated (all scores transformed to z-scores for comparison).

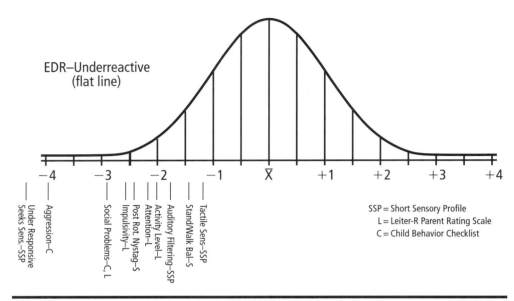

Figure 13.7. Stevie's pretreatment scores on assessments.

EDR–Underreactive
(flat line)

−4 −3 −2 −1 X̄ +1 +2 +3 +4

Under Responsive
Seeks Sens.–SSP

Aggression–C

Social Problems–C, L

Post Rot. Nystag–S
Impulsivity–L

Attention–L
Activity Level–L

Auditory Filtering–SSP

Stand/Walk Bal–S

Tactile Sens.–SSP

SSP = Short Sensory Profile
L = Leiter-R Parent Rating Scale
C = Child Behavior Checklist

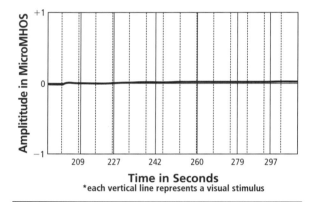

Figure 13.8. Sample from Stevie's pretreatment electrodermal reactivity recording.

Stevie demonstrated a hyporeactive "flat-line" profile on EDR (see Figure 13.8). Children with sensory modulation dysfunction sometimes exhibit this type of EDR recording. It shows no amplitude and no peaks and thus no habituation. Behavioral hypotheses regarding "shutdown" reactions might be valid, although the objective data related to the meaning of the flat-line profile in children with SMD is still under investigation. Additional research is required to evaluate the neurophysiologic and behavioral correlates of this profile.

Though hyporeactive in vestibular and proprioceptive processing, Stevie demonstrated mild sensory defensiveness in tactile and auditory systems. Certain clothing textures bothered him, and he was uncomfortable with grooming tasks (washing face, combing hair, cutting nails). He became fidgety and giggly during the tactile tests on the SIPT and had more difficulty attending to those subtests than others. His mild sensitivity to touch and auditory sensation were also reflected in his SSP scores (Tactile Sensitivity −1.33 SD; Auditory Filtering −1.7 SD).

Emotions

Scores on the Leiter–P and CBCL concurred with the information from Stevie's parents' interview. Stevie had pronounced difficulties in emotion regulation, particularly in social situations (CBCL Social Problems −3 SD; Leiter–P Social Abilities −2.5 SD). Stevie's parents reported that his aggression seriously affected his school and home life (CBCL Aggressive score −4 SD) (see Figure 13.7). He fought with peers at school and in the neighborhood. Agemates were terrified of Stevie and avoided him. If not supervised, Stevie would bite, push, and kick his sister. He had difficulty transitioning between activities and situations, becoming angry and aggressive. His "short fuse" and low frustration tolerance put his parents in a constant state of hypervigilance in case he "blew up." When upset, he stuttered and could not perform simple tasks. Stevie's parents could not separate Stevie's manipulative behaviors from true functional disabilities.

Attention

Stevie showed poor attention accompanied by hyperactive, impulsive behavior (Leiter–P Activity Level −2 SD; Impulsivity −2.5 SD; Attention −2.2 SD) (see Figure 13.7). Stevie was constantly in motion, seeking intense vestibular and proprioceptive input, which distracted him from attending to tasks for more than a minute. In school, his teachers viewed him as hyperactive and disorganized (teacher rating on Leiter–P of −3 SD on Activity Level and Organization). During his occupational therapy evaluation, Stevie needed repeated cues to focus on tasks. He had difficulty listening, and needed instructions repeated often. When overwhelmed, he demonstrated difficulty completing a thought or explanation.

Stevie's Intervention

Stevie's Goal Attainment Scale Objectives

1. to improve ability to self-regulate emotions, resulting in consistent emotions from day to day

2. to increase social participation at home and school by decreasing aggressive behavior with peers and siblings

3. to improve ability to transition between activities and settings

4. to increase self-confidence and improve abilities to perform age-expected tasks by helping him to self-regulate during tasks requiring skill

5. to improve parents' understanding of difficulties and behaviors and provide tools for parents to use when unregulated behavior occurs

Direct Therapy

Stevie had direct occupational therapy using a sensory integration frame of reference twice a week for 8 of his 10 weeks (16 of 20 sessions, the typical number of visits approved by managed care). After that time, his course of intervention changed to once-a-week direct therapy, alternating home and school intervention/consultation.

In Stevie's first therapy session, he resisted entering the occupational therapy clinic, using inappropriate and aggressive language and attempting to hit, bite, and kick his therapist. Clearly, therapy was just like any other new transition to Stevie. His therapist used his reactions to transitioning into therapy therapeutically. In the beginning of the therapy sessions, she focused on helping Stevie learn tools to self-regulate and adapt to this change.

The *task* of blowing bubbles mesmerized Stevie. The therapist utilized the component of *predictability* as Stevie sat blowing bubbles, keeping the door open so he could see into the clinic and watch his therapist playing with the toys and equipment. Eventually, Stevie edged into the clinic area and hesitantly tried a few activities, selecting deep pressure activities (being picked up and squeezed, rolling on a large air mattress, and being buried with weighted pillows). When Stevie's first session was over, he was eager to return.

At his second session, Stevie easily entered the occupational therapy clinic. The therapist again consciously selected *predictability* as a therapeutic tool, having Stevie play only those games he'd played in his first session for half of the second session. Though Stevie resisted anything new, the therapist used *sensation* to ready Stevie for new challenges. Lifting Stevie up and providing firm hugs helped him calm and lessened his resistance to new activities. A safe, *fun* place was clearly essential to Stevie, although his therapist made small changes in the *environment* each week that allowed incremental challenges to the difficulty of *tasks.*

By the third week (sessions five and six), Stevie had identified the clinic as a secure place, and his *relationship* with his therapist permitted him to try challenging activities. For example, using pretend play and having Stevie control the situation, the therapist could engage Stevie in pretend war games that allowed him to express his aggressive tendencies. The therapist showed Stevie how to control his outbursts by using sensory techniques such as deep pressure and proprioception for calming.

On frequent occasions, an upsetting experience at home or demands in his *culture* (e.g., visiting his grandparents, going to a frenetic birthday party) caused aggressive outbursts and increased resistance in the subsequent occupational therapy session. The therapist tried to reenact many of these scenarios during therapy and led Stevie through several alternative outcomes. One parent was always present in the clinic, so his parents also became familiar with alternative strategies for interacting and preventing his aggression, which seemed to calm effectively with sensory input in vestibular and proprioceptive domains.

By week five (10th session), Stevie easily transitioned in and out of therapy even when changes to routine or upsetting events occurred at home before his therapy session. He was also able to begin *self-monitoring* when he began to get out of control, obtaining what he needed to reorganize himself (e.g., chewing bubble gum or rubber tubing, jumping activities, and fast movement). His behavior and mood became somewhat more consistent at home and school, but even after 5 weeks of direct intervention twice a week, his emotional intensity at school and home was still a significant issue.

In direct therapy, the therapist noticed that "heavy work" in oral motor activities had a significant calming effect. Eating is such a common, everyday activity occurring not only during mealtimes but also during snacks, so Stevie's therapist and parents devised an intensive oral motor program that encouraged Stevie to eat foods that were crunchy and chewy and foods that required "work," such as sucking pudding and gelatin through a straw.

At the review session halfway through the 20 sessions, Stevie's parents and therapist agreed that Stevie still needed the intensity and direct support that the clinic environment was able to offer him. By the eighth week, the therapist and parents agreed that Stevie would benefit from a few consultation visits. His therapist used these visits to get a better idea of which *external dimensions* disorganized Stevie.

Stevie was one of those children who need such sensory intensity that direct intervention is the best way to satisfy their needs. With a child like Stevie, it can take 20 sessions or more to provide what the child needs. Stevie communicated that he was this type of child by continuing to seek

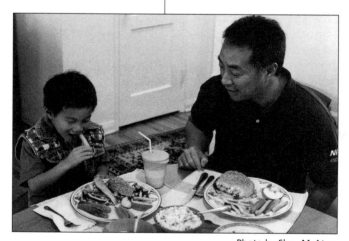

Photo by Shay McAtee.

Figure 13.9. Providing a crunchy, chewy, texture-full sensory diet improved Stevie's behavior dramatically at mealtime.

intense vestibular and proprioceptive input throughout his first 16 sessions. He never seemed to "get enough" input, yet intense movement activities often overwhelmed Stevie, causing aggression. The therapist had to provide structure and proprioceptive input consciously and continually by selecting *tasks* and structuring the *environment* to help Stevie maintain control. Roughly one-third of each session consisted of training Stevie's parents to reason through and identify activities that provided the "just-right" intensity while still affording the structure that Stevie required.

Home Consultation

Once Stevie's therapist understood his internal needs and Stevie was able to transition into and participate in therapy without constant aggressive outbursts, parents and therapist collaborated on ways to incorporate these intervention strategies into daily routines. During the therapist's visit to Stevie's home in the 17th session, Stevie's parents and the therapist devised a plan to use the family's unfinished basement as a playroom for Stevie. The parents purchased a minitrampoline at a thrift store and made an air mattress by roping together inner tubes from Stevie's dad's garage business. Stevie's mother fashioned a huge pretend boat filled with blankets and pillows. They made plans to construct an indoor tire swing so Stevie could give himself the intense movement he craved, even though it was winter. Stevie's parents and therapist also developed a springtime plan to add a spinning swing and a climbing rope to the outside swing set.

Stevie's parents had seen immense changes in Stevie during the therapy sessions after movement and proprioceptive input began, so they were willing and creative in making accommodations at home. Because the therapist had trained them to understand *why* these adaptations could help Stevie, they began to realize that many of Stevie's aggressive behaviors were a result of sensory modulation dysfunction rather than an attempt to manipulate his parents. When his parents began to provide Stevie with the intensity of movement and proprioceptive information that he consistently sought, Stevie was able to handle transitions better and his aggression decreased considerably.

Outcomes of Intervention for Stevie

Stevie's changes during the 20 sessions of occupational therapy were immense, as reflected in scores on some of his tests (see Figure 13.10), yet Stevie was a child who wasn't "done" after the 20 sessions. Even *he* could articulate his feelings and said, "I feel better, a lot more in control." The largest and most meaningful changes were evident on Goal Attainment Scaling, and Stevie's parents discussed these improvements with the therapist in the parent exit interview. Stevie's parents were thrilled that he now could eat dinner with the family, show affection to his grandparents, and (usually) sit through a church service (while chewing vigorously—but quietly!). Although significant, life-changing improvements had taken place, the therapist recommended continuing occupational therapy to focus on improving peer relations, refining skills, and developing additional home program routines and activities.

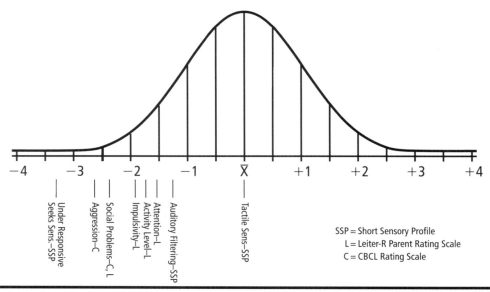

Figure 13.10. Stevie's posttreatment outcome scores.

EDR was undderreactive but did demonstrate some reactivity.

Conclusions and Discussion Points

The Ecological Model of SMD, in combination with the STEP-SI clinical reasoning framework, are useful tools for structuring and organizing the assessment, intervention, and clinical reasoning processes of occupational therapists who work with children who demonstrate SMD. The case studies demonstrate not only the usefulness of this approach but also its effectiveness. Several key factors regarding this approach are:

- **Importance of considering external and internal dimensions of the model.** Children with SMD can have atypical interactions in both *external and internal dimensions.* It is important to consider each element of the Ecological Model of SMD in evaluating and treating SMD. Therapists often receive referrals for emotional and attentional problems that occur in natural settings. These emotion, attention, and sensation problems often distinguish children with SMD from children with other types of sensory integration problems.

- **Difficulty in therapy sessions.** Children with SMD frequently demonstrate severe aggression, withdrawal, or other social/emotional disturbances, making direct therapy challenging. Developing a strong therapeutic alliance or relationship with both the parents and the child is vital to be able to use the trust the child and parents have in the therapist to help the child try new activities. Helping parents understand and articulate the underlying sensory processing problems that cause or contribute to the child's extreme behavior problems is essential to generalize the interventions outside the direct service setting. Once parents observe the changes in their child in center-based therapy, they frequently are willing to make more changes at home. In the authors' experience, the more the parents actively participate during the therapy, the more confident they become in adapting environments, tasks, and relationships at home and in natural settings in the community. This participation must be much more than being in the room observing the child and therapist; it should involve active problem solving by the parents.

- **Importance of family-centered care.** The parents of children with SMD sometimes feel guilty about being a bad parent and might have been accused by well-meaning relatives, friends, and neighbors of "spoiling" their child. They frequently hear, "Don't worry so much; he will grow out it," or "There's nothing wrong, you're overreacting." When parents receive a diagnosis for the problem, along with written, website, audiotape, or videotape information about the condition, their own ability to cope with the child often increases dramatically. The authors encourage development of their clinic's lending library with as many adult learning tools as possible so parents can check out materials that fit their learning styles. Whenever possible, the authors also help arrange parent-to-parent networking for support.

- **Importance of parent-to-parent networking.** To protect their children, families sometimes disengage from extended family, neighbors, and friends and do not receive the personal support they need. However, once the problem is diagnosed and parents understand that their children's difficulties are not their "fault," they can be more assured when explaining their child's problems to others. The more information parents have and can actually articulate, the better prepared they can be to advocate for their child. Therapists can consider training parents to talk knowledgeably about their child's condition as an active part of the therapeutic process.

- **Importance of using a clinical reasoning approach to intervention.** Using specific techniques and lists of sensory integration intervention ideas is a much easier way to treat children than the time-consuming process of using clinical reasoning to determine plan and implement intervention. However, it is the authors' contention that the only effective sensory integration intervention is occupational therapy focused on quality-of-life issues, using an ongoing process of clinical reasoning to design intervention. Using these guidelines, the therapist first sets a specific goal for each activity, subsequently questions whether the activity accomplished the goal, then thinks through what he or she could have done differently before or during the activity to increase the gains provided by the activity. Each success or failure of a specific activity should invoke a follow-up question by the therapist (e.g., This activity succeeded because . . . ? Consequently, I can make the activity more challenging by . . . ?; or, This activity failed because . . . ? Consequently, I can support the child to be successful by . . . ?) This is a challenging approach for the treating therapist. The process is an active, ongoing evaluation process moment to moment rather than a more passive, routines-based approach to intervention.

- **Importance of a multidisciplinary approach.** Because the sensory problems of SMD can lead to extreme behavioral and emotional dysregulation, collaboration with other professionals is critical in designing and implementing interventions for SMD. Occupational therapists understand the contribution of the sensory processing dimension and how it affects the other internal and external dimensions but may not be comfortable dealing with family issues that result, such as differences of opinion between parents in how to cope with the child's challenges. Although it may be difficult to find a counseling professional who is competent in family systems and who also understands SMD, it is critical to incorporate the expertise of other professionals, such as psychologists, behaviorists, and learning specialists for interventions with the array of complex issues that arise in treatment of SMD.

- **Difficulty determining duration and focus of intervention.** Determining the duration and focus for intervention is challenging, particularly if the number of sessions is limited (e.g., by a managed-care system). Often children make huge initial gains but then show slower gains through home programs, school programs, and in natural community settings. Not all third-party payers are willing to support nondirect types of interventions outside the clinic, and not all interventionists feel comfortable with intervention outside of a direct-service setting. Deciding the amount and type of therapy needed and explaining and justifying these decisions to insurance companies and other professionals (doctors, teachers, other therapists), although frustrating, is critical.

- **Importance of continuing research in SMD.** Only recently has the professional literature begun to describe sensory modulation dysfunction. Practicing clinicians desperately need rigorous study designs to provide empirical data related to this disorder. Only through implementing and reporting well-controlled, rigorous studies will investigators be able to answer questions such as, Is SMD a valid syndrome? Does occupational therapy help ameliorate the condition? What are the underlying mechanisms in the disorder?

Acknowledgments

We would like to acknowledge the tremendous support of Dr. Marshall Haith, who reviewed this manuscript and provided consultation on the Ecological Model of SMD constructs. In addition, our laboratory director, Jude McGrath, and research assistants Kelly Church, Julie Bonnell, and Todd Ognibene devoted countless hours gathering data for this chapter. This complex work could not be completed without the dedication of the other treating occupational therapists on our research team: Sharen Trunnell, Nicki Pine, Robin Seger, Lisa Waterford, Becky Greer, and Julie Butler; the support of Dr. Dennis Matthews, Director of Pediatric Rehabilitation at The Children's Hospital. We appreciate the mentorship of Julie Wilbarger, Sharen Trunnell, and Tracy Stackhouse in development of the intervention model discussed in this chapter; and the special assistance of Robin Seger with Kamon's Goal Attainment Scale. Finally, we appreciate the contribution of Judy Benzel, who provided administrative support for this and other projects.

Primary funding for this work was provided by the Wallace Research Foundation. Additional support has been provided by a NIH Career Award to the first author (# 1 K01 HD01183-01). The overhead was supported in part by a grant from Maternal and Child Health (MCH grant # MC J 08941301).

References

Achenbach, T.M. (1991). *Manual for the Child Behavior Checklist/4-18 and 1991 Profile.* Burlington, VT: University of Vermont, Department of Psychiatry.

Altman, J.S., & Mills, B.C. (1990). Caregiver behaviors and adaptive behavior in home care and daycare. *Early Child Development and Care, 62,* 87–96.

Ayres, A.J. (1972). *Sensory integration and learning disorders.* Los Angeles: Western Psychological Services.

Ayres, A.J. (1989). *Sensory Integration and Praxis Tests.* Los Angeles: Western Psychological Services.

Cermak, S.A. (1991). Somatodyspraxia. In A.G. Fisher, E.A. Murray, & A.C. Bundy (Eds.), *Sensory integration: Theory and practice* (pp. 137–170). Philadelphia: F.A. Davis Company.

Chen, W.J., Faraone, S.V., Biederman, J., & Tsuang, M.T. (1994). Diagnostic accuracy of the Child Behavior Checklist scales for attention-deficit hyperactivity disorder: A receiver-operating characteristic analysis. *Journal of Counseling and Clinical Psychology, 62*(5), 1017–1025.

Cohn, E., Miller, L.J., & Tickle-Degnen. (2000). Parental hopes for therapy outcomes: Children with sensory modulation disorders. *American Journal of Occupational Therapy, 54*(1), 36–43.

DeGangi, G.A., DiPietro, J.A., Greenspan, S.I., & Porges, S.W. (1991). Psychophysiological characteristics of the regulatory disordered infant. *Infant Behavior and Development, 14,* 37–50.

Douhitt, V.L. (1992). A comparison of adaptive behavior in gifted and non-gifted children. *Roeper Review, 14,* 149–151.

Dunn, W. (1997). The impact of sensory processing abilities on the daily lives of young children and their families: A conceptual model. *Infants and Young Children, 9*(4), 23–25.

Dunn, W. (1999). *The Sensory Profile: Examiner's manual.* San Antonio, TX: The Psychological Corporation.

Dunn, W., & Brown, C. (1997). Factor analysis on the Sensory Profile from a national sample of children without disabilities. *American Journal of Occupational Therapy, 51*(7), 490–495.

Dunn, W., & Westman, K. (1997). The Sensory Profile: The performance of a national sample of children without disabilities. *American Journal of Occupational Therapy, 51*(1), 25–34.

Elliott, S.N., & Busse, R.T. (1992). Review of the Child Behavior Checklist. In J. Kramer & J.C. Conoley (Eds.), *Mental measurements yearbook* (Vol. 11, pp. 166–169). Lincoln, NE: Buros Institute of Mental Measurement.

Frick, S., Gjesing, G., Harkness, L., Hickman, L., Kawar, M., Shellenberger, S., Lawton-Shirley, N., Wilbarger, J., Wilbarger, P., & Williams M.S. (in press). Complementary tools for intervention. In A.C. Bundy, S.J., Lane, & Murray, E.A. (Eds.), *Sensory integration: Theory and practice* (2nd ed.). Philadelphia: F.A. Davis

Hanft, B.E., Miller, L.J., & Lane, S.J. (2000). Toward a consensus in terminology in sensory integration theory and practice: Part 3: Observable behaviors: Sensory integration dysfunction. *Sensory Integration Special Interest Section, 23*(3), 1–4.

Jensen, P.S., Wantanabe, H.K., Richters, J.E., & Roper, M. (1996). Scales, diagnosis, and child psychopathology: Comparing the CBCL and the DISC against external validators. *Journal of Abnormal Child Psychology, 24*(2), 151–168.

Kiresuk, T., & Sherman, R. (1968). Goal attainment scaling: A general method of evaluating comprehensive mental health programs. *Community Mental Health Journal, 4,* 443–453.

Lane, S.J., Miller, L.J., & Hanft, B.E. (2000) Toward a consensus in terminology in sensory integration theory and practice: Part 2: Sensory integration patterns of function and dysfunction. *Sensory Integration Special Interest Section, 23*(2), 1–3.

Macmann, G.M., Barnett, D.W., Burd, S.A., & Jones, T. (1992). Construct validity of the Child Behavior Checklist: Effects of item overlap on second-order factor structure. *Psychological Assessment, 4*(1), 113–116.

March, J. (1997). *Multidimensional Anxiety Scale for Children.* New York: Multi-Health Systems, Inc.

March, J.S., Parker, J.D.A., Sullivan, K., Stallings, P., & Conners, C.K. (1997). The Multidimensional Anxiety Scale for Children (MASC): Factor structure, reliability, and validity. *Journal of American Academy of Child and Adolescent Psychiatry, 36*(4), 554–565.

Mattingly, C. (1991). The narrative nature of clinical reasoning. *American Occupational Therapy Association, 45*(11), 998–1005.

Mattingly, C., & Fleming, M.H. (1994). *Clinical reasoning: Forms of inquiry in a therapeutic practice.* Philadelphia: F.A. Davis Company.

McIntosh, D.N., Miller, L.J., Shyu, V., & Dunn, W. (1999). Development and validation of the Short Sensory Profile. In W. Dunn (Ed.), *The Sensory Profile: Examiner's manual.* San Antonio, TX: The Psychological Corporation.

Miller, L.J. (1982, 1988). *Miller Assessment of Preschoolers.* San Antonio, TX: Psychological Corporation.

Miller, L.J. (1989). *Developing norm-referenced standardized tests.* Binghamton, NY: The Haworth Press, Inc.

Miller, L.J. (1993). *First STEP.* San Antonio, TX: Psychological Corporation.

Miller, L.J., & Lane, S.J. (2000). Toward a consensus in terminology in sensory integration theory and practice: Part 1: Taxonomy of neurophysiological processes. *Sensory Integration Special Interest Section Quarterly, 23*(1), 1–4.

Miller, L.J., McIntosh, D.N., McGrath, J., Shyu, V., Lampe, M., Taylor, A.K., Tassone, F., Neitzel, K., Stackhouse, T., & Hagerman, R. (1999). Electrodermal responses to sensory stimuli in individuals with Fragile X syndrome: A preliminary report. *American Journal of Medical Genetics, 83*(4), 268–279.

Miller, L.J., Wilbarger, J.L., Stackhouse, T.M., & Trunnell, S.L. (in press). Use of clinical reasoning in occupational therapy: The STEP-SI Model of sensory modulation dysfunction. In A.C. Bundy, S.J. Lane, & E.A. Murray (Eds.), *Sensory integration: Theory and practice* (2nd ed.). Philadelphia: F.A. Davis Company.

Mooney, K.C. (1984). Review of the Child Behavior Checklist. In D. Keyser & R. Sweetland (Eds.), *Test critiques* (Vol. 1, pp. 168–184). Kansas City, MO: Westport Publications, Inc.

Ottenbacher, K.J., & Cusick, A. (1990). Goal attainment scaling as a method of clinical service evaluation. *American Journal of Occupational Therapy, 44*(6), 519–525.

Parham, L.D., & Mailloux, Z. (1996). Sensory integration. In J. Case-Smith, A.S. Allen, & P.N. Pratt (Eds.), *Occupational therapy for children* (3rd ed., pp. 307–355). St. Louis, MO: Mosby-Year Book, Inc.

Parker, J.D.A., & March, J.S. (1997). *Structure of the Multidimensional Anxiety Scale for Children (MASC): A confirmatory factor analytic study.* Manuscript submitted for publication.

Roid, G.H., & Miller, L.J. (1997). *Leiter International Performance Scale—Revised.* Wood Dale, IL: Stoelting Company.

Rosenbaum, P., Saigal, S., Szatmari, P., & Hoult, L. (1995). Vineland Adaptive Behavior Scales as a summary of functional outcomes of extremely low birthweight children. *Developmental Medicine and Child Neurology, 37,* 577–586.

Sparrow, S.S., Balla, D.A., & Cicchetti, D.V. (1984). *Manuals for the Vineland Adaptive Behavior Scales.* Circle Pines, MN: American Guidance Service, Inc.

Wechsler, D. (1991). *Wechsler Intelligence Scale for Children—Third edition.* San Antonio, TX: The Psychological Corporation.

Voelker, S.L., Shore, D.L., & Brown-More, C. (1990). Validity of self-report of adaptive behavior skills by adults with mental retardation. *Mental Retardation, 28,* 305–309.

Wilbarger, P., & Wilbarger, J.L. (1991). *Sensory defensiveness in children aged 2–12: An intervention guide for parents and other caretakers.* Santa Barbara, CA: Avanti Educational Programs.

Description of Assessments Used in Evaluation of SMD at the STAR Center at The Children's Hospital in Denver, CO

The *Child Behavior Checklist* (CBCL; Achenbach, 1991) measures social and emotional behaviors based on parent reports. The CBCL is widely used and its construct, content, and criterion validity are well established (Chen, Faraone, Biederman, & Tsuang, 1994; Elliott & Busse, 1992; Jensen, Wantanabe, Richters, & Roper, 1996; Macmann, Barnett, Burd, & Jones, 1992; Mooney, 1984). The CBCL subtests Withdrawn, Anxious/Depressed, Thought Problems, Aggressive, and Social Problems assess emotions; the Attention subtest assesses behaviors in the attentional domains.

Goal Attainment Scale: Using a system such as Goal Attainment Scaling (GAS) that is sensitive to individual variation is critical in SMD because symptoms vary widely (Ottenbacher & Cusick, 1990). A GAS is constructed for each child based on the parent(s)' priorities and goals on a five-point scale:

1	2	3	4	5
decline from current level	current level	expected outcome of intervention	better-than-expected outcome	long-term goal

At outcome, a GAS final score is calculated that represents the child's change (Kiresuk & Sherman, 1968). Appendix 13-D presents a sample goal from one child's GAS.

The *Leiter International Performance Scale—Revised* (Leiter–R; Roid & Miller, 1997) includes several well-standardized rating scales that include domains of attention emotion, and sensation. The Leiter–R parent rating subtests of Adaptation, Social Abilities, Mood/Confidence, and Energy/Feelings assess emotions, and the subtests Attention, Activity Level, and Impulse Control assess behaviors in the attentional domain.

The *Sensory Profile* (SP; Dunn, 1999) is a parent report measure of functional behaviors associated with abnormal responses to sensory stimuli, motor tasks, and emotions. Dunn and colleagues nationally standardized 125 items that fall into eight domains and nine factors (Dunn & Brown, 1997; Dunn & Westman, 1997).

A short version of the SP, the *Short Sensory Profile* (SSP; McIntosh et al., 1999), evaluates only sensory aspects of functional performance to discriminate specifically between children who are typically developing and those with SMD. The SSP construction, reliability, and validity, detailed elsewhere (McIntosh et al., 1999), demonstrate that the SSP adheres to recognized standards of reliability and validity (Miller, 1989). The SSP includes seven factors (subtests) and uses a scoring system based on the cumulative frequency distribution of the national standardization sample, transformed into z-scores. We used a conservative criterion to qualify children as SMD in our research project: total score < -3 SD, or scores on two or more subtests < -2.5 SD, or one subtest score < -4 SD. We analyzed performance in sensory processing to identify *sensitivities* (i.e., Taste/Smell, Movement, Visual/Auditory, and Tactile Sensitivity subtests), *sensory seeking* (Under-Responsive/Seeks Sensation subtest), and *hyporeactivity* (i.e., Low Energy/Weak subtest).

The *Vineland Adaptive Behavior Scales* (Sparrow et al., 1984) is the most frequently used norm-referenced scale of adaptive performance in published research. The Vineland is validated by many studies for accurate discrimination (.40–.70) of abnormal daily living skills (Altman & Mills, 1990; Douhitt, 1992; Rosenbaum, Saigal, Szatmari, & Hoult, 1995; Voelker, Shore, & Brown-More, 1990). In this study, we used the socialization abilities and daily living skills subtests to measure social participation and functional abilities.

The *Multidimensional Scale for Children* (March, 1997) is a norm-referenced anxiety scale, valid in separating children with and without anxiety disorders (classification accuracy 87%). The reliability is also excellent (.79–.93) (March, 1997; Parker & March, 1997).

To measure intelligence, the *Wechsler Intelligence Scale for Children–III* and/or the *Wechsler Preschool and Primary Scale of Intelligence* are administered (Wechsler, 1991).

Parents' Priorities, Resources, and Goals: Clinicians conduct semistructured, open-ended narrative interviews of parents prior to designing a child's intervention program. A qualitative study of interview themes noted five areas in which parents hoped for therapy changes: for their child they wanted to see (a) social participation, (b) self-regulation, and (c) perceived competence; for themselves, they wanted (a) tools to help their child regulate him- or herself and (b) feelings of competence about living with a child with SMD (Cohn, Miller, & Tickle-Degnen, 2000).

SMD Behavior
During Testing Checklist

Observations made during (name of test administered) _____

Behavior	Extreme Reaction	Moderate Reaction	Mild Reaction	Normal Reaction
Response to Sensory Stimuli				
Silliness or giggling during tactile tests	3	2	1	0
"Shutting down" during tactile tests	3	2	1	0
Withdrawal from or aversive reaction to tactile stimuli	3	2	1	0
Bothered by shield touching body	3	2	1	0
Bothered by having shield occlude vision	3	2	1	0
Complaints of feeling ill during or after PRN/spinning	3	2	1	0
Continues to spin on PRN board after test is administered	3	2	1	0
Distracted by items in visual field	3	2	1	0
Unable to keep eyes closed	3	2	1	0
Aversive response to routine noise	3	2	1	0
Distracted by outside noise	3	2	1	0
Attempts by the Child to Self-Regulate				
Excessive movement (rocking, bouncing in seat, tipping chair)	3	2	1	0
Puts things in or around mouth (food/nonfood)	3	2	1	0
Heavy or hard poking, pounding, slapping when responding	3	2	1	0
Needs more than typical number of breaks during testing	3	2	1	0

Behavior	Extreme Reaction	Moderate Reaction	Mild Reaction	Normal Reaction
Behavioral Disorganization				
Restless, fidgety, impulsive grabbing	3	2	1	0
Inability to stay seated	3	2	1	0
Overly talkative	3	2	1	0
Impulsive responses to test items	3	2	1	0
Poor focus on tasks, needs redirection	3	2	1	0
Lack of persistence, needs cues to persist	3	2	1	0
Difficulty entering or transitioning into testing room	3	2	1	0
Somatic Responses to Testing Situation				
Repeatedly requests to go to the bathroom	3	2	1	0
Complains excessively of being thirsty or hungry	3	2	1	0
Complains of being tired even though reportedly well rested	3	2	1	0
Complains of headache/stomachache/eyes hurt/not feeling well	3	2	1	0
Yawning	3	2	1	0

1. Observed but no modification by therapist needed to continue testing reliably
2. Interfered with testing; but with therapist's intervention and modification could continue test reliably (note modifications made)
3. Had to discontinue testing or felt performance was unreliable

Other Comments:

Parent Interview for Children With SMD

Child's name: _____

Child's ID #: _____

Parent's name: _____

Interview date: _____

Parent Interview

1. Tell me about [child's name: _____]. I especially want to hear about the kinds of things that you enjoy about [child: _____], what are his or her gifts and talents; what are his or her strong points.

2. What has led you to seek occupational therapy services for [child: _____]? (If necessary: what have you noticed about [child's: _____] development that concerns you?)

3. What do you know about sensory processing that has led you to seek occupational therapy for your child?

4. Tell me about [child's: _____] abilities in:

    daily care activities

    playing

    making friends

    following directions

    communicating

    regulating his or her behavior:

    aggression

    anxiety

    activity level

    attention span

    sleep patterns

    self-esteem/confidence

5. Tell me what you notice about [child's: _____]:

    reactions to sounds

    reactions to lights and other visual stimuli

    reactions to being touched

    reactions to smelling things

    reactions to moving in space

6. Tell me about your pregnancy, delivery, and [child's: _____] early history.

7. Tell me about [child: _____] prior hospitalizations or medical problems.

8. Tell me about [child's: _____] previous therapeutic interventions.

9. Tell me a little about who is in your family. What do you enjoy about your family the most?

10. Tell me what a typical day is like with your child.

11. (If in school) What is school (preschool) like for [child: _____]? Is there anything that you would like to see changed about his or her school situation or the way he or she behaves or learns at school?

12. What are the barriers in [child's: _____] world to his or her successful participation in meaningful activities?

13. What things do you think might help [child: _____] to participate in those activities?

14. Has [child: _____] had any traumatic experience that might affect his or her interventions?

15. What kind of equipment and/or toys do you have at home that [child: _____] enjoys playing with? What kinds of activities does [child: _____] do after school and on weekends?

16. What are your expectations and/or hopes for therapy? (Or what is it about [child: _____] that you are hoping will change?)

Sample Goal Attainment Scale for Kamon

Name: Kamon

D.O.B.: 11/26/94

Age: 3 years 6 months

Sample Goal Attainment Scale for Kamon

*	Goal	1	2	3	4	5
1	Increase ease of and tolerance for dressing activities, (decreasing parent's involvement and the amount of time he needs to get dressed) by decreasing tactile defensiveness in body and head	Refuses to dress self/must be dressed by adult	Often has oppositional behaviors in dressing; sometimes can complete dressing in 2 hours if given assistance and redirection from an adult	Able to complete age-expected dressing activities within one hour; given preparatory sensory diet activities by an adult with prior set up and cues	Able to complete age-expected dressing activities within 30 minutes if given preparatory sensory diet activities with prior set up and occasional cuing by adult	Able to set up dressing, obtain sensory diet activities as needed, and complete age-expected dressing activities within 15 minutes
2	Increase ability to attend family events by increasing tolerance for everyday noises (decreasing auditory defensiveness)	Demonstrates behavioral distress for an hour after he is taken from situations where everyday noises occur	Removes self from noisy everyday situations (e.g., shuts door when hairdryer is running; avoids groups of children & parties)	Able to remain in presence of everyday group-type noise for an hour if an adult directs a sensory diet routine prior to & during the event	Able to remain in group situation for 2 hours in the presence of everyday noise after directed by adult to complete a routine sensory diet ahead of time	Able to remain in noisy group situation for 3 or more hours seeking self-selected sensory diet activities as needed
3	Increase ability to self-regulate and decrease tantrums at home especially when arriving home from school	Tantrums 10–20 times per day. Has a tantrum every day when arrives home from school even with sensory diet and behavioral interventions	Tantrums 5-10 times per day at home, especially when returning home from school or other outing	Tantrums 3–5 times per day & only 2–3 times per week directly after school; given adult-directed routine sensory diet 4 times a day & with special attention to sensory diet on the way home & immediately after getting home	Tantrums 1–2 times per day, only once per week directly after school; given adult-directed daily routine sensory diet and verbal encouragement to seek appropriate sensory tools after school	Tantrums once-twice per week, rarely directly after school; given adult-directed routine sensory diet. Beginning to seek his own sensory diet to help him remain regulated when returning home
4	Increase ability to play with other children by decreasing aggression that occurs when he "smells" others, or their normal, child-like movement and touch come unexpectedly	Becomes combative during all play times with peers, so much so that friends no longer ask him over to play	Difficulty maintaining relationships with children his age. Identifies certain sensory aspects of children as the reason (e.g., "she smells" or "he touches me too hard")	Can have a friend over and participate in an age-appropriate manner for 1 hour if prepared by parent using sensory diet tools and parent supervises directly, suggesting sensory play as needed for regulation	Occasionally becomes combative during a play time with friend at home, but accepts parent-suggested sensory diet activities. Can play with supervision and sensory tools as needed for 2 hours	Can play for more than 2 hours independently without aggressive outbursts; seeks sensory diet activities for calming without parent cues when starting to feel aggressive
5	Improve praxis and perform age-appropriate fine motor tasks during school and play	Refuses participation in any fine motor tasks	Refuses to participate in most fine motor tasks or play with other children when fine motor skill is required	Engages in fine motor play for 5–10 minutes given preparatory sensory diet activities to hands and arms and a choice of two tasks	Engages in fine motor play for 10–20 minutes given short sensory diet preparation & a choice of two tasks	Engages in fine motor play for 30 minutes or more with sensory diet activities suggested by parent or teacher; beginning to seek own sensory activities to prepare for fine motor tasks

*Parents' priority for goals

14

Sensory Integration With High-Risk Infants and Young Children

Roseann C. Schaaf, M.Ed., OTR/L, FAOTA

Marie E. Anzalone, Sc.D., OTR, FAOTA

Sensory integration principles and practice have become widely accepted by professionals working with infants and young children (Stallings-Sahler, 1998). This chapter extends the application of sensory integration principles and practice with this population, beginning with a consideration of the unique challenges and opportunities of infancy and early childhood. The second section describes a model for viewing infant behavior from a sensory integrative and developmental perspective. This model focuses on the dynamic interplay between sensory responsivity and behavioral organization in infants and young children. The third section of this chapter presents a framework for assessment of infants and young children. This framework suggests a combination of formative and summative information to glean a holistic picture of the child's behavior within the context of the family. Finally, the chapter suggests principles for intervention according to sensory integration theory and presents a three-pronged approach to intervention, one that considers the child's needs as well as the impact of the social and physical environment on the child's behavioral competence.

The Unique Opportunities and Challenges of Infancy and Early Childhood

The resiliency and rapid physical maturation of the infant and young child present an opportunity for developmental neurological change unmatched in any other stage of life. The child's rapid rate of developmental maturation creates an exceptional opportunity for the experiences of early childhood to shape future capabilities. The skills the child acquires during development influence future capabilities. For example, in terms of motor development and praxis, the child "learns how to learn" motor skills through the initial formation of a sensorimotor body scheme and acquisition of motor milestones, as depicted in Figure 14.1.

Children who are unable to experience and respond to the richness of their environments effectively

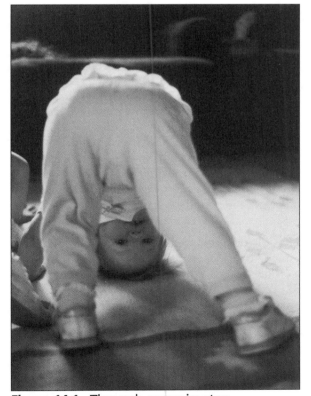

Figure 14.1. Through sensorimotor experiences, the child develops body scheme and motor skills.

because of inadequate abilities to process sensory information run the risk of missing foundational life experiences. A child needs an enriched physical environment, a responsive social environment, and opportunities for successful adaptive responses to this enrichment. The importance of this need for sensory input and social interaction poses a unique challenge. Caregivers and therapists must provide optimal experiences that extend the limits of the child's potential without exceeding his or her tolerance during infancy and early childhood. This optimal zone of challenge and stimulation is the "just-right challenge" (Ayres, 1972, 1979) or the "zone of proximal development" (Vygotsky, 1978) where challenge meets opportunity to extend developmental competence, where the child is able to succeed, but only with effort and support. During these challenges, the processes of sensory integration—the organization of sensory information for use—take place.

Another important consideration when applying sensory integration principles with high-risk infants and young children is that the first 2 years of life are a period during which primary attachment relationships form (Ainsworth, 1991; Bowlby, 1969). These early relationships (see Figure 14.2) serve as the foundation for social and affective development throughout life. The most important affective relationship—that between child and parent—is influenced to a great extent by the child's ability to process and respond to sensory input. The sensory input received during early nurturing and caregiving is one of the most significant factors in the formation of these relationships (Ayres, 1972; Field, 1995; Montague, 1971; Stern, 1985). Any breakdown in this process because of inadequate sensory processing, inability to modulate sensory stimuli, inadequate caregiving, or chaotic or inconsistent environmental supports can disrupt important social and affective processes. The match or goodness-of-fit (Thomas & Chess, 1977; Zeitlin & Williamson, 1994) between the child and the caregiver, as well as the affordances of the physical and social environments, are crucial determinants of the child's development. Any therapeutic intervention during the first years of life must involve the family or a primary caregiver. The therapist's involvement with the family will affect not only how the parents interpret their child's behavior but also how the parents interact with the child.

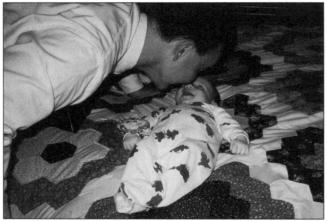

Figure 14.2. Interaction and reciprocity between parent and child are critical to the development of primary attachment relationships.

Finally, the infant's and young child's physiological state of arousal and the impact of arousal on behavioral adaptation are major considerations at this age and stage of development. Infants are in the process of developing self-regulation to achieve physiological homeostasis (Greenspan, 1992; Porges, 1993; Porges, McCabe, & Yongue, 1982). Their behavioral responsiveness to sensory input is often unpredictable. The infant's ability to adapt to the naturally occurring changes in environmental stimuli is an important factor in the development of self-regulation. Given the relatively unstable physiological state of infants and young children, it is easy to overstimulate or overarouse them with stimuli that might not be overwhelming to an older child. Temperature changes, simple position changes, or an increase in visual or auditory input, for example, can trigger changes in the physiological state of the infant. These state changes are reflected in extremes in behavioral arousal, increased heart or respiratory rate, or gastrointestinal reactions (e.g., hiccups or spitting up). Changes in arousal can also result in disorganized behaviors (e.g., inconsolable crying) or avoidance behaviors (e.g., visual avoidance to shut out extraneous stimuli). Assessment of infants' behavioral adaptation, therefore, must include an appreciation of their physiological state and regulatory abilities as they adapt to environmental changes. Als' (1986) theory of synactive development clearly articulated the need to consider the infant's physiological reactivity, motoric and behavioral responsivity, state of arousal, and interactive organization (or disorganization) relative to sensory challenges and changes. This chapter presents evidence that the principles of synactive development, as applied to infants and young children, are consistent with sensory integration theory as first described by Ayres (1972). Through the combination of sensory integrative and synactive theoretical foundations, the therapist can understand the behaviors of infants and young children more accurately and thereby plan more meaningful interventions. Although physiological factors are most obvious in neonates, these factors continue to influence infants and toddlers. Therefore it is important to consider the physiological factors with these older children as well.

A Model for Viewing the Infant From the Sensory Integration Perspective

Sensory integration theory is a useful framework for structuring observations of infants' and young children's behaviors and capabilities and interpreting their implications. The theory, by definition, necessitates consideration of both intrinsic and extrinsic factors that influence behavior. Figure 14.3 depicts the intrinsic and extrinsic factors affecting infants and young children. Intrinsic factors consist of the "four As" (arousal, attention, affect, and action), sensory responsivity, and self-regulation. These intrinsic factors are interrelated and therefore influence each other. For example, a child's ability to process and respond to sensory information (the child's *sensory responsivity*) is an intrinsic factor that influences the child's arousal level, affect, attention, and action, as later sections in this chapter will discuss. Similarly, sensory responsivity is an important determinant of self-regulation. Extrinsic factors such as the demands, opportunities, and goodness-of-fit between the social and physical environments are also important determinants of sensory integrative-based behaviors.

According to this model of infant behavior, the ability to process sensory input and respond to it is a core intrinsic factor and therefore occupies the center of the model. Sensory responsivity affects and is affected by the infant's arousal level, attention, affect, and action (the four As). A ring, or filter, around the central core in Figure 14.3 depicts the important interrelationship between sensory responsivity, the four As, and self-regulation. Self-regulation refers to the child's ability to maintain regulated states of arousal in the face of changing environmental demands and challenges. In a noisy room, for example, a tired child with adequate self-regulation might turn his or her head away from the crowd and begin to suck vigorously on a pacifier in an attempt to maintain regulation during this

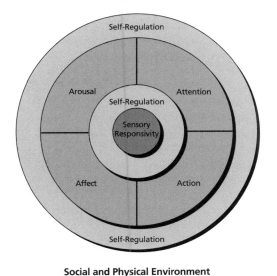

Figure 14.3. Model of infant behavior based on sensory integration and self-regulation.

sensory experience. In contrast, a child with poor self-regulation might become over-stimulated and disorganized. Accordingly, sensory responsivity and self-regulation are interrelated aspects of the child's behavioral expression: the child's responsivity and ability to maintain a regulated state in a changing sensory environment are interdependent. Responsivity and self-regulation, in turn, have a significant influence on arousal, attention, affect, and action, and vice versa (as illustrated in Figure 14.3).

The preceding examples illustrate the relationship among arousal (crying or calm state), attention (organized or disorganized), affect (e.g., the negative emotion conveyed by crying versus the calm of a suckling child), and action (e.g., bringing hand to mouth for sucking). This example also demonstrates how all four components interrelate to produce an organized response to a sensory event. In combination, the intrinsic factors illustrated in Figure 14.3 guide and direct the child's purposeful activity or occupation.

The final component of the model consists of the extrinsic factors, the social and physical environments, which also play a significant role in the child's behavioral expression. The outside rim of Figure 14.3 represents these factors. The physical environment includes the objects and spaces that the child experiences in the course of daily life. The social environment encompasses the caregiving relationship, parental style, and the ability of the social partner to modulate interaction in response to the infant's communicative cues. Extrinsic factors also include the goodness-of-fit between the child and the environment. Goodness-of-fit refers to the match between the child's needs and abilities and the environmental demands and supports (Thomas & Chess, 1977; Zeitlin & Williamson, 1994). Extrinsic factors determine the challenges and supports available to the child as he or she develops sensory integrative competence.

Taken in whole, this model demonstrates that the young child's behavior is a complex interplay of intrinsic and extrinsic factors that affect behavioral expression and resultant interactions. The role of therapeutic intervention, then, is to determine which of these factors is in need of remediation to optimize function. Therapeutically, the challenge is to utilize the interplay between the child's intrinsic abilities and the environment during naturally occurring functional activities. The therapist must improve the goodness-of-fit between the child and his or her physical and social environments to create and modify "just-right challenges" for the child that will promote growth and development.

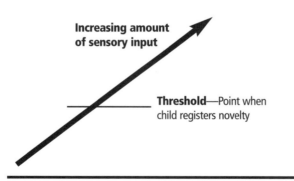

Figure 14.4. Sensory threshold.

Note. From *Helping Infants and Young Children Interact With Their Environment: Improving Sensory Integration and Self-Regulation,* by G. G. Williamson and M. E Anzalone, 2001, Washington, DC: Zero-to-Three. Reprinted with permission.

Sensory Responsivity

One of the most important aspects of sensory processing is sensory responsivity, the ability to regulate the response to sensory input. This concept is not new. Ayres (1972, 1985) used the term *sensory registration* to refer to the initial awareness of sensory input. Other authors subsequently elaborated on sensory registration to include the concept of *sensory threshold,* the individual set point at which the person detects and responds to sensory information (Dunn, 1997; Williamson & Anzalone, 1997). Figure 14.4 illustrates the sensory threshold, the point at which the child registers novel sensory input. Below this threshold, the child is unaware of the sensory input (i.e., the child has not yet noted any change or novelty in the sensory environment).

However, the sensory threshold is not a discrete, stationary point at which the child detects a stimulus of a given intensity, duration, or frequency. Rather, threshold is dynamic and variable, influenced not only by the child's inherent set point but also by a variety of intrinsic and extrinsic factors. Some of these factors include the accumulation of sensation over time and the sensory modality, intensity, and location of the stimulus.

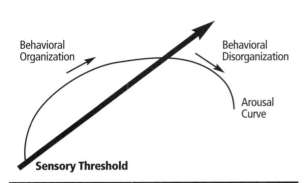

Figure 14.5. The sensory threshold interacts with the arousal curve to determine behavioral response and organization.

Note. From *Helping Infants and Young Children Interact With Their Environment: Improving Sensory Integration and Self-Regulation,* by G. G. Williamson and M. E Anzalone, 2001, Washington, DC: Zero-to-Three. Reprinted with permission.

Sensory Threshold and Behavioral Organization

Other factors affecting the sensory threshold are sensory and affective experiences, the perceived importance of the stimulus, the child's expectations regarding the stimuli, present activity level, and level of arousal. Figure 14.5 depicts the relationship among state of arousal, sensory threshold, and the resultant behavioral response (behavioral organization versus disorganization) (Posner & Boies, 1971; Williamson & Anzalone, 1997). As arousal increases, behavioral disorganization improves until a point at which the individual exceeds his or her ability to cope with the sensory input. At this point, behavioral disorganization occurs. In addition, the child's sensory threshold influences both arousal and the subsequent response, as depicted in Figure 14.5. A child with a low sensory threshold will become disorganized more readily than the child with a high sensory threshold.

A Continuum of Responsivity

Figure 14.6 depicts two distinct categories of sensory responsivity, children with low threshold (increased sensitivity) and children with high threshold (decreased sensitivity) (Dunn, 1997; Williamson & Anzalone, 1997, in press). Children who have very low sensory thresholds do not require much sensory input to reach the point of sensory registration, and therefore it is easy for sensation to overstimulate them. Behaviorally, these children are often sensorily defensive or overresponsive to sensory input (Ayres, 1979; Knickerbocker, 1980; Wilbarger & Wilbarger, 1991).

Although therapists and researchers have paid much attention to children with low thresholds and resultant hyperresponsivity, it is also important to consider children at the opposite end of the continuum, those with high threshold. Children with high sensory thresholds require greater-than-normal levels of input to register and orient and, as a result, are behaviorally hyporesponsive. Children with a high threshold sometimes appear to be disengaged or to have a flattened affect. Often, as a result of their passivity, they also elicit less stimulation from the environment even though they require more.

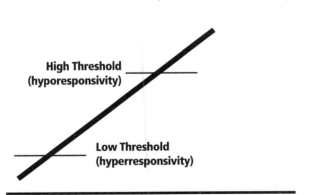

Figure 14.6. Sensory threshold: A continuum of responsivity.

Note. From *Helping Infants and Young Children Interact With Their Environment: Improving Sensory Integration and Self-Regulation,* by G. G. Williamson and M. E Anzalone, 2001, Washington, DC: Zero-to-Three. Reprinted with permission.

Both of these conditions (high and low threshold) represent extreme situations at either end of the continuum. Most young children are able to modulate their sensory threshold or their behavioral responsivity to sensation and remain in the midrange of this continuum. The child who has a problem modulating his or her behavioral response often has difficulty with arousal, attention, affect, and action as well. The goal of intervention, then, is to increase or decrease sensory responsivity, to regulate the behavioral response, or to widen the range for adaptive responses by adapting the physical and/or social environment to improve the goodness-of-fit between each child's innate sensory responsivity and the environmental challenges (see the section on Basic Principles of Sensory Integrative Intervention for Infants and Young Children, later in this chapter).

Sensory threshold is a dynamic and variable concept. Response to sensory input is under the influence of the child's current level of arousal, previous sensory and affective experiences, the child's current engagement in goal-directed activity, and the perceived importance of the stimuli and expectations. For example, an infant's tolerance of light touch might be significantly different if he or she is overtired and stressed, in contrast to when the child is rested.

Second, the child's ability to recover or return to a baseline level of arousal after the sensory event is an important factor affecting behavioral responsivity. Many children with tactile or sensory defensiveness take more time to recover from sensory events than children who are not tactually or sensorily defensive (Williamson & Anzalone, 2001). The prolonged recovery time means that the child remains in an overaroused and disorganized state for a longer period.

Given this dynamic and variable nature of behavioral responsivity and sensory threshold, it is useful to conceptualize threshold as a range of responsivity (not a single point) that varies both among and within individuals. This range (Figure 14.7) is based on multiple intrinsic and extrinsic factors, as discussed earlier. The wider the range, the greater the possibilities for the child to maintain a regulated, behaviorally organized state and produce organized, adaptive responses.

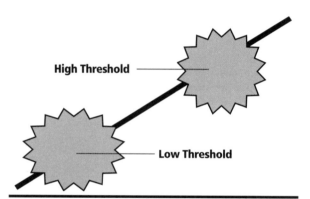

Figure 14.7. Sensory threshold: Range of behavioral responsivity.

Although the concept of sensory threshold can help to illustrate the child's sensory modulation, it does not explain the resultant behavior. Some children will act in accordance with their threshold; others will attempt to compensate for their threshold (see Table 14.1) (Dunn, 1997; Williamson & Anzalone, 1997, in press).

Table 14.1. Sensory Profiles and Behavioral Response*

| Behavioral Response | Low Threshold ← → High Threshold | |
	(Increased sensitivity)	(Decreased sensitivity)
Acts in accordance with threshold	Hyperresponsive	Hyporesponsive
Attempts to counteract threshold	Sensory Avoider	Sensory Seeker

*Note. From *Helping Infants and Young Children Interact With Their Environment: Improving Sensory Integration and Self-Regulation,* by G. G. Williamson and M. E Anzalone (2001), Washington, DC: Zero-to-Three. Reprinted with permission.

Children with low threshold who act in accordance with their threshold are *hyperresponsive*. They have high levels of arousal and an inability to focus attention, exhibit predominantly negative or stressed affect, and engage in action that seems impulsive or defensive. In contrast, children with low threshold who are attempting to counteract their threshold will engage in *sensory-avoidant* behaviors. Their protective adaptations help them to modulate their state of arousal most of the time, but attention is often hypervigilant as they attempt to avoid sensory overload. Affect is frequently fearful or anxious, and action is constrained because these children withdraw from a wide variety of sensorimotor experiences at a time when most children are exploring their environments.

Children with high thresholds also present in two different behavioral profiles: hyporesponsive and sensory seeking. *Hyporesponsive* children act in accordance with their threshold and, as a result, frequently seem disengaged from their environment because they do not register and orient to the typical sensory experiences. These children tend to have decreased states of arousal, show a prolonged latency to attaining focused attention, exhibit a flattened affect that discourages social interaction, and seem passive and sedentary. In contrast, the *sensory seeker* is a child with a high threshold who attempts to counteract or regulate that threshold by actively pursuing excitatory sensory input. The sensory seeker often exhibits heightened arousal but can also be labile because it is difficult for this child to achieve sensory homeostasis. These children frequently become overstimulated and disorganized (see Figure 14.5). Attention in the sensory seeker is often brief and poorly modulated. Affect is variable within each child, ranging from flat to frenzied depending on the status of the sensory threshold and behavioral organization. These children gear their action toward increasing sensory input and sometimes tend toward risk taking and impulsivity.

It is particularly important to discern whether a child has a low threshold and is sensory avoidant or has a high threshold (hyporesponsive) and has not yet attained threshold. Both of these types of children can appear to be disengaged from the environment, but for opposite reasons. The focus of intervention is very different for each type of child. Intervention for the low-threshold, sensory-avoidant child involves decreasing sensory input while encouraging engagement in adaptive behavior; intervention for the hyporesponsive child involves providing arousing sensory input grounded in adaptive behavior. The best way to discriminate between these two very different types of children is to decrease sensory input. For the sensory-avoidant child, decrease of sensory input should result in behavioral organization. In the hyporesponsive child, a decrease of sensory input should produce no further disorganization.

Behavioral Organization: The Four *A*s

One way of understanding and describing the behaviors that reflect sensory integration and regulation in young children is to describe infant functioning and sensory-related behaviors in terms of the four *A*s of infancy: arousal, attention, affect, and action (Williamson & Anzalone, 2001; Lester, Freier, & LaGasse, 1995). Each of these processes requires regulation within each *A* for optimal functioning, and that regulation has a mutual regulatory influence on each of the other processes. For example, the ability to maintain attention is dependent on maintenance of a quiet, alert state of arousal; that attention, in turn, can influence the ability to accomplish an adaptive action successfully. Sensory modulation, or threshold, as discussed previously in this chapter, influences this regulatory process and is in turn influenced by it.

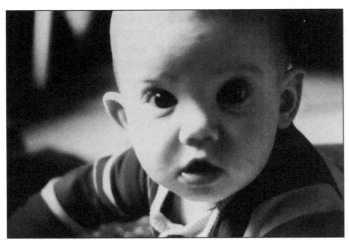

Figure 14.8. The quiet alert state, optimal arousal for learning and interaction.

Arousal

Arousal refers to the ability to maintain and transition between different sleep and wake states (Berg & Berg, 1979). Neonates often demonstrate the six states of arousal: deep sleep, light sleep, drowsiness, quiet alert, active alert, and crying. Observation of these states is an important part of many clinical assessments and observation approaches in neonatal intensive care units (Als, 1982; Brazelton, 1984). The ability to regulate state behavior is often one of the first signs of recovery in a high-risk infant; conversely, difficulty with such regulation is one of the earliest signs of problems (Als, 1989; Lombroso & Matsumiya, 1985). The baby in Figure 14.8 exemplifies the quiet alert state, in which the infant is organized and in a state of optimal arousal for learning and interaction.

The need to observe state does not end with the neonatal period. State of arousal continues to influence (and be influenced by) the perception and interpretation of sensory input long after the infant attains stable sleep-wake patterns. For example, the touch that might be acceptable to a toddler during a drowsy or quiet alert state can be aversive when the child is stressed or in an active alert state.

Attention

Attention is the ability to focus selectively on a desired stimulus or task. Most children are able to sustain focused attention best in a quiet alert state. Three factors influence attention in the young child: alertness (maintaining the quiet alert state), selection (choosing what to attend to and the ability to shift between several foci), and allocation (the amount of time a child can attend to a stimulus and the amount of effort inherent in maintaining that focus). It is also important to recognize that infants can have a preference for certain modalities (e.g., one child might calm and orient to a visual target; another will calm and orient to a music box or the mother's voice).

It is not unusual for a young child who is having sensory integration or self-regulatory problems to be able to attend to input in only one modality at a time. Adding another sensory modality induces behavioral disorganization. For example, a child might be able to smile and look at his or her parent only if the parent does not speak. When an auditory stimulus accompanies the visual stimulus, however, the child can become overstimulated. An older child might be able to attend to independent free play in preschool, but only when the music is not playing.

Although clinicians tend to think about attention in terms of duration of attention span, it is also important to consider threshold's effect on attention. A young child whose threshold is exceeded (usually the child with a low threshold or sensory defensiveness) might actively avoid sensory input (e.g., the child who uses active gaze aversion during face-to-face social interaction, or the child who hides under the table during free play in toddler group). In contrast, the child with a high threshold will be inattentive and nonresponsive because he or she has not yet oriented to salient stimuli in the environment.

Affect

Affect is one of the most important aspects of behavior in high-risk infants and young children. Affect is the emotional component of behavior and involves not only the affective response to sensory input but also the socially based emotions that occur in the context of social relationships (Holloway, 1998). As with children of any age who have difficulties with sensory modulation, infants with sensory modulation problems often have atypical, heightened, or depressed affective responses to sensory input. With infants and young children, however, these atypical responses can influence the formation of primary attachment relationships (Stern, 1985) or disrupt the children's ability to be influenced by the social environment not only because of their atypical response but also because of how parents might interpret these responses (Holloway). For example, Julie is tactually defensive and irritable and stiffens when held or cuddled. Her mother, Helen, describes Julie as "not liking her." In response, Helen tends to leave Julie alone and quiet rather than disrupt her tenuous equilibrium with interaction and additional sensory input. This results in decreased opportunities for important nurturing, social interaction, and reciprocity.

Action

Action, the final *A,* is the ability to engage in adaptive goal-directed behavior (Anzalone, 1993). Motor abilities are the foundation for action, but action is much more complex than just moving. Action involves the organization of perceptual and cognitive contributions to adaptive, goal-directed behavior. Muscle tone, strength, and the asymmetrical tonic neck reflex are motor; play is action. Strength, muscle tone, and other components of motor maturation are necessary to play; however, having age-appropriate motor control does not give one the ability to interact adaptively with and explore the environment. In infants, the interaction between motor maturation and the capacity to use that ability in the context of play and exploration is an exciting process to observe (Figure 14.9).

Ayres (1985) described praxis as encompassing three interdependent steps, which are useful in understanding action in infants:

- ideation (formulating the goal based upon perception of environmental affordances)

- motor planning (figuring out specifically how to accomplish the goal; involves cognitive problem solving and sensorimotor awareness of the body that underlies that plan)

- execution (actually carrying out the planned action)

Adequate sensory integration is necessary for all components of praxis. For example, to form a goal, one must notice and orient to novelty and be motivated to explore the environment. If a child perceives the environment as overstimulating and threatening, the child will be more likely to avoid the environment than to explore it. Similarly, if the child does not process the tactile and proprioceptive feedback obtained from motor activities optimally, he or she will not develop a body scheme adequate to support motor planning.

The four *As* provide a useful way of contrasting the observed behaviors in each of the four profiles presented in Table 14.1 (Williamson & Anzalone, 1997, 2001). Table 14.2 summarizes these behavioral profiles.

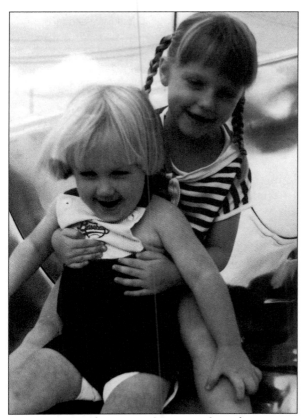

Figure 14.9. Play, as action, requires the organization of perceptual, cognitive, sensory, and motor skills.

Table 14.2. Sensory Responsivity's Effect on Behavior

Behavioral Response	Sensory Responsivity			
	Hyperresponsive (low threshold)	**Sensory Avoidant (low threshold)**	**Hyporesponsive (high threshold)**	**Sensory Seeking (high threshold)**
Arousal	Usually high	Attempts to modulate arousal, so often in quiet state	Usually decreased arousal	Arousal heightened but labile
Attention	Inability to focus attention; distractible	Hypervigilant, needing to "scan" for sensory threats	Inattentive or has a latency to attend; often misses opportunities because of latency	Poorly modulated attention; attends to sensory yield, not other affordances
Affect	Predominantly negative affect	Fearful or anxious; when older, can be demanding	Restricted or flat affect; can appear depressed	Affect is variable but can become overexcited with excess sensory input
Action	Impulsive reaction; can seem aggressive	Constrained, avoids developmentally appropriate exploration	Passive; tends to watch action but not engage	Action is geared primarily to gaining sensation; can be impulsive and take excess risks

Note. From *Helping Infants and Young Children Interact With Their Environment: Improving Sensory Integration and Self-Regulation,* by G. G. Williamson and M. E Anzalone, 2001, Washington, DC: Zero-to-Three. Reprinted with permission.

Problem Setting: Assessment of High-Risk Infants and Young Children With Sensory Integrative Dysfunction

Sensory integration is not about gaining new skills or motor milestones but rather about the process by which the child attains them and how he or she uses those newly gained abilities to interact dynamically with the environment. The process of assessment, then, is about describing the quality of performance, not merely providing insight into the developmental level of that performance.

This section outlines a two-fold assessment process using both formative and summative strategies (Anderson, Ball, & Murphy, 1975) to guide the therapist in a valid and comprehensive evaluation of function and dysfunction in sensory integration in infants and young children. Both formative and summative assessment strategies provide insights into the acquisition of developmental skills and abilities. Summative strategies provide insight into the skills a child already has. These assessments are useful in detecting developmental delay or providing criteria regarding evolving skills. Most standardized developmental assessments are of this type (e.g., *Bayley Scales of Infant Development II,* Bayley, 1993; *First STEP,* Miller, 1993; *Mullen Scales of Early Learning,* Mullen, 1984, 1989).

In contrast, formative assessment strategies describe the "how" of performance. Therapists frequently use formative measures as part of ongoing assessment during intervention, but such assessments are also very useful in describing the quality of performance. The qualitative aspect of performance is what underlies the four *As* discussed previously. To assess the qualitative aspects of performance, one must observe the child in an ongoing activity and capture the uniqueness and dynamics of his or her performance. Merely administering a standard set of items does not provide the flexibility necessary for summative assessment. Instead, the clinician must look at the child within a context and describe the child's performance, the environmental challenges, and the goodness-of-fit between the two.

Unfortunately, few standardized tools provide the appropriate type of structure for assessment of sensory integrative abilities or disabilities in infants (see *Functional Emotional Assessment Scale,* Greenspan, 1996; DeGangi & Greenspan, in press; and the *Early Coping Inventory,* Zeitlin, Williamson, & Szczepanski, 1988, for two exceptions), and none provide all of the information necessary to describe sensory integrative functioning in the young child. Therefore, therapists should combine summative and formative strategies with systematic observation and data gathering from the family and others involved with the child to gain a comprehensive, holistic picture of the child's sensory integrative strengths and needs.

This process is interactive and reflective, guided by the therapist's clinical reasoning. The therapist will gather information from many sources, then thoughtfully reflect on the information, synthesize it using a theoretical perspective, and refine the findings into an intervention plan that considers all areas of need. Although the initial assessment will shape the starting point for intervention, assessment is an ongoing process that continually alters and modifies the intervention plan and process. Frequently therapists are part of an interdisciplinary team of medical, educational, and therapeutic professionals who work together with the family to provide input into the child's areas of strength and need. It is important that the entire team cooperate in influencing and coordinating the target areas for assessment (Greenspan & Meisels, 1996).

The factors that shape the occupational therapy assessment include the needs of the child, the needs and desires of the family, and the philosophy and mission of the setting and/or the funding source. For example, in an early intervention setting, the child's need to function in a learning environment, in conjunction with the needs and wants of the family, will shape the therapist's assessment and ultimately form the Individualized Family Service Plan (IFSP). In a hospital environment, the factors shaping assessment are the medical needs, the child's length of stay, and the discharge environment. For community-based programs, influences on the nature of the assessment include the philosophy and mission of the organization, the nature of child and family needs, and the skills and theoretical approach of the clinician. In any case, it is important that the therapist consider the environment(s) in which the child must function; the primary medical, nutritional, and developmental demands and challenges; and family expectations. This will ensure a comprehensive yet collaborative approach that is in keeping with the program's stated goals.

Regardless of the setting, an important component in a comprehensive assessment is the family narrative. As explained in chapter 11 of this text, the narrative provides a mechanism by which to understand the child's problems in the context of his or her unique situation. In the case of the infant and the young child, the narrative is the family's story, including the parents' hopes and dreams for their child as well as their family values, routines, and rituals (Burke & Schaaf, 1997). The narrative can give the therapist insight into the child's occupational roles in the context of the family environment. This narrative also provides a way of understanding how the sensory integrative process might be influencing these roles or the roles of others within the family. Questions about the child's daily routines elicit information about the child's areas of strength and need. Queries regarding the family's daily activities and leisure pursuits can uncover facets of the family's interests and occupations and the nature of the child's integration and interaction with them. Observation of the family during daily activities furnishes insight into the workings of the family, the goodness-of-fit between the child and his or her family, and how effectively he or she functions as a member of the family.

The Components of Assessment

Assessment of infants and young children with potential sensory integrative dysfunction must consider three major components: the child, the physical environment, and the social environment (including family and peers) (Schaaf & Mulrooney, 1989b). Assessment that includes all of these components provides comprehensive information regarding specific strengths and needs that underlie function and serves as a guide for intervention. (For an in-depth review of standardized and nonstandardized assessment instruments that address these areas, consult the several texts that provide detailed descriptions or overviews of assessment information: Asher, 1996; Case-Smith, Allen, & Pratt, 1996; King-Thomas & Hacker, 1987; Schaaf & Davis, 1992). Appendix 14-A gives an overview of the instruments that are useful for assessing the three components of a sensory integrative evaluation.

As stated earlier, it is important to use a combination of formative tools (which measure specific levels of sensory processing development) and summative or qualitative assessments (which provide information about *how* the child's sensory processing influences behavior). Both formative and summative strategies should consider the child within the context of the family and physical environments, thereby evaluating not only the child's sensory needs and abilities but also how those needs and abilities might be influencing occupational behavior and social interactions.

Assessment of the Child

When assessing the child's strengths and needs using a sensory integrative framework, consider the child's responsivity to various types of sensory inputs; his or her ability to modulate input under various demands; his or her ability to self-calm after periods of disorganization, as well as the types of self-calming the child uses; and the quality and intensity of sensory input that are organizing and disorganizing to the child. Of utmost importance is how these factors influence the child's ability to function effectively in his or her occupational roles. How does responsivity to sensory input affect the ability to play or develop attachment with the caregiver? How does sensory modulation affect regulatory behaviors such as sleeping and eating? How does sensory modulation affect the regulation of the four *A*s? How does regulation of the four *A*s affect sensory modulation? How does the parent's interaction style match the child's sensory needs (i.e., what is the goodness-of-fit)? How does the child's sensory threshold affect his or her ability to engage in self-care and play activities? In what ways does the child's play reflect sensory preferences? The answers to these and similar questions, gathered through a combination of formative and summative strategies, are of prime importance in the assessment process.

It has become increasingly obvious that evaluators must frame the child's sensory integrative needs within the context of functional behavior (Coster, 1998; Dunn & Westman, 1997; Fisher, Murray, & Bundy, 1991; Schaaf & Burke, 1992). The sensory integrative process provides a way of understanding dysfunction as well as individual differences in style. Therapists need to interpret sensory integrative difficulties in light of whether or not they create problems for the child in his or her daily occupations or actions (Coster, 1998). For example, assessment of a child with slight problems in sensory modulation that do not interfere with play or social relationships might provide some insight into preferences and performance but might not indicate specific intervention unless the sensory modulation dysfunction is interfering with the child's ability to function at home or in the classroom. If, on the other hand, the sensory modulation problem is interfering with the child's ability to function optimally, assessment results would recommend intervention and parent education. Evaluating both the sensory issues and the functional sequelae, if any, of the sensory dysfunction ensures that the therapists and the caregivers clearly understand the sensory integrative needs of the child in terms of the child's developmental and functional behaviors and lends validity and acceptance to this approach. However, because standardized assessment tools do not usually address this type of information, therapists will need to consider combining standardized child-based quantitative assessment with qualitative observation and history taking. (Refer to Appendix 14-A for a listing of many of the currently available assessments that address sensory processing in infants and young children.) Appendix 14-B provides the *Sensory Integration Observation Guide*, an interview tool that is useful for ascertaining the parent's perspective regarding salient behaviors associated with sensory processing function and dysfunction in infants and young children.

A sensory history is also a useful method for gathering information regarding the child's early and current development and behaviors that might give clues about his or her sensory processing. It is important to obtain information about pre-, peri-, and postnatal development and medical and developmental history, as well as information regarding the child's current behaviors related to each sensory system (visual, auditory, olfactory, tactile, proprioceptive, and vestibular) and praxis.

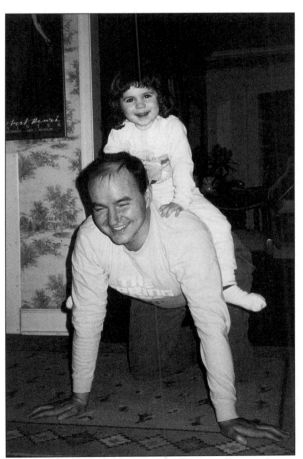

Figure 14.10. Observation of play allows the therapist to observe the child's responses to sensory input in an unstructured environment.

Contemporary parent-interview instruments with strong validity and reliability address the manifestation of sensory integrative dysfunction in a child's daily life activities. The *Sensory Profile* (Dunn, 1999) and the *Evaluation of Sensory Processing* (LaCroix, Johnson, & Parham, 1997) are two such instruments. Both of these instruments are promising new assessments that have the potential to assess the child's sensory processing and its influence on and expression in occupational activities.

Observing the child during structured and unstructured activity can be helpful in understanding each child's unique responses to sensory input. For example, a component of the *Bayley II*, the Infant Behavior Record (Bayley, 1993), provides a system for documenting qualitative components of performance during standardized testing that might have a sensory integrative basis. Observation of unstructured play situations (Figure 14.10) is particularly helpful. Play is an activity that reflects the child's underlying developmental and sensory processing abilities and needs. When observing a child in a play context, it is important to observe not only the child but the sensory demands of the environment and the dyadic or social interaction in which the child is performing (Burke, 1998; Burke & Schaaf, 1997; Schaaf & Burke, 1992, 1997; Schaaf, Merrill, & Kinsella, 1987).

Finally, excellent formalized assessments that provide the opportunity for examining sensorimotor skills and making inferences about sensory integration are the *Miller Assessment for Preschoolers*

(Miller, 1982, 1988), the *Test of Sensory Functions in Infants* (DeGangi & Greenspan, 1989), and the *First STEP* (Miller, 1993). (See Appendix 14-A for a brief review of these and other assessments.)

Assessment of the Physical Environment

Assessment of the physical environment includes an evaluation of the nonhuman factors in the environment that support, challenge, or counteract the child's occupational functioning relative to his or her unique sensory needs. When interviewing parents, therapists should include questions that address the physical objects in the environment, such as toys and play spaces. Are developmentally appropriate toys available for the child? Are there opportunities for many different types of sensory input? Does the child exhibit toy or play preferences that reveal his or her self-regulatory strategies? Does the environment produce sensory overload by having too many inappropriate toys or too much noise and activity? Is the child's play space safe? Simple yet effective strategies for adjusting the play spaces and objects for the child can have a profound and long-lasting effect on the child's ability to play competently and effectively. (Appendix 14-A lists assessments that focus specifically on the physical environment.)

Assessment of the Social Environment

Assessment of the social environment includes an evaluation of caregiver-child interactions, such as those during play as depicted in Figure 14.10. When examining interaction, it is important to evaluate the abilities of both the child and the partner, along with the goodness-of-fit between the child and his or her social partners. Although there are no instruments that evaluate specifically how the child's sensory processing affects the interaction between the caregiver and the child, a few instruments measure caregiver-child interactions (see Appendix 14-A). Once again, the therapist must utilize a clinical reasoning process rooted in sensory integration theory to make inferences and interpretations about the caregiver-child interactions and the effect of the child's sensory processing on these interactions. Greenspan and DeGangi's *Functional Emotional Assessment Scale* (DeGangi & Greenspan, in press; Greenspan, 1996) evaluates the child's behaviors using a sensory integrative and social-emotional framework. Through systematic observation and rating of the caregiver-child behaviors during play, this scale also examines the caregiver's behaviors, including availability, interest, attachment, and interactions with the child.

Several other assessments of the social environment, specifically of the family and/or caregiver, are available. Many of these provide information regarding the caregivers' or family's strengths, needs, ability to identify these needs, and/or their ability to cope with the potential stress involved in raising a child with special needs (Schaaf & Davis, 1992). (Appendix 14-A summarizes the assessments focused on the family.)

Shaping Outcomes: Organizing Assessment Data Into an Intervention Plan

In the final stage of the assessment process, a therapist organizes the information into a meaningful description of how the child's sensory needs are affecting his or her occupational behavior, then outlines an intervention plan to build on areas of strength and improve areas of need. Figure 14.3, a model of infant behavior, gives a framework within which to organize intervention on three different (but not mutually exclusive) levels:

1. helping parents to *understand* their infant

2. facilitating *goodness-of-fit* between the infant and his or her environment

3. *remediating* the underlying sensory processing and self-regulation problems and/or their behavioral expression in terms of the four *A*s as necessary

This three-pronged approach to intervention allows the therapist to plan a course of intervention that will address specific areas of need and build on areas of strength in the context of naturally occurring events within the family. Integration of therapeutic activities into daily routines provides the repetition and reinforcement of learning necessary to bring about developmental change and establish a foundation for the formation of developmentally appropriate affective relationships (Holloway, 1998). Table 14.3 presents a useful method for synthesizing this information and organizing the assessment data into an intervention plan. This system helps the therapist to identify the key issues related to sensory processing dysfunction (i.e., parents' ability to read cues, goodness-of-fit, responsivity/threshold, self-regulation, individual sensory systems, and the four As,), then determine the best focus of intervention. With infants and young children, the focus of intervention will frequently be the parents in the

Table 14.3. Organizing Assessment Data for Intervention

Component	Questions for Intervention	Promote organization or disorganization?	Intervention Implications
Parents	Ability to read cues Insight into child's difficulties Synchrony or reciprocity Ability to scaffold		
Goodness-of-fit	Social environment Physical environment		
Child's Sensory Processing: State of the nervous system and threshold	Hyperresponsive Sensory Avoider Hyporesponsive Sensory Seeker Mixed		
Child's Sensory Processing: Self-regulation	Arousal (including sleep/wake) Activity level Recovery or calming		
Child's Sensory Processing: Specific sensory systems	Tactile Vestibular Visual Proprioceptive Auditory Olfactory Temperature Oral Pain		
Child's Sensory Processing: Sensory-based behavioral organization	Arousal Attention Affect Action		
Summary			
Intervention Focus	Parent:	Goodness-of-Fit:	Child:

home environment; however, each situation brings with it a unique combination of environmental, social, and intrinsic strengths and areas of need.

Helping Parents Understand Their Infant

One of the most useful aspects of a sensory integrative frame of reference in working with the infant and young child is that it helps to clarify behaviors that are otherwise puzzling to parents. Sensory integration theory supplies a language for translating behaviors (e.g., tactile avoidance or feeding difficulty) into a manageable and neutral context. For example, many parents interpret tactile-avoidant behaviors such as unwillingness to cuddle as having an emotional basis ("I am not a good mother") rather than a sensory basis ("My child doesn't like *touch*"). Parents also tend to interpret some sensory integrative symptoms in terms of willfulness, being "bad," or just being "disinterested." Helping parents understand the sensory basis of their child's behavior can have a tremendous impact on the parents as well as on the child.

Sensory-avoidant behaviors, sensory-based feeding difficulties, arousal modulation problems, and other sensory-based behavioral problems can disrupt the important nurturing and attachment relationship of the early years of life. For example, parents might describe the child who still does not sleep through the night at 2 years of age as a "difficult" or "manipulative" child, when actually the child's poor self-regulation and sensory hyperresponsivity prevent him or her from remaining in a sleep state for long periods. Often, the most effective intervention is to help the parents identify behaviors that might have a sensory basis, understand the cues that the child is giving regarding his or her sensory preference, state of arousal, or readiness for interaction, and develop reciprocal and supportive interactions with their child (Brazelton, 1990; Holloway, 1998; Williamson & Anzalone, 2001). This approach provides an essential foundation for the type of collaborative relationship between clinician and parent that is essential for family-centered care (Hanft, 1989).

Facilitating Goodness-of-fit Between Child and Environment

Facilitating goodness-of-fit between the infant and the environment is also an important consideration when working with infants and young children. Gorski (1983) used the term *environmental medicine* to describe the essential match in neonatology between the environment and the child. He believed that medical intervention for the young premature infant was not the treatment of illness but rather the treatment of a child who was in the wrong environment (the nursery instead of the uterus). Similarly, the therapeutic challenge is to find the correct match between environmental inputs (social and/or physical) and the child's sensory processing capabilities that will allow the infant to flourish.

Many approaches to intervention grew from Gorski's (1983) view of the infant. Most notable was Als' (1982, 1989) synactive theory of development, which addressed the delicacy and resiliency of the infant's developing nervous system and the stress that medical care places on it. Sensory integration theory provides a clearly articulated and valid way of extending this concept beyond the nursery. Sensory integration theory, unlike models of neonatal development, helps therapists to understand the role of goodness-of-fit not just in terms of reactive behaviors but also in terms of exploratory and complex behaviors such as play. For example, sensory integration theory helps explain how and why a child with hypersensitivity avoids playful (i.e., sensory-generating) interactions with peers. The challenge for the therapist is to understand not only how each child's unique self-regulatory responses affect his or her sensory responsivity and sensory preferences, but also how the demands and stresses of the physical and social environments influence behavioral organization.

An understanding of self-regulation, sensory responsivity, and environmental influences becomes the foundation for intervention with the infant and the young child. Intervention focuses on creating a supportive environment for the child's evolving self-regulatory abilities, to prevent the development of significant maladaptive behavior patterns. This approach assumes that each individual has the potential to function optimally in an environment with adequate sensory experiences that are matched to the individual's needs, including a caregiver who is responsive to subtle communicative cues. Observation of the child's behavior (the four As) and the extrinsic factors affecting behavior becomes the basis for guiding intervention strategies. Sarah's case study is an example of using intervention strategies that focus on facilitating the fit between the child and the social and physical environment and helping the parent to understand her child.

Case Study: Sarah

Sarah was a healthy, premature infant referred to occupational therapy at 10 months of age for excessive fussiness and difficulty with sleeping and eating. The first stage of the assessment involved observation of the interactions between Sarah and her mother, Mrs. L. It was evident that Sarah's *arousal* level was variable and extreme, with frequent changes from drowsiness to eventually inconsolable crying. She was physiologically unstable with frequent spitting up and significant color changes. Her *attention* was not available for social interaction or even momentary fixation on her mother's face because of her physiological instability. Rather than orienting toward her mother during attempts at interaction, Sarah turned away and arched her back. Her *affect* was predominantly negative and stressed. Her *actions* were completely disorganized and avoidant in nature, with jerky movements and predominant hyperextension of the neck and trunk.

At first glance, Sarah seemed to be a child with hyperresponsivity and minimal to no self-regulatory capacity. However, it became evident that there was a significant mismatch between Sarah's sensory responsivity and her social and physical environment. Mrs. L.'s comforting style did not match Sarah's sensory needs. Mrs. L. used high-intensity sensory input during her interactions with Sarah, such as a high-frequency arrhythmic voice, light touch on the abdomen and face, bouncing (vestibular input), and visual looming (close face-to-face contact). The strategies that Mrs. L. used in attempting to comfort Sarah, although typical of most parent-child interactions, were overstimulating to Sarah. They did not promote self-regulation but instead produced disorganized behavior. Each one of Sarah's protestations was followed by an increase, not a decrease, in sensory input. Sarah's mother was using common parenting strategies that might help calm and organize another child but were overstimulating and disorganizing to Sarah because of her hypersensitivities.

The therapist coached Sarah's mother to change the sensory environment from multisensory stimulation to a stable visual stimulus (Mrs. L.'s quiet face looking at Sarah), stopping all other input (auditory, vestibular, and tactile). As a result, Sarah was able to orient to this low-sensory demand, calm herself, and maintain a quiet alert state for about 3 minutes while sustaining her attention to her mother's face. She even began to flirt and smile. Her affect was now positive and her actions were goal-directed. Her movements became less jerky and better controlled.

As therapy continued, Sarah's mother began to introduce low levels of combined input with Sarah (e.g., holding her *and* looking at her). Mrs. L. also learned strategies to help Sarah calm during periods of distress, such as providing a pacifier to suck on in a low-stimulus environment, swaddling Sarah and speaking to her softly, or slow rocking with swaddling.

In this example, the dramatic change did not occur directly through increasing Sarah's capabilities (although her sensory processing capabilities did improve over time with this graded input) but in response to finding a match or goodness-of-fit between Sarah's capabilities and her social and physical environments. Helping Mrs. L. to understand Sarah's communicative cues that reflected her sensory needs and the type of environment that Sarah needed to maintain organization and express her capabilities became the focus of intervention. Sarah's mother was able to reinterpret Sarah's arching and turning away as communication, Sarah's way of showing overstimulation. Reduction in the sensory environment resulted in increased orienting, focusing, and social interaction. This seemingly simple and low-intensity intervention occurred within the context of the family and produced immediate and significant improvement that might offset longterm difficulties.

Direct Sensory Integrative Intervention With the Child

The final focus of intervention is the one that frequently comes to mind first—specific remediation of the sensory processing dysfunction. As illustrated with Sarah's case, not all children require more intensive and individualized therapy. However, when indirect methods are not possible or do not achieve the desired results, more specific direct intervention might be necessary. For all children, but especially for infants and young children, clinicians and caregivers must constantly recognize the power of sensory input. It is often a decrease in the sensory input, not an increase that will help the child to organize behavior for adaptive responses. Activities that provide proprioceptive and firm tactile inputs (such as swaddling and vigorous sucking) and resistive activities (e.g., pushing a baby carriage or pulling or carrying pillows from the couch to use for jumping or landing) are very effective in eliciting engagement and attention.

When discussing direct remediation of sensory integrative deficits, it is important to distinguish sensory *integration* from sensory *stimulation*. Sensory stimulation refers to providing or imposing sensory input *on* the child who is not necessarily actively engaged. Sensory integration, in its purest sense, involves active engagement of the child in self-directed, meaningful activities—"adaptive responses"—to promote integration and organization of sensation for use. Although infants might not be able to self-direct activity in the traditional sense, they are constantly telling the adults in their world about their needs and wants through nonverbal communicative cues and gestures, as in the example of Sarah. Learning to read and respond to the language of infants and young children is an essential aspect of the sensory integrative process. By learning to recognize, read, and respond to those cues, therapists, parents, and caregivers gain insight into the child's interests, wants, and needs.

Choosing activity(s) that will provide the "just-right challenge" during direct sensory integrative intervention involves a complex clinical reasoning process. The therapist must consider several factors: the clinical profile as outlined in Table 14.1, the child's motivation, the family, and their priorities. It is also important to consider the sensory challenges and affordances available in the intervention environment as a therapeutic tool: How flexible is the environment? How can one make it novel or change the sensory richness?

It is essential to include the family in any intervention plan with a young child. Consequently, the clinician must observe the parent-child interaction, one aspect of which is the goodness-of-fit between the parent's style and routines and the child's sensory needs. Often the occupational therapist's role with the young child is to utilize the parent-child dyad and work to expand the parent's understanding, observation, relationship, and communication with the infant. The aim is to foster reciprocity between the infant and the parent.

The next goal is to modify the physical environment or manipulate the sensory input that the child is seeking or receiving. Modification of environment requires appreciation of multiple properties of that sensory input: type, intensity, duration, location, and frequency. The clinician also needs to consider the child's sensory threshold and whether he or she is acting in accordance with or compensating for this threshold. How wide, narrow, or changeable is the child's threshold range? What sensory modalities are arousing, calming, organizing, or disorganizing for *this* child? What properties of that sensory input (type, intensity, duration, location, frequency) might influence the child's sensory threshold, self-regulation, and organization? Finally, what available toys, equipment, and other environmental factors (including social) must clinicians and caregivers modify to influence the environmental affordances available to the infant (i.e., expand, limit, or clarify the possibilities for action in the physical environment)?

Basic Principles of Sensory Integrative Intervention for Infants and Young Children

Based on all of these factors, the therapist must determine the start point for intervention. First, clinicians must respect the infant's sensory responsivity and work within the child's tolerance and needs, recognizing that the child requires time to integrate and respond to sensory input (Ayres, 1972; Koomar & Bundy, 1991). With infants, it is important to modify input slowly and very conservatively.

It is also important to keep in mind that, for the infant and very young child, sensory integration intervention more often will involve *decreasing* the amount of input rather than *increasing* it. One useful concept for designing intervention that focuses on modifying sensation is that of *sensory diet* (Wilbarger, 1995; Williams & Shellenberger, 1996). The goal of the sensory diet is to provide a well-balanced variety of sensation, much as a balance of food is the basis of a good nutritional diet. The therapist must find the sensory inputs (modalities and qualities) that promote organization and integration, then gradually work to expand the child's ability to respond to these sensations adaptively (rather than maladaptively). Following the theoretical foundations of sensory integration, the effects of sensory input are most dramatic when the child engages in meaningful activity (Ayres, 1972, 1979, 1985). Therefore, the optimal sensory diet is one that is grounded in the child's daily routines or embedded in meaningful activity such as play. The general recommendation is not to impose sensory input on the child but rather to use creative and artful shaping and maximizing of the environmental affordances for play, parent-child interactions, or skill development.

When working with infants, clinicians must be very be careful about instituting changes in the basic sensory inputs. Sensations that are organizing for an older child can be overwhelming for a very young child. A good example is rotary vestibular input. Spinning, combined with an adaptive goal, can be a useful tool for a preschool or school-aged child with hyporesponsivity. However, spinning is generally *far too stimulating* for the young child, whose developing motor and physiological systems cannot tolerate the intensity of that type of vestibular input. The authors strongly recommend that therapists use suspended equipment very cautiously when working with infants and young children. More effective, vestibular-based activities are those that are part of the child's typical environment, such as "riding horsy" on the parent's knee for vestibular input; water play during bath time, followed by towel drying with firm pressure; sucking juice from a sipper cup or push pop; controlled roughhousing with parents or siblings; playing in a ball pit; rolling in or over a carpeted barrel; playing in an inflated, suspended tire swing for a toddler; or piling up couch pillows and jumping onto to them. Such activities allow for controlled sensory input, engagement, and initiation from the child and occur within a playful context. For some children, something as simple as playing in prone or creeping over a sofa pillow on the floor can be either an overwhelming sensory threat or a just-right challenge. There are a number of sensory-based activities available in the mainstream market for infants and young children that clinicians can incorporate into the therapeutic session or the home, such as tactile blankets, inflatable rolls, a large ball to bounce on, and a variety of tactile-based manipulative and oral toys. For the child who requires more intensive intervention to remain focused and calm, equipment such as a front-carrying snuggle pack can be helpful.

It is imperative that therapists and parents be aware of the signs of autonomic instability in infants. These signs include color changes, digestive system changes (i.e., spitting up, bowel movements, hiccups), flushing, perspiring, gagging, crying, anxiety, or sudden increase or decrease in arousal levels. These signs indicate an increase in the child's stress and signal the need to simplify or discontinue the activities.

Another central principle of sensory integration intervention is that the activities be child-directed and intrinsically motivated. This might seem problematic when considering the limited initiation or ideation of the young child, but by redefining the concept of *child-directed* for this age, more possibilities become apparent. Therapists must become cognizant of and skilled in observing the child's communicative intent. Young children are communicating constantly with adults. Sometimes that communication is clear, as in the crying of a child who is hungry, or the eager pointing at a favorite toy that is out of reach. More often, the communication is subtle, as in the quiet gaze of a shy child toward his or her mother when a stranger approaches. It is easy to misunderstand the communication, such as the gaze aversion of a child who needs a break before continuing to engage in social interaction. If therapists become skilled observers, the communicative intent of most children becomes evident, and activities that tap into their intrinsic motivation emerge. The challenge then becomes recognizing those cues and translating them into adaptive, goal-directed activities designed to promote the child's development. In other situations, motivational intent is not so different from that of older children. Infants and young children will often look or gesture toward a desired activity, smile or laugh in anticipation, and most importantly, persist in those activities that are meaningful and organizing for them.

One powerful motivator for the young child is novelty. All children are motivated towards novel stimuli. Although the motivation is consistent, the ability to explore that novelty is variable. In a child with limited ideation, poor motor control, or immature developmental motor abilities, exploration of novelty might consist of nothing more than mouthing a toy or visually exploring it. If mouthing is consistent with the developmental level of the child, it is important that the therapist recognize its importance as an exploratory strategy as well as a source of important sensory input. It is equally important for the therapist to move the child on to more advanced skills, when the timing is right, by reintroducing novelty.

The final factor essential to intervention with the young child is recognition of the power of play as a motivator and as a means of enhancing ideation and expanding the ability to tolerate and utilize sensory input for adaptive behavior. Many reviews of play and playfulness are available both within and outside of the occupational therapy literature (see, for example, Chandler, 1997; Lindner, 1993; Parham & Fazio, 1997; following sidebar, Using Play With Young Children).

Using Play With Young Children

- Social or physical play might be the most appropriate type of play. Acknowledge that object play in young children prior to the development of language and pretense is primarily exploratory in nature. As such, play is frequently associated with neutral as opposed to positive affect and is somewhat constrained by the object. This presents challenges to the therapist attempting to work on affective components of self-regulation, in which case social or physical play might be a more appropriate focus than object play for intervention.

- Use sensory-enriched objects for the child to explore, striking a balance between novelty and focused, prolonged exploration. Each toy presents distinct challenges for each child. A toy that is overstimulating for one child might be boring for another. Be aware that toys themselves, as well as the objects and people in the environment, produce affordances for adaptive behaviors. It is the appropriateness of the toy, object, and/or environment, matched with the child's state of arousal, interest, sensory needs, and capabilities, that creates successful affordances through play.

- Engage parents in play with the child, keeping in mind that preliminary research with children who are developing typically has indicated that mothers define *play* and *teaching* differently (Anzalone, 1994). When asked to play, mothers structured the environment (e.g., organized, added, or removed toys; positioned toys closer to the child), but when asked to teach, they structured the task (i.e., showed the child what to do). The challenge in utilizing play with the young child is to find ways to structure the environment for both the child and the parent in such a way that play becomes possible and self-directed.

Summary

There is no specific prescription for sensory integration intervention with the infant or the young child who has a sensory integrative dysfunction. Rather, it is a complex, evolving process that considers the child's sensory needs, the parent's interaction style, and the occupational roles and behaviors of the child within the context of the guiding principles of sensory integration theory. Following a systematic formative and summative assessment and observation of the child's sensory processing (intrinsic factors) and the social and physical environmental needs and supports (extrinsic factors), the therapist develops an intervention plan to reflect the family's goals and the child's occupational roles. Intervention considers both the intrinsic factors (sensory responsivity, self-regulation, and the four *A*s) and extrinsic factors (goodness-of-fit between the child and the social and physical environments) that affect the child's behavioral expression.

The primary focus of intervention with the infant and the young child is to assist the parent to read, interpret, and act on the child's cues and to facilitate the goodness-of-fit between the social and physical environment and the child's sensory needs. As a second phase, direct intervention considers not only the sensory input (modality and properties) but also the child's threshold and self-regulatory capacity while constantly modifying environmental affordances to promote engagement and action. Finally, the child's intrinsic motivation, interest, enjoyment, and active participation in the activity are significant factors for activity choice and effectiveness. The challenge for the therapist is to utilize a solid clinical reasoning process to constantly shape and reshape intervention that assists the child and family in being successful.

References

Abibin, R. (1986). *Parenting Stress Index* (2nd ed.). Charlottesville, VA: Pediatric Psychology Press.

Ainsworth, M.D.S. (1991). Attachment and other affectional bonds across the life cycle. In C.M. Parkes, J. Stevenson-Hinde, & P. Marris, (Eds.), *Attachment across the life cycle*. London: Tavistock/Routledge.

Als, H. (1982). Toward a synactive theory of development: Promise for the assessment and support of infant individuality. *Infant Mental Health Journal, 3*, 229–243.

Als, H. (1986). A synactive model of neonatal behavioral organization: Framework for the assessment of neurobehavioral development in the premature infant and for support of infants and parents in the neonatal intensive care environment. *Physical and Occupational Therapy in Pediatrics, 6*, 3–53.

Als, H. (1989). Self-regulation and motor development in preterm infants. In J. Lockman & N. Hazen (Eds.), *Action in social context. Perspectives on early development* (pp. 65–97). New York: Plenum Press.

Als, H., Lester, B.M., Tronick, E., & Brazelton, T.B. (1981). *Assessment of preterm infant behavior. Manual for the naturalistic observation of newborn behavior (preterm & fullterm)*. Boston, MA: The Children's Hospital.

Anderson, S.B., Ball, S., & Murphy, R.T. (1975). *Encyclopedia of educational evaluation*. San Francisco: Jossey-Bass.

Anzalone, M.E. (1993). Sensory contributions to action: A sensory integrative approach. *Zero to Three, 14*(2), 17–20.

Anzalone, M.E. (1994). *Mother-infant play: Developmental level, quality, and style*. Unpublished doctoral dissertation, Boston University.

Asher, I.E. (1996). *Occupational therapy assessment tools: An annotated index* (2nd ed.). Bethesda, MD: American Occupational Therapy Association.

Ayres, A.J. (1972). *Sensory integration and learning disorders*. Los Angeles: Western Psychological Services.

Ayres, A.J. (1979). *Sensory integration and the child*. Los Angeles: Western Psychological Services.

Ayres, A.J. (1985). *Developmental dyspraxia and adult-onset apraxia*. Torrance, CA: Sensory Integration International.

Ayres, A.J. (1989). *Sensory Integration and Praxis Tests*. Los Angeles: Western Psychological Services.

Bayley, N. (1969). *Manual for the Bayley Scales of Infant Development*. San Antonio: The Psychological Corporation.

Bayley, N. (1993). *The Bayley Scales of Infant Development* (2nd ed.). San Antonio, TX: The Psychological Corporation.

Berg, W.K., & Berg, K.M. (1979). Psychophysiological development in infancy: State, sensory function, and attention. In J. Osofsky (Ed.), *Handbook of infant development* (pp. 238–317). New York: J. Wiley and Sons.

Berge, T., & Lerine, I. (1965). The imitation of gestures: A technique for studying the body schema and praxis of children three to six years of age. *Clinics in Developmental Medicine, 18*, 116.

Berk, R.A., & DeGangi, G.A. (1983). *DeGangi-Berk Test of Sensory Integration*. Los Angeles: Western Psychological Services.

Bowlby, J. (1969). *Attachment and loss: Vol. 1. Attachment*. New York: Basic Books.

Bradley, R., & Caldwell, B. (1979). Home Observation for Measurement of the Environment (HOME): A revision of the preschool scale. *American Journal of Mental Deficiency, 84,* 235–244.

Brazelton, T.B. (1984). *Neonatal Behavioral Assessment Scale* (2nd ed.), *Clinics in Developmental Medicine, No. 88.* Philadelphia: J.B. Lippincott.

Brazelton, T.B. (1990). Saving the bathwater. *Child Development, 61,* 1661–1671.

Burke, J.P. (1998). Play: The life role of the infant and young child. In J. Case-Smith (Ed.), *Pediatric occupational therapy and early intervention* (2nd ed., pp. 189–206). Boston: Butterworth-Heinemann.

Burke, J., & King-Thomas, L. (1989). The environment of the child: Assessment considerations, treatment/intervention implications. *The AOTA Practice Symposium Program Guide.* Bethesda, MD: The American Occupational Therapy Association, Inc.

Burke, J.P., & Schaaf, R.C. (1997). Family narratives and play assessment. In L.D. Parham & L.S. Fazio (Eds.), *Play in occupational therapy for children* (pp. 67–85). St. Louis: Mosby.

Case-Smith, J., Allen, A.S., & Pratt, P.N. (1996). *Occupational therapy for children* (3rd ed.). St. Louis: Mosby.

Chandler, B. (1997). *The essence of play: A child's occupation.* Bethesda, MD: American Occupational Therapy Association, Inc.

Coster, W.J. (1998). Occupation-centered assessment of children. *American Journal of Occupational Therapy, 52,* 337–344.

Darling, R. (1989). Parent Needs Survey. In M. Seligman & R. Darling (Eds.), *Ordinary families, special children: A systems approach to childhood disability.* New York: Guilford Press.

DeGangi, G.A., & Greenspan, S. (1989). *Test of Sensory Function in Infants.* Los Angeles: Western Psychological Services.

DeGangi, G., & Greenspan, S.I. (in press). *The Functional Emotional Assessment Scale: Revised version and reliability studies.* Bethesda, MD: Interdisciplinary Council on Developmental and Learning Disorders.

DeGangi, G., Poisson, S., Sickel, R., & Wiener, A. S. (1995). *Infant and Toddler Symptom Checklist.* Tucson, AZ: Therapy Skill Builders.

Dunn, W. (1997). The impact of sensory processing abilities on the daily lives of young children and their families: A conceptual model. *Infants and Young Children, 9,* 23–35.

Dunn, W. (1999). *Sensory Profile.* San Antonio, TX: Therapy Skill Builders.

Dunn, W., & Westman, K. (1997). The Sensory Profile: The performance of a national sample of children without disabilities. *American Journal of Occupational Therapy, 51,* 25–34.

Dunning, H.D. (1972). Environmental occupational therapy. *American Journal of Occupational Therapy, 26,* 292–298.

Dunst, C.J., Cooper, C.J., Weeldreyer, J.C., Snyder, K.I.D., & Chase, J.H. (1988). Enabling and empowering families: Principles and guidelines for practice. In C.J. Dunst, C.M. Trivette, & A.G. Deal (Eds.), *Children's health care* (p. 151). Cambridge, MA: Brookline Books.

Field, T.M. (1995). *Touch in early development.* Mahwah, NJ: Lawrence Erlbaum Associates.

Fisher, A.G., Murray, E.A., & Bundy, A.C. (Eds.) (1991). *Sensory integration: Theory and practice.* Philadelphia: F.A. Davis Co.

Gorski, P.A. (1983). Premature infant behavioral and physiological responses to caregiving interventions in the intensive care nursery. In J.D. Call, E. Galenson, & R.L. Tyson (Eds.), *Frontiers in infant psychiatry* (pp. 256–263). New York: Basic Books, Inc., Publishers.

Greenspan, S. (1992). *Infancy and early childhood: The practice of clinical assessment and intervention with emotional and developmental challenges.* Madison, CT: International Universities Press.

Greenspan, S.I. (1996). Assessing the emotional and social functioning of infants and young children. In S.J. Meisels & E. Fenichel (Eds.), *New visions for the developmental assessment of infants and young children* (pp. 231–266). Washington, DC: Zero to Three.

Greenspan, S.I., & Meisels, S.J. (1996). Toward a new vision for the developmental assessment of infants and young children. In S.J. Meisels & E. Fenichel (Eds.), *New visions for the developmental assessment of infants and young children* (pp. 11–26). Washington, DC: Zero to Three.

Hanft, B.E. (1989). *Family-centered care: An early intervention resource manual.* Rockville, MD: American Occupational Therapy Association.

Hanft, B., & Place, P.A. (1996). School observation—Environment. In *The consulting therapist: A guide for OTs and PTs in the schools* (pp. 145–147). San Antonio, TX: Therapy Skill Builders.

Holloway, E. (1998). Early emotional development and sensory processing. In J. Case-Smith (Ed.), *Pediatric occupational therapy and early intervention* (2nd ed., pp. 167–187). Boston: Butterworth-Heinemann.

Holroyd, J. (1987). The Questionnaire on Resources and Stress: An instrument to measure family response to a handicapped member. *Journal of Community Psychology, 2,* 92–94.

Jirgal, D., & Bouma, K. (1989). A sensory integration observation guide for children from birth to three years of age. *Sensory Integration Special Interest Newsletter, 12*(2), 5.

King-Thomas, L., & Hacker, B.J. (1987). *A therapist's guide to pediatric assessment.* Boston: Little Brown.

Knickerbocker, B.M. (1980). *A holistic approach to the treatment of learning disorders.* Thorofare, NJ: Slack, Inc.

Koomar, J.A., & Bundy, A.C. (1991). The art and science of creating direct intervention from theory. In A.G. Fisher, E.A. Murray, & A.C. Bundy (Eds.), *Sensory integration: Theory and practice* (pp. 251–314). Philadelphia: F.A. Davis Company.

LaCroix, J., Johnson, C., & Parham, L.D. (1997). The development of a new sensory history: The evaluation of sensory processing. *Sensory Integration Special Interest Section Newsletter, 20,* 3–4.

Lester, B.M., Freier, K., & LaGasse, L. (1995). Prenatal cocaine exposure and child outcome: What do we really know. In M. Lewis & M. Bendersky (Eds.), *Mothers, babies, and cocaine: The role of toxins in development* (pp. 19–40). Hillsdale, NJ: Erlbaum.

Lindner, T.W. (1993). *Transdisciplinary play-based intervention: Guidelines for developing a meaningful curriculum for young children.* Baltimore: Brookes.

Lombroso, C., & Matsumiya, Y. (1985). Stability in waking-sleep states in neonates as a predictor of long-term neurologic outcome. *Pediatrics, 76,* 52–63.

Miller, L.J. (1982). *The Miller Assessment for Preschoolers.* Littleton, CO: The Foundation for Knowledge in Development.

Miller, L.J. (1988). *Miller Assessment for Preschoolers.* San Antonio, TX: The Psychological Corporation.

Miller, L.J. (1993). *First STEP.* San Antonio, TX: The Psychological Corporation.

Montague, A. (1971). *Touching: The human significance of the skin.* New York: Columbia University Press.

Moos, R.H., & Moss, B.S. (1988). *Family Environment Scale Manual.* Palo Alto, CA: Consulting Psychologists Press.

Mullen, E. (1984). *Mullen Scales of Early Learning.* Cranston, RI: T.O.T.A.L. Child, Inc.

Mullen, E.M. (1989). *The Infant Mullen Scales of Early Learning: AGS revision.* Circle Pines, MN: American Guidance Service, Inc.

Parham, D.L., & Fazio, L.S. (Eds.). (1997). *Play in occupational therapy for children.* St. Louis: Mosby.

Porges, S.W. (1993). The infant's sixth sense: Awareness and regulation of bodily processes. *Zero to Three, 14*(2), 12–16.

Porges, S.W., McCabe, P.M., & Yongue, B.G. (1982). Respiratory-heart rate interactions: Psychophysiological implications for pathophysiology and behavior. In J. Cacioppo & R. Petty (Eds.), *Perspectives in cardiovascular psychophysiology* (pp. 223–264). New York: Guilford Press.

Posner, M.I., & Boies, S.J. (1971). Components of attention. *Psychological Review, 78,* 391–408.

Provost, B., & Oetter, P. (1993). The Sensory Rating Scale for Infants and Young Children: Development and reliability. *Physical and Occupational Therapy in Pediatrics, 13*(4), 13–35.

Schaaf, R.C., & Burke, J.P. (1992). Clinical reflections on sensory integration and play. *Sensory Integration Special Interest Section Newsletter, 15,* 1–2.

Schaaf, R.C., & Burke, J.P. (1997). What happens when we play? A neurodevelopmental explanation. In B. Chandler (Ed.), *The essence of play: A child's occupation* (pp. 79–106). Bethesda, MD: American Occupational Therapy Association, Inc.

Schaaf, R.C., & Davis, W. (1992). Promoting health and wellness in the pediatric disabled and "at-risk" population. In R. Levine & J. Rothman (Eds.), *Prevention practice: Strategies for physical therapy and occupational therapy.* Philadelphia: W.B. Saunders.

Schaaf, R.C., Merrill, S.C., & Kinsella, N. (1987). Sensory integration and play behavior: A case study of the effectiveness of occupational therapy using sensory integrative techniques. *Occupational Therapy in Health Care, 4,* 61–75.

Schaaf, R., & Mulrooney, L. (1989a). *Environmental Observation Guide.* Unpublished guidelines.

Schaaf, R.C., & Mulrooney, L.L. (1989b). Occupational therapy in early intervention: A family-centered approach. *American Journal of Occupational Therapy, 43,* 745–754.

Stallings-Sahler, S. (1998). Sensory integration assessment and intervention with infants. In J. Case-Smith (Ed.), *Pediatric occupational therapy and early intervention* (2nd ed., pp. 223–254). Boston: Butterworth-Heinemann.

Stein, R.E.K., & Reissman, C.K. (1979). The development of the Impact on Family Scale. Preliminary findings. *Medical Care, 18,* 465–472.

Stern, D.N. (1985). *The interpersonal world of the infant.* New York: Basic Books.

Thomas, A., & Chess, S. (1977). *Temperament and development.* New York: Brunner/Mazel.

Vygotsky, L.S. (1978). *Mind in society: The development of higher psychological processes.* Cambridge, MA: Harvard University Press.

Wilbarger, P. (1995). The sensory diet: Activity programs based on sensory processing theory. *American Occupational Therapy Association Sensory Integration Special Interest Section Newsletter, 18*(2), 1–4.

Wilbarger, P., & Wilbarger, J.L. (1991). *Sensory defensiveness in children aged 2–12: An intervention guide for parents and other caretakers.* Santa Barbara, CA: Avanti Education Programs.

Williams, M.S., & Shellenberger, S. (1996). *How does your engine run?: A leader's guide to the Alert Program for Self-Regulation.* Albuquerque, NM: Therapy Works, Inc.

Williamson, G.G., & Anzalone, M.E. (1997). Sensory integration: A key component of the evaluation and treatment of young children with severe difficulties in relating and communicating. *Zero to Three, 17,* 29–36.

Williamson, G.G., & Anzalone, M.E. (2001). *Helping infants and young children interact with their environment: Improving sensory integration and self-regulation.* Washington, DC: Zero to Three.

Zeitlin, S., & Williamson, G.G. (1994). *Coping in young children: Early intervention practices to enhance adaptive behavior and resilience.* Baltimore: Paul H. Brookes.

Zeitlin, S., Williamson, G.G., & Szczepanski, M. (1988). *Early Coping Inventory.* Bensenville, IL: Scholastic Testing Service.

Additional Readings

Als, H. (1981). *Manual for the naturalistic observation of newborn behavior (preterm and fullterm infants).* Boston: The Children's Hospital.

Bledsoe, N.P., & Shepherd, J.T. (1982). A study of reliability and validity of a preschool play scale. *American Journal of Occupational Therapy, 36,* 783–788.

Dunn, W., & Brown, C. (1997). Factor analysis on the Sensory Profile from a national sample of children without disabilities. *American Journal of Occupational Therapy, 51,* 490–495.

Knox, S. (1974). A play scale. In M. Reilly (Ed.), *Play as exploratory learning* (pp. 247–266). Beverly Hills, CA: Sage.

La Croix, J.E. (1993). *A study of content validity of the sensory history questionnaire.* Unpublished master's thesis, University of Southern California, Los Angeles.

Lindner, T. (1990). *Transdisciplinary play-based assessment: A functional approach to working with young children.* Baltimore: Brookes.

14A Selected Assessment Instruments

Child

Assessment/ Author	Method	Target Population	Yield/Description	Standardization
Assessment of Preterm Infant Behavior (Als, Lester, Tronick, & Brazelton, 1981)	Behavior checklist and scale	Preterm infants	Assesses function and integration of five systems: 1. physiological 2. motor 3. state 4. attention/ interactive 5. regulatory	• Normed on 38 newborns in Boston Children's Hospital • No reliability studies, but educational training sessions are conducted to ensure reliability • Predictive validity • Criterion validity
Bayley Infant Behavior Record (Bayley, 1969)	30-item rating scale	2 to 30 months	Ratings are based on behaviors exhibited during motor and mental scales tests. Examines personality and temperament variables such as attention span, persistence, endurance, and activity level.	No psychometric information on this section of the Bayley Scales of Infant Development
DeGangi-Berk Test of Sensory Integration (Berk & DeGangi, 1983)	Screening, 3-point scale	3 to 5 years	Screens sensorimotor functions: 1. postural control 2. bilateral motor integration 3. reflex integration	• Not standardized, validated on a sample of 3- to 5-year-old children using the criterion groups validation model • Internal consistency .67–.82 • Interrater reliability between .67–.79 for subtests besides reflex integration • Test-retest reliability .85–.96 Domain and construct validity
First STEP (Screening Test for Evaluating Preschoolers) (Miller, 1993)	Screening, performance-based checklist and rating	2 years 9 months to 6 years 2 months	Identifies preschool children at risk for developmental delays. Five domains: 1. cognitive 2. communication 3. motor 4. social/emotional 5. adaptive behavior	• Norm referenced • Split half reliability .71–.92 • Test-retest reliability .85–.93 • Interrater reliability for classification agreement .81–1, for scaled scores .77–.96 • Content, construct, criterion, concurrent, and face validity
Functional Emotional Assessment Scale (DeGangi & Greenspan, in press; Greenspan, 1996)	Play observation	7-month-old to 3-year-old children who experience problems with self-regulation, communication, or social relatedness, and/or multiproblem families	Yields information about parent/child play interaction for three types of toys/play: 1. Symbolic-play toys 2. Tactile-play toys 3. Vestibular situations	None available
Imitation of Gestures (Berge & Lerine, 1965)	Screening scores reported as pass, fail, or incomplete	3 to 6 years	Examines body scheme and motor planning	Normative sample of 489 children

Child (continued)

Assessment/ Author	Method	Target Population	Yield/Description	Standardization
Infant Toddler Symptom Checklist (DeGangi, Poisson, Sickel, & Wiener, 1995)	Screening checklist	7 to 30 months	Examines predispositions towards developing sensory integration disorders, attention deficits, emotional behavioral problems, and learning difficulties	• Criterion referenced • Sampled on 154 infants typically developing and 67 infants with regulatory disorders • No reliability studies • Construct validity • Concurrent validity studies showed low correlations between checklist scores and other infant tests, indicating the distinct nature of the checklist.
Miller Assessment for Preschoolers (Miller, 1982, 1988)	Screening	2 years 9 months to 5 years 8 months	Designed to identify children with later school-related problems. Screens: 1. cognitive 2. language 3. perceptual 4. motor	• Standardized on 1200 children developing typically • Test-retest reliability .72–.94 • Interrater reliability .978 • Content, criterion, and construct validity
Mullen Scales of Early Learning (Mullen, 1984)	Performance scales	0 to 36 months 15 to 68 months	Four scales assess areas of strength/ weakness and learning style: 1. visual receptive organization/visual discrimination, sequencing, organization, and memory 2. visual expressive organization, unilateral and bilateral hand skills 3. language receptive organization, comprehension, verbal/spatial awareness 4. language expressive organization, verbal ability	• Concurrent validity • Test-retest reliability .83–.98 • Interrater reliability .99
Newborn Individualized Developmental Care and Assessment Program (NIDCAP) (revised) (Als, 1986)	Checklist based on observation of behavior and the context in which it occurs	Newborns at high risk for developmental compromise	Systematic naturalistic observation of the infant in the nursery or home offers information about the infant's response to environmental input and caregiver routine. Measures: 1. autonomic/visceral 2. state 3. motor 4. attention	• Sample of 40 low-birth-weight infants in NICU • Completion of training criteria needed to administer test Interrater reliability >.85 • Concurrent and predictive validity
Sensory Integration and Praxis Tests (Ayres, 1989)	Battery of standardized performance tests	4 years to 8 years 11 months	Assesses praxis and sensory processing and integration of vestibular, proprioceptive, tactile, kinesthetic, and visual systems.	• Standardized Users must undergo certification training • Interrater reliability .94–.99 • Content validity • Concurrent validity
Sensory Integration Observation Guide (Schaaf, Anzalone, & Burke)	Behavioral rating scale using a 5-point Likert scale	0 to 3 years	Parent report regarding infant sensory responsiveness on four factors: 1. tactile-kinesthetic 2. vestibular-proprioceptive 3. adaptive motor 4. regulatory	None available

Child (continued)

Assessment/Author	Method	Target Population	Yield/Description	Standardization
Sensory Profile (Dunn, 1999)	Parent rating scale using a 5-point Likert scale	3 to 10 years (infant version being developed)	Measures behavioral statements. Arranged into eight categories: 1. auditory 2. visual 3. taste/smell 4. movement 5. body position 6. touch 7. activity level 8. emotional/social	None available
Sensory Rating Scale for Infants and Young Children (Provost & Oetter, 1993)	Parent rating scale using a 5-point scale	Form A: 0 to 9 months Form B: 9 to 36 months	Parent rating scale regarding the degree of sensitivity children have to various types of sensory stimulation: 1. touch 2. movement and gravity 3. hearing 4. vision 5. taste/smell 6. temperament	• Internal consistency reliability Form A: .83 Form B: .90 • Interrater reliability within 1 point: .86 • Content validity
Test of Sensory Function in Infants (DeGangi & Greenspan, 1989)	Screening rating scale (designed for use in conjunction with other standardized comparative developmental scales)	4 to 18 months	Measures sensory processing responsivity in five domains: 1. Tactile deep pressure 2. Visual tactile integration 3. Adaptive motor 4. Ocular motor 5. Responsivity to vestibular stimuli	• Criterion referenced • Interrater reliability .88–.99 • Test-retest reliability .64–.96 • Best results between 7 and 18 months • Domain and criterion validity

Environment

Assessment/ Author	Method	Target Population	Yield/Description	Standardization
Checklist of Environmental Factors (Burke & King-Thomas, 1989)	Guided observation checklist	Designed for, but not limited to, environments of children 0 to 5 years	Qualitative data about physical, emotional, and social aspects of the environment	None reported
Environmental Observation Guide (Schaaf & Mulrooney, 1989a)	Guided observation	Designed for, but not limited to, environments of children 0 to 5 years	Descriptive data about physical and social environment related to child's strengths and needs	None reported
Environmental Questionnaire (Dunning, 1972)	Semistructured interview	Environment of adult psychiatric outpatients. Revision available for adults with mental retardation in the community. Also might be useful for families with young children when requiring more information about parents'/caregivers' environmental interactions.	Descriptive information about the individual's preferences and the environment. Contains questions about the physical, social, and task environments. Information can suggest possibilities for modification.	• Reliability not reported • Face validity • Some construct validity
Family Needs Scale (Dunst, Cooper, Weeldreyer, Snyder, & Chase, 1988)	Self-rating scale, 41 items	Families with special-needs children	Provides information regarding family's identified needs. Also assists families to clarify their concerns and to define the nature of their needs.	• Split half reliability .96 • Criterion validity
Home Observation for Measurement of the Environment (HOME) (revised) (Bradley & Caldwell, 1979)	Observation and interview allow rater to complete a checklist	Home environment of families with children 0 to 6 years (two versions: one for infants to 3 years, one for 3 to 6 years)	Total and subscale scores describing household environment. Measures environmental influences that facilitate or inhibit various behaviors. Looks at quality and quantity of social, emotional, and cognitive support available to children in the home environment. Examines factors that facilitate or limit play.	• Standardized on families from New York and Little Rock • Kuder-Richardson reliability estimate of .89 for total scores and estimates of subscale reliabilities from .38–.89 • Test-retest reliabilities of subscales range from .24–.77 • Face, concurrent, and predictive validity
School Observation- Environment (Hanft & Place, 1996)	Guided environmental observation	School children	Observation of general environment, sensory environment, and a particular environment	None reported

Family

Assessment/ Author	Method	Target Population	Yield/Description	Standardization
Early Coping Inventory (Zeitlin, Williamson, & Szczepanski, 1988)	Systematic observation and 5-point rating scale	Infants 4 to 36 months of age	Measures a range of coping effectiveness. 54 items in three categories: 1. Sensorimotor organization 2. Reactive behavior 3. Self-initiated behavior	• Interrater reliability .80–.94 • Content and construct validity
Family Environment Scale (Moos & Moss, 1988)	Questionnaire (true/false); 90 questions	Families including single-parent and step-families	Score indicates each family member's view of his or her environment. Measures the social-environmental characteristics of all types of families. Measures family relationships (support, expression of feelings, and conflict), personal growth of family and family members, and system maintenance (organization and control of family life).	• Normative data on subscale of Form R were compiled for 500 distressed families and 1125 typical families • Internal consistency reliability between .61–.78 on subscales • Test-retest between .52–.89 • Construct validity
Impact on Family Scale (Stein & Reissman, 1979)	Structured interview, 24-item questionnaire	Mothers of children with chronic illnesses (ages of children not specified)	A measure of the variability of impact of chronic illness in a child on the family Looks at five conceptual areas: 1. Financial 2. Social/family 3. Personal strain 4. Mastery 5. Sibling strain	• Internal reliability .72–.86 for each subscale, .88 for overall
Parent Needs Survey (Darling, 1989)	Self-report survey	Families with children with special needs	Information regarding the needs of families in areas such as treatment needs for the child, formal and informal support for the family, eliminating competing family needs, and needs for information	None available
Parenting Stress Index (Abibin, 1986)	Questionnaire/ rating scale, self-report	Families with 0- to 3-year-olds with disabilities/ special needs Parent-child systems under stress or in high-risk situations	Information to determine specific stress factors related to dysfunctional parenting. Helps parents understand importance of creating positive environment. "At-risk" screening tool for parent-child relationships.	• Standardized on 534 parents who visited a small pediatric clinic in central Virginia • Internal consistency for Child domain score .89 • Parent domain score .93 • Total stress score .95 • Construct, concurrent, predictive, discriminant, and factorial validity
Questionnaire on Resources and Stress for Families (Holroyd, 1987)	Self-administered 285-item true/false questionnaire	Families with a member who is ill or has a disability	Measures stress and coping in families caring for ill relatives and examines events/factors influencing the family. Uses 15 scales, covers three domains: 1. Personal problems for responders 2. Family problems 3. Problems for patient/ill family member	• Limited normative data • Kuder-Richardson internal consistency .96 for long form and .79 for short form • Content validity

Name of Child: _____ Date: _____

Person Interviewed: _____

Date of Birth: _____ Chronological Age: _____

Number of Weeks Gestation: _____ Adjusted Age: _____

Interviewer: _____

Directions: Best use is with infants 0 to 12 months of age.

Ask the parent(s)/caregiver(s) each question and wait for a response. If you need additional information to determine the frequency or quality of a behavior, use the probes. Record significant information in the space below each question to describe the baby's behavior.

Determine the frequency rating of the behavior based on the information presented by the parent/caregiver.

Key:

   1 = Never: The child never demonstrates the behavior.

   2 = Almost Never: The child demonstrates the behavior 1–3 times out of 10.

   3 = Sometimes: The child demonstrates the behavior 4–6 times out of 10.

   4 = Almost always: The child demonstrates the behavior 7–9 times out of 10.

   5 = Always: The child always demonstrates the behavior.

---

1. Does the baby like to be held and tend to mold to his or her body into
   the adult holding him or her?   (TK) _____

   Probes: Does the baby: Arch or stiffen his or her body when held? Pull or
   push away when held? Cry when held? Snuggle in when held? Prefer some
   adults over others (e.g., your calm sister versus your physical brother)?

   Describe the baby's reaction when held:

2. Is the baby comfortable being moved?   (VP) _____

   Probes: Does the baby: Become irritable when passively moved in space?
   Become irritable when body position is changed? Cry or appear to look
   fearful when moved in space? Tolerate being turned upside down or
   moved around in a circle? Smile and/or giggle when bounced around?

   Describe the baby's reaction to imposed movement:

3. Does the baby have movement games or favorite songs (e.g., pat-a-cake
   or peek-a-boo) with others and anticipate these special interactions?   (AM) _____

   Probes: Does the baby: Avoid interactions with others (e.g., turn away
   or cry)? Actively participate during interactions with others? Watch when
   others attempt to interact with him or her?

   Describe the baby's reaction to interaction with others:

---

*Note. Adapted with permission by R. Schaaf, M. Anzalone, and J. Burke from "A sensory integration observation guide for children from birth to three years of age," by D. Jirgal and K. Bouma, 1989, *Sensory Integration Special Interest Newsletter, 12*(2), 5.

4. Does the baby initiate new play situations? (AM) _____

   Probes: Does the baby: Prefer novel or familiar play situations? Notice new toys? Notice familiar toys? Touch and explore the toys for a period of time? Turn/glance away from toys? Bang toys? Manipulate toys? Use many different strategies to play with toys?

   Describe the baby's play:

5. Does the baby put toys in the mouth to play? (TK) _____

   Probes: Does the baby: Avoid putting toys in the mouth? Gag when toys are put in the mouth? Overstuff toys into the mouth? Cry when toys are put in the mouth? Chew on toys when toys are placed in the mouth? Smile/laugh when toys are in the mouth?

   Describe the baby's behavior when putting a toy in his or her mouth:

6. Does the baby use only his or her fingertips when manipulating toys? (AM/TK) _____

   Probes: Does the baby: Extend fingers to drop a toy placed in his or her hand? Cry when toys are placed in his or her hand? Close hands to avoid having a toy placed in the hand? Actively hold on to a toy for an extended period of time (e.g., 1 to 2 minutes)? Attempt to reach for or grab toys?

   Describe what the baby does with toys:

7. Does the baby use two hands together to play with toys (e.g., switch an object from one hand to the other and cross the midline)? (AM) _____

   Probes: Does the baby: Use one hand or the other but avoid play with the hands together? Reach across his or her body to grab a toy? Bang toys together? Bang on the floor with only one hand? Appear to use only one hand when playing? Avoid certain kind of toys that provide a specific type of sensory input (e.g., bunny toy)?

   Describe what the baby does with his or her hands when toys are presented:

8. Does the baby eat food? If yes, does the baby accept a variety of textures when they are introduced at an appropriate age? (TK) _____

   Probes: Does the baby: Refuse to eat? Cry when textured foods are introduced? Have food preferences, like/dislikes?

   Describe the baby's reaction to textured foods:

9. Does the baby appear comfortable with more than one stimulus (or information from more than one sensory modality) at one time? (R) _____

   Probes: Does the baby: Appear to "tune out" if more than one stimulus is presented at a time? Fall asleep if more than one stimulus is presented at a time? Cry if more than one stimulus is presented at a time?

   Describe the baby's reaction to stimuli (e.g., toys, pictures).

10. Does the baby appear to enjoy all types of stimulation
(e.g., music, vision, or touch)? (R) _____

   Probes: Does the baby: Avoid certain kinds of toys that provide a specific
   type of sensory input (e.g., bumpy toys)? Appear to enjoy fuzzy, soft, and
   textured objects? Appear to enjoy brightly colored objects? Appear to enjoy
   objects with contrasting colors? Like "busy" pictures? Like "plain" pictures?
   Do you as a caregiver have difficulty determining the baby's preference for
   sensory input?

   Describe the baby's sensory stimulation preferences:

11. Does the baby move easily from one position to another
(e.g., belly to back or sit to crawl) in play? (VP/AM) _____

   Probes: Does the baby: Appear to prefer to stay in one position
   and avoid moving to different positions (especially prone)? Fall
   frequently when attempting to change position? Cry or otherwise
   signal parent/caregiver when he or she wants to change position?

   Describe the baby's reaction to movement produced by him- or herself,
   and describe the baby's movement:

12. Did the baby sleep through night after the first 6 weeks? (R) _____

   Probes: Does the baby: Constantly cry when put to bed? Sleep for
   short periods of time (15 minutes or fewer), then wake again? Sleep
   for long periods of time? Stay awake for only short periods of time
   (20 to 30 minutes) each day?

   Describe the baby's sleep habits and patterns:

13. Is the baby easy to get to sleep? (R) _____

   Probes: Does the baby: Fall asleep in many places (e.g., crib, bassinet,
   car seat, baby carrier)? Can the baby fall asleep without being rocked,
   cuddled, or gently bounced? Need long periods rocking, cuddling, or
   gentle bouncing (e.g., 30 minutes or more)?

   Describe the baby's going-to-sleep routines, including how you put the
   baby to sleep:

14. Does the baby calm easily after being upset and crying? (R) _____

   Probes: Does the baby: Continue to cry when rocked, hugged, cuddled, or
   bounced gently? Is the baby easily distracted when upset? Continue to cry
   for extended periods of time (e.g., 1 hour or more)?

   Describe how you calm the baby when he or she is upset:

15. Does the baby touch and explore different textured toys (e.g., a smooth rattle or a bumpy squeak toy)? (TK) _____

    Probes: Does the baby: Extend his or her fingers to drop a toy placed in his or her hand? Cry when textured toys are placed in the hand or touch the face? Close his or her hands to avoid having a toy placed in the hand? Actively hold the toy for extended periods of time (1 to 2 minutes)? Does the baby attempt to reach for and grab textured toys?

    Describe the baby's reaction when texture toys/objects are placed in the hand:

16. Does the baby like (tolerate) laying/sitting/playing on different textured surfaces (e.g., blanket, rug, sand, grass, water)? (TK) _____

    Probes: Does the baby: Cry when placed on textured surfaces? Stiffen the body or arch the back when placed on textured surfaces? Withdraw arms/legs when touched by a texture? Extend arms/legs when touched by a texture?

    Describe the baby's reaction when placed on or touched by different textures:

17. For babies who are 6 months of age or older: If the baby loses his or her balance, do the arms extend in the correct direction to protect the baby from falling over? (VP) _____

    Probes: Does the baby: Fall frequently? Extend the arms at all (delayed or no reaction)? Appear to demonstrate fear when falling? Stiffen/arch his or her body? Flex arms/legs when falling?

    Describe the baby's reaction to unexpected movement:

18. **Examiner:** Comment on the parent/caregiver behavior and the interaction with the child. Briefly describe the baby's behavior and the parents'/caregivers' responses to the different types of behavior the baby demonstrated.

    _____
    _____
    _____

19. Is parent/caregiver information consistent with the examiner's observations? Explain.

    _____
    _____
    _____

20. Additional comments:

    _____
    _____
    _____

Analysis/Interpretation

Summarize the infant's sensory preferences and regulatory and adaptive motor skills by checking the descriptor that best fits the child's behavior.

TK (Tactile-Kinesthetic)
- ☐ Seeks
- ☐ Avoids
- ☐ Fluctuates

VP (Vestibular-Proprioceptive)
- ☐ Seeks
- ☐ Avoids
- ☐ Fluctuates

AM (Adaptive Motor)
- ☐ Engages in
- ☐ Needs prompts
- ☐ Avoids

R (Regulatory)
- ☐ Regulates independently
- ☐ Needs assistance to self regulate

Sensory Integration and Visual Deficits, Including Blindness

SUSANNE SMITH ROLEY, M.S., OTR

COLLEEN SCHNECK, SC.D., OTR, FAOTA

Children with disabilities commonly have diagnosed or undiagnosed visual deficits or impairments. This sensory loss or distortion profoundly affects the individual's interpretation of sensory information not only from vision but from other sensory channels as well. Interpretation of environmental information is essential for adaptive interactions within the physical and social environments. Sensory integration provides a framework for understanding the complexities of functional vision. The sensory integration frame of reference also serves as a model for explaining how visual deficits and impairments contribute to difficulties in the ease and joy of participating in everyday life and how the individual might compensate in the absence or distortion of vision.

The Holistic Nature of Vision

The importance and complexity of vision is apparent not only from the volumes of literature on this topic but also from the amount of neural tissue (in humans and non-human primates) that is involved in the processing of visual information. In fact, the optic nerve alone contains more than one million fibers (Kandel, Schwartz, & Jessell, 1991). Ayres (1972) originally described vision as being so important that the word *perception* typically meant visual perception. She discussed visual perception as an end product, contributing to the complex function of form and space perception.

During normal development, vision assists in the investigation of one's surroundings or contextual environment, understanding of temporal conditions, and determination of one's location relative to objects in space. Vision reinforces much of what a child learns through other sensory channels (Baker-Nobles & Rutherford, 1995). Functional vision develops through a complex array of experiences that provide intersensory information and associations. Through the developmental process, vision becomes a specialized sensory channel in the mature system that supplies a myriad of details about the distant environment. A person can look at a rose and, in addition to seeing its color, size, and shape, remember how it smells, recall the softness of the petals, and bring to mind its weight and texture. This ability to associate other sensory data with qualities learned through vision alone is the product of sensory integration.

Vision, the process of using light energy for interpreting environmental data, is the fast track to dynamic interrelationships within the social and physical environments. Daily and seasonal light cycles affect visceral functions (such as hunger and menstruation) that an individual perceives through interoceptors. Orienting, localizing, and tracking functions work in concert with proprioceptive systems for feedforward postural and ocular control. Cognitive visual components contribute

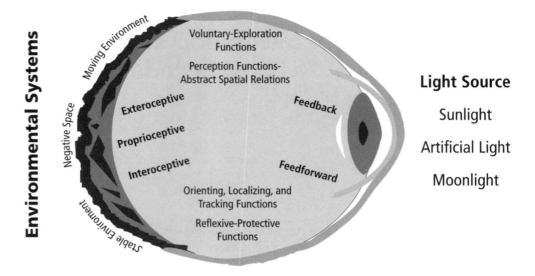

Environmental Systems

Moving Environment

Negative Space

Exteroceptive

Proprioceptive

Interoceptive

Stable Environment

Voluntary-Exploration
Functions

Perception Functions-
Abstract Spatial Relations

Feedback

Feedforward

Orienting, Localizing, and
Tracking Functions

Reflexive-Protective
Functions

Light Source

Sunlight

Artificial Light

Moonlight

Figure 15.1. The dynamic process of vision

Vision is the process of using light energy for interpreting environmental data. Light cycles are interpreted, influencing interoceptive functioning. Orienting, localizing, and tracking functions work in concert with proprioceptive systems for feedforward postural and ocular control. Cognitive visual components contribute refined exteroceptive data to the perception of itneracting systems of the individual with the stable and changing spatial and temporal aspects of environment.

refined exteroceptive data to the perception of interacting systems of the individual with the stable and changing spatial and temporal aspects of the environment (see Figure 15.1).

The most important contribution of vision is the rapid, constant perceptual availability of the detailed contextual framework of the social and physical environment. No other sensory system can replace this capability. Because of vision's far-reaching capacity as a distance sensor, it dominates the construction of the sensory context, the picture of the environment individuals develop in their mind's eye. With a glance, vision allows the individual to perceive the dynamic interactions of changing elements within the framework or context of the more stable elements in the environment. Cognitive understanding and predictability of systems unfold as a consequence of this perception. According to Moore (as cited in Okoye, 1997), vision is the most important sense for survival. Its functions include spatiotemporal orientation, anticipation, adaptation, and support for learning, memory, and recall.

The internalization of the visual spatial context, along with the constant scanning for changes within the environment, give the individual an ability to anticipate, plan, monitor, and correct interactions within the environment. Vision effectively facilitates anticipation and, consequently, planning, which predicates adaptation to and manipulation of the environment (Moore, cited in Okoye, 1997). Likewise, vision provides immediate feedback to guide the accuracy of interactions. How individuals receive and then perceive sensory information from the environment determines how effectively they will respond to situations. This anticipation of information further gives humans the ability to adapt to the ever-changing environment (Warren, 1994). Therefore, adaptation depends on the integration of sensory information, of which vision is a powerful organizer. Adaptation allows one not only to survive the environment but also to act upon it, manipulate it, and improve one's existence. Humans have adaptively created a culture catering to visual cues (such as road signs, exit signs, and gender signs on public restrooms), consequently making our lives dependent on light sources that make visual reception possible. Cognitively, vision contributes to spatial orientation, memory, and visual imagery, supplying perceptual images of vivid details and their context.

Visual Components

Zaba (1984) defined vision as the total process responsible for the reception of visual stimuli and cognition that uses visual data. Reflexive eye movements regulate light reception. As a result of light perception, vision occurs. Vision requires the processes of extracting and organizing information from the environment, the visual-receptive component (Solan & Ciner, 1986), and the ability to interpret what the individual sees and then use that information, the visual-cognitive component (see Table 15.1). These two components are essential to all aspects of functional vision. The visual-receptive component is primarily related to reflexive-protective functions (see Table 15.2), and orienting, localizing, and tracking functions (see Table 15.3). The visual-cognitive component is primarily related to voluntary exploration functions (see Table 15.4) and abstract spatial relations (see Table 15.5).

Warren (1993) presented a developmental framework for the evaluation and treatment of visual perceptual deficits in adults with acquired brain injury that Schneck (1998) generalized to pediatric populations. Warren's hierarchy of visual skill levels blends the visual-receptive and visual-cognitive components. Each skill level is dependent on integration of the skill level preceding it, therefore problems in skill levels lower on the hierarchy contribute to problems in skills higher on the hierarchy (Schneck, 1998).

Table 15.1. Components of the visual system

Visual-Receptive Component	Visual-Cognitive Component
Oculomotor control	Attention
Fixation	Memory
Pursuit eye movements	Visual discrimination
Saccadic eye movements	Recognition
Visual fields	Matching
Visual acuity	Categorization
Visual skills	Form perception
Accommodation	Constancy
Binocular vision	Visual closure
Convergence/divergence	Figure-ground
Orientation	Visual imagery Spatial perception Position in space Depth perception Topographical scanning

Table 15.2. Reflexive-protective functions

Function	Definition	Deficit
Accommodation	The ability of each eye to compensate for a blurred image; refers to the process used to obtain clear vision to focus on an object at varying distances.	Problems with acuity Blurred vision
Teaming and automatic conjugate eye movements	The vestibular-ocular pathways control reflexively in response to head movement and position in space. These pathways enable the eyes to remain fixed on a stationary object while the head and body move	Blurred vision with head movement Double vision Difficulty controlling eye movements during head movements
Distance and movement detector	Automatic visual scanning of the environment.	Poor adjustment to moving objects
Light/dark/brightness perception	Dependent on pupillary constriction and pineal gland function for diurnal cycles	Difficulty adjusting from dark to light areas and vice versa

Table 15.3. Orienting, localizing, and tracking functions

Function	Definition	Deficit
Acuity	The capacity to discriminate the fine details of objects in the central visual field (20/20 = the ability to perceive as small an object as an average person can perceive at 20 feet)	Blurred vision Difficulty seeing at either close or far ranges Misses details of environment at either close or far ranges
Tracking, gaze stability, and fixation	Includes saccades and smooth pursuits	Loses place when reading Turns head with eye movement Loses place on page
Regulation of eye position relative to head position	Oculomotor control through cranial nerves III, IV, and VI, which work in concert with neck proprioceptors and vestibular receptors	Moves whole body when looking at something
Spatial orientation of body within environment	Vestibular proprioceptive awareness of body scheme relative to environmental space	Difficulty knowing where body is in space relative to objects and other people
Laterality and directionality	Knowing spatial concepts such as up/down, right/left, back/front	Difficulty with right and left on self and others
Depth perception	Ability to see in three dimensions	Difficulty negotiating surfaces
Visual-auditory integration	Ability to orient to the distant environment	Difficulty coordinating sound and visual localization of data from the same or different sources

Table 15.4. Voluntary-exploratory functions

Function	Definition	Deficit
Volitional scanning and gaze shifting	Voluntary ability to look around and back and forth within a visual field	Poor eye contact Difficulty with visual orientation
Visual attention and memory	The ability to focus cognitively on a specific set of points in the visual field and remember them in context	Poor ability to recognize, store, or retrieve visual information
Visual discrimination	The ability to detect features such as color, texture, shape, and size of stimuli for recognition, matching, and categorization	Poor ability to recognize, match, and catagorize visual information Difficulty detecting same and different
Learning, memory, recall for colors, details	Visual information stored so that it can be used for comparison in the future	Difficulty recalling visually presented material, remembering directions, and relating details viewed sequentially
Visual surround and global relationships	Visual awareness of environmental context	Poor ability to sustain attention to the larger environment
Visual-tactile-motor integration	Ability to gauge distance and intensity of interaction with the skin	Difficulty writing Difficulty locating objects tactually
Visual-manual and visual-motor activities	Coordination of head, neck, eye, and body movements with auditory and touch information Visual guidance of fine and gross motor activities	Poor control of refined hand skills
Orientation of objects Visual-spatial relationships	Awareness of two- and three-dimensional view and their relationships to other objects	Poor ability to provide orientation and sequential order visually
Serial processing of stimuli	Ability to scan in a sequential fashion	Difficulty integrating the central and peripheral visual information
Visual figure-ground	Ability to recognize foreground from background Comprehension of context	Over- or underattention to details, misses the relevant information
Communication: symbolic language recognition	Visual recognition of gestural and symbolic communication	Difficulty reading body language, written symbols
Quick localization	Rapid movement of the eyes while maintaining focus	Poor rapid location of objects, especially during movement

Table 15.5. Perception functions—abstract spatial relations

Function	Definition	Impairment
Cohesion	Ability to detect groups or relationships through the proximity and spatial orientation of its parts	Difficulty understanding the necessity of maintaining proximity with the group
Boundaries	Ability to perceive the edge of a person, group, or thing. This can include the distance at which someone is comfortable during a personal encounter or the possible distance that something can move.	Difficulty respecting other people's space Difficulty understanding the location and trajectory of something that moves Difficulty planning movements relative to other objects or people
Consistency	Ability to anticipate the limits of movement through a space or a group	Bumps into things frequently
Spatial continuity	Ability to locate and track a path between two points	Difficulty planning and following routes between locations

Functional Vision Deficits

Because functional vision develops through a complex array of intersensory information and associations, visual deficits encompass a wide array of difficulties in accessing and utilizing sensory information (Ballinger, 1995) (see Tables 15.2 through 15.5). Vision loss and visual perceptual disorders can hinder a child's ability to manipulate the environment, slow the rate of development, and precipitate functional problems.

Skilled movement is dependent on and necessary for visual perception. Body movement and exploration of the environment are dependent on visual abilities (Hellerstein & Fishman, 1987). With the loss of vision comes delay or lack of self-propelled mobility in the infant (Fraiberg, 1977). Children with environmental deprivation or deprivation of typical motor exploration of the environment can have visual perceptual deficits that remain undetected. The lack of mobility further causes deprivation of postural control, spatial monitoring, and sensory feedback and also contributes to poor sensory feedback, sensory defensiveness, and problems with the acquisition of skills in all occupational performance areas (Baker-Nobles, 1990).

Tables 15.2 through 15.5 define aspects of functional vision and possible related deficits. Deficits in visual function include the processing of light, accommodating to changes in the visual field, detecting and discriminating visual images, and comprehension of the abstract properties of spatial relationships. These visual deficits can occur in children with and without other disabilities. Children who have no known visual deficit can exhibit functional visual deficits. In contrast, even children with diagnoses of blindness sometimes possess inexplicable functional vision abilities.

Visual Dysfunction in Children With Disabilities

Types and Incidence of Visual Dysfunction

Because of the complexity of the visual system and its contribution to function, there are hundreds of disorders that are associated with visual problems in young children. A visual impairment results from problems in any part of the visual apparatus, including the outer layers of the eye, the lens, the retina, the extraocular muscles, and the brain. The ICIDH-2 (World Health Organization, 2000) lists several areas in which impairment of function in the visual system occurs. Pathology of the eye and related structures, such as optic atrophy and cataracts, can result in loss of functional vision. Deficits can also occur in visual-sensory functions, visual acuity, visual field, quality of vision, and sensations of the eye and adjoining structures. Clinicians define visual impairment in terms of functional changes, which include visual acuity and ocular mobility. Visual deficits affect a person's access to the sighted culture and can profoundly limit an individual's ability to engage in meaningful and purposeful occupation in the context of social and physical environments.

Approximately 50 to 64 children per 100,000 have serious visual impairments, and at least another 100 children per 100,000 have less serious difficulties (Davidson, 1992). Estimates of 40% to 70% of preschool children with visual impairments have additional disabilities. A large percentage of children with disabilities also have visual impairments (Rogow, 1992).

Coexisting Disorders in Children With Disabilities

The most common coexisting disabling diagnoses in children with developmental disabilities who have visual dysfunction include cerebral palsy, Down syndrome, spina bifida, head injury, Attention-Deficit/Hyperactivity Disorder, learning disabilities, and prematurity (Downing-Baum, 1995). Teplin (1995) further included mental retardation, Autistic Disorder, seizure disorders, emotional disabilities, and hearing impairments in the list of coexisting disabilities in children with visual dysfunction. Visual dysfunction can be difficult to diagnosis and sometimes remains unnoticed because of the attention given to the coexisting diagnosis.

There is enormous variability in the visual disorders or impairments in children with developmental disabilities (Chen & Dote-Kwan, 1994). Among the less serious visual problems in infancy and childhood are refractive errors, strabismus, and amblyopia. Refractive errors occur when there is deviation in the course of the light rays as they pass through the eye, preventing sharp focus on the retina. Refractive errors that require glasses are present in approximately 20% of typically developing children, and this percentage is even higher in children with developmental disabilities (Rogow, 1992). However, only a few children with refractive errors have significant visual impairments not corrected by glasses. Strabismus is present in 3% to 4% of all children; however, it is much more common in children with disabilities (Batshaw & Perret, 1992). (See Table 15.6 for a description of refractive errors.)

Table 15.6. Refractive errors

Type of Refractive Error	Impairment
Myopia (nearsightedness)	Sees most clearly at close range
Hyperopia (farsightedness)	Sees most clearly at a distance (except in the case of high hyperopia, where both distances can be blurry)

Vision Impairment and Blindness

Vision impairment is a term that describes a wide variety of problems in any part of the visual apparatus. Some of these problems can produce blindness. Professionals define blindness as visual acuity of less than 20/200 or a visual field of less than 20 degrees using both eyes with correction by glasses (Colenbrander & Fletcher, 1995). Blindness can result from illness or injury to the eye, the optic nerve, or the brain. Cataract, retinopathy of prematurity, retinal disorders, and glaucoma are common causes of serious visual impairment in the United States (Table 15.7).

Table 15.7. Common causes of visual impairment and blindness in children

Condition	Description
Anophthalmos	Absence of the eyeball
Cataract	Any opacity in the eye's lens that can lower visual acuity depending on its size and location
Cortical visual impairment	Loss of ability to interpret visual cues due to central nervous system damage
Glaucoma	Excess accumulation of intraocular fluid, which causes pressure on the retina and damage to the nerve fibers
Optic nerve hypoplasia or dysplasia	Irregularity or damage of the optic nerve; often coexists with hormonal and/or metabolic disorders
Retinoblastoma	Cancerous growth on the eyeball typically requiring surgical removal of the eyes
Retinopathy of prematurity or retrolental fibroplasia	Neonatal administration of oxygen, which causes abnormal growth of blood vessels in the eyes of some infants, leading to scarring and retinal detachment

In the United States, blindness and serious visual impairment occur in approximately 2 to 10 children per 10,000 population, with 75% of all children with diagnosed vision loss retaining some functional vision (Teplin, 1995). Congenital visual impairments can result from inherited conditions (e.g., congenital cataracts), chromosomal abnormalities (e.g., Down syndrome), or congenital infections (e.g., rubella). Inherited conditions are responsible for approximately half of all congenital and later-onset blindness. Perinatal events, such as retinal damage in premature infants (retinopathy of prematurity), can also cause visual defects. Postnatal causes include trauma (e.g., severe shaking), infection (e.g., cellulitis, *toxocara canis*), and connective tissue diseases (e.g., Marfan's syndrome). Strabismus can result in amblyopia or progressive loss of vision in one eye.

Central visual inattention or cortical blindness is a common cause of visual impairment in infants who have sustained brain damage (e.g., from intraventricular hemorrhage). Cortical blindness results from damage to the visual cortex, usually in association with widespread damage to other parts of the cerebral cortex, and frequently occurs with other developmental disorders (e.g., cerebral palsy, developmental delay) (Eken, de Vries, van der Graaf, Meiners, & van Nieuwenhuizen, 1995) (Figure 15.2). Children with cortical visual impairment have varying degrees of functional vision loss due to their inability to process the visual information. Most children with this diagnosis are unable to interpret some or all visual data as meaningful.

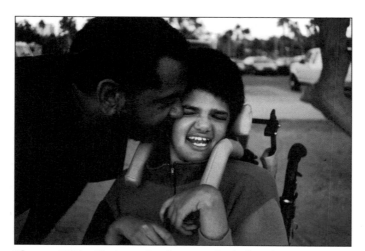

Figure 15.2. Sierra, who has cortical visual impairment, uses primarily auditory and tactile perceptions when relating socially, given her abilities and her functional limitations resulting from hydrocephalus and cerebral palsy.

Role of Sensory Integration in Vision

Levels of Sensory Processing

Vision plays a profound role in the nature and development of perception. There are three primary categories of sensory perception that provide individuals with spatial and temporal information (Kandel et al., 1991): *interoception*, *proprioception*, and *exteroception*. (See Table 15.8 for a description of these levels.)

Orientation to inner space occurs via *interoceptive* information and is essential for the formation of accurate ideas about how one literally feels inside one's body.

Table 15.8. Visual contribution to complex function by levels of perception

Level of Sensory Processing	Function	Visual Contribution
Interoception	Cycling behaviors such as eating, sleeping, and hormonal	Light/dark
Proprioception	Awareness of body position and movement in space	Visual monitoring of body in context
	Postural control	Visual feedback for precise movements
	Postural responses	Visual monitoring of self and environment
	Body scheme	Vision matched with somatosensory data
	Body image	Visual memory
	Body concept	Visual memory
	Ocular control	Reception and interpretation of visual field, saccades, visual closure, stability of images
Exteroception	Visual discrimination	Spatial, temporal details of objects, people, and environment
	Tactile discrimination	Spatial and detail reference
	Auditory discrimination	Spatial and detail reference
	Auditory awareness and use of language	Detection and interpretation of nonverbal or gestural language
	Olfactory and gustatory discrimination	Provides feedback for accuracy of judgment and aesthetics
	Monitoring environment	Provides near and distant context and detail
Intersensory Interactions	Awareness of body boundaries	Visual memory and feedback
	Praxis	Spatial context, visual data for feedforward and feedback
	Transition movements	Spatial memory or map, concrete details, stable information source unlike auditory, which is transient
	Interpret relationships between environmental systems	Capability to discern near and far, context, and anticipation of movement trajectory
	Attention, emotion, and creative expression	Visual memory; aesthetics of color, form, and dimension; spatial relationships

Interoception is important in identifying hunger, sleepiness, need to toilet, illness, and location of pain, and in discriminating subtle internal feelings. Interoceptive data allow the individual to identify the location of sensations in viscera and organs. Visual data contribute to interoceptive processing through the perception of light cycles and their effects on daily, monthly, and yearly rhythms (Kandel et al., 1991).

The second level of sensory processing is *proprioception,* encompassing vestibular and proprioceptive sensation. These sensations, in conjunction with vision, are essential for formation of body scheme, guiding direction and force of movement, postural control, stability and orientation, acquiring knowledge about body movements, and interactions between body parts during movement as well as while stable. At this level, vision is an important contributor to functional knowledge obtained from the vestibular/proprioceptive systems, providing the rapid data needed for feedforward anticipatory responses, especially for the control of posture and movement (Ayres, 1972).

Mechanisms inside the body work continuously to maintain homeostasis, although individuals barely notice interoceptive signals unless these signals inform the individual to keep the body healthy and safe. Proprioceptors fire constantly, also predominantly unconsciously, to maintain and monitor body position and movement in space relative to gravity. In addition, individuals utilize exteroception for interactions with things and people beyond the body.

Exteroception, the third level of sensory processing, encompasses primarily auditory and visual data working in conjunction with somatosensory, olfactory, and gustatory input to orient the self in space and in relation to others or objects in space (Streri, 1993). The most dynamic exteroceptive experiences originate through the pairing of auditory and visual data. Audition and vision are the only senses that perceive far beyond the body's boundaries. Exteroception provides the primary data sources for receiving precise information about both the content and the context of current interactions.

The combination of sensory data from the three levels provides a sense of one's own body boundaries and of the outer world. This information is important in the development of the self-concept. The skin creates the boundaries of the self, and the vestibular/proprioceptive systems yield information about the body's location in space relative to the earth's gravitational pull. In conjunction with the visual and auditory systems, an individual is able to detect his or her own body position relative to both static and moving environments. The knowledge of one's boundaries, one's location, and how either the self or the world is moving, interact to form perceptions of physical reality within a spatial context. The spatial context is the background for the action sequences that operate through time. Consequently, an individual makes choices of exploring or not exploring and begins planning the activities in which he or she will engage.

Intersensory Interactions

The visual system works as a part of the dynamic system of intersensory interactions that motivate, guide, and correct behavior. Of all the senses, vision, when it is available, is the unifying system that integrates all other systems and enables individuals to learn about, interact with, and survive in the world (Moore, as cited in Okoye, 1997).

Warren's (1993) model, described previously, is useful when determining vision deficits within the visual system. However, in the context of daily life, vision provides information in conjunction with all the sensory systems. Skeffington (1963) recognized that vision is more than light coming from the physical environment, entering the eye, then becoming transformed into an external phenomenon. He believed that vision could not be separated from the total individual, nor from any of the sensory

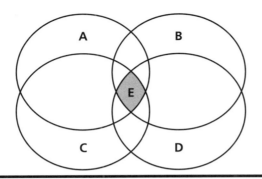

Figure 15.3. Skeffington model of vision.

A, Antigravity: coming to terms with gravity to move. *B,* Centering: ability to locate objects in space. *C,* Identification: ability to focus on information, to refine and discriminate detail, and to save that information in the brain. *D,* Speech audition: ability to communicate through speech and gesture and to use hearing. *E,* Vision: interweaving of all these modalities (*A* through *D*).

Note. From *The Skeffington Papers,* Series 36, #2 (p. 11), by A.N. Skeffington, 1963, Santa Ana, CA: Optometric Extension Program. Copyright 1963 by Optometric Extension Program. Reprinted with permission.

systems, because it is integrated into all human performance. He proposed a model that describes the visual process as the meshing of audition, proprioception, kinesthesia, and body sense with vision. Four connecting circles represent this interaction, each denoting one important subsystem (see Figure 15.3). The core, where each circle connects with the others, is *vision*. It is obvious from this model that visual cognition does not result from vision alone but rather from combining visual skills with all the other sensory modalities, especially the auditory, tactile, proprioceptive, and vestibular systems. As such, in sighted individuals, vision is the most complex and dominant of all the sensory systems.

Titcomb, Okoye, and Schiff (1997) further elaborated on Skeffington's model and described vision as more than 20/20 sight, defining it rather as a total action system. "The total action system refers to the blending of proprioceptive, vestibular, and visual processing in a dynamic system of data processing that summates new visual and motor input, compares it to previously stored data, then, in the twinkling of a millisecond, instructs one's body how to react appropriately, be it with hand,

foot, leg, or total body" (p. 6). This is consistent with Ayres' findings (1972) that visual perceptual difficulties rarely occur in isolation from postural, ocular, and somatosensory disabilities. The classic work of Held and Hein (1963) demonstrated the link between active movement and visual perception. There is no debate that vision is linked not only to other sensory information and processing but also to the resulting perceptual and adaptive responses. It is precisely this linking of vision with other sensory processing and action systems that makes sensory integration theory applicable to individuals with visual impairment.

Other studies concur with Skeffington's (1963) early proposals as well as those made by Titcomb et al. (1997). Damasio (1989) and Thelen and Smith (1994) demonstrated that although there is a primary organization of separate modalities, there is also an expansive interconnectivity of sensory systems. Stein and Meredith (1904) found brain processing of sensory information to be fundamentally multimodal and interactive. Their evidence that the superior colliculus is a site at which modality-specific experiences occur suggests that this intersensory interaction is a continuous intermeshing of the senses. These authors found that the topographic map of visual space in the cat superior colliculus consists primarily of multisensory neurons that fire in response to auditory, somatic, and visual stimulation, which suggests that the brain activity for seeing does not involve vision alone. An example of this interaction is the capacity to know where to look when one hears a sound.

Maintenance of head position is an example of how the senses work together. The angle of the head influences the way individuals process sound for hearing (Blauert, 1994). The angle of the head is also relevant to the stimulation of specific semicircular canals in the vestibular system and the activation of the ocular musculature (Herdman, 1994). These then interact with the neck proprioceptors to provide head movement and stability or mobility of the body. Something as simple as a person's head position alters the processing of sound, movement, and vision.

The clinical implications of the structure, function, and interaction of sensory systems are enormous. For example, individuals with blindness often hold their heads in excessive neck flexion. If Blauert's (1994) work on spatial hearing is correct, this head position will have consequences not only on postural ocular control and perception of the body's alignment in space but also on relating hearing to visual or perceptual images of space and spatial relationships.

Dan

Dan provides an example of the adaptive use of intersensory interactions. His eyes were removed shortly after birth because of retinoblastoma. Although Dan does not have vision, he is able to use other sensory systems effectively to compensate for his vision loss. His lack of visual data does not hinder him in participating meaningfully in a sighted world. Instead, Dan uses intersensory associations in the absence of vision. He utilizes his acute sense of hearing to obtain a sense of his surroundings. With a technique called echolocation, he is able to use a series of clicks or whistles to calculate the size of objects and the distance between objects. The sound reflects off the objects, and he is able to navigate at relatively fast speeds, even on a bicycle. The auditory feedback provides information from three-dimensional space at near and far distances. His vestibular sense tells him where gravity is pulling him and whether or not he is sustaining an upright posture. His proprioceptors promote rapid accommodations of all his muscles and limbs in order to maintain his balance and prevent falling. His memory, cognitive, and praxis abilities supply the attention and sequencing of his actions necessary to sustain this complex activity without the aid of visual feedforward or feedback. Dan and other capable individuals who are blind must be able to use their other sensory systems effectively to compensate for their vision loss.

Dan, although blind, is competent and independent. He has many hobbies and interests and is not afraid to try new things. He rides a bike quite well, and he could possibly fly a plane due to the instrumentation, but he has not tried it. Dan does not consider himself disabled any more than someone who wears glasses. He acknowledges, however, that his brain must have compensated early for its lack of vision through neuroplastic changes.

Analysis of Space

Ayres (1972) identified four closely interrelated functions essential to survival: (a) perception of gravity and motion through space, (b) extraocular muscle control, (c) locomotion and postural responses and proprioception relative to them, and (d) visual perception of space. In addition, Ayres cited Gernandt's view of space perception that also stressed a multisensory source. Gernandt considered the ocular system, the vestibular system, and sensations from muscles, joints, viscera, and skin to be interdependent and acting as an equilibration triad with the duty of keeping the body regulated and positioned in space (Ayres, 1972). Ayres emphasized the importance of the learned ability to attribute meaning to the sight of the body-space environment as an end product of adaptive motor responses.

Dr. Ayres discussed form and space perception as an idea, a cognitive process based primarily on vision. She was the first to highlight the contributions of the vestibular/proprioceptive and tactile sensations to the development of the functional use of form and space perception (Ayres, 1972, 1979; Fisher, Murray, & Bundy, 1991). Many investigators continue to neglect these hidden senses in the analysis of visual processing (Morrongiello, 1994). Additionally, theorists frequently attribute the complexity of the interactive nature of the sensory data to cognitive analysis rather than the sensory integrative processes.

Praxis

Vision contributes substantially to praxis. As mentioned previously, visual information is the fastest data individuals can access about the world. Vision provides the information for maximum feedforward processing in a given interaction due to vision's specificity of information in both near and far spatial contexts. Individuals also use visual data for rapid feedback so that even during action, they can modify a plan and alter it to ensure success. Visual information interacts with linguistic data to provide a sequential and organized understanding and planning of ideas and actions. The visual and language systems can be anticipatory in musing, visualizing, and discussing plans in the past, present, or future. The human mind can organize ideas into a sequence of potential interactions that it can then rehearse, play, replay, and reorganize.

Vision contributes to the speed of performance of projected action sequences. By definition, these projected action sequences are dependent on feedforward information as the environment or the individual moves. As the individual speeds up, feedforward becomes more critical. In addition, vision supplies the feedback information necessary especially for initial learning of events or space. Once learning has taken place, other sensory systems can take over the action, leaving the visual system free to guide more novel interactions and perform its anticipatory role in feedforward action plans.

Transitions are difficult for children who do not have efficient access to feedforward action systems. Transitions consist of passage from one form, state, style, or place to another. Appropriate visual monitoring of the environment for context, movement, and verbal and nonverbal communication is necessary in adaptive anticipation, planning, and navigation of transitions. Transitions require a complex array of abilities—not just vision, but also access to past memories, anticipation of future actions, adaptation to current circumstances, praxis, and comprehension of language. Transitions also require the ability to understand and anticipate the trajectory of change of the people and the environment with which the individual is interacting.

The human environment includes gravity, people, and objects in constantly changing dynamic patterns. Monitoring the moving environment and anticipating, planning, and adapting one's own interactions relative to stable and moving environments are most efficient when an individual has good postural control and access to vision to plan, monitor, and maintain control (see Figure 15.3).

Visual Impairment, Blindness, and Sensory Integration

Although visual impairment and blindness are disabling conditions, individuals such as Dan show that if the remaining sensory systems are working well, there are alternatives to vision in the formation and use of perceptions. Children who are blind from infancy will make sensory associations and form perceptions through their experiences that do not include vision. These children have little awareness of the meaning of blindness or sightedness. Only later in development will some of these children develop the capacity to understand the experiences that are reserved for the sighted.

When there is a lack of or distorted vision, the brain compensates for the lack of vision by reallocating the neural tissue typically allotted to vision (Kraemer, 1992). In the example described previously, Dan is able to utilize information sources other than vision to develop, maintain, and advance his competencies. His perspective is that his ability to do everything he can't see and integrate all other sensory information has made it possible for him to do whatever he wants to do. Dan is not functionally disabled from his vision loss, because he has adequate sensory integration and praxis in conjunction with a healthy mind and body.

Intersensory associations are obvious contributors to perception, but their contributions to motor abilities might be less obvious. Intersensory associations form perceptions that allow individuals to be competent participants in an ever-changing environment requiring constant temporal-spatial adaptation. Sensory integration is essential to temporal and spatial perceptions that precipitate temporal-spatial adaptive responses. Vision not only supplies rapid differentiated information to the feed-forward motor centers but also provides the ongoing feedback necessary to recalibrate the execution of the motor responses.

Michael

Michael is a young adolescent with a diagnosis of cerebral palsy. In addition, he is blind due to retinopathy of prematurity. In contrast to Dan, Michael has problems functionally because of some neuromotor and cognitive impairments as well as his inability to compensate for his blindness using other sensory systems. Although he has good social skills and is well liked, Michael has functional limitations that affect his ability to perform even routine daily occupations. He is not able to open a potato chip bag, a soda can, or a door. He cannot climb onto or off of a swing, nor does he want to. He cannot dress himself independently, and his table manners are poor. He puts his hands in his food and places whole sandwiches into his mouth without taking bites.

Michael is an endearing but fearful boy, emotionally labile and fully dependent on his caregivers. As an infant and toddler, Michael was difficult to work with in occupational and physical therapy. He complained of pain if someone moved his joints. He did not tolerate postural challenges against gravity. He did not appear to learn from repetition of activities. He cried when challenged. By the age of 2, he was seeing a physical therapist once a month for consultation. He learned to walk with the aid of a walker by age 5, and he continued to use the walker until recently. As he enters adolescence, some of his behaviors that were tolerable when he was a child, such as rubbing another person's arm over and over again, are no longer acceptable. He has a perception of himself as incapable of doing almost anything independently. His fearful dependence for most functional activities thwarts his struggle for independence.

Dan is Michael's orientation and mobility instructor. Dan insists that blind individuals must experience the world kinesthetically in order to learn about the environment. Due to Michael's sensory integrative deficits that coexist with the blindness and cerebral palsy, Michael has avoided the very activities that might serve to aid in the development of perceptions and action plans. With Dan's encouragement, Michael has experienced many activities of daily living, such as opening cans, walking on uneven surfaces, and dressing himself. Dan has allowed Michael to try, fail, and try again. Using a mentorship model, Dan has provided opportunities for Michael to play with boys his own age or older by participating in games such as laser tag. Dan has begun to address activities of daily living by breaking the activities down into minute steps and guiding Michael through touch and hearing into the environment where he has been afraid. This approach has been highly successful, and Michael is beginning to attempt activities at which he had previously thought he would fail. However, Dan expresses frustration that there are too many activities that Michael needs to learn, for Dan to teach them one at a time.

Evaluation for sensory integrative-focused occupational therapy found that Michael exhibited profound deficits in postural control leading to over-whelming insecurity with movement. He had sensitivity to proprioceptive sensations and did not appear to be able to discriminate his movements through proprioceptive feedback. He processed information slowly, which made it difficult for him to interpret vestibular data for effective postural control, leading to difficulty with postural accommodations and righting and equilibrium reactions. He had extremely poor praxis. He did not initiate novel schemes of action, remember how to do things he had tried before, or attempt to follow complex sequences of activities. Michael's therapist decided he could benefit from occupational therapy utilizing a sensory integrative approach in order to provide the foundation for meaningful participation in age-appropriate occupations.

Michael's therapist recommended twice-weekly occupational therapy, once in school and once in a specialized clinic setting. Michael participated in consultation and intervention in the classroom one time per week for approximately 6 months, at which time the team determined that Michael would benefit more from twice-weekly sessions within the clinic environment.

Michael's primary goals for occupational therapy included the following:

1. **Increase spatial awareness and comfort in moving his body through space.** This goal required that Michael have an increased vestibular and proprioceptive awareness of his own body's position and better control over the movements of his body in space. He was completely dependent on feedback, mostly from a caregiver. He did not utilize feedforward processes *effectively* in his interactions. He needed to learn all of his activities in a slow kinesthetic fashion. At the point at which he learned a skill, he needed to practice it to increase his speed of performance. When he could achieve the goal and perform a skill rapidly, he was utilizing feedforward information. The therapist also encouraged Michael to monitor his own feedback channels. Auditory feedback worked well for Michael. Wearing hard shoes that made loud noises and using a hand-held clicker when he walked allowed his own movements to produce auditory feedback.

2. **Increase tactile discrimination in order to refine his ability to manipulate objects with his hands.** This goal required that Michael begin to orient to specific tactile cues and textures that he encountered discriminitively. For example, when preparing a peanut butter sandwich, he needed to refrain from dipping his hands into the peanut butter and instead use utensils and guide his knife with his left hand while holding it in his right hand. He learned to measure the water level in the glass with his left hand while pouring with his right hand, and find the location of the padlock keyhole with one hand, then turn the key to open the lock.

3. **Enhance bilateral integration skills so that he could successfully use his hands cooperatively.** This goal required that Michael begin to have a global awareness of his body in space and his body parts relative to each other. He needed to be able to know where both of his hands were and how they were moving in order to open a can of soda. He also needed to have a measure of laterality in order to hold the can in his left hand while manipulating the tab with his right hand. He needed to be aware of the

spatial orientation of the can at all times in order to not spill the soda. Additionally, he needed to gauge proprioceptively how much force to utilize to hold the can, flip the top, and stabilize the can once the top gave way.

4. **Increase automatic righting and equilibrium reactions.** Michael had delayed postural reactions to tilt. He could not navigate a curb successfully. He was unable to weight shift and balance effectively to raise one foot up to step up the curb. In addition, the strength on one leg was currently insufficient to bring his body weight up to the curb. Therefore, one of Michael's goals was that he would tolerate movement on swinging equipment in a linear plane in order to elicit postural sway and tilt reactions opposing the direction of the tilt in a timely fashion. In therapy, he worked on weight shifting and balancing in sitting. Making accommodations with his trunk helped when he needed to balance on one foot long enough to raise the other foot when stepping off a curb.

5. **Increase hand strength.** Michael did not use his hands in a functional manner, such as for opening doorknobs. He did not have finger isolation or refined grasp patterns. He showed a tenuous grasp on utensils and preferred to finger feed. When he used a spoon, he did not guide with his left hand, and the food fell off prior to getting it to his mouth. Hanging from a trapeze in therapy, using a full grasp with opposing thumb to support his body weight helped to improve Michael's grasp. He began to trust his hand strength, holding on to the trapeze for 10 seconds while he lifted his feet off the mat. He continued to need guidance in appropriate grasp for the trapeze bar.

Progress Report

Michael's mother was thrilled at the progress he made after receiving occupational therapy in addition to his orientation and mobility training with Dan. After 12 months of occupational therapy using a sensory integrative approach combined with some neurodevelopmental techniques and skill training in

Table 15.9. Analysis of components contributing to functional deficits for Michael

Functional Deficits	Sensory Integrative Contributions	Contributions From Other Areas
Walking independently	Vestibular/proprioceptive awareness	Cerebral palsy, blindness
Finding his way to his classroom	Tactile-proprioceptive spatial awareness	Cognition, memory, blindness
Standing still	Proprioceptive awareness, balance	Poor tactile sensation, clonus, cerebral palsy, blindness
Using a Brailler	Tactile discrimination, muscle tone, postural stability	Cognition, memory, motivation
Opening a door	Muscle tone, muscle strength, motor planning, spatial awareness	Motivation, dependence
Stepping off a curb	Bilateral integration, proprioceptive awareness	Security, cognition, cerebral palsy

activities of daily living, Michael was much happier and less dependent. He began to have an easier relationship with his fulltime aide. His sister found Michael to be a more enjoyable playmate. He took some risks and asserted his independence in daily tasks. Dan took Michael riding on the back of a tandem bike, and he was able to stay on and enjoy the ride most of the time.

There was still much Michael could not do. However, his willingness to try opened up a new world for Michael and his family. Table 15.9 shows an analysis of the components contributing to Michael's functional deficits. Table 15.10 is an analysis of Michael's abilities according to the International Classification of Disability and Health (ICIDH-2, World Health Organization, 2000).

Commonalities Between Individuals With Blindness and Autistic Disorder

Researchers have noted relationships in the behaviors of individuals with visual impairment and Autistic Disorder (Chase, 1972; Gense & Gense, 1998). Similarities exist in the development of physical, language, cognitive, and social skills; response to sensory information; ability to relate to people or the environment (i.e., use of objects/toys, social interaction, and stereotypic behaviors), and impaired verbal/ nonverbal language or social communication (Wing, 1976). Although children with Autistic Disorder have difficulty with oculomotor control (Rosenthall, Johannsson, & Gilberg, 1988), these comparisons of behaviors are striking, considering that a significant strength in those with Autistic Disorder is visual processing (Parham, Mailloux, & Smith Roley, 1998) compared to the obvious visual loss in those with blindness.

Children with other diagnoses, such as retinopathy of prematurity, exhibit a variety of behaviors that are sometimes similar to the behaviors seen in Autistic Disorder. Children with Autistic Disorder have notable difficulties with praxis (Parham et al., 1998) and processing sensory information (Ritvo & Freeman, 1978). Disorders in sensory processing and praxis are possibly the reason these two separate and distinct diagnostic groups exhibit similar behaviors.

In the authors' clinical experience, children with optic nerve hypoplasia show the most similarities to children with Autistic Disorder. Children with optic nerve hypoplasia have difficulty with motivation, eating, and thermal regulation in addition to blindness. These similarities might reflect underlying commonalties, such as the ocular nerve's relationship to the hypothalamus.

Until there is further evidence of the presence of Autistic Disorder in individuals with visual impairment and blindness, clinicians and other professionals must use caution in applying the diagnosis of Autistic Disorder to children with visual impairment and blindness. Without further knowledge about the etiologies and nature of Autistic Disorder and the ramifications of prematurity, loss of vision, and the interrelationship of each sensory system and its contribution to the development of other sensory systems and subsequent function, applying a diagnosis of Autistic Disorder to an individual with blindness is conjecture.

Culver

Culver was a 3-year-old boy who was totally blind as a result of retinopathy of prematurity. He was born at 24 weeks gestation. He had severe expressive language difficulty. Culver attended a special preschool for children with visual impairment and blindness. Sometimes during the day he screamed, shouted, and banged his head. If he was restrained, he would hit his head on the floor or the person restraining him, in a rage. He self-

Table 15.10. Multilevel analysis of Michael's abilities

Profile Analysis	Impairment	Activity	Participation	Environment Social/Physical
Level of Function	Retinopathy of prematurity 26 weeks gestation Cerebral palsy	Engages in activity with maximum assistance	Good attachments to family, friends, and caregivers	Loving, consistent family Well-liked by all care-givers and other students
Characteristics	Blind—no light vision Neuromotor deficits Clonus Cognitive impairment	Finger feeds self Dresses and toilets self Mobile with cane and guide Difficulty maintaining balance, especially on uneven surfaces Does little activity other than routine daily care	Extremely passive Resists actively engaging in anything Will sometimes try an activity if he likes the person engaging him	Full-time aide in school Mother supports all aspects of his care
Strengths	Healthy	Ambulatory Good receptive and expressive language Listens to stories and music on tapes and CDs	Engaging with social language Kind to everyone Uses social skills to obtain help from familiar individuals	Friendly, sociable, empathic Remembers schedule of events past and future well
Difficulties	Ocular ennucleation Poor proprioceptive awareness Poor spatial awareness Poor praxis Poor vestibular awareness Diminished tactile sensitivity Gravitationally insecure	Cries easily Perceives difficulty before trying Difficulty figuring out how to do anything unfamiliar Resists motor engagement of any kind Cannot generalize skills	Feels lost when he is not with someone even for short periods Does not like change	Cannot operate alone Highly dependent on others

stimulated through rocking, stroking his lips, masturbating, or jumping. Culver was high strung and had temper tantrums that did not seem to relate to environmental events. Although he communicated primarily nonverbally, he could say some words that were easily intelligible, such as *mom, bye-bye,* and *no.* His teacher suggested that he might be autistic because of his antisocial and self-stimulatory behaviors.

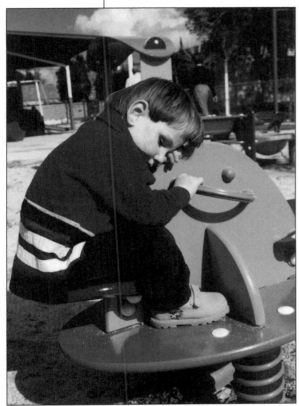

Figure 15.4. Culver takes a break on the bouncing daisy

Culver did not have functional language, although his receptive language was quite good. Caregivers tended to lead Culver to different places by holding his hand, and forced him to sit and do things that he did not choose. His angry outbursts typically occurred after being led through a series of activities from which he could not get away. Hitting his head appeared to be directly related to his frustration with not being able to effect a change in his environment through the communication channels to which he had access.

Culver responded well to occupational therapy and became angry if the therapist did not take him immediately to the clinic area when he heard her voice. He showed sensory-seeking behaviors that were predominantly proprioceptive, and he became much more organized after long periods of high bouncing on the bungee swing. He craved deep-pressure tactile input and vestibular stimulation (Figure 15.4). He tired with the activities that were predominantly low intensity in the classroom environment. The therapist also suggested that Culver's teacher remove Culver to the occupational therapy clinic area whenever he became upset and hit his head. He calmed as soon as he entered the clinic environment and asked for activities that provided him with deep pressure or heavy work (proprioception). This procedure worked well and diminished the head hitting considerably. The therapist also recommended speech and language therapy that would include signing and assistive technology.

Although Culver demonstrated behaviors similar to those seen in children with Autistic Disorder, he was not autistic. The common features with Autistic Disorder were severe language disorder, severe perceptual disorder, sensory seeking behaviors, poor modulation of sensory information from the environment, and poor imitation and praxis. His blindness and language delays in conjunction with his proprioceptive discrimination difficulties and poor modulation limited options to explore the world and vary his interactions. He did not have sufficient complexity in his play to vary his opportunities to meet his sensory needs appropriately. His frustration with his inability to feel in control of his life effectively yielded behaviors that were angry and inappropriate.

Table 15.11. Multilevel analysis of Culver's abilities

Profile Analysis	Impairment	Activities	Participation	Environment Social/Physical
Level of Function	Retinopathy of prematurity, Grade V 24 weeks gestation Bronchiopulmonary dysplasia	Engages in activities with maximum assistance and direction	Attached to his mother Attached to OT aide Aware of other children in class Rejects other children's advances Father alienated, minimally involved	Family support is present but disorganized Teacher dislikes and fears Culver due to unpredictable aggression Extended daycare daily
Characteristics	Blind—no light vision Mobility limited Has receptive language No expressive speech	Finger feeds self Assists in dressing Uses diapers Mobile, but quality poor Throws self around Poor orientation in space	Unpredictably aggressive Extreme frustration with lack of ability to control his environment effectively Seeks out what he enjoys, rejects everything else	Bangs on walls of mom's apartment, causing other tenants distress Limited interactions with people
Strengths	Healthy	Eats well Loves rough physical play Seeks out interactions he enjoys Strong-willed, determined	Indicates likes and dislikes with caregivers through gestures	OT is available when he becomes distressed His mother loves him, roughhouses with him frequently
Difficulties	Ocular ennucleation Poor proprioceptive awareness Poor spatial awareness Poor praxis Diminished sensitivity to touch Disordered modulation of vestibular stimulation	Self-stimulatory when left alone, rocking, masturbating, jumping, mouth flicking Needs one-on-one direction and assistance during activities and transitions Limited functional mobility Transitions, changes difficult	Difficult to control at circle time or field trips Poor spatial awareness of body, others, and environment Aggressive reactions to behavioral interventions	Not understood by majority of individuals interacting with Culver Speculations regarding cognitive impairment and Autistic Disorder as additional diagnoses when negative behaviors emerge

Assessment of Children With Visual Impairment and Blindness

Children with visual impairment and blindness are difficult to assess using standardized measures. There currently are no standardized sensory integrative assessment tools for indivi-duals with visual impairment.

Often it is necessary to rely on clinical observations of component functions. It is possible to make informal assessment of sensory processing functions, relationships to space, and the interactions of self and objects in space and time. (See chapter 12 in this text, Assessment of Sensory Integration and Praxis, for further information.)

Ramifications of Severe Visual Impairment and Blindness

Attachment

Fraiberg (1977) was the first to identify attachment as a serious concern in children with blindness. An important component in attachment is the social interaction between the child and the parent. Bruner (1990) discussed the concept of intersubjectivity that arises out of the child's ability to interact and predict the other's experience in a social interaction. Research with primates showed that monkeys are able to participate in mutual gaze (Povinelli & Eddy, 1996). Infants with visual impairment might not develop refined intersubjectivity because they are not able to monitor their actions visually and do not have the capacity to sustain contact with their caregivers at a distance. Alternative sensory conditions (e.g., sustaining tactile or verbal contact) can address this difficulty by maintaining the connections (see Figure 15.5). Without this contact, the infant can have a perception of being physically and emotionally disconnected. Later, the child's language might reflect a lack of reciprocity that the child learned through the early nonverbal dialogue with the caregivers (Sacks, Kekelis, & Gaylord-Ross, 1988).

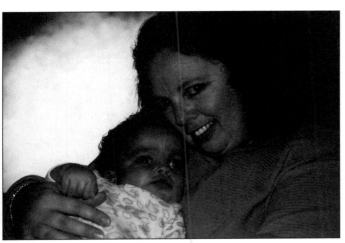

Figure 15.5. Logan and his mother nourish their relationship through touch.

Exploratory Behavior

Even when children with low vision or blindness accomplish motor milestones within relatively similar time frames compared to their sighted peers, their ability to explore with the same intensity is often diminished. Unlike sighted children, individuals with visual impairment frequently need encouragement to find and explore the larger environment outside of their immediate body-centered space. Caregiving tends to be more intensive, at times restricting the child from getting into things as a sighted child might do. This results in essential deprivation of typical motor experiences.

Sensory modulation difficulties are also common in individuals with visual impairment. Such individuals tend to restrict their interactions with the environment that would provide certain types of stimulation and instead over-engage in activities that provide other qualities of sensations.

Ideation and praxis are also of concern here. Watching what others are doing provides ideas about what to do. Inadequate experiences in creating novel ways to manage the environment can limit ideation, especially in early childhood. Additionally, lack of vision to guide and provide feedback to action plans can limit motor planning. Children will have a limited repertoire of activities in which they engage.

Postural Control

Postural control and ease of mobility are concerns for individuals with visual impairment and blindness. Lack of or distorted vision appears to affect the vestibular/proprioceptive systems that contribute to tonic postural control. In the absence of vision, the vestibular/proprioceptive systems require additional stimulation to keep operating well. In these cases, individuals tend to move constantly in order to maintain their tonic postural control. Additionally, when the individual is moving through space, information from vestibular/proprioceptive information must be accurate to indicate spatial orientation to gravity, alignment against gravity, and ongoing activation and automatic calibration of equilibrium and righting responses.

Fine Motor Development

Visual impairment frequently affects fine motor development because fine motor skills depend heavily on visual monitoring. Loss or distortion of vision compromises visual motor skills as well. The individual can use compensatory sensory data through the tactile system to guide fine motor skills. Tactile and proprioceptive information contributes to muscle tone in the fingers. Tactile spatial orientation is essential to perceiving the details of objects. Tactile sensitivity must allow repeated touch contact. Researchers have noted that absence or distortion of vision severely limits the level of complexity of visual manual skills (Fraiberg, 1977). Feedback from the tactile and proprioceptive systems does not provide enough data regarding the context in which the action takes place while the action is in motion.

Stereotypic Behaviors

Stereotypic behaviors, often called blind mannerisms, occur frequently in children with blindness and visual impairment. The most common of these behaviors are eye poking, self-rocking, and sometimes hand flapping (Fraiberg, 1977). Baranek (1998) and Baranek, Foster, and Berkson (1997) have discussed stereotypic behaviors in children with developmental delays and proposed that the constructs of stereotopies include repetitive motion patterns, object manipulations, behavioral rigidities, and tactile defensiveness. These types of behaviors also occur in a large number of children with visual impairment and blindness. These stereotypic behaviors appear to be sensory-seeking in nature, perhaps as a compensation for vision loss. Self-rocking might be a way to obtain vestibular input in the absence of being able to run through space, eye poking might provide proprioception and a light source for individuals without access to vision, and hand flapping could also be a way to obtain proprioceptive sensation.

In addition to the constructs proposed by Baranek, the authors of this chapter hypothesize that stereotypic behavior patterns emerge due to severely limited repertoires of movement and behavior. Difficulties with praxis limit the variety of movement options available to the individual who is blind. In an effort to self-calm, increase pleasurable sensations, move without being able to watch others to gain the ideas for movement, and/or generate new and adaptive movement options, the individual tends to revert to habitual patterns of movement even when those movements fail to provide the desired outcome.

Language

The content and style of language in most children with visual impairment differ from sighted children's language in grammar and syntax (Kekelis, 1988). Many factors contribute to these contextual language issues for this population.

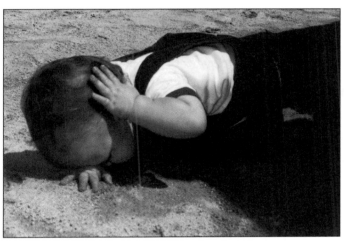

Figure 15.6. Andrew listens to his surroundings.

Competing auditory stimuli can obscure the location of objects or identification of voices. A child without vision might pay attention by holding very still, poking an eye, and listening intently, looking almost as if asleep (body language that, in an individual with sight, looks like indifference, boredom, sleepiness, or illness) (see Figure 15.6). A child might limit his or her dialogue to be able to pay attention to the location of people and objects in the surroundings.

The social context of language is predominantly visual in sighted individuals. Visual perception cognitively connects people to each other through social referencing, providing important predictive clues about the behavior of others (Povinelli & Eddy, 1996). Shared visual experiences often provide the foundation for contextual dialogue. Typical early language development originates from visual monitoring and patterns of mutual gaze (Povinelli & Eddy). In fact, eye contact is a form of intentional communication (Bretherton & Bates, 1979). Following another's line of gaze and predicting not only that person's actions but also thoughts allows for smooth social interchanges. A result of these early shared exchanges is the establishment of visually based gesturing for communication (Povinelli & Eddy).

Not only is social dialogue visually loaded, the English language also uses visual references to describe perceptual imagery from multisensory sources. The culture expects individuals without sight to learn the language of individuals with sight. Those with visual impairment must infer qualities of objects they cannot see using proprioceptive, tactile, or auditory information, which leaves much to the imagination. Commonly used phrases such as "Look at this" implies that two people have shared visual images that will be perceptually cohesive. People often express qualifiers in visual-spatial terms such as, "No, the blue one" or "It's the one over there next to the lamp." Children without access to vision from an early age will not have the benefit of eye contact, imitation of facial gestures, mutual gaze, intentional gaze shifting for initiation of interactions, the contextual perception of visual images, or activation of perception based on visually based language. Vision provides a depth of information that the individual cannot obtain through even a combination of other sensory channels.

The language of children with blindness contains more dialogue that is self-referencing (Kekelis, 1988). They talk about thoughts and activities that they engage in to the exclusion of dialogue about other people or contextually appropriate events. Given the loss of the most primary exteroceptor, their perceptions are skewed toward knowledge more at a body-centered level. This might account for the compromised ability to engage reciprocally in dialogue about another's activities or the qualities of activities and events outside of the individual.

Language and play often encompass sequences of activities that are visual and spatial in nature that an individual who has limited sight might not understand. Vision provides access to information about a broader set of relationships external to the individual. For a sighted child, "Let's go play on the swing" will result in looking at an entire playground of equipment, only one option of which is the swing. A child with blindness or severe visual impairment can only conjure an image of a swing, limiting the knowledge that enriches verbal dialogue.

Although language deficits occur most often in individuals with hearing impairment, clinicians must not overlook these deficits when working with individuals who have visual impairment and blindness. The contributions of vision, oculomotor control, and social and spatial referencing to social language are enormous. Visual impairment and blindness provide significant challenges to the development of functional language.

Occupational Performance

Visual distortion or loss in individuals with sensory integration deficits affects all aspects of daily living, play skills, and learning. Observing children's play skills often provides insights into their future capabilities to relate creatively and joyfully with the social and physical environments.

Lack of vision often compromises participation in independent activities of daily living. For example, children sometimes have difficulty choosing socially appropriate combinations of clothing and putting them on in the correct orientation and sequence. Preparing meals, selecting the correct dollar bill denomination, and finding one's way with public transportation present challenges for the individual with blindness.

Using Sensory Integration Intervention Principles With Children With Visual Impairment and Blindness

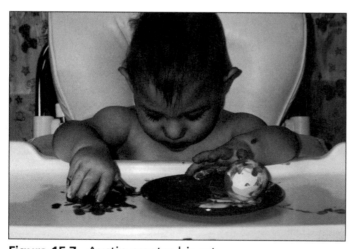

Figure 15.7. Austin creates his art.

Physical interaction with the environment builds the intersensory perceptions necessary for participating in occupations (see Figure 15.7). When an individual has a sensory loss, the therapist considers the contributions of other sensory channels for function to optimize learning and diminish the impact of the sensory loss. Based on the assumption that other sensory experiences will help compensate for a sensory loss, sensory integration therapy provides opportunities for people with visual impairments to do what they cannot see. Interventions focus on providing enrichment in appropriate activities so that the individual can be adaptive. An appropriately enriched sensory environment is so important for development when vision is lost or absent that all contexts of these individuals' daily lives must include the recommended activities.

During intervention, the clinician takes into account the typical contributions of vision to function. If there is a deficit in an area of development, the therapist examines the most important sensory systems underlying that function. Although most functions rely on multisensory processing, certain sensory systems are more important for specific functions than others. In selecting activities during intervention, clinicians must consider the connections between available sensory channels for learning and choose activities that facilitate development of perception, using the sensations that substitute for vision during the different tasks and activities.

The following paragraphs give examples of some major functional areas and their primary sensory connections. The therapist working with children who have visual impairment and blindness needs to engage these children in activities that include specific sensory experiences to enhance discriminative and supportive perceptual functions. For example, a baby who cannot see his or her mother must touch the mother's face and be carried throughout the house to understand the mother's emotional tone, where she is, and where they are going. Consequently, the tactile, vestibular, and auditory systems are paramount in the baby's ability to learn about the external environment. To develop the baby's abilities to participate well socially, the therapist targets activities providing these sensations in ways that the baby can enjoy.

Postural control depends on the information from the vestibular, proprioceptive, and visual systems. In the absence of vision, the individual must depend more heavily on auditory feedback for spatial orientation related to postural alignment. Gross motor skills rely greatly on visual and proprioceptive sensory data. In the absence of vision, the individual must use both proprioceptive and vestibular information to guide and control gross motor interactions. Echolocation is a style of orientation through auditory feedback. Learning this type of orientation aids in the ability to travel for those with low or absent vision.

Fine motor and precision activities require both tactile and visual information (Streri, 1993). An individual with absence or distortion of vision must recruit the proprioceptors to assist in fine motor control. The somatosensory system therefore is critical in the development of finely skilled movements in the absence of vision.

Clinicians can facilitate praxis using somatosensory activities in conjunction with the fine-tuning of auditory perception. An individual with loss of vision can use the auditory system for anticipation of events in the outside world and for adaptation to the external environment. Development of fine discrimination through the auditory system is important in establishing strategies for differentiation between people, distance, and systems within the context in which the child finds him- or herself.

Cognitive/spatial conceptual development and social language require auditory and visual information. In the absence of vision, the tactile and vestibular systems play a much larger role. The spatial mapping that will take place requires far more participation through the proprioceptive system.

Clinicians can approach modulation through sensory means also. Multiple factors contribute to regulatory difficulties in this population. At the most basic level, regulating diurnal cycles through light detection affects sleep patterns. Lack of sufficient sleep can create anxiety and irritability in addition to sensory sensitivity. Providing calming and rhythmic activities aids in self-regulatory behaviors. Early exposure to painful procedures creates a sensitivity to a variety of tactile experiences. Therefore, caregivers and professionals need to promote engagement in tactually based activities that the child enjoys. During interventions for such problems as restrictive food choices or poor eating habits, sensitivity on the part of the therapist and family is necessary so as not to create further reactivity.

Use of body-centered sensations and active engagement in activities for alerting and calming is an effective approach to intervention. Multiple opportunities for swinging and rocking, obtaining deep pressure, and doing heavy work activities through jumping, climbing, and hanging will have a regulatory effect. When the visual system and vestibular/proprioceptive systems are not working well, a child will often seek such activities to obtain comfort with the feeling of his or her own body in space and move-

Table 15.12. Diagnosis: Retinoblastoma

Presenting Problem	Underlying Difficulties	Intervention Strategies
Literacy	Blindness	Use orientation and mobility training procedures Provide literacy training, especially Braille and technology utilizing sound and Braille
Mobility	Sustaining static upright postures	Provide enhanced vestibular/proprioceptive information through active self-initiated play and movement Provide opportunities for swinging in prone to enhance posture
Self-care	Auditory and tactile discrimination refinement	Provide tactile activities to train and enhance stereognosis Encourage practice with and adaptation of methods, tools, and/or environment
Body concept	Development of good body scheme	Provide opportunities for jumping, climbing, hanging, pushing, and pulling in order to enhance body awareness
Orientation to space	Confidence in moving through space/spatial mapping	Train and enhance echolocation abilities
Enculturation into sighted world	Knowledge and awareness of the sighted physical and social world	Provide opportunities for socialization Provide social skills training for expectations by the sighted community, such as color matching, proximity during conversation, etc.

Table 15.13. Diagnosis: Retinopathy of prematurity

Presenting Problems	Underlying Difficulties	Intervention Strategies
Delayed motor milestones, speech acquisition, physical independence	Depends upon the grade of retinal detachment. Grades IV and V are severely visually impaired/blind	Educational strategies Developmental activities
Difficulty with handling, feeding, and attachment	Low muscle tone with poor postural stability: often too much extension in upper extremities with high guard position	Use neurodevelopmental treatment techniques to enhance appropriate movement patterns Stimulate active tonic flexion
Sensitivity to sounds and touch, irritability, difficulty calming	Difficulty with transitional movements, especially trunk accommodations	Build balance reactions in trunk
Eye poking and rocking	Balance reactions limited to straight planes of movement	Provide enhanced vestibular/proprioceptive/visual sensations through play on swinging equipment
Frightened of tactual exploration	Tactile and auditory defensiveness is common	Reduce sensory defensiveness through modulation techniques
Frightened of movement through space	Check for gravitational insecurity	Address gravitational insecurity if present

Table 15.14. Diagnosis: Optic nerve damage (hypoplasia, dysplasia, degeneration, etc.)

Presenting Problems	Underlying Difficulties	Intervention Strategies
Feeding disorders, especially restrictive in trying new foods, regulating hunger and satiation Temperature regulation disturbances	Difficulty with regulation of homeostatic mechanisms that influence feeding, sleeping, toileting, motivation, etc.	Use sensory modulation techniques Use rhythm and music activities Provide proprioceptive activities Encourage heavy work
Sleep disturbances	Regulatory disorder	Spend time in natural light Provide full-spectrum indoor lighting
Autistic-like features, especially in the style of stereotypic behaviors	Modulation disorder Sensory seeking/avoiding	Introduce novel activities through multisensory approaches and routine
Poor social adaptability	Poor ideation and praxis Poor modulation	Increase awareness of social routines Provide cues to body position and others' perspectives
Withdrawn and unmotivated	Poor discrimination of the environment	Provide enriched sensory environment in all areas of life
Poor use of hands for functional tasks	Tends to restrict exploration to own body or immediate environment Poor fine motor skill development	Encourage weight bearing on palmar surface Expose to vibration and multiple textures
Poor posture	Low muscle tone	Increase vestibular input, especially linear, vertical, and rotary as tolerated
Echolalic, perseverative, self-centered language	Poor play skills	Modeling; role playing; clear, slow, and simple language usage

Table 15.15. Diagnosis: Dual or multiple sensory impairment (i.e., deaf and blind)

Presenting Problems	Underlying Difficulties	Intervention Strategies
Lack of language development	Auditory and visual impairment	Teach alternative communication methods Use hand-over-hand kinesthetic approaches
Pounds on things	Proprioceptive seeking	Provide strong proprioception and vibration as tolerated
Poor posture, holds head in unusual positions	Difficulty with postural control, especially head and trunk control	Provide movement in inverted plane unless the child has a shunt Provide linear vestibular input in prone or upright
Poor motor skills acquisition	Tactile irregularities; can be overly sensitive, underresponsive, or both, depending on the texture and how it is encountered	Use as many tactile cues as possible to train motor skills Reinforce with vibration as tolerated
Hits head	Frustration Poor communication Behavior disorder	Provide increased heavy work/proprioception and vestibular activities Articulate feelings for the child
Difficulty with language and socialization	Poor play skills	Use role playing, modeling Provide assistance with expressive language

Table 15.16. Diagnosis: Cortical visual impairment

Presenting Problems	Underlying Difficulties	Intervention Strategies
Often encountered with wide range of medical and neurological deficits	Damage to neurological centers in or related to the visual cortex	Multidisciplinary approach is vital
Concomitant cognitive deficits are typical	Lack of interpretation of retinal data	Provide supports in all areas of activities of daily living
Usually frank motor involvement	Might have ocular motor skills intact but cannot use this information to guide function	Be cautious of erratic visual stimulation; it can cause seizures
Language delays usually severe	Can have concomitant auditory processing deficits and neuromotor deficits	Provide as many opportunities for pleasant interpersonal touch as possible
Socialization difficulties	Lack of social responsiveness	Teach play

Table 15.17. Diagnosis: Visual spatial deficits

Presenting Problems	Underlying Difficulties	Intervention Strategies
Fine motor delays	Poor integration of vestibular/ proprioceptive/visual data	Classic sensory integrative techniques will be effective
Gets lost easily	Poor lateralization Poor spatial mapping	Enhance bilateral integration and head, neck, and eye control with upper limb and body movements Use orientation and mobility techniques
Lack of awareness of others relative to themselves	Poor imitation skills, body scheme, body image, and spatial awareness	Enlist classroom support in environmental modifications Provide opportunities for movement, heavy work, and tactile play during the school day; in other words, take body-centered sensory breaks throughout the day
Poor hand skills	Poor visual praxis	Use specific fine motor development programs
Poor reading and math abilities	Poor oculomotor skills Poor visual perception	Consult with developmental optometrist
Difficulty sitting still and staying in seat	Poor ability to hold positions	Provide dynamic seating assistance
Attention deficits	Poor concentration	Increase sensory awareness through provision of increased relevant sensory information
Wanders	Poor perception of abstract spatial relationships and boundaries (see Spelke, 1990)	Enhance muscle tone in flexor musculature for holding in place Orient to boundaries of the group

ment through open space. Providing activities that aid in sensory modulation, including teaching self-regulation through appropriate activities, becomes increasingly important as the child matures.

Tables 15.12 through 15.17 list the common clinical findings in individuals with visual impairment within diagnostic categories and describe possible intervention strategies that therapists can utilize in intervention.

Sticking Points

During evaluation and intervention of children with visual impairment and blindness, therapy sometimes seems to falter and stall. The following questions outline the types of analyses a therapist can use to examine the sticking points and develop a new intervention approach.

1. What aspects of the child's difficulties in age-appropriate, meaningful participation stem from the visual impairment? What deficits are typical for this population with visual impairment or blindness?

2. How do the other sensory channels develop relative to the visual loss? Is there enhanced sensory reception and interpretation, or has the loss of visual data produced subsequent deficits in other sensory channels (especially auditory)?

3. Is it possible to extinguish self-stimulatory behaviors, especially those providing visual stimulation (e.g., eye poking, proprioception given lack of fast body

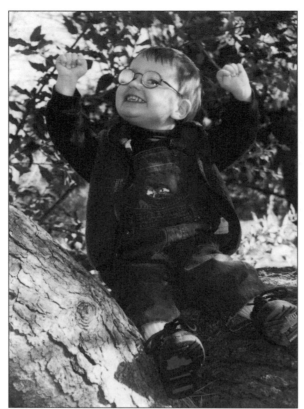

Figure 15.8. Vejas enjoys the moment.

movements, or vestibular input given lack of visual data and active fast movements through the environment)?

4. How do you teach a child about external space when the child cannot see or feel distance?

5. How do you teach a child relative spatial relationships when the child's visual information is absent or distorted?

6. What is the best way for the child to gain knowledge about the dynamic contexts in which this child needs to operate?

Understanding space through nonvisual sensory input is essential, as is understanding praxis in organizing interactions and movement over time through space. Maximizing an individual's potential for perception using the full complement of senses can help the person reach the goal of participating meaningfully and becoming functionally independent (see Figure 15.8). The application of sensory integrative theory and intervention can make enormous contributions to this special population.

Acknowledgments

The authors extend sincere appreciation to the children and families of the Blind Children's Learning Center (BCLC) Gabrielle Hass, past executive director of BCLC, and to the Crayton family, Maureen, Tommy, Sierra, Evan, and Logan.

Works Cited

Quotation on page 323 from "Introduction to the Dynamic Process of Vision" by R.E. Titcomb, R. Okoye, and S. Schiff (1997) in *Functional Visual Behavior: A Therapist's Guide to Evaluation and Treatment Options* have been reprinted with permission by The American Occupational Therapy Association.

References

Ayres, J. (1972). *Sensory integration and learning disorders*. Los Angeles: Western Psychological Services.

Ayres, A.J. (1979). *Sensory integration and the child*. Los Angeles: Western Psychological Services.

Baker-Nobles, L. (1990). A multisensory approach to developing the use of residual vision for quality movement. *Occupational Therapy Practice, 1*(4) 23–33.

Baker-Nobles, L., & Rutherford, A. (1995). Understanding cortical visual impairment in children. *American Journal of Occupational Therapy, 49,* 899–903.

Ballinger, B. (1995). Visual influences in the learning process. *Sensory Integration Special Interest Section Newsletter, 23,* 1.

Baranek, G.T. (1998) Sensory processing in persons with autism and developmental disabilities: Considerations for research and clinical practice. *Sensory Integration Special Interest Section Newsletter, 21*(2), 1–3.

Baranek, G.T., Foster, L.G., & Berkson, G. (1997). Tactile defensiveness and stereotyped behaviors. *American Journal of Occupational Therapy, 51,* 91–95.

Batshaw, M.L., & Perret, Y.M. (1992). *Children with disabilities: A medical primer* (3rd ed.). Baltimore: Paul H. Brookes Publishing Co.

Blauert, J. (1994). *Spatial hearing: The psychophysics of human sound localization.* Cambridge, MA: MIT Press.

Bretherton, I., & Bates, E. (1979). The emergence of intentional communication. In I. Uzgiris (Ed.), *New directions for child development* (Vol. 4). San Francisco, CA: Jossey-Bass.

Bruner, J. (1990). *Acts of meaning.* Cambridge, MA: Harvard University Press.

Chase, J.B. (1972). *Retrolental fibroplasia and autistic symptomatology.* New York: American Foundation for the Blind.

Chen, D., & Dote-Kwan, K. (1994). *Starting points: Instructional practices for young children whose multiple disabilities include visual impairment.* Los Angeles: Blind Children's Center.

Colenbrander, A., & Fletcher, D. (1995). Basic concepts for low vision rehabilitation. *American Journal of Occupational Therapy, 49,* 865–876.

Damasio, A.R. (1989). Time-locked multiregional retroactivation: A systems-level proposal for the neural substrates of recall and recognition. *Cognition, 33,* 25–62.

Davidson, P.W. (1992). Visual impairment and blindness. In M.D. Levine, W.B. Carey, & A.C. Crocker (Eds.), *Developmental and behavioral pediatrics* (2nd ed., pp. 102–154). Philadelphia: W.B. Saunders.

Downing-Baum, S. (1995, June 15). Exercises in pediatric vision therapy. *OT Week, 9,* 20–22.

Eken, P., de Vries, L.S., van der Graaf, Y., Meiners, L.C., & van Nieuwenhuizen, O. (1995). Haemorrhagic-ischaemic lesions of the neonatal brain: Correlation between cerebral visual impairment, neurodevelopmental outcome and MRI in infancy. *Developmental Medicine and Child Neurology, 37*(1), 41–55.

Fisher, A.G., Murray, E.A., & Bundy, A. (1991). *Sensory integration: Theory and practice.* Philadelphia: F.A. Davis.

Fraiberg, S. (1977). *Insights from the blind.* New York: Basic.

Gense, M., & Gense, D.J. (1998, November). Identifying autism in children who are blind/visually impaired. Lowenfeld-Akeson Intervention Symposium: Autism and the Visually Impaired Child. California School for the Blind, Fremont, CA.

Held, R., & Hein, A. (1963). Movement-produced stimulation in the development of visually guided behavior. *Journal of Comparative and Physiological Psychology, 56,* 872–876.

Hellerstein, L., & Fishman, B. (1987). Vision therapy and occupational therapy: An integrated approach. *Sensory Integration Special Interest Section Newsletter, 10*(3), 4–5.

Herdman, S.J. (1994). *Vestibular rehabilitation.* Philadelphia: F.A. Davis.

Kandel, E.R., Schwartz, J.H., & Jessell, T.M. (1991). *Principles of neural science* (3rd ed.). Connecticut: Appleton & Lange.

Kekelis, L.S. (1988). Peer interaction in childhood: The impact of vision in childhood. In S. Sacks, L. Kekelis, & R. Gaylord-Ross (Eds.), *The social development of visually impaired students* (pp. 1–28). San Francisco, CA: San Francisco State University.

Kraemer, G.W. (1992). A psychobiological theory of attachment. *Behavioral and Brain Sciences, 15*(3), 493–511.

Morrongiello, B.A. (1994). Effects of colocation on auditory-visual interactions and cross-modal perception in infants. In D.J. Lewkowitz & R. Lickliter (Eds.), *The development of intersensory perception: Comparative perspectives* (pp. 235–263). Hillsdale, NJ: Lawrence Erlbaum Associates.

Okoye, R. (1997). Neuromotor prerequisites of functional behavior. In M. Gentile (Ed.), *Functional visual behavior: A therapist's guide to evaluation and treatment options* (pp. 55–86). Bethesda: MD: American Occupational Therapy Association.

Parham, D., Mailloux, Z., & Smith Roley, S. (1998). Sensory processing and praxis in high-functioning children with autism. Montreal, Canada: Presentation *World Federation of Occupational Therapy Conference.*

Povinelli, D.J., & Eddy, T.J. (1996). What young chimpanzees know about seeing. *Monographs of the Society for Research in Child Development, 61*(3, Serial No. 247).

Ritvo, E.R., & Freeman, B.J. (1978). Current research on the syndrome of autism: Introduction. The National Society for Autistic Children's definition of the syndrome of autism. *Journal of the Academy of Child Psychiatry, 17,* 565–575.

Rogow, S.M. (1992). Visual-perceptual problems of visually impaired children with developmental disabilities. *Review, 25*(2), 57–64.

Rosenthall, J., Johannsson, E., & Gilberg, C. (1988). Oculomotor findings in autistic children. *Journal of Laryngeal Otology, 102,* 435–439.

Sacks, S., Kekelis, L., & Gaylord-Ross, R. (Eds.) (1988). *The social development of visually impaired students.* San Francisco, CA: San Francisco State University.

Schneck, C.M. (1998). Intervention for visual perceptual problems. In J. Case-Smith (Ed.), *Occupational therapy: Making a difference in the school system.* Bethesda, MD: American Occupational Therapy Association.

Skeffington, A.N. (1963, November). *The Skeffington Papers,* Series 36, #2 (p. 11). Santa Ana, CA: Optometric Extension Program.

Solan, H.A., & Ciner, E.B. (1986). *Visual perception and learning: Issues and answers.* New York: SUNY College of Optometry.

Spelke, E.S. (1990). Principles of object perception. *Cognitive Science, 14,* 29–56.

Stein, B., & Meredith, A. (1904). Multisensory integration. In A. Diamond (Ed.), The development and neural bases of higher cognitive functions. *Annals of the New York Academy of Sciences, 608,* 51–65.

Streri, A. (1993). *Seeing, reaching, touching.* Cambridge, MA: MIT Press.

Teplin, S.W. (1995). Visual impairment in infants and young children. *Infants and Young Children, 8*(1), 18–51.

Thelen, D., & Smith, L.B. (1994). *A dynamic systems approach to the development of cognitions and action.* Cambridge, MA: MIT Press.

Titcomb, R.E., Okoye, R., & Schiff, S. (1997). Introduction to the dynamic process of vision. In M. Gentile (Ed.), *Functional visual behavior: A therapist's guide to evaluation and treatment options* (pp. 3–53). Bethesda: MD. American Occupational Therapy Association.

Warren, M. (1993). A hierarchical model for evaluation and treatment of visual perceptual dysfunction in adult acquired brain injury. Part 1. *American Journal of Occupational Therapy, 47,* 42–54.

Warren, M. (1994). Visuospatial skills: Assessment and intervention strategies. *AOTA self-study series: Cognitive rehabilitation.* Rockville, MD: American Occupational Therapy Association.

Wing, L. (1976). *Early childhood autism* (2nd ed.). New York: Pergamon Press.

World Health Organization. (2000). *ICIDH-2: International classification of disability and health. Prefinal draft.* Geneva, Switzerland: Author.

Zaba, J. (1984). Visual perception versus visual function. *Journal of Learning Disabilities, 17,* 182–185.

Sensory Integration
and the Child With Cerebral Palsy

Erna Imperatore Blanche, Ph.D., OTR, FAOTA

Bonnie Nakasuji, M.A., OTR

Occupational therapy intervention for the child with cerebral palsy (CP) has undergone many transformations during the last decades. In the 1940s and 1950s, intervention focused on the use of braces, stretching, and functional activities. During that time, occupational therapy highlighted independence in activities of daily living (New York Occupational Therapists, 1953, 1954), the construction of adaptive equipment (Zimmerman, 1957), the acquisition of play skills (Robinault, 1953), and the importance of perceptual motor skills (Robinault, 1954).

Towards the late 1950s and early 1960s, the Bobath approach, based on the integration of reflexes and the development of postural control, entered the occupational therapy literature (Fiorentino, 1966) and became a popular intervention approach with which to address the movement deficits in children with CP. Consequently, a focus on the development of motor milestones through the integration of reflexes and the development of postural reactions replaced the earlier focus on play and perceptual motor skills (Fiorentino, 1966).

During this same time, Jean Ayres worked with children with CP. As a young therapist, Ayres addressed the motor execution deficits of children with CP, in some cases with limited success (A.J. Ayres, personal communication, May, 1984). This limited intervention success led her to question whether the functional deficits of these children with CP were indeed due to the motor execution disorder. The questions she formulated in the 1950s about the sensory basis of movement disorders contributed to her growing interest in researching sensory processing disorders as the basis of movement disorders in children with learning disabilities in the 1960s (A.J. Ayres, personal communication, May, 1984). Ayres devoted the rest of her career to unraveling sensory integration (SI) disorders in children with learning difficulties and never returned to answer her original questions about the nature of the functional deficits in children with CP. However, by identifying sensory processing disorders as the basis of functional problems for some children, she paved the road for others to apply these principles to children with neuromotor disorders. Ayres was ahead of her time in suggesting the possibility of sensory processing disturbances as the root of many motor characteristics present in children with CP.

Until recent years, the traditional classification of CP, initially based on the motor dysfunction, warranted an intervention approach that focused on motor performance. Current theories of motor behavior support the notion that movement and sensation are related and that intervention does not need to address them separately. Investigators now recognize that children with CP exhibit sensory as well as motor deficits (Lesny, Stehlik, Tomasek, Tomankova, & Havlicek, 1993; Moore, 1984). In fact, the presence of sensory processing deficits in children with CP has gained empirical support throughout the last 20 years (Cooper, Majnemer, Rosenblatt, & Birnbaum, 1995; Lesny et al. 1993; Wann, 1991; Yekutiel, Jariwala, & Stretch, 1994), and many practitioners have addressed these deficits in intervention (Blanche, Boticelli, & Hallway, 1995; Blanche & Burke, 1991; DeGangi, 1990a,b,c; Windsor, 1986).

Despite the recognition of sensory processing deficits in children with CP, understanding the nature of those deficits and the expected outcomes of SI intervention with this population needs refinement. This chapter focuses on increasing current information on the sensory processing deficits exhibited by children with CP and describes specific intervention techniques that address some of the SI deficits presented by children with CP.

Clinical Picture of Sensory Processing Deficits in the Child With CP

Many children with CP exhibit sensory processing and praxis disorders that often impose greater functional limitations on these children than the movement disorder itself. Intervention that does not consider a sensory processing disorder but rather treats the problems as disorders in motor execution usually has limited success. This section describes the sensory processing deficits presented by children with CP, examining the impact of these deficits on performance.

There is ample material in the literature describing tactile and proprioceptive deficits in children with CP; however, the literature documents vestibular deficits minimally or not at all. The tactile processing deficits in children with CP might be the direct result of injury to an area in the central nervous system or might be secondary to the neuromotor deficits (Moore, 1984). Secondary deficits could result from impairment of peripheral nerves due to spasticity and abnormal positioning (Dellon, 1997) and/or from decreased sensory experiences (Blanche & Burke, 1991; Moore, 1984; Sugden & Keogh, 1990). Peripheral nerve compression can be the cause of sensory loss when there is a marked difference in sensation between the different parts of the body. In that case, surgery and sensory re-education sometimes relieve the impairment to the peripheral nerve (Dellon, 1997). On the other hand, when there is a generalized deficit in somatosensory processing, then SI intervention principles can improve functional performance. Studies focusing on somatosensory deficits in children with CP conclude that (a) tactile deficits in the hands are more common in children with spasticity than in children with athetosis (Yekutiel et al., 1994), (b) the intensity of the tactile deficit is not related to age or cognitive abilities (Yekutiel et al., 1994), and (c) tactile processing deficits are common in children with hemiplegia (Van Heest, House, & Putnam, 1993) and can affect both sides (Cooper et al., 1995).

The tactile and kinesthetic deficits that the literature most often identifies include deficits in tactile discrimination, pressure sensitivity, proprioception, sense of directionality, two-point discrimination, stereognosis, and grip force (Eliasson, Gordon, & Forssberg, 1991, 1995; Kenney, 1963; Lesny et al., 1993; Van Heest et al., 1993; Yekutiel et al., 1994).

Proprioceptive/kinesthetic deficits that children with CP present are difficult to diagnose because of the accompanying tactile perception and motor control deficits (Cooper et al., 1995; Eliasson et al., 1991, 1995).

Investigators have done little or no research on other sensory processing deficits, such as sensory modulation deficits and vestibular processing disorders, most likely because it is difficult to differentiate the symptoms of these disorders from the neuromotor deficit. Vestibular processing disorders include poor registration of vestibular input, sensitivity to movement experiences, and gravitational insecurity (Blanche et al., 1995).

General Principles of Assessment and Intervention

The assessment of sensory processing and praxis in the child with CP is a difficult task because many of the behavioral characteristics associated with sensory processing disorders in children without neuromotor disorders can stem from the neuromotor disorder in children with CP. One rule of thumb for identifying sensory processing disorders in children with CP is to suspect the presence of a sensory processing dysfunction when a child responds atypically to intervention strategies that address movement disorders. In such a case, SI theory is useful in identifying, classifying, and addressing the sensory processing disorder. In addition, most assessment tools that clinicians have traditionally used to assess sensory processing and praxis abilities presuppose little or no neuromotor involvement and therefore have little validity for children with motor impairments.

Identification of Sensory Processing Disorders

The identification of sensory modulation disorders in children with CP is particularly difficult, and such disorders often remain unnoticed, even when the disorders affect the child's motor performance as much as or more than the neuromotor dysfunction. For example, registration and modulation disorders commonly affect muscle tone, postural control, and interaction with the environment, all of which are areas of concern for children with CP. The questions listed below can help the therapist identify registration and modulation disorders that might indicate sensory processing deficits in children with CP.

Tactile Defensiveness or Hyperresponsiveness to Tactile Input*

Does the child:

1. object to being handled when not wearing clothes?
2. struggle against being held? (Parham & Ecker, 2000)
3. avoid being messy (mouth as well)?
4. object to light touch applied with a cotton swab? (Baranek & Berkson, 1994)
5. object to having stickers applied on the skin? (Baranek & Berkson, 1994)
6. avoid getting his or her hands in finger paint, paste, sand, mud, glue, or other messy materials? (Parham & Ecker, 2000)
7. startle easily when being touched lightly or unexpectedly by others?
8. push the therapist's hand away from his or her body?
9. rub or scratch a part of the body that has been touched? (Dunn, 1999)

Poor Tactile Discrimination and/or Hyporesponsiveness

Does the child:

1. fail to localize/respond when touched?
2. mouth objects?
3. enjoy having hair brushed?
4. enjoy being handled or touched?
5. fail to notice when clothing is twisted on his or her body? (Dunn & Westman, 1997)

continued on p. 348

---

6. fail to recognize when hands or face are messy? (Dunn, 1999)

7. like vibration (manual vibration)?

Processing of Proprioceptive Input

Does the child:

1. bite or chew on nonfood objects (clothing, toys, etc.)?

2. pinch and hit others or self?

3. lean into the therapist's hands during therapeutic handling techniques?

4. fail to adjust the body in response to changes in position?

5. exhibit decreased, increased, or fluctuating postural tone?

6. grind his or her teeth? (Parham & Ecker, 2000)

Processing of Vestibular Input

Hyperresponsiveness to Gravity and/or Movement

Does the child:

1. object to being moved backward in space even when the trunk and head are supported?

2. express fear/anxiety when placed on the large therapy ball?

3. object to having the feet leave the supporting surface or the ground?

4. overreact when moved in space?

5. become fearful of bouncing or swinging? (Parham & Ecker, 2000)

6. dislike sudden or quick movement?

Hyporesponsiveness to Movement

Does the child:

1. enjoy being moved and/or rocked passively?

2. fail to increase extensor tone when linear movement is provided?

3. seek opportunities to fall without regard to his or her safety? (Dunn, 1999)

4. fail to notice or react when moved in space?

5. not seem to get dizzy when others usually do? (Parham & Ecker, 2000)

6. like to be roughhoused or moved with more intensity than other children?

7. enjoy being held upside down during play, even for short periods of time?

8. If the child has the motor abilities, does the child like to twirl and spin? or does he/she like to be twirled and spun passively?

A yes answer to any of these questions is suggestive of sensory processing deficits.

Note: Unless otherwise noted, questions in this list are adapted from *Combining neurodevelopmental treatment and sensory integration principles* (p. 45), by E. Blanche, T. Botticelli, and M. Hallway, 1995, Tucson, Arizona: Therapy Skill Builders. Copyright 1995 by Therapy Skill Builders. Adapted with permission.

Other assessments that are useful in identifying sensory processing disorders include the *Sensory Profile* (Dunn, 1999) and the *Sensory Integration and Praxis Tests* (SIPT; Ayres, 1989). When using the *Sensory Profile,* it is helpful to analyze the parent's answers to each question (raw data) in addition to focusing on the interpretation of the total score and section scores obtained from this assessment tool. The SIPT is of some use when testing children with mild forms of CP. Ayres included reports on 10 cases of children with CP when she first standardized the SIPT. This small group of children had low scores on most of the SIPT subtests. Some of the lower scores reported were on the tactile discrimination tests.

Sensory Systems

In reference to the assessment of individual sensory systems, with the exception of standardized assessment focusing on visual perception, there are few objective measurement tools that successfully evaluate specific tactile and kinesthetic processing in children, much less children with CP. Somatosensory examinations often are less useful with children with CP because these instruments rely on the children's processing verbal instructions and producing verbal responses, two areas in which this population can experience impairments. The areas most commonly evaluated by somatosensory tests are vibration, touch, pain, temperature, sharp-dull discrimination, texture discrimination, stereognosis, and two-point discrimination. Thibault, Forget, and Lambert (1994) evaluated the intrarater reliability with healthy children on four tests of tactile and proprioceptive processing: touch-pressure measurement with the Semmes Weinstein monofilaments, vibration perception with the tuning fork, thermal discrimination with the Minnesota Thermal Disks, and kinesthesis with the Bairstow and Laszlo instrument. Thibault et al. concluded that all four measurements were reliable and that clinicians could use them to test children with neuromotor disorders. On the other hand, because two-point discrimination and stereognosis are often affected when all other tactile functions exhibit impairment, many researchers choose to limit the sensory examination to these two tests (Yekutiel et al., 1994).

Evaluation of vestibular processing can also prove to be difficult. Practitioners traditionally evaluate vestibular functions with clinical observations of postural control, oculomotor control, and emotional responses to changes of body position relative to movement and gravity. However, the existing neuromotor disorder affects postural control and oculomotor control skills; consequently, the evaluation of processing vestibular input relies on careful observation of changes in level of arousal and emotional responses. Differentiating vestibular processing deficits (such as gravitational insecurity) from postural control deficits in the child with CP can be a complex task that requires that the examiner understand the child and the demands of the environment (Blanche et al., 1995). For example, a child who is anxious when moved backward on the large therapy ball even when he or she can adjust his or her position in response to the change in the supporting surface might be gravitationally insecure. However, under the same circumstances, a child who throws him- or herself back when postural control fails is not exhibiting signs of gravitational insecurity.

Motor Planning Disorders

Motor planning is the ability of the brain to conceive of, organize, and carry out a sequence of unfamiliar actions as necessary when learning new skills (Ayres, 1979). Evaluation of motor planning skills in children with CP is complex. Differentiating motor planning deficits from signs of a neuromotor disorder depends on discerning whether the motor control deficits that a child presents are due to the absence of movement components or the inability to utilize these movement components in a variety of novel situations. The absence of movement components can indicate a neuromotor dysfunction. The presence of a movement component the child uses in one situation but is unable to use in other similar but novel situations can indicate motor planning deficits. For example, a child who is unable to figure out how to get off a piece of equipment, even when he or she is able to climb onto it, might have motor planning problems. On the other hand, a child with spastic diplegia who is able to describe what his or her body needs to do to get off but cannot actually get on or off a piece of equipment independently might not have motor planning deficits.

Motor planning correlates closely to sensory processing in that it requires the ability to use feedback and feedforward loops when performing a novel motor act (Ayres, 1972; Fisher, 1991). Individuals use feedback mechanisms to correct motor actions and feedforward mechanisms prior to the reception of the peripheral feedback. Feedforward mechanisms utilize sensorimotor maps of previous interactions with the environment to anticipate the outcome of an action in the present (Bly, 1996). Feedback and feedforward mechanisms complement each other (Bly, 1996). Feedforward mechanisms generally function prior to the performance of the action, whereas feedback mechanisms provide the information about the action during or after its execution (Fisher, 1991). For the feedforward mechanisms to develop, the individual must have experienced and practiced a specifically related motor act in the past. Feedforward mechanisms require adequate processing of vestibular and proprioceptive input (Fisher, 1991) that operate, for example, in postural control and in planning interactions within the environment. According to Bly, the Bobaths empirically identified feedforward as postural preparations. Feedforward mechanisms also play a role in motor planning actions that require management of space and time. Feedforward mechanisms come into play when the individual needs to organize an action that requires speed, whereas feedback mechanisms operate in actions that require constant monitoring. In the clinic, the child who moves slowly and has difficulty anticipating the movements of an object in space (e.g., a ball) might have difficulty with feedforward mechanisms, therefore utilizing and relying more on feedback mechanisms to monitor most actions. Conversely, the child might have less access to feedback in addition to or instead of feedforward. The child who has difficulty with actions that do not require anticipating movement in space (e.g., climbing on a piece of equipment) also might have difficulties with feedback.

Children with CP often have impaired feedforward mechanisms with which to organize actions, because the mechanisms develop from atypical experiences of abnormal or compensatory movement patterns (Bly, 1996). In addition, not only do these children have abnormal feedback and feedforward mechanism experiences derived from the motor performance, they can also exhibit sensory processing deficits that further distort the feedback interpretation derived from the motor act. These sensory processing deficits also affect the feedback produced by the activities the child performs during the intervention session. Sensory processing deficits decrease the child's ability to use the sensory input to create and develop accurate motor programs that the child can later utilize as representations for actions. In other words, these children have feedback and feedforward mechanism deficits that are secondary to the motor deficits, as well as primary sensory processing disorders that might be as much the root of the motor dysfunctions as the neuromotor disorder itself. These sensory processing deficits often interfere with the child's ability to respond optimally to intervention geared to address the neuromotor deficit.

Bly (1996) suggests that therapists can utilize SI principles with the child who has CP to increase or decrease the sensory feedback. Specifically, clinicians can use SI with these children to address the sensory processing dysfunction underlying feedback/feedforward mechanisms and motor planning dysfunction (Blanche et al., 1995). Therefore, understanding SI principles can be useful when addressing the initial stages of learning new motor skills. When a child is learning a motor component, the therapist who understands SI principles can identify the child's sensory needs and provide meaningful sensory feedback. Once the child masters the skill's motor components, the child can string them together in the performance of novel tasks. For example, the types of sensory input that increase feedback include touch and proprioception through the use of resistance. When the child is learning novel tasks, the clinician can use SI to advance the child from slow and feedback-dependent execution to speed-dependent, active performance of motor-planned tasks.

It is possible to combine SI with neurodevelopmental treatment (NDT) principles during the intervention. NDT principles work best when working on feedback and feedforward mechanisms in postural sets or preparations. SI principles are most effective on feedback and feedforward mechanisms in motor planning actions with objects in space and time. In some cases, the child might have acquired the postural set and the movement components necessary for an action but cannot utilize these movement components in an action that requires motor planning.

In summary, the lack of valid and reliable assessment tools highlights the need for careful analysis of sensory processing skills in the child with CP. This careful analysis originates in a solid understanding of the neuromotor disorder and the sensory processing disorders underlying the child's functional limitations. See the list included in the section on Identification of Sensory Processing Disorders for a general guide to assessment of sensory processing disorders in children with CP.

Specific Sensory Processing Deficits Presented by Children With CP

It is possible to confuse neuromotor dysfunctions with the sensory processing and praxis impairments exhibited by children with CP. This section describes the specific sensory processing deficits and possible intervention strategies for children with CP, based on the literature review and the authors' clinical expertise. Table 16.1 provides a guideline of behaviors that suggest sensory processing impairments. Individual sensory processing impairments that can be masked by motor impairments are:

1. motor planning disorders observed in children with hemiplegia
2. sensory registration and/or modulation disorders affecting the response to intervention in children with spastic quadriplegia
3. gravitational insecurity increasing the functional limitations in children with spastic diplegia
4. sensory processing disorders associated with cerebellar ataxia
5. sensory processing disorders associated with athetosis
6. sensory processing disorders associated with hypotonia

Describing the SI and praxis dysfunction in connection with a specific classification of CP does not imply that these dysfunctions always coexist. Instead, the authors have linked the specific sensory processing and praxis disorders to the individual neuromotor classifications of CP because it is possible to confuse the sensory processing disorder these children present with the neuromotor limitations.

Table 16.1. Neuromotor and Related Sensory Processing Dysfunctions by Diagnostic Classifications of Cerebral Palsy

Diagnostic Classification	Neuromotor Limitations	Sensory Processing Deficits That May be Masked as Motor Deficits	Traditional Intervention of the Motor Dysfunction	Sensory-Based Principles to Apply To Intervention
Hemiplegia	• Unilateral movement disorder that affects both sides • Asymmetry of posture, movements • Bilateral coordination difficulties • Weakness in involved extremities, distal weakness	• Bilateral tactile and proprioceptive deficits that can contribute to severe praxis deficits • Sensory dormancy • Sensory defensiveness • Visual perceptual difficulties, particularly visuospatial relations	• Improve postural control • Increase symmetrical motor functions • Improve bilateral motor coordination • Increase weight-bearing and weight-shifting ability on the involved side • Strengthen the involved side	• Improve tactile discrimination • Increase registration and modulation of vestibular and proprioceptive sensory input • Interpret the speed of movement and timing of the motor act needed to respond to anticipated changes in the environment (projected action sequences) • Initiate movement sequences • Improve motor planning skills and organization of behavior in a larger spatiotemporal environment (see chapter 10 in this text)
Mild-moderate spastic quadriplegia	• Increased muscle tone throughout the entire body, UE more than LE • One side can have greater motor compromise than the other	• Sensory registration deficits (vestibular and proprioceptive sensory systems) • Sensory dormancy • Sometimes sensory modulation difficulty • Hyperresponse to tactile input • Tactile discrimination problems • Visual motor deficits	• Improve postural head control • Increase active/passive ROM • Increase ability to weight bear • Improve positioning and posture • Improve strength	• Improve registration of sensory input, particularly of vestibular/proprioceptive sensory input (e.g., intense swinging, work against gravity, joint compression) • Improve modulation of tactile input • Modulate state of arousal, which can affect muscle tone, focus and attention, emotional readiness, and intrinsic motivation to act on the environment • Address postural control and postural tone—primarily extensor tone and integration of oculomotor control—with head control and movement experiences
Spastic diplegia	• Bilateral movement disorder • Spasticity more evident in the lower extremities • Decreased postural tone and postural control in the trunk	**Vestibular processing disorders:** • Fear of movement, gravitational insecurity • Decreased response to linear vestibular input **Tactile processing disorders:** • Decreased or increased response to tactile input during handling • Tactile discrimination problems such as 2-point discrimination/stereognosis **Proprioceptive processing disorder:** • Delayed or decreased response to handling due to inadequate processing of proprioceptive input **Visual motor and nonmotor visual perceptual difficulties**	• Improve bilateral coordination • Increase active/passive ROM • Increase weight-bearing ability • Improve posture • Increase strength	• Increase registration/modulation of vestibular, tactile, and proprioceptive sensory input • Improve ability to tolerate movement and changes of position • Increase ability to tolerate variety of tactile input including during handling

Table 16.1. Neuromotor and Related Sensory Processing Dysfunctions by Diagnostic Classifications of Cerebral Palsy *(continued)*

Diagnostic Classification	Neuromotor Limitations	Sensory Processing Deficits That May be Masked as Motor Deficits	Traditional Intervention of the Motor Dysfunction	Sensory-Based Principles to Apply To Intervention
Ataxia	• Decreased stability in the trunk • Decreased postural tone • Wide base of support during ambulation • Poor balance • Poor co-contraction around joints	• Sensory registration deficits • Decreased proprioceptive and vestibular feedback from active movements • Sensory modulation difficulties of vestibular sensory input	• Strengthen trunk • Improve proximal stability • Improve balance • Improve midrange control	• Increase registration of sensory input, particularly of proprioceptive and vestibular sensory input • Facilitate attention and active participation and engagement in purposeful tasks and, ultimately, functional performance. • Improve motor planning skills and organization of behavior in a larger spatiotemporal environment (see chapter 10 in this text)
Athetosis	• Lack of stability in the trunk and the extremities • Use of atypical synergies (tonic reflexes) to obtain control • Decreased postural tone and postural control	• Decreased response to vestibular and proprioceptive input • Tactile processing deficits • Sensory modulation deficits	• Head/neck/trunk control • Weight bearing • Functional use of extremities • Decrease influence of reflexes • Improve head/neck/trunk control • Improve postural control • Increase strength/endurance • Improve modulation of sensory input	• Improve registration of vestibular/proprioception • Improve modulation of sensory input, particularly tactile sensory input • Hypotonia • Decreased head and trunk control • Decreased muscle tone throughout trunk and extremities • Poor co-contraction around joints • Generalized proprioceptive defensiveness often associated with generalized modulation difficulties of many sensory systems including tactile, vestibular, auditory, visual, gustatory, and/or olfactory • Can demonstrate extremes in arousal level, fluctuating between states of hypervigilence to coping by "shutting down" through sleeping

Spastic Hemiplegia and Motor Planning Disorders

Children with hemiplegia exhibit unilateral motor disorders that affect both sides of the body. These motor disorders influence ambulation and symmetrical use of the trunk and the upper extremities. Along with the motor dysfunction, children with hemiplegia often exhibit a variety of sensory processing disorders, including modulation and discrimination deficits. The intervention during the first years of life emphasizes motor development. However, after the child becomes an independent ambulator, some of the most functionally limiting conditions involve motor planning deficits and proprioceptive feedback contributing to problems with coordinated and smooth motor control. Motor planning deficits then affect a child's ability to negotiate obstacles in the environment, develop a variety of strategies to solve a task, time the motor action, and anticipate actions in space and time.

Many children with CP present motor planning disorders. However, these problems become more evident in children who exhibit less severe neuromotor deficits, such as children with hemiplegia. The literature seldom describes motor planning deficits in children with hemiplegia. However, the literature does report bilateral tactile and kinesthetic discrimination deficits (Bolanos, Bleck, Firestone, & Young, 1989). Because tactile and kinesthetic discrimination deficits tend to coexist with motor planning deficits (Ayres, 1972, 1985, 1989), it is possible that motor planning deficits exhibited by children with hemiplegia relate as much to the tactile processing disorder as to the neuromotor disorder.

It is important to address motor planning skills as soon as the child has gained control over the motor components of movement necessary to move independently through space. Initially, NDT or other intervention techniques that focus on the development of movement components are useful. SI theory can take a more important role in intervention as the child learns to utilize the movement components in tasks that require motor planning and the use of tools. The following case study is an example of a motor planning deficit that is common in children with hemiplegia.

Case Study: Motor Planning Disorder—Spastic Hemiplegia

Joe

Joe was a 6-year-old boy who was born 2 months prematurely weighing 4 pounds 4 ounces. Joe was found to have a right hemiplegia when he was 6 months old. From the age of 6 months until he was 18 months, he received weekly home-based occupational therapy utilizing primarily an NDT approach. He learned to walk at 18 months of age. At that point, therapists used a combination of both NDT and SI frames of reference to address Joe's needs.

Joe was shy, quiet, and distractible, yet cooperative and obedient. He rarely initiated an interaction with the environment. When he moved, his actions were clumsy and not timed adequately. He often tripped and bumped against the equipment. Joe became more disorganized when there were many children playing in the gym. In those situations, he appeared to freeze, unable to choose or engage in an activity. He usually waited for instructions on what to do or simply watched the other children play.

Joe's sensory processing deficits included decreased tactile discrimination skills, poor hand manipulation skills, and poor motor planning. He enjoyed games that provided moderately intense vestibular input, including rotary movement, but after awhile he appeared hyperresponsive to the movement.

Joe evidenced motor planning difficulties in his difficulty with multistep activities, both within a gross motor context such as negotiating an obstacle course as well as in a fine motor context such as completing a simple craft. It was easier for him to perform multistep activities if there was at least one familiar step within the motor sequence, the therapist facilitated his movements, he received verbal instructions for each step, or he could model another child. And even when Joe had mastered all the movement components necessary to perform a motor task, he was unable to duplicate and combine the same movement components to perform another purposeful sequence.

Occupational therapy focused on addressing the sensory processing needs that seemed to contribute to difficulties with organizing behavior and maintaining an optimal level of arousal. The intervention sessions included activities that provided tactile, vestibular, and proprioceptive experiences, such as moving through tight spaces, swinging, resisted movement, and applied joint compression techniques. These activities had the purpose of increasing Joe's level of arousal, attention to task, and awareness of his body in space. Joe improved markedly in his ability to stay focused on the task at hand. Within 6 months, he initiated actions more frequently, contributed to the organization of motor mazes, and negotiated more than half of the steps of a multistep task independently.

The therapist added weight to a thumb abductor splint to give Joe increased sensory feedback from that hand and to position his thumb for fine motor activities. Hand manipulation skills, particularly bilateral tasks, improved proportionately with his ability to grasp with his more involved right hand. The tactile and proprioceptive input provided in the intervention appeared to increase the use of his right hand as a spontaneous assist.

Although Joe remained a shy child, he demonstrated more self-confidence. He was independent in most aspects of self-care, including managing clothing fastenings (such as buttons) and tying his shoes. He used his right hand as a spontaneous stabilizer for such activities as cutting with scissors, pulling off marker tops, opening zippered plastic lunch bags, and opening and inserting the straw of boxed drinks. Most importantly, he was more physically spontaneous and more willing to participate in group activities with his friends. For the first time in his life, he started participating in sports, including soccer and swimming, broadening his recreational options and social opportunities.

Spastic Quadriplegia and Generalized Registration Deficits

Traditionally, the intervention techniques clinicians have used with children with CP have focused on the facilitation of movement through handling. The success of such handling relies in part on the child's intact feedback mechanism. Facilitation through handling is useful in the initial stages of treating young children with severe neuromotor deficits, because these children have difficulties obtaining and sustaining postural control or initiating movement independently. In recent years, the emphasis on facilitation and the use of feedback has shifted to the use of feedforward mechanisms and the need to encourage the initiation of active or proactive movement (Bly, 1996). However, encouraging proactive movement requires motivation to act on the environment, which is often limited or absent in children who exhibit poor registration of sensory input (sensory dormancy). Consequently, identifying overall decreased arousal level and sensory dormancy becomes pivotal in the intervention of movement dysfunction.

Sensory dormancy is present in children with a variety of neuromotor disorders. Children with CP with mild to moderate spastic quadriplegia, who might or might not be able to ambulate independently, often manifest sensory dormancy. This poor registration of sensory input affects the child's functional and interactive abilities in the motor, cognitive, and socioemotional areas. Sensory defensiveness might or might not be part of the clinical picture.

It is common for children who exhibit generalized decreased sensation and decreased arousal level to seek tactile, proprioceptive, and vestibular experiences. Children with mild quadriplegia who also exhibit sensory dormancy similarly need the same input. Because of the physical limitations, they sometimes do not seek this input appropriately, which requires the clinician to take a more active role in providing input. A general guideline for the therapist providing proprioceptive input is to observe the child's tonal fluctuations after the activity. Although spasticity and atypical posturing tend to increase during active resistive movements with these children, increased resistance and bombardment of somatosensory input tend to decrease the posturing of upper extremities and increase the active functional engagement of the upper extremities.

When one views the dysfunctional movement pattern presented by these children primarily as a *movement disorder,* the decreased patterning response to the intervention seems unusual. However, if one considers the dysfunctional movement pattern as primarily a sensory processing disorder affecting overall level of arousal, increased active use of the upper extremities might be an expected result of increased sensory experiences. It is possible that the increased tone and posturing sometimes observed in these children might be an attempt to gain proprioceptive awareness of that part of the body. Providing input reduces this need, which produces a decrease as well in the tone and posturing. An additional hypothesis combining motor and sensory-based explanations suggests that the added sensory input increases the proximal tone in the trunk, thereby decreasing the need for increasing muscle tone by fixing distally.

For example, Chris, a 5-year-old boy who had received primarily traditional occupational therapy and physical therapy intervention, often engaged spontaneously in a game in which he threw himself back onto some pillows from a standing position. The therapist, realizing that Chris was probably seeking sensory input, incorporated increased sensory input into the intervention. Encouraging Chris to push himself on the floor while prone on the hammock swing produced elongation between the scapula and humerus, facilitated by upper extremity traction and weight bearing. In similar cases in which the child receives massive amounts of deep pressure and proprioception (such as when rolling down an incline, bouncing on a ball, or sliding down a ramp), the posturing of the motorically more involved upper extremity often decreases.

In summary, one important contribution of SI to the intervention of the child with CP is in helping to discover the child's best sensory channels through which to modulate optimally the level of arousal and function. By providing input through the appropriate sensory channels for that child, sensory processing can contribute significantly to the intervention success of children with CP, intervention traditionally concerned with, for example, postural control, muscle tone, and function.

Case Study: Generalized Sensory Registration Disorder—Spastic Quadriplegia

Raul

Raul was born after a 26-week gestation with a birth weight of 1 pound, 11 ounces. Raul required 2 months of ventilator support for bronchopulmonary dysplasia. A neurological examination revealed brisk reflexes and increased tone of all four extremities. His difficulties were diagnosed as delayed motor development secondary to CP and spastic quadriparesis, and he went home to the care of his parents when he was almost 3 months of age. Intervention utilizing an NDT approach began when he was 6 months old. By 13 months of age, he was not sitting, rolling over, or lifting his head in prone.

By the time Raul was 4 years of age, he was able to sit in a chair with a posterior pelvic tilt but was unable to move into or out of it. When presented with activities, Raul tended to increase traction of the upper extremity flexors, which made smooth bilateral movements difficult. Raul displayed very little motivation to move or to challenge himself. He would often collapse and whine, appearing helpless.

The greatest challenge for the therapists working with Raul was to obtain and maintain his attention and to procure his cooperation at each step of a task. Even when the intervention environment was modified to limit distractions (e.g., intervention in isolated rooms, glasses with peripheral blinders), keeping Raul focused was extremely difficult.

Raul's parents' primary concern for their son was that he be able to ambulate functionally and independently with a walker and be more independent in dressing. Continuing an NDT approach seemed appropriate in meeting these goals to help Raul maintain proper posture and to improve his mobility and quality of movement. The therapists soon realized that Raul's inability to attend and focus hindered progress in developing skills in functional activities. Because Raul did not appear aware of movement, the therapist incorporated rigorous vestibular input to the intervention regimen at the beginning of each session. Raul loved the movement. It enhanced his alertness and therefore his ability to cooperate with the functional aspects of his intervention session. Although Raul's initial response to this sensory input was an increase in abnormal flexor patterning of extremities, the therapist positioned him appropriately so she could continue to include movement in his intervention.

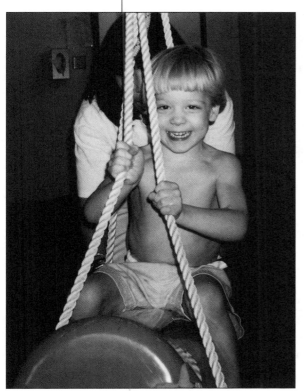

Figure 16.1. Positioning the child while providing proprioceptive and vestibular input that can influence postural alignment, visual attention, and arousal level.

Combining the NDT approach (focusing on decreasing abnormal posturing) with an SI approach (focusing on facilitating appropriate arousal level) continued to be a balancing challenge. Over time, as Raul was able to cooperate better with the instructions the therapist gave during the intervention, atypical patterns decreased. Facilitation and physical support while Raul was on a moving swing provided both proprioceptive and vestibular input. This resulted in improved postural alignment and mobility, a decrease in the frequency and intensity of muscular traction, and improved visual attention and arousal level (Figure 16.1). These skills set the foundation from which to build specific skills such as functional ambulation and self-dressing.

Spastic Diplegia and Gravitational Insecurity

The motor disorders that children with spastic diplegia typically present include spasticity more evident in the lower extremities, decreased postural tone, poor postural control in the trunk, and a bilateral movement disorder. Most children with spastic diplegia exhibit signs of atypical sensory processing abilities that often influence functional performance. Tactile processing dysfunctions in two-point discrimination and stereognosis frequently occur. Children with spastic diplegia often exhibit visual perception deficits as well.

Closely related to visual perception of space is the child's ability to integrate visual, proprioceptive, and vestibular information necessary to feel comfortable and safe while moving or being moved in space. Some children with spastic diplegia exhibit difficulties in integrating these sensory experiences and do not respond typically to intervention approaches designed to address the neuromotor disorder by imposing movement. These children have a tendency to avoid moving out of the midline, exhibit increased postural tone in the shoulder girdle and neck area, have increased trunk flexion, and can become anxious when the therapist or caregiver facilitates movement. Such children sometimes prefer to be placed in sitting rather than in supine or prone, and they either avoid the standing position or stand in a noncorrectable crouched position with a tendency to fix for stability rather than use active extension against gravity. Frequently, practitioners attribute these tendencies to the neuromotor disorder. However, in some cases, sensory modulation deficits contribute significantly to the disorder or can even be the root of the disorder.

The sensory processing deficits underlying the above-mentioned difficulties include gravitational insecurity (GI) and/or hyporesponsiveness to proprioceptive and vestibular input. GI is an excessive level of anxiety and distress caused by inadequate modulation or inhibition of sensations from gravity receptors of the vestibular system (Ayres, 1979) and/or a perceived threat from vestibular and proprioceptive sensory input or position in space (Fisher, 1991). GI increases the child's tendency to avoid moving away from the midline or center of gravity. The child with GI prefers to sit, lie down, or stand.

In an attempt to gain control, the child with GI tends to decrease the degrees of freedom of movement by fixing proximally, which can result in increased maintained elevation of the shoulders and maintained co-contraction of the shoulder girdle musculature. This pattern of fixing increases muscle tension and proprioceptive feedback.

It is possible to interpret the sensory processing disorder underlying this fixing pattern as decreased control over movement and treat it as a movement problem. In such a scenario, the therapist would facilitate the child's movements, creating a more threatening situation for the child. In these cases, in an attempt to avoid the lack of control created by the imposed movement, the child would increase muscle tension and, in time, slowly reduce the available repertoire of movement even more. Therapists can confuse this increased muscle tension with spasticity and lack of motor control.

In addition, during the intervention, the clinician might place the child on surfaces high off the ground to facilitate movement, thus creating an even more challenging situation. Frequently, when the child is close to the ground, he or she utilizes a greater variety of movement components and/or greater range of movement that do not appear to be available when the child is farther away from the ground.

Successful intervention approaches incorporate linear vestibular and proprioceptive input. For example, when a child is bouncing on a ball with both feet firmly planted on the floor, there is an observable decrease in fixing patterns. Vibration and shaking also can contribute to a decrease in fixing and an active use of available components of movement.

Case Study: Gravitational Insecurity—Spastic Diplegia

Matt

Matt was born prematurely and was referred for physical and occupational therapy at 18 months of age, soon after receiving a diagnosis of CP, spastic diplegia. His parents described him as an irritable child who was often difficult to console. Matt was beginning to pull himself to stand, and by 22 months, he was walking. Flexion patterns dominated much of his posture and extremities, with the hips also adducted and internally rotated and ankles in valgus. During therapy sessions, use of the therapy ball or suspended equipment to strengthen his truck and facilitate appropriate weight bearing and weight shifting caused Matt to become quite distressed, which increased proximal fixing. He also refused to play on any equipment that was unstable and did not want to climb or be lifted onto even stable therapeutic structures. Learning to dress himself was particularly hard. He had trouble crossing his arms to pull his shirt sleeve and tended to fix proximally at the shoulder girdle when his weight shifted during pants dressing.

Early in the intervention process, Matt avoided the use of suspended or moving equipment unless fully supported. His progress was slow. Over time, the intervention expanded to include grounded vestibular input or a combination of vestibular and proprioceptive sensory input (pushing himself while prone in the hammock swing or on the scooter board, rolling himself prone over the top of a slowly moving barrel, riding a therapy ball with handles). He began to tolerate weight-bearing activities while on suspended equipment, especially when combined with proprioceptive sensory input and linear movement. He especially liked tandem bouncing on the therapy ball with handles, which resulted in decreased proximal fixing. Trunk rotation and frequency of spontaneous crossing of midline increased. Bilateral and functional hand use improved, as well as ease with dressing and writing, thus increasing his self-confidence and interest in completing tasks independently. Intrinsic motivation replaced gravitational insecurity as the influential factor directing physical and occupational therapy goals and the intervention. Matt's willingness to cooperate with other difficult tasks also increased, thereby proportionately influencing the breadth and rate of his progress overall.

Cerebellar Ataxia and Vestibular/ Proprioceptive Processing Disorders

The motor disorders exhibited by children with ataxia include decreased stability in the trunk, decreased postural tone, and the need for a wide base of support during ambulation. The sensory deficits include decreased proprioceptive feedback during movements.

Some children with ataxia also present with registration and modulation deficits that often impose greater functional limitations than the motor disorders associated with the ataxia. The sensory processing disorders in children with ataxia can affect interaction and movement in space or coexist with other diagnoses such as Autistic Disorder.

When the intervention focuses too much on the facilitation of motor control, these children learn to rely on external facilitation rather than to utilize their own intrinsic need to move. In some cases it is necessary to prompt them with a proprioceptive and tactile cue to initiate the action. Once they have initiated the action, they are able to complete it independently, suggesting that the motor control to carry over the activity is there. The therapist needs to assess these children's dependence on facilitation or external prompting to initiate the movement, and communicate to adults and caregivers about the importance of diminishing this overdependence.

Case Study: Registration/Modulation of Vestibular/Proprioceptive Disorder—Ataxia

Helen

Helen, 3½ years old, had an evaluation at the school where she attended an integrated special preschool day class. The evaluation described her muscle tone as low. She was able to sit in a regular chair at the table with assistance to stay seated.

Helen used her left hand primarily but not exclusively. Grasp on the pencil was awkward (palmar, too high), with only a beginning inclusion of fingers in the grasp and poor grading of pressure (increased). She was unable to use regular scissors, preferring to use those that were spring-loaded. Helen had difficulty with coordinated muscle activation, proximal stability, and midrange control. Standing balance was poor, although she was able to walk independently. She required some assistance on uneven surfaces and when maneuvering around a challenging environment such as a cluttered room or a playground with children running around. She was able to pick up objects from the floor by holding onto the table or wall and locking her knees.

Helen appeared to have trouble with sensory registration of somatosensory and vestibular input. She often dropped items she was holding in her hand, especially if offered something else or while reaching for another object when she already had something in each hand. She did not demonstrate tactile defensiveness and enjoyed playing with play dough and finger paint and getting messy. When given an opportunity to swing, Helen became quite anxious and was comfortable swinging only when sitting in an adult's lap.

During intervention, Helen wore a weighted vest and the SPIO lycra compression garment (Hylton & Allen, 1997) to increase deep pressure and proprioceptive input. Both approaches, combined with weight-bearing and heavy work activities, helped to increase proximal stability of the trunk. On the days that she did not wear the compression garment, she fell more often. Within 6 months of the initiation of therapy, Helen had made many gains. She pushed and pulled herself while standing on a platform swing and engaged in more challenging tasks. For example, she was able to swing independently while throwing beanbags at a target.

At one point, Helen began to seek proprioception with fine motor tasks by engaging in activities that provided proprioceptive input, such as rolling play dough with a rolling pin, squeezing clothes pins, and pulling apart locked toys. Fine motor planning improved. The parents purchased both the weighted vest and Neoprene pants, which she wore at school. After 6 months of intervention, her teacher reported that Helen was more physically active and confident and appeared to be more autonomous in initiating interaction with her peers.

Athetosis and Registration Disorder of Proprioceptive/Vestibular Input

Children with athetoid CP exhibit decreased stability in the trunk and the extremities, decreased postural tone and postural control, and poorly coordinated movements. They tend to use atypical synergies of movement, including tonic reflexes, to obtain control. Children with athetosis often respond well to increased amounts of vestibular, tactile, and proprioceptive input, suggesting sensory processing disorders in these areas.

Case Study: Registration Disorder of Proprioceptive/Kinesthetic and Vestibular Sensory Input—Athetosis

Bobby

Bobby had received extensive occupational and physical therapy intervention since infancy. At 5 years of age, Bobby was totally dependent for all needs. He did not have adequate head or trunk control to sit without support or to move independently. He was very bright, with at least age-level receptive language ability but severely limited expressive language ability. Bobby communicated "yes" by raising his eyes and "no" by shaking his head. Self-initiated communication with others included only prolonged eye contact ("I want to tell you something," "I want your attention") and crying ("I do not like this," "I am frustrated").

Poorly coordinated movements hindered Bobby's ability to use his hands functionally for any activity. He preferred to have his upper extremities firmly secured (e.g., in the troughs of his wheelchair) to control extraneous movements. His supports in the wheelchair included head support, shoulder straps, lateral trunk supports, a hip stabilizer, and feet secured to the foot rests.

At first, independence in mobility and communication were the functional priorities in Bobby's intervention. Bobby, who was eager to be independent, worked very hard during the intervention session. He made steady but slow progress with a traditional intervention approach. His rate of progress changed, however, when his therapist realized that Bobby participated in several family outings that included intense sensory input. Bobby's father, an avid recreational athlete, frequently used adapted equipment to take Bobby water skiing and downhill snow skiing. Bobby's family described him as a "thrill seeker."

The therapist introduced intense sensory input to Bobby's intervention. For example, in the clinic, intense swinging successfully facilitated head/trunk control and encouraged weight bearing over upper extremities (Figure 16.2). In addition, Bobby wore a tight-fitting neoprene suit during his therapy sessions to add deep pressure and proprioceptive input. The increased pressure and resistance that the suit offered increased Bobby's head and postural

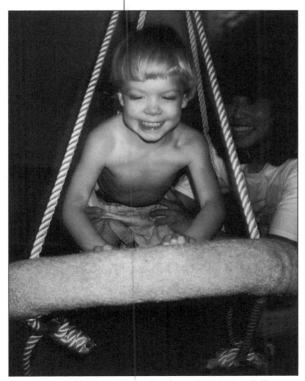

Figure 16.2. Riding a platform swing while weight bearing over the upper extremities.

control and decreased proximal and distal extraneous movements. The impact functionally was dramatic as he became able to maneuver himself independently in a trunk-supported walker and activate the hand controls on a motorized wheelchair, and began using a head wand to press the keys on a computer. In Bobby's case, it was obvious that the added input helped him organize his movements and attain some of the functional goals.

Hypotonia and Generalized Proprioceptive Defensiveness

Some children with hypotonia also experience sensory defensiveness that often goes unrecognized. Sensory defensiveness has a greater impact in these children because it includes the proprioceptive system. Such children will demonstrate proprioceptive defensiveness when they are placed in weight-bearing positions or when adults move their joints passively. Under these conditions, children sometimes exhibit distress and intolerance to the stimulus. This extreme form of defensiveness can be part of an over-all defensiveness pattern. Children who exhibit proprioceptive sensitivity often calm down with linear vestibular input as long as their body parts are not moved in relation to each other. They also sometimes exhibit poor interactive skills, although the neuromotor impairment often receives the most attention.

Case Study: Generalized Proprioceptive Defensiveness—Hypotonia

Kyle

Kyle began occupational therapy intervention when he was 18 months old. The initial visits in his home consisted of the therapist sitting in one room while a distressed Kyle and his mother sat in another. Kyle demonstrated extreme sensory defensiveness of tactile, vestibular, auditory, and proprioceptive input. Occupational therapy intervention gradually improved his ability to accept sensory input, including playing in the beans, swinging if positioned securely, and shaking rattles. He continued to resist any activity in the prone position or with his feet on the ground when the therapist provided facilitation so Kyle could gain control over his movements.

Around his sixth birthday, Kyle's weight-bearing tolerance suddenly increased, along with progress in gross motor development. By the time Kyle turned 7 years of age, he was taking facilitated steps with a walker. His therapist began to set more advanced goals to utilize this added proprioceptive tolerance in fine motor development, particularly with tools such as a spoon and crayons.

Summary and Conclusions

Children with CP and other impairments in neuromotor functions often exhibit concurrent sensory processing dysfunctions that sometimes impose greater limitations than the neuromotor disorder. These impairments in sensory processing and praxis can masquerade as impairments in the neuromotor system. The descriptions of the most common combinations of neuromotor and sensory processing disorders in this chapter are by no means an exhaustive list. SI intervention techniques for children with CP can affect the following components of behavior and movement:

- arousal level, which can affect muscle tone, focus and attention, emotional readiness, and intrinsic motivation to act on the environment

- postural control and postural tone, primarily extensor tone and integration of oculomotor control with head control and movement experiences

- interpretation of the speed of movement and timing of the motor act needed to respond to anticipated changes in the environment (projected action sequences)

- initiation of movement sequences
- motor planning skills in a larger spatiotemporal environment (see chapter 10 in this volume, Praxis and the Organization of Behavior in Time and Space, by Blanche & Parham)
- active participation and engagement in purposeful tasks and, ultimately, functional performance

References

Ayres, J. (1972). *Sensory integration and learning disorders.* Los Angeles: Western Psychological Services.

Ayres, J. (1979). *Sensory integration and the child.* Los Angeles: Western Psychological Services.

Ayres, J. (1985). *Developmental dyspraxia and adult-onset apraxia.* Torrance, CA: Sensory Integration International.

Ayres, J. (1989). *Sensory Integration and Praxis Tests.* Los Angeles: Western Psychological Services.

Baranek, G., & Berkson, G. (1994). Tactile defensiveness in children with developmental disabilities: Responsiveness and habituation. *Journal of Autism and Developmental Disorders, 24(4),* 457–471.

Blanche, E., Botticelli, T., & Hallway, M. (1995). *Combining neurodevelopmental treatment and sensory integration principles.* Tucson, AZ: Therapy Skill Builders.

Blanche, E., & Burke, J. (1991). Combining neurodevelopmental and sensory integration approaches in the treatment of the neurologically impaired child: Parts 1 and 2. *Sensory Integration International Quarterly, 19(2),* 1–6.

Bly, L. (1996). What is the role of sensation in motor learning? What is the role of feedback and feedforward? *Neurodevelopmental Treatment Association Network, 5(5),* 1–7.

Bolanos, A., Bleck, D., Firestone, P., & Young, L. (1989). Comparison of stereognosis and two-point discrimination testing of the hands of children with cerebral palsy. *Developmental Medicine and Child Neurology, 31,* 371–376.

Cooper, J., Majnemer, A., Rosenblatt, B., & Birnbaum, R. (1995). The determination of sensory deficits in children with hemiplegic cerebral palsy. *Journal of Child Neurology, 10(4),* 300–309.

DeGangi, G. (1990a, January). Perspectives on the integration of neurodevelopmental treatment and sensory integrative therapy, Part 1. *Neurodevelopmental Treatment Association Newsletter,* 1–4.

DeGangi, G. (1990b, March). Perspectives on the integration of neurodevelopmental treatment and sensory integrative therapy, Part 2. *Neurodevelopmental Treatment Association Newsletter,* 1–6.

DeGangi, G. (1990c, May). Perspectives on the integration of neurodevelopmental treatment and sensory integrative therapy, Part 3. *Neurodevelopmental Treatment Association Newsletter,* 1–5.

Dellon, A.L. (1997). *Somatosensory testing and rehabilitation.* Rockville, MD: American Occupational Therapy Association.

Dunn, W. (1999). *Sensory Profile.* San Antonio, TX: Therapy Skill Builders.

Dunn, W., & Westman, K. (1997). The Sensory Profile: The performance of a national sample of children without disabilities. *American Journal of Occupational Therapy, 51(1),* 25–34.

Eliasson A.C., Gordon A., & Forssberg, H. (1991). Basic co-ordination of manipulative forces of children with cerebral palsy. *Developmental Medicine and Child Neurology, 33,* 661–670.

Eliasson, A.C., Gordon, A., & Forssberg, H. (1995). Tactile control of isometric fingertip forces during grasping in children with cerebral palsy. *Developmental Medicine and Child Neurology, 37,* 72–84.

Fiorentino, M. (1966). The changing dimension of occupational therapy. *American Journal of Occupational Therapy, 20,* 251–252.

Fisher, A. (1991). Vestibular-proprioceptive processing and bilateral integration and sequencing deficits. In A.G. Fisher, E.A. Murray, & A.C. Bundy (Eds.), *Sensory integration: Theory and practice* (pp. 71–107). Philadelphia: F.A. Davis.

Hylton, N., & Allen, C. (1997). The development and use of SPIO Lycra compression bracing in children with neuromotor deficits. *Pediatric Rehabilitation, 1*(2),109–116.

Kenney, W.E. (1963). Certain sensory defects in cerebral palsy. *Clinical Orthopedics 27,* 193–195.

Lesny, I., Stehlik, A., Tomasek, J., Tomankova, A., & Havlicek, I. (1993). Sensory disorders in cerebral palsy: Two-point discrimination. *Developmental Medicine and Child Neurology, 35,* 402–405.

Moore, J. (1984, May). The neuroanatomy and pathology of cerebral palsy. In *Selected Proceedings from the Barbro Salek Memorial Symposium,* 3–60.

New York City Occupational Therapists. (1953). Feeding suggestions for the training of the cerebral palsied. *The American Journal of Occupational Therapy, 7*(5), 199–204.

New York City Occupational Therapists. (1954). Dressing techniques for the cerebral palsied child. *The American Journal of Occupational Therapy, 8*(1), 8–11.

Parham, J.D., & Ecker, C. (2000). *Evaluation of Sensory Processing (ESP-V4).* Unpublished manuscript.

Robinault, I.P. (1953). Occupational therapy techniques for the preschool hemiplegic— Toys and training. *The American Journal of Occupational Therapy, 7*(5), 205–207.

Robinault, I.P. (1954). Perception techniques for the preschool cerebral palsied. *The American Journal of Occupational Therapy, 8*(1), 3–7.

Sugden, D.A., & Keogh, J.F. (1990). Cerebral palsy. In H.G. Williams (Ed.), *Problems in movement skills development: Growth, motor development and physical activity across the life span* (pp. 1–39). Columbia, SC: University of South Carolina Press.

Thibault, A., Forget, R., & Lambert, J. (1994). Evaluation of cutaneous and proprioceptive sensation in children: A reliability study. *Developmental Medicine and Child Neurology, 36,* 796–812

Van Heest, A.E., House, J., & Putnam, M. (1993). Sensibility deficiencies in the hands of children with spastic hemiplegia. *The Journal of Hand Surgery, 18*(2), 278–281.

Wann, J. (1991). The integrity of visual-proprioceptive mapping in cerebral palsy. *Neuropsychologia, 29*(11), 1095–1106.

Windsor, M.M. (1986). Incorporating sensory integration principles into treatment of children with cerebral palsy. *American Occupational Therapy Association Developmental Disabilities Special Interest Section Newsletter, 9,* 3–4.

Yekutiel, M., Jariwala, M., & Stretch, P. (1994). Sensory deficits in the hands of children with cerebral palsy: A new look at assessment and prevalence. *Developmental Medicine and Child Neurology, 36,* 619–624.

Zimmerman, M.E. (1957). Analysis of adapted equipment. *The American Journal of Occupational Therapy, 11*(4), 229–235.

Sensory Integrative Principles in Intervention With Children With Autistic Disorder

Zoe Mailloux, M.A., OTR, FAOTA

Autistic Disorder has gained attention over the past 20 years as scientific discoveries advance knowledge of it. The *Diagnostic and Statistical Manual* (fourth edition) (*DSM-IV*; American Psychiatric Association, 1994) includes Autistic Disorder in the diagnostic category of Pervasive Developmental Disorders (PDD). The PDD category includes four other related disorders in addition to Autistic Disorder: Rett's Disorder, Childhood Disintegrative Disorder, and Asperger's Disorder, as well as PDD-NOS (not otherwise specified), a classification for individuals who display some but not all of the characteristics of Autistic Disorder. Although each of these specific diagnoses involves defining characteristics, Autistic Disorder is the most common of the diagnoses under the PDD classification and the most widely recognized.

Definitions and Incidence

Professionals consider Autistic Disorder a *spectrum disorder,* meaning that the symptoms can vary from mild to severe and the behaviors that accompany Autistic Disorder appear very different among individuals who share this diagnosis. The reported incidence varies; the current numbers from the Center for Disease Control are up to $2/1000$ (Boyle, Bertrand, & Yeargin-Allsop, 1999). The diagnosis of Autistic Disorder is applicable when there is evidence of problems in social interactions and communication or when stereotyped patterns of behavior exist. Specifically, at least 6 of the following 12 symptoms must be present for an individual to qualify for a diagnosis of Autistic Disorder, with at least 2 symptoms from the social interaction category and 1 each from the communication and stereotyped patterns of behavior areas.

Social interaction deficits:
- marked impairment of nonverbal behaviors
- failure to develop age-appropriate peer relationships
- lack of spontaneous seeking to share interests and achievements with others
- lack of social or emotional reciprocity

Communication deficits:
- delay in or lack of spoken language
- marked impairment in conversational skills in verbal individuals
- stereotyped and repetitive use of language
- lack of spontaneous age-appropriate pretend or social imitative play

continued on p. 366

Current Research

In considering Autistic Disorder from a sensory integrative perspective, it is helpful to examine the current research findings on the neurologic underpinnings of Autistic Disorder and on the effects of deficits in imitation and planning of action. Autopsy studies (Bauman, 1991; Bauman & Kemper, 1994; Kemper & Bauman, 1993) have provided important insights about anatomical abnormalities in individuals with Autistic Disorder. These researchers have found consistent abnormalities in the number and size of cells within the limbic system, particularly in the amygdala and hippocampus. The amygdala is responsible for many aspects of emotion and behavior, and the hippocampus participates significantly in learning and memory. Bauman and Kemper (1994) reviewed previous studies showing that damage to the amygdala correlates to withdrawal from social contact; compulsive, indiscriminate association of objects; decreased ability to attach meaning to situations; poor eye contact; increased temper tantrums in novel situations; and changes in responsivity to sensory stimuli. Hippocampal damage results in hyperactivity, stereotyped behavior, and difficulty with novel stimuli. Both structures appear necessary for memory, in particular, declarative or representational memory that involves processing sensory information, facts, and previous experiences in order to generalize and integrate information for learning. In a study comparing neuropsychological task performance by children with Autistic Disorder to children with Down syndrome and children who were developing typically, Dawson, Meltzoff, Osterling, and Rinaldi (1998) also found evidence of involvement in the medial temporal lobe and related structures of the limbic system. Of particular note was their finding that specific tasks associated with rule learning linked to amygdala and hippocampal functions correlated highly with all symptom domains for the children with Autistic Disorder but not for the two comparison groups.

Autopsy studies (Bauman & Kemper, 1994) and magnetic resonance imaging (MRI) studies (Courchesne, 1987, 1989, 1991) have demonstrated the presence of abnormalities in the cerebellum in individuals with Autistic Disorder, although there are differences in the specific abnormalities found on autopsy versus MRI. Courchesne and his colleagues suggested that the cerebellar abnormalities present in Autistic Disorder might interfere with the ability to shift attention in an efficient manner (Courchesne et al., 1993). Bauman and Kemper (1994) postulated that cerebellar abnormalities play a role in modulation of emotions, mental imagery, anticipatory planning, some aspects of attention, and some aspects of language processing. Their research also revealed specific damage to the posterior inferior region of the cerebellum, which has direct connections to the vestibular system, although the vestibular apparatus itself did not appear to be impaired (Bauman, 1996). This finding might be especially relevant to the role of the cerebellum in providing inhibitory input to brainstem structures (Kandel, Schwartz, & Jessell, 1995). Atypical inhibition might be involved in oversensitivity to

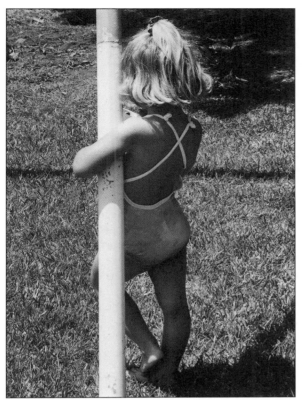

Photo by Shay McAtee.

Figure 17.1 Children with Autistic Disorder often show early signs of deficits in sensory processing and social responsivity.

certain sensory input, such as stimulation of the gravity receptors. Other important findings by Kemper and Bauman (1993) include evidence that the neurologic abnormalities found in individuals with Autistic Disorder occur prior to 30 weeks gestation. These results suggest that the predisposition for Autistic Disorder develops prior to birth and lend support to early intervention, when there is the greatest potential for influencing developing neural structures.

Research exploring deficits in imitation, arousal, and attention in relation to problems in social interaction and communication also have contributed to understanding Autistic Disorder from a sensory integration perspective. Dawson and her colleagues (Dawson, 1988; Dawson & Adams, 1984; Dawson & Lewy, 1989a, 1989b) proposed that the neurologic deficits present in Autistic Disorder are associated closely with the observed impairments in imitation, arousal, and social responsiveness. In a similar track, Smith and Bryson (1994) suggested that problems in imitation in individuals with Autistic Disorder are part of an information-processing deficit rather than a social dysfunction. They suggested further analysis of "nonsocial limitations on the autistic individual's ability to act and to comprehend actions of others" (p. 270).

In a retrospective study of home videotapes of children who later received diagnoses of Autistic Disorder, Baranek (1999) found early signs of dysfunction in visual orientation/attention, response to name, mouthing of objects, and social touch aversion. These findings suggested that children with Autistic Disorder show early indications of atypical sensory processing and social responsivity (Figure 17.1).

Research specific to the relationship between sensory processing and social skills, including imitation, has used the *Sensory Integration and Praxis Tests* (SIPT; Ayres, 1989) with matched samples of children with and without Autistic Disorder (Parham, Mailloux, & Smith Roley, 2000). The children with Autistic Disorder in this study demonstrated significantly low scores on all tests of praxis, as well as poor tactile, vestibular, and proprioceptive sensory processing compared to children who were developing typically. The children with Autistic Disorder had particular difficulty with the SIPT Oral Praxis subtest, which requires imitation of mouth and facial movements. Parham et al. hypothesized that the implications of these sensory disorders and motor planning deficits include an impact on social skill and the development ability to function in a social arena. That is, poor sensory processing associated with impaired motor planning abilities in children with Autistic Disorder might be a link between their problems in imitation and related social reciprocity. For example, problems with oral praxis might explain the difficulty some individuals with Autistic Disorder have in interpreting facial expressions and gestures. Inability to perceive somatosensory feedback from facial and oral structures adequately and, in turn, limited ability to formulate the often-subtle motor plans that enable facial expression severely limit the basis for social exchange from a very early age. This conclusion is consistent with the following explanation offered by Dawson et al. (1998).

Children with autism have difficulty imitating the motor actions of others, especially deferred imitation. A failure to participate in social imitative interactions may preclude the development of other social skills, such as social reciprocity and empathy. (p. 1283)

Relevance of Sensory Integrative Theory to Autistic Disorder

In chapter 1, Spitzer and Roley present Ayres' view of the importance of multisensory integration and discuss her use of the term *sensory alchemy* to describe the process of experiencing and interpreting a variety of sensations as a means for feeling safe and comfortable, for learning about the world, and for forming an effective view of oneself. Their examples of obstacles faced by children with developmental disabilities in participating in the typical sensory experiences of childhood are particularly relevant for the child with Autistic Disorder. Dr. Ayres was acutely aware of the applicability of sensory integrative theory to the diagnosis of Autistic Disorder. As professionals began to understand this disorder better during the 1970s, Ayres (1979) clearly described the sensory disorders accompanying Autistic Disorder. The sections that follow address the application of sensory integration concepts to occupational therapy for the child with Autistic Disorder, reviewing the presenting problems and considering the assessment, intervention, and community integration aspects of practice.

Presenting Problems

Difficulty in registration of meaningful sensory input is often one of the most disabling and commonly observed aspects in children with Autistic Disorder. Inability to cope with sensation can also lead to "overload" and "shutdown" which interferes with the child's ability to process incoming input, which produces an appearance of lack of registration. Adults with Autistic Disorder who have communicated about these conditions have exquisitely described both the pain and the confusion that accompany the inability to register sensory input in a meaningful way (Grandin, 1995; Stehli, 1991; Williams, 1994). Children with Autistic Disorder often have heightened sensitivities not only to the sensory qualities inherent in various experiences and environments but also to basic variations in place and time. Children with Autistic Disorder can demonstrate a great deal of variability in their abilities and reactions. Jessica's case illustrates this point.

Jessica

Jessica was a 3-year-old girl with Autistic Disorder who demonstrated extreme swings in her tolerance for sensory experiences. On some days, she enjoyed going to the park with her mother, playing in the sand at preschool, or attempting new swings during her occupational therapy sessions. On other days, Jessica barely could tolerate the light coming in through the blinds in her room or the motion of a car ride. In-depth medical testing revealed severe allergies that were affecting Jessica's breathing to the point of interrupting her sleep cycles. Her variations in sensory responses were the first clues that Jessica was experiencing some level of internal disruption. Once her doctors discovered her problems with allergies, observations of her reactions to sensory experiences helped to determine when new episodes of allergies were occurring, in addition to how well she was responding to medication.

Because of the condition Ayres (1979) referred to as *gravitational insecurity*, stimulation of the gravity receptors in situations such as having the head tilted backward or moving

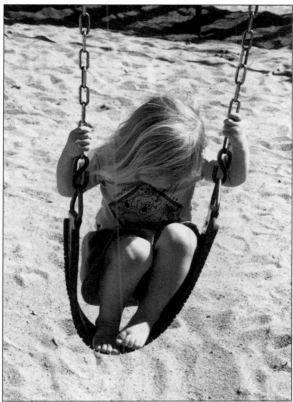

Photo by Shay McAtee.

Figure 17.2. Children with Autistic Disorder commonly show both sensory seeking and sensory avoidance behavior.

across uneven surfaces can create significant feelings of anxiety and fear for children with Autistic Disorder. In response, these children commonly show both sensory-seeking and sensory-avoidance behaviors in relation to movement (Figure 17.2). Movement seeking frequently takes the form of rocking or rhythmic motions (usually considered to be calming or organizing to the child) or twirling and swinging motions (usually considered to be alerting and activating). Professionals often categorize these behaviors as "self-stimulatory" and "nonpurposeful." Analyzed in this way, it is not uncommon for behavioral strategies to aim at extinguishing the behaviors.

Many children with Autistic Disorder also demonstrate problems in processing tactile information. Some children react defensively to touch and textures; other children either don't register much of this type of input or fluctuate between over- and underresponding. Reacting defensively to tactile information leads to discomfort during self-care tasks such as tooth brushing, hair washing and combing, dressing, and eating. Some children with Autistic Disorder experience extreme limitations in acceptance of foods, and textures often are a critical factor in the choice of food. Limited development of hand skills and utensil use in children with Autistic Disorder can stem from an inability to tolerate a variety of tactile experiences in play and craft activities, because these experiences are significant in the typical progression of manual dexterity (Exner, 1996). Additionally, because tactile processing is an important aspect in connecting to others on an emotional level and participating in social situations, the social withdrawal seen in most children with Autistic Disorder commonly has a tactile component. Sitting at circle time, standing in line, and negotiating games on the playground can involve human contact that is intermittent and unpredictable. For the child with Autistic Disorder who experiences tactile sensitivity and who has difficulty reading environmental cues that normally help an individual know what to expect next, these situations are likely to create anxiety and discomfort.

Researchers generally consider children with Autistic Disorder to be "visual learners" (Grandin, 1995), and strengths in visual memory and visual manipulation of objects are common. However, there are elements of visual stimuli that can be confusing or overwhelming for the child with Autistic Disorder. When Temple Grandin, a woman with Autistic Disorder and a well-known author and speaker on the topic of Autistic Disorder, visited an occupational therapy clinic that utilized a sensory integration approach, she described an aversive feeling she had to the brightly colored overhead beams. She commented that, being much taller that the children who used the therapy gym, she felt as though the beams were coming down on her head (personal communication, 1988). She also described the visual difficulties she often has using a computer screen but noted that she is better able to use a laptop computer where there is less distance between the keyboard and the screen (Grandin, 1995, 1997). Irlen (1991) reported that some children with Autistic Disorder experience scotopic sensitivity syndrome and are helped significantly by lenses that reduce symptoms such as light sensitivity, vibration of letters on the page, and difficulty sustaining visual attention. There is a close neural relationship between the visual and vestibular systems, and some of the visual disturbances described in Autistic Disorder might relate to the interactions between these two systems (e.g., coordination of head and eye movements and maintenance of a stable visual field when the head is moving).

Children with Autistic Disorder often demonstrate auditory processing problems as well. At times they can give the impression of being deaf or hard of hearing, yet some children with Autistic Disorder experience certain sounds as painful and unable to tune out irrelevant noises. Celebrations such as birthday parties can be particularly troublesome for these children because of the quality of spontaneous noise (balloons popping, children singing, and so forth). Participation in the community, such as walking through a shopping mall, attending a school assembly, watching a movie in a theater, or attending a sporting event, can be irritating, due in part to the levels and quality of sounds. Emphasizing the degree to which sound sensitivity can occur in individuals with Autistic Disorder, Stehli (1991) gave the example of a child who described rain as sounding like machine gun fire. The following vignette provides an example of sound sensitivity.

> ### Carlos
>
> Carlos was a 10-year-old boy with a diagnosis of Asperger's Disorder. He attended a regular-education, third-grade class with the support of a speech pathologist, an occupational therapist, a resource teacher, and an inclusion specialist. Carlos demonstrated extreme sensitivities to the sensory components of everyday occurrences in the school setting. The quiet work time was most difficult, because Carlos was sensitive to subtle sounds such as rustling of paper, pencil lead moving across a page, and clearing of throats. The louder sounds on the playground and during less structured class time were not as disturbing. Carlos also found himself distracted by some of the visual stimuli on the walls and outside the classroom windows. The light touch of classmates brushing by him as they moved around the room could also be irritating on some days. The occupational therapist helped Carlos and his teachers recognize which sensory experiences were most bothersome and develop strategies for coping with them. These included changing his seat assignment to reduce visual, tactile, and auditory stimulation; wearing ear phones or ear muffs during quiet work time; and leaving the classroom to go to the resource room for "regrouping" breaks during the day.

Many children with Autistic Disorder experience difficulties in aspects of praxis in association with their other sensory processing disorders (Dawson & Adams, 1984; Parham et al., 2000; Smith & Bryson, 1994). Of particular note is a common difficulty in ideation. Ayres (1979) described atypical ideation in children with Autistic Disorder:

> There is a part of the brain that is concerned with the desire to initiate behavior, to respond to sensory stimuli, to do something new or different. This part of the brain has an energizing effect; it says, "Do it!" . . . Like the system that registers sensations, the "I want to do it" system is working poorly in the autistic child. (pp. 127–128)

Problems in ideation probably account for a great deal of the trouble children with Autistic Disorder demonstrate relative to quality of play, because ideation is fundamental to the creative nature of play behavior (Mailloux & Burke, 1997). Ideation and planning of action are essential in all novel activities. The difficulty that children with Autistic Disorder routinely have with these functions would be likely to make

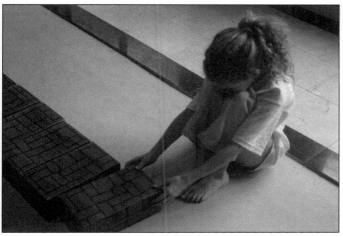

Figure 17.3. Ideational dyspraxia present in Autistic Disorder can be a factor in the tendency to favor sameness and routines.

new or novel activities confusing and anxiety producing. Thus, the deficits in ideation present in Autistic Disorder can be a factor in the tendency to favor sameness and routines (Figure 17.3). Without the sensory processing foundations and neural substrates necessary to facilitate skill acquisition in actions that initially require ideation and planning, many tasks will continue to require motor planning long after they should be habitual. However, children with Autistic Disorder often excel once a motor plan becomes a motor skill. This dichotomy of exquisite motor skills for some tasks and extreme inability to initiate other tasks can be confusing for families and professionals attempting to help these children learn new skills. The starting point for facilitating praxis is recognizing that the natural inquisitiveness that drives exploration and the sensory foundations that enable imitation are limited in children with Autistic Disorder. Jonah's story illustrates this point.

Jonah

Jonah flitted from one piece of equipment to another when he entered the therapy clinic. Although he appeared to seek intense sensory experiences, his interactions with toys, equipment, and people appeared largely nonpurposeful. When his therapist presented a new piece of equipment, he usually showed fleeting visual regard but did not show signs that he had any ideas about how to use the equipment. Jonah's therapist helped him with the most simple forms of purposeful action. Because he enjoyed joint traction, she helped him to hold his weight from a trapeze swing. It took several sessions for Jonah to know consistently how to position himself to hold his weight and swing from a trapeze. Once he mastered this skill, however, he automatically assumed a swinging posture when his therapist presented the trapeze. Having helped Jonah achieve this simple adaptive response, the therapist was then able to help Jonah build a larger repertoire of meaningful, playful, and satisfying activities that included the trapeze and increasingly complex ways of planning actions that incorporated its use.

Assessment

Although people typically think of assessment as the initial step in the intervention process, it is almost always an ongoing process. This is especially true when working with children who have Autistic Disorder, for whom a myriad of internal and external mechanisms influence function. Therefore, although a separate section in this chapter covers intervention to illustrate salient points, assessment actually continues throughout whatever type of intervention plan is in effect. Because the range of abilities in children with diagnoses of Autistic Disorder is so broad, finding the appropriate means for evaluation can be challenging. However, regardless of the functional level of the child, it is likely that measures of sensory integration will be relevant for understanding how the child perceives, relates to, and copes with the surrounding world.

Skilled observation always will be an important part of assessing sensory integration in children with Autistic Disorder, because so many children with this diagnosis cannot tolerate standardized tests and it is not possible for testing alone to determine fully all aspects of sensory integration. Kientz and Miller (1999) produced an overview of observational assessments of children with Autistic Disorder in the school setting that included aspects of sensory integration based on an ecological model. Clinical observations that therapists commonly utilize as a part of assessments using a sensory integrative approach (University of Southern California/Western Psychological Services, 1999) are also quite useful for the child with Autistic Disorder. Observations of praxis can occur at school, at home, and in the community, as well as in specialized therapy centers. Parham (1987) described means of evaluating praxis in young children through observation. She suggested observation of spontaneous play with toys, reactions to novel equipment, degree of anticipatory action, randomness versus goal-directed activity, and initiation of actions, stating that all are relevant for assessing this ability in children with Autistic Disorder, in conjunction with tests or when standardized testing is not possible.

Sensory histories and questionnaires also provide important insight into aspects of sensory processing that are not always apparent through direct testing. A large body of research is developing on the *Sensory Profile* (Dunn, 1994, 1999; Dunn & Westman, 1997). Use of this instrument with children whose disabilities have been diagnosed as Autistic Disorder uncovered sensory processing deficits (Ermer & Dunn, 1997; Kientz & Dunn, 1997). Other investigators have used the *Evaluation of Sensory Processing* (Johnson, 1996; LaCroix, 1993; LaCroix, Johnson, & Parham, 1997; VerMaas, 1999) with children with Autistic Disorder. Preliminary research on this instrument suggests that parents of children with Autistic Disorder rate their children significantly differently compared to parents of typically developing children in every sensory domain (VerMaas). These studies further underscore the importance of considering how sensory processing and sensory modulation affect the daily life routines of children with Autistic Disorder. These tools are especially helpful in introducing the concepts of sensory registration, modulation, and processing. Evaluations such as the *Sensory Profile* and *Evaluation of Sensory Processing* are also helpful for enlightening parents about the underlying mechanisms of many of the behaviors they observe in their children.

Jonathon

Jonathon was a 4-year-old child who was resistant to having his teeth brushed and his face washed. Morning and evening routines had become extremely problematic. His parents initially viewed his reactions as possible noncompliance, avoidance of human contact, or a simple lack of self-care skills. As they completed the sensory questionnaire and considered related questions regarding reactions to many types of sensory experiences, they began the process of analyzing Jonathon's responses from a new perspective. They began to understand the sensory aspects of Jonathon's reactions and were better able to develop strategies that helped increase Jonathon's level of comfort, as well as their own tolerance for the situation.

The SIPT (Ayres, 1989) offers the most sophisticated measure of sensory integration. These tests are appropriate for children within the standardized age range (4-0 to 8-11 years) and who are considered to have intelligence within the normal range. The study by Parham et al. (2000) indicated that children with Autistic Disorder typically demonstrate significant difficulty with praxis in addition to disorders in sensory perception. In that study, all of the tests of the SIPT discriminated significantly between children who were developing typically and children with Autistic Disorder in the high-functioning range. The pattern of sensory integrative dysfunction seen in the children with Autistic Disorder highlighted particular difficulties in somatosensory-based praxis, bilateral integration, sequencing, and some aspects of vestibular function, in contrast to relative strengths in visual perception.

> ### Melissa
>
> Melissa was a 6-year-old girl with a diagnosis of Autistic Disorder in the high-functioning range. Melissa demonstrated good cooperation at school and above-age-level academic performance. Her mother was most concerned about her shyness and lack of social involvement. During administration of the SIPT, Melissa paid close attention and appeared to give her best effort throughout the testing. Once the praxis tests had started, she began to demonstrate significant trouble, but she continued to attempt each item. Finally, without warning, she burst into tears during the Sequencing Praxis Test. These tests clearly represented an area of function that was overwhelming for Melissa. Her quiet cooperation and high academic performance masked some of her struggles at school, because she did not stand out during class. However, her dyspraxia severely limited her ability to plan actions necessary to participate in social play.

Although the SIPT will not be appropriate for all children with Autistic Disorder, the study by Parham et al. (2000) suggests that clinicians should consider these areas of sensory integration in the assessment process for children with this diagnosis.

Intervention

Some principles of sensory integration theory that guide the intervention process are tailor-made for the child with Autistic Disorder. For example, Ayres' (1972, 1979) principles of utilizing controlled and meaningful sensory experiences to elicit adaptive responses provide an appropriate starting point for application of sensory integration theory to Autistic Disorder. Addressing the ability to register sensory input and attach meaning to it is often an important focus in applying this framework to understanding and planning intervention for children with Autistic Disorder. Spitzer and Smith Roley give an extensive description of the adaptive response concept in chapter 1 of this text. A therapist working with a child with Autistic Disorder often will use controlled sensory input to elicit the simplest adaptive responses. Demonstrating registration and attaching meaning to sensory experiences might be the first adaptive responses elicited when clinicians use the sensory integrative approach in intervention planning for the child with Autistic Disorder. Randy's profile provides an example of this point.

> ### Randy
>
> Randy was a 4-year-old child who responded favorably to having gentle pressure applied to the top of his head. When a teacher or his parent provided this sensory experience, Randy generally became calmer and more organized. In turn, he also often showed a better ability to orient toward other people in his environment and to make eye contact. Children with Autistic Disorder seem to register this type of proprioceptive input in a meaningful way more frequently than many other types of sensation. The simple adaptive response of making eye contact opens the door of possibility for attention and interaction in a variety of ways. For Randy, this simple sensory-based intervention often helped him to avoid further agitation and encouraged greater participation in the activity at hand within his environment.

Other central principles of the sensory integration approach require greater adaptation for the child with Autistic Disorder. Perhaps the most striking example of adaptation relates to the importance of inner drive and child-directed activity within the sensory integrative framework. The child with Autistic Disorder who has dysfunction in the neural substrates for sensory perception, attachment of meaning, drive, and initiation of purposeful action is likely to demonstrate diminished inner drive for purposeful interaction, limited ideation, and impaired planning and participation in new or novel activities. Thus, an initial step in the intervention process is to establish a means for engaging the child in activity that is meaningful. The following example illustrates this point.

Lisa

Lisa was a 5-year-old child with Autistic Disorder who tended to stand alone on the playground and engage in self-stimulatory behavior such as hand flapping, jumping, and some body rocking. When Lisa encountered toys or swinging and climbing equipment, she tended to run from place to place without showing intent to interact. Lisa's self-stimulatory behavior suggested that she might be seeking vestibular, proprioceptive, and visual sensory experiences. Lisa's therapist believed that helping her to associate a play experience (such as swinging) with a sensory need she was seeking might elicit more purposeful action and less self-stimulatory behavior that was generally isolating for Lisa. Although Lisa did not initiate getting on a swing herself at first, once her therapist placed her on a swing and showed her how to propel it herself, the sensory experience seemed especially gratifying and Lisa began independently to seek play activities that involved swinging.

As an entrée into the therapeutic process, orchestrating meaningful sensory experiences might be the most direct way to develop rapport with the child with Autistic Disorder. Just as disturbances of sensory registration, perception, and modulation are hallmarks of Autistic Disorder, so too is the power that sensory experiences can have on children with this diagnosis.

Patrick

One day, a young boy named Patrick, who had been found to have Autistic Disorder and who exhibited limited language and eye contact, came to an occupational therapy appointment with A. Jean Ayres. Without using verbal language, she sat down next to him on the mats. He showed no interest in her or in the many enticing pieces of play equipment around him. Dr. Ayres picked up a piece of satin and firmly rubbed his arms and legs with the material as she carefully monitored his face for a reaction. He looked straight at her and smiled and said "more." She later said that she felt that Patrick bonded with her at that instant. In every subsequent therapy session, he came directly to her, seemingly ready to play (author's personal observation, circa 1979).

The first phase of many occupational therapy intervention plans for children with Autistic Disorder begins with individual therapy sessions in an environment offering a variety of equipment and activities that will provide safe, purposeful, and satisfying sensory experiences (Figure 17.4). The purpose of this phase of intervention is often two-fold: to provide the types of sensory experiences that will have the most organizing and productive effect, and to analyze this process in depth so that the therapist can offer appropriate activities throughout the environments in which the child lives. The latter idea, that part of the purpose of individual therapy is to develop carryover activities and experiences for the child, is especially pertinent for the child with Autistic Disorder. Although therapeutic intervention can be very effective in lessening symptoms and increasing functional abilities, many individuals with

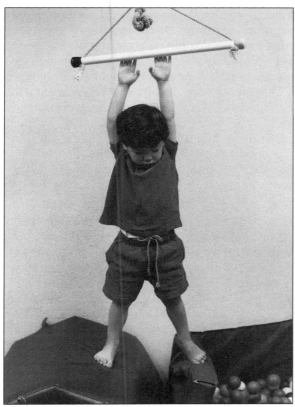

Figure 17.4. Many occupational therapy intervention plans for children with Autistic Disorder begin with individual therapy sessions in an environment offering a variety of equipment and activities that will provide safe, purposeful, and satisfying sensory experiences.

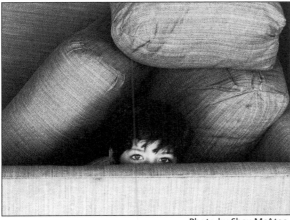

Figure 17.5. Deep pressure is often helpful in preparing the child with Autistic Disorder for other challenging sensory or social experiences.

Autistic Disorder have sensory needs that will require attention throughout their lifespan.

There are many examples of sensory-based activities and equipment that children can use as part of their daily routines. Rocking chairs and rocking horses, gliders, hammocks, slings, and oscillating platforms are often useful, in therapy settings as well as in homes and schools, for allowing regular availability of these sensory experiences. Intense rotary or linear movement carries more potentially disorganizing or overloading effects and is less likely to be sought by the child with Autistic Disorder if appropriate movement experiences are consistently available in the child's environment. Swings, teeter totters, merry-go-rounds, skates, bicycles, and scooters can provide more socially and age-appropriate means for receiving rotary and linear sensory input.

It is easy to work proprioceptive input and deep pressure into daily activities by having the child sleep with a weighted blanket, carry heavy objects such as groceries or laundry, bake with dough and stir thick mixtures while cooking, and sit in beanbag chairs or pillows. Children often achieve better tolerance for a variety of tactile experiences through a combination of activities aimed at normalizing reactions in the touch system and strategies to prepare for and cope with those situations that evoke defensive reactions. Proprioceptive input and deep pressure is often helpful in preparing the child with Autistic Disorder for tactile experiences (Figure 17.5). For example, facial and gum massage helps prepare some children for activities such as tooth brushing and feeding.

Gradual introduction of textures and varieties of tactile stimuli is also a common approach. Stretch fabrics such as lycra and spandex provide touch pressure that is often very appealing to the child with Autistic Disorder and can be quite calming (Figure 17.6). Parents and teachers can incorporate stretch-fabric hammocks, swings, capes, and blankets into activities at home and school.

Auditory training, an approach still being studied, employs application of modulated sounds, usually through headphones, for a specified number of sessions. There are several types of auditory training programs currently under investigation (Edelson, 1997). This approach shares some of the principles of sensory integration theory in that it aims at normalizing response to specific sensory (i.e., auditory) input. Further research on this

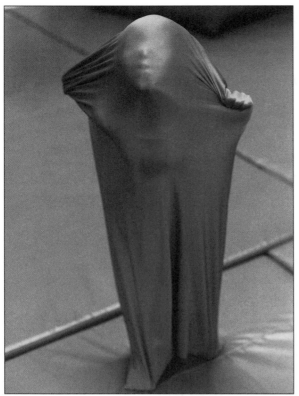

Photo by Shay McAtee.

Figure 17.6. Stretch fabrics provide touch pressure that is often very appealing and calming to the child with Autistic Disorder.

approach might eventually lead to therapeutic activities that incorporate auditory desensitization in specified ways. At this time, occupational therapists commonly utilize a variety of auditory input during therapeutic activities to help children with Autistic Disorder develop better tolerance. Therapists can incorporate auditory tapes, musical instruments, whistles, and environmental sounds into play activities to reduce reactions. Again, coping strategies are also an important means for addressing sensitivities that do not diminish with intervention. Introducing earplugs, head phones, or techniques such as covering one's ears can be helpful in teaching a child to "get through" auditorily painful experiences.

Therapists can enhance praxis in therapy through selected therapeutic activities aimed at improving sensory processing and facilitating abilities such as initiation, sequencing, bilateral coordination, timing, and imitation. On a broader level, being able to interpret sensory cues and plan actions within one's environment forms an important foundation for functioning within a social context. Like language, praxis allows humans to interact with one another. Accordingly, in the same way that disruption in the ability to use language in a typical way interferes with social reciprocity, so too do inefficient practice capabilities. Therefore, enhancing praxis through therapeutic intervention is an important component of the intervention process as part of a broader goal to facilitate social participation.

Utilizing a Sensory Framework to Build a Meaningful Social Environment

As described above, the sensory integrative disorders that are inherent to Autistic Disorder will interfere with socialization as defined by the common cultural norms. Utilization of a sensory integrative approach can assist in improving toleration for and satisfaction in social arenas. This is achieved both through enhancing abilities for the child with Autistic Disorder and working to make environments more appropriate and comfortable. Although children with Autistic Disorder characteristically do not show the typical drive to interact socially with other children, this is not equivalent to lacking a desire to interact. The anxiety and confusion that come with the disabling conditions that define Autistic Disorder might be masking the desire to interact. Therefore, an important means of facilitating socialization for the child with Autistic Disorder is to diminish the factors that would most likely lead to anxiety and confusion. Ways in which the occupational therapist can be especially helpful include helping peers, teachers, and parents, as well as the child, to understand those things that will be irritating and those things that will be organizing for the child.

Assessment, Intervention, and Measurement of Outcome Continuum: Case Example

Occupational therapists routinely address the social and physical environmental contexts in which their patients function as important variables in the intervention planning process. Those who work with children with Autistic Disorder and apply the sensory integration framework with this population must consider these contexts carefully because of the significant and long-term impact of this disorder. Application of a sensory integrative approach offers the opportunity to empower parents with an important function in the assessment and intervention phases of therapy. The following case example demonstrates the role of the family and the broad-range implications of utilizing a sensory integrative intervention approach for a child with Autistic Disorder.

Austin

Austin was a 3-year-old boy whose Autistic Disorder was diagnosed at age 2 by a developmental psychologist. He had a 5-year-old brother who was developing typically, except for some speech and language delays. Austin's mother was an occupational therapist who directed a therapy unit in a rehabilitation hospital, and his father was an engineer. A state agency for developmental disabilities referred Austin for an occupational therapy evaluation.

Austin, like many children with Autistic Disorder, had significant trouble performing tasks according to specific standardized criteria. Therefore, evaluation consisted of nonstandardized testing that relied heavily on clinical observations designed to evaluate use of objects, responses to sensory stimulation, postural reactions and balance, motor planning and other aspects of coordination, eye movements, interactions with family members and the therapist, and spontaneous play. Additionally, Austin's parents completed a sensory history questionnaire and provided additional information about his development and typical behavior patterns at home, in the classroom, and in the community. An occupational therapist evaluated Austin's comfort level in the world, his overall independence, and his current developmental skill level. The assessment also included recognition of those objects, people, and environmental qualities that helped Austin to transition and feel supported in various situations. As is commonly optimal in evaluating children with Autistic Disorder, the therapist observed Austin over several visits, in a variety of settings, and in the presence of familiar people. The therapist also contacted other significant people in Austin's life, such as behaviorists, childcare providers, and teachers, to gather information about his performance in different settings.

Austin was 2 years 6 months at the time of his occupational therapy evaluation. His family was just beginning to cope with what it meant to have a diagnosis of Autistic Disorder. Initial assessment and dialogue with Austin's family indicated that he demonstrated immature play skills, delayed fine motor and self-care development, poor motor planning and organization of behavior, sensory defensiveness, and sensory-seeking behavior. Because of Austin's age, his significant delays, and his intense sensory needs, the occupational therapist recommended intervention.

Austin began receiving occupational therapy that emphasized a sensory integrative approach. He received therapy at a private clinic two times per week, for an hour each session, with his mother or childcare provider attending most sessions. At home, his mother began observing his behavior with greater insight, and she shared what she saw with Austin's therapist in each of the occupational therapy sessions. Together, Austin's mother and therapist analyzed his behavior from a sensory integrative perspective and started to make adjustments in his home life. Austin's mother's level of participation in his occupational therapy sessions allowed for spontaneous sharing of information between the therapist and the family, which led to greater understanding of Austin's needs by both the therapist and the family. Early on, Austin's father also visited therapy to share his perspective. Because of his work situation, he was not able to come to Austin's sessions on a regular basis but was particularly good at finding ways to be involved. The occupational therapist clearly chose a method of communication that met the needs of the family. This was invaluable in communicating effectively about the child's progress, response to therapy, and successes and challenges in the clinic, at home, at preschool, and in the community. Austin's mother facilitated the communication by bringing in videotapes of Austin at home and in behavior therapy.

The initial phase of Austin's intervention plan involved extensive analysis of his sensory processing and motor planning abilities. Austin's therapist and parents monitored Austin's reactions to controlled, systematic exposure to sensory experiences to create a plan that included daily sensory experiences, recommendations for environmental modifications, and individualized therapeutic intervention. The therapist worked with the family to create environments that Austin would experience as soothing, to help him achieve an ideal state for learning and participating in meaningful occupations. In Austin's case, opportunities to participate in pleasurable sensory activities at home were a key component for helping his family begin to organize their day. For a period of time when Austin was not able to stay asleep at night, his parents allowed him to sleep in a suspended net swing. Although this is somewhat atypical in the western culture, giving Austin this opportunity allowed him and his family to obtain sufficient sleep. After several months, Austin no longer needed the net swing to sleep at night and used it only for swinging and naps. Both in the clinic and at home, Austin's therapist and parents encouraged him to meet his sensory needs through a variety of activities. This gave the therapist and Austin's mother insight into what Austin found pleasurable and meaningful. The goal of this aspect of intervention was to gather information about what was necessary in creating a comfortable and organizing environment for Austin and to identify ways for his family to adapt certain daily routines to provide Austin with satisfying sensory experiences throughout his day.

As mentioned previously, a key to using a sensory integrative approach effectively in occupational therapy is to guide the child through activities that challenge his or her ability to process sensory input in a way that allows organized and successful adaptive responses to the varying demands of daily life. For Austin, it became clear that large doses of vestibular and proprioceptive input in activities were important for him to become organized enough to tolerate daily life activities and to focus on challenging tasks. Much of his early therapy consisted of trying a variety of swinging, jumping, hanging, and climbing activities that appeared to calm and satisfy him. His therapist introduced these activities in ways that not only met his basic sensory needs but also challenged his ability to imitate, sequence, and time his actions. When Austin was calmed following or during movement and deep pressure activities, the therapist began to introduce fine motor activities that had previously been frustrating. These sensory channels opened doors to Austin's ability to learn, first by helping him to achieve an optimal state for attempting new skills. Second, the utilization of multisensory experiences facilitated meaning of activity (e.g., combining tactile and visual input to attach meaning to objects). Finally, the use of selected sensory experiences normalized aspects of his sensory processing, which allowed participation in activities that led to skill development (e.g., manipulation of a variety of textures to enhance finger and hand skills).

Consideration of what motivates the child plays an important role in selecting activities. For Austin, certain mechanical toys were intriguing. Although there was a tendency for him to become "fixated" on these toys, they also provided a means to entice him to try novel equipment or new ways of moving through space. As he was able to tolerate, then enjoy, a greater repertoire of play activities, he was no longer limited to these select toys.

Frequent parent and team meetings for transition planning are also invaluable in the process of helping families feel informed and develop a sense of empowerment. Austin's transition-planning meetings were critical in fostering good communication between all the professionals in Austin's life and identifying when to make changes in intervention. During these meetings, the team used problem-solving strategies to facilitate a greater degree of purposeful, organized behavior and successful community involvement for Austin. In these meetings, Austin's mother was able to share with the team the family's priorities, and the team shared their view of Austin's abilities and style of learning. A collaborative approach by all the team members was especially helpful for Austin's overall intervention plan, as was the team's responsibility in respecting the cultural, religious, and financial values and constraints of the family.

Choosing appropriate learning and therapy settings is a significant decision for families of children with special needs, especially for children with Autistic Disorder who display unique responses to variations in environments. In Austin's case, he began occupational therapy on a one-to-one basis in a private therapy clinic and later began participating in an early intervention group program that included occupational therapy using a sensory integrative approach. After his third birthday, he began attending a special education program. The team decided that he would benefit most by continuing to receive occupational therapy, with sessions once per week in the classroom and once per week in the therapy clinic. The team based this decision on the changing expectations for Austin now that he was entering the school setting. Therapy in the classroom would facilitate generalization of skills for Austin, and the activities with the equipment at the clinic would continue to provide the appropriate intensity of sensory input needed for optimal growth and development of critical processes within his young nervous system. The team's plan was that in the near future, a therapist would visit the community gym he and his brother attended for private lessons, replacing Austin's need to continue to receive therapy in a specialized clinic setting.

Austin's family and his teachers and therapists believe he is on a road that will take him toward meaningful occupation and social participation. However, continued collaboration, planning, analyzing, and advocating will be necessary to make sure this occurs.

Comparing Sensory Integration to Other Approaches

Occupational therapists often use sensory integrative techniques in combination with other intervention strategies to address the needs of the child with Autistic Disorder. Clinicians frequently combine play and developmentally based approaches with sensory integration theory in a complementary manner to assess and treat the child with Autistic Disorder. Social stories (Gray, 1994) and floor time (Greenspan & Wieder, 1998) are two examples of specific social/play-based approaches that blend naturally with the sensory integrative perspective.

Educator Carol Gray (1994) developed "social stories" to help children with Autistic Disorder cope with challenging social situations. This technique involves writing stories with or for the child to help develop strategies for specific situations. For example, a social story for a young child whose mother has had a new baby might include pages with snapshots of the baby and the client, and simple, written strategies for coping with the challenges that will accompany having a new baby in the house; many of which involve sensory issues. An example for a child who has auditory sensitivity might be "What can Josh do when the baby cries? He can cover his ears. He can look at a book. He can play with his trains." "Sometimes Josh will need to wait while Mommy feeds the baby. What can Josh do? He can watch a video. He can play with his cars. He can sit next to Mommy and the baby. Josh is a big brother for the baby!"

Floor time is an approach developed by child psychiatrist Stanley Greenspan (Greenspan & Wieder, 1998) to help parents and child development specialists facilitate play and social skills. This approach also blends nicely with sensory integration, because sensorimotor-based activity is such a natural enhancer of play for the young child.

Behavioral approaches are usually a part of the overall intervention plan for children with Autistic Disorder, and occupational therapists routinely participate in behavior management plans. However, some behavioral approaches are less congruent with sensory integration principles. For example, there are some inherent differences between behavior management techniques and sensory integration. One difference in these two approaches is the emphasis that sensory integration theory places on the neurological aspect of behaviors. For example, if a child demonstrates behaviors such as head banging, spinning, rocking, or hand flapping, application of a sensory integrative framework would lead to seeking an understanding of the behavior from a neurological view. Often stereotypical behaviors such as these provide certain types of sensations that are comforting to the child. Rather than purely extinguishing the behavior, a therapist with a sensory integration perspective would probably attempt to find a more appropriate way for the child to obtain the sensation he or she is seeking. Participating in therapeutic activities that involve swinging, jumping, and other movement sensations often diminishes the need for socially inappropriate actions such as rocking back and forth.

Another variation between sensory integration and the behavioral approach relative to Autistic Disorder relates to the way in which clinicians teach new skills. Some behavioral approaches tend to emphasize a highly structured and repetitive approach to elicit responses from the child. This type of interaction is probably dependent on the rote aspects of memory that are more apt to be intact in the child with Autistic Disorder and is likely to be successful in teaching a child to respond to particular stimuli in specified ways. Sensory integrative intervention focuses on processing of information and emphasizes planning abilities in novel circumstances, to develop a wider repertoire of capabilities in a variety of situations. The focus of sensory integration intervention is to stimulate parts of the brain that research has shown to have some structural abnormalities. This is the reason clinicians often emphasize this approach with younger children whose nervous systems are still actively developing. This approach attempts to increase function in those parts of the brain that manage novelty or encourage other structures within the nervous system to develop this function. Occupational therapists utilizing a sensory integrative approach with children with Autistic Disorder will, therefore, want to be cognizant of the differences between interpretations of behaviors and typical plans for intervention. Compromise and cross education will often help professionals to develop broader views and collaborate to create effective strategies in their intervention planning.

Long-Term Planning

It is important to remember that children with Autistic Disorder have life-long needs. Changes in programs, living situations, and family life can have profound effects on individuals with Autistic Disorder. Physiological changes that occur during periods such as puberty can also alter organization and function significantly (Ayres & Mailloux, 1983). Well-developed intervention programs can help families to anticipate and prepare for challenges that will occur over the lifespan.

Although many families feel that they would like their child to receive occupational therapy "forever," this is rarely necessary. The ability to be successful with less direct support from intervention programs is a significant step for a child with Autistic Disorder; however, parents can feel abandoned while wondering if they have the necessary tools to cope with new challenges as they arise. Parents are more likely to have positive views about changes or reductions in therapy if they feel prepared, supported, empowered, informed, and confident about their skills to deal with the challenges that lie ahead. Families need to have—and perceive that they have—the resources they need to continue to help their children as they believe best.

As a child begins to seem ready for less direct intervention, the therapist can improve the chances of a successful transition for both the child and the family by refining home programs and documenting strategies for use at home, at school, and in the community. It is important for the family to know where to find resources for the future. Using a sensory integrative model with children who have life-long needs enables families and individuals to gain a better understanding of their behavior and sensory needs and create routines that promote organized and goal-directed behavior, as well as modify environments to provide pleasure, comfort, security, and safety. It is only when these basic needs are met that an individual can participate in meaningful occupations.

Conclusion

Atypical sensory processing is a central aspect of Autistic Disorder spectrum disorders. The sensory integrative approach, utilized within a comprehensive occupational therapy program, provides a critical feature of service for the child with Autistic Disorder. Continued research will expand the understanding of this disorder and the most effective means for planning intervention programs. Twenty years ago, Dr. Ayres stated the following:

> The objective of therapy for the autistic child is to improve the sensory processing so that more sensations will be effectively "registered" and modulated, and to encourage the child to form simple adaptive responses as a means of helping him to learn and to organize his behavior. . . . As we continue to treat autistic children, we shall find out more about their neurologic problems and develop ways of "reaching" their brains with sensory experience. (1979, p. 130)

Dr. Ayres' words ring true today, and ongoing research continues to support her hypotheses about many neurologically based disorders, including Autistic Disorder. From her early lead, the importance of sensory integration for the child with Autistic Disorder continues to gain recognition and pertinence.

Works Cited

References

American Psychiatric Association. (1994). *Diagnostic and statistical manual of mental disorders* (4th ed.). Washington, DC: Author.

Ayres, A.J. (1972). *Sensory integration and learning disabilities.* Los Angeles: Western Psychological Services.

Ayres, A.J. (1979). *Sensory integration and the child.* Los Angeles: Western Psychological Services.

Ayres, A.J. (1989). *Sensory Integration and Praxis Tests.* Los Angeles: Western Psychological Services.

Ayres, A.J., & Mailloux, Z. (1983). Possible pubertal effect on therapeutic gains in an autistic girl. *American Journal of Occupational Therapy, 37*(8), 535–540.

Baranek, G.T. (1999). Autism during infancy: A retrospective video analysis of sensory-motor and social behaviors at 9–12 months of age. *Journal of Autism and Developmental Disorders, 29*(3), 213–224.

Bauman, M. (1991). Microscopic neuroanatomic abnormalities in autism. *Pediatrics, 87,* 791–796.

Bauman, M.L. (1996). *Current research and clinical practice in autism.* Conference presentation at the Center for Pediatric Therapy, Miami, FL.

Bauman, M.L., & Kemper, T.L. (1994). Neuroanatomic observation of the brain in autism. In M.L. Bauman & T.L. Kemper (Eds.), *The neurology of autism* (pp. 119–145). Baltimore: Johns Hopkins University Press.

Boyle, C.A., Bertrand, J., & Yeargin-Allsop, M. (1999). Surveillance of autism. *Infants and Young Children, 12,* 75–78.

Courchesne, E. (1987). A neurophysiological view of autism. In E. Shopler & G. Mesibov (Eds.), *Neurological issues in autism* (pp. 285–324). New York: Plenum.

Courchesne, E. (1989). Neuroanatomical systems involved in infantile autism: The implications of cerebellar abnormalities. In G. Dawson (Ed.), *Autism: Nature, diagnosis and treatment* (pp. 119–143). New York: Guilford Press.

Courchesne, E. (1991). Neuroanatomic imaging in autism. *Pediatrics, 87,* 781–790.

Courchesne, E., Townsend, J.P., Akshoomoff, N.A., Yeung-Courchesne, R., Press, G.A., Murakami, J.W., Lincoln, A.J., James, H.E., Saitoh, O., Egaas, B., Haas, R.H., & Schreibman, L. (1993). A new finding: Impairment in shifting attention in autistic and cerebellar patients. In S.H. Broman & J. Grafman (Eds.), *Atypical cognitive deficits in developmental disorder: Implications for brain functions* (pp. 101–137). Hillsdale, NJ: Lawrence Erlbaum.

Dawson, G. (1988). Cerebral lateralization in autism: Clues to its role in language and affective development. In D.L. Molfese & S.J. Segalowitz (Eds.), *Brain lateralization in children: Developmental implications* (pp. 437–461). New York: Guilford Press.

Dawson, G., & Adams, A. (1984). Imitation and social responsiveness in autistic children. *Journal of Abnormal Child Psychology, 12,* 209–226.

Dawson, G., & Lewy, A. (1989a). Arousal, attention and the socioemotional impairments of individuals with autism. In G. Dawson (Ed.), *Autism: Nature, diagnosis and treatment* (pp. 49–74). New York: Guilford Press.

Dawson, G., & Lewy, A. (1989b). Reciprocal subcortical-cortical influences in autism: The role of attentional mechanisms. In G. Dawson (Ed.), *Autism: Nature, diagnosis and treatment* (pp. 144–173). New York: Guilford Press.

Dawson, M., Meltzoff, A., Osterling, J., & Rinaldi, J. (1998) Neuropsychological correlates of early symptoms of autism. *Child Development, 69*(5), 1276–1285.

Dunn, W. (1994). Performance of typical children on the Sensory Profile. *American Journal of Occupational Therapy, 48,* 967–974.

Dunn, W. (1999). *The Sensory Profile.* San Antonio, TX: Therapy Skill Builders.

Dunn, W., & Westman, K. (1997). The Sensory Profile: The performance of a national sample of children without disabilities. *American Journal of Occupational Therapy, 51,* 25–34.

Edelson, S. (1997). Basic information about auditory integration training (AIT) [Online]. Available: http://www.autism.org/ait.html.

Ermer, J., & Dunn, W. (1997). The Sensory Profile: A discriminant analysis of children with and without disabilities. *American Journal of Occupational Therapy, 52,* 283–290.

Exner, C. (1996). Development of hand skills. In J. Case-Smith, A.S. Allen, & P.N. Pratt (Eds.), *Occupational therapy for children* (pp. 268–306). St. Louis: Mosby.

Grandin, T. (1995). *Thinking in pictures.* New York: Bantam Doubleday Dell Publishing Group.

Grandin, T. (1997). A personal perspective on autism. In D.J. Cohen & F.R. Volkmar (Eds.), *Handbook of autism and pervasive developmental disorders* (2nd ed., pp. 1032–1042). New York: John Wiley & Sons.

Gray, C. (1994). *Comic strip conversations.* Arlington, TX: Future Horizons.

Greenspan, S.I., & Wieder, S. (1998) *The child with special needs: Encouraging intellectual and emotional growth.* Reading, MA: Addison Wesley.

Irlen, H. (1991). Reading by the colours: Overcoming dyslexia and other reading disabilities through the Irlen method. New York: Avery Publishing Group.

Johnson, C. (1996). A study of a pilot sensory history questionnaire using contrasting groups. Unpublished master's thesis, University of Southern California, Los Angeles.

Kandel, E.R., Schwartz, J.H., & Jessell, T.M. (1991). *Principles of neural science* (3rd ed.). Norwalk, CT: Appleton & Lange.

Kemper, T.L., & Bauman, M.L. (1993). The contributions of neuropathologic studies to the understanding of autism. *Behavioral Neurology, 11,* 175–187.

Kientz, M.A., & Dunn, W. (1997). A comparison of the performance of children with and without autism on the Sensory Profile. *American Journal of Occupational Therapy, 51,* 530–537.

Kientz, M. and Miller, H. (1999). Classroom evaluation of the child with autism. *School System Special Interest Section Quarterly,* 6(1), 1–4.

LaCroix, J.E. (1993). *A study of content validity using the Sensory History Questionnaire.* Unpublished master's thesis, University of Southern California, Los Angeles.

LaCroix, J., Johnson, C., & Parham, L.D. (1997). The development of a new sensory history: The evaluation of sensory processing. *Sensory Integration Special Interest Section Quarterly, 20,* 3–4.

Mailloux, Z., & Burke, J.P. (1997). Play and the sensory integrative approach. In L.D. Parham & L.S. Fazio (Eds.), *Play in occupational therapy for children* (pp. 112–125). St. Louis: Mosby-Year Book.

Parham, L.D. (1987). Evaluation of praxis in preschoolers. In Z. Mailloux (Ed.), *Sensory integrative approaches in occupational therapy* (pp. 23–36). New York: The Haworth Press.

Parham, D., Mailloux, Z., & Smith Roley, S. (2000). Sensory processing and praxis in high functioning children with autism. Paper presented at Research 2000, February 4–5, 2000, Redondo Beach, CA.

Smith, I.M., & Bryson, S.E. (1994). Imitation and action in autism: A critical review. *Psychological Bulletin, 116*(2), 259–273.

Stehli, A. (1991). *The sound of a miracle: A child's triumph over autism.* New York: Bantam Doubleday Dell Publishing Group.

University of Southern California/Western Psychological Services. (1999). *From interpretation to intervention* (Course handouts).

VerMaas, J.R. (1999). *Parent ratings of children with autism on the Evaluation of Sensory Processing.* Unpublished master's thesis, University of Southern California, Los Angeles.

Williams, D. (1994). *Somebody, somewhere: Breaking free from the world of autism.* New York: Times Books.

18

The Effects of Deprivation on Processing, Play, and Praxis

SHARON A. CERMAK, ED.D., OTR, FAOTA

For a young child, living in an impoverished environment (such as an orphanage, institution, multiple foster placements, or poverty) results in a greater risk for poor health, including malnutrition, stunted growth, behavioral problems, and developmental delay. Recently, professionals and parents have observed signs of sensory integration dysfunction in institutionalized and post-institutionalized children. These behaviors impede a child's ability to learn, play, socialize with and relate to caregiver and peers, and function independently. Recent research on the effects of institutionalization indicates that, although not all children from institutions show problems in sensory integration, as a group these children are at significant risk. Although young children are no longer institutionalized in the United States, there are still hundreds of thousands of young children throughout the world being raised in orphanages and institutions. Examination of the effects of institutionalization has theoretical and practical relevance for several reasons. This chapter describes the factors in orphanage life that contribute to developmental delays and discusses the importance of stimulation, both human and environmental. The chapter also reviews the outcomes of children adopted from Romania, along with discussion of potential for recovery.

What is happening now with children in orphanages in other countries reflects the history of orphanages in the United States. As with such institutions in many other countries, very few of the children in these orphanages were really orphans. A large majority had at least one parent, usually the mother. The father was often absent or incapacitated by injury, illness, alcohol, or lack of work. A woman did not usually send all of her children to an orphanage; rather, she might send one or two for whom she could not provide.

During the Great Depression of the 1930s, approximately 144,000 children were in orphanages (Jones, 1993). In 1936, the principal child-caring institution in Kentucky reported that on most of the wards, two children were sleeping in every bed, with some children sleeping on the floor (Jones). In 1964, there were still 77,300 children residing in 1,483 institutions for dependent and neglected children (Provence, 1967).

In the United States, there are thousands of children in the current foster care system, many of whom are experiencing multiple placements with multiple caregivers. Many are undergoing abuses not unlike children in orphanage environments (Perry, 1993a, 1993b). Because of the many problems with the foster care system in the United States, some politicians have suggested reinstituting orphanages in this country. It is important to be aware of the effects of institutional care for young children.

Additionally, the number of international adoptions is increasing. From 1984 to 1994, there were 8,195 intercountry adoptions. In 1996, American parents adopted 11,340 children from outside the United States (Albers, Johnson, Hostetter, Iverson, & Miller, 1997). To date, more than 18,000 children adopted from Eastern European countries, where institutional care is prominent for children whose parents cannot care for them, currently live in the United States.. Many of these children are experiencing long-term delays and require professional intervention. The following letter is from a woman who adopted a child, Andrea, who spent the first 10 months of her life in an orphanage. This letter highlights some of the difficulties facing many adopted children and their families.

I thought completing a Romanian adoption was hard—it was nothing compared to living with Andrea. Andrea has many problems, the most difficult being sensory integration. Currently our main issue is getting Andrea to eat. She is now 17 months old and still will not put anything in her mouth. She would rather starve herself to death than eat a piece of food.

Andrea is a very unhappy child. It is very hard for me to understand how such a young baby could be so discontented. She whines and cries constantly. I never know if she is sick, cold, hot, hungry or what her problem could be; I just never know with Andrea because nothing really makes her happy. She does not like to be held for comfort—she is not a cuddly baby; she is more like a 17-month-old loner.

Everyone told us "Andrea will outgrow this; love and attention is all she needs."

I don't see an end in sight and I feel as if my family life as I once knew it is over. No one ever told us about the damaging effects orphanage life causes.

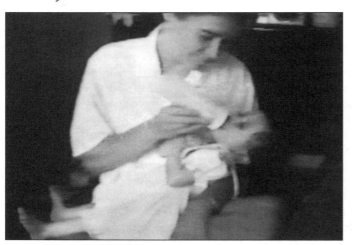

Figure 18.1. Andrea being fed by her mother during the first week with her family.

Factors Needed for Development

Child development is a dynamic process of growth, maturation, and change. Several factors are important to child development: adequate nutrition, social stimulation or interaction, "tender, loving care," and active exploration of the environment. Each of these factors, if adequate, contributes to health development. Deficits (or absence) of these factors can lead to social and developmental issues.

Nutrition plays a critical important role in development. Studies have shown a consistent association between maternal undernutrition and low birth weight in infants (Meyers & Chawla, 2000). These researchers have also found breast feeding to be important. Recent evidence suggests that breast milk contains nutrients essential for optimal brain development. Randomized clinical trials indicated that the composition of milk (expressed breast milk versus formula) fed to premature infants affects their cognitive development (Meyers & Chawla). In a metanalysis of 20 studies of infants and toddlers, Anderson, Johnstone, and Remley (1999) found that even when factors such as social class were taken into account, breast-fed infants demonstrated better cognitive and motor development than formula-fed infants. These effects were most pronounced among low-birth-weight infants.

Researchers noted a positive correlation between the number of calories available to toddlers and scores on language and nonverbal measures of cognitive skills that developed later (Latham, 1997; Sigman, McDonald, Neumann, & Bwibo, 1991).

Researchers have also found that protein malnutrition decreases playfulness, exploratory activities, motivation, and arousal, and increases apathy (Frank & Zeisel, 1988). Galler (1993) conducted a longitudinal study with children in Barbados who were malnourished in their first 2 years of life. Galler found that with adequate nutrition, these children caught up in height and weight, but they showed long-term attentional and behavioral deficits. Teachers and parents reported attention problems in 60% of the previously malnourished children compared with 15% of controls. Moreover, subsequent generations exhibited many of these behavioral effects (Galler & Ross, 1998).

Another major influence on a child's development is social stimulation or interaction. Vygotsky (1978) argued that adults and older children socially mediate young children's early cognitive development by helping infants and toddlers to master tasks that are in the zone of proximal development. Bradley, Caldwell, Rock, and Harris (1986) found that responsive caregiving and maternal involvement with a child in the first year correlated to cognitive development at 3 years.

Children learn through active exploration of the environment, by playing and manipulating materials. There is empirical evidence that availability of stimulation materials or toys, variety of stimulation, responsivity of stimuli, and physical restrictiveness all influence development. Bradley et al. (1986) found positive correlation between variety in stimulation at 6, 12, and 24 months, and intelligence scores at 3 and 4½ years. Field (1994) emphasized that an interesting, organized physical environment and a responsive human environment are critical for infant development.

Because orphanages and institutions often are deficient in nutrition, "tender, loving care," social stimulation, and opportunities for environmental exploration, it is not surprising that institutionalization results in significant delay in children. The following section, based on research between the 1900s and the 1960s, describes life in an orphanage and its effects on aspects of development.

Institutionalization: The Effects of Deprivation

Early Work

Provence and Lipton (1962) studied 75 children over a period of time and described the conditions in an orphanage: "As one walked along the halls to reach the rooms where the infants and children lived, . . . an unusual degree of quietness was an outstanding feature. It seemed incredible that 75 children . . . were living here" (Provence & Lipton, p. 25).

In describing the care of the infants, Provence and Lipton (1962) stated that "Care is of necessity routinized and is only occasionally related to the needs of a particular infant at a given moment" (p. 19). As a result, the infant doesn't have the opportunity to learn about what and who brings comfort or pleasure.

In 1953, Bowlby reported that an institutional environment can contribute to sleep disturbances, lack of appetite, delayed language development, and poor concentration. Bowlby concluded that infants under 6 months who had been in an institution for some time presented a well-defined picture with the following characteristics:

- listlessness
- emaciation and pallor
- relative immobility
- quietness

- unresponsiveness to stimuli like a smile or coo
- indifferent appetite
- failure to gain weight properly despite the ingestion of adequate diets
- frequent stools
- poor sleep
- an appearance of unhappiness
- proneness to febrile episodes
- absence of sucking habits

There is extensive research on the effects of institutionalization on development. Studies of institutionalized children conducted in the United States, England, and other countries from the 1900s through the 1960s have shown that maternal and environmental deprivation in orphanages results in delays in the children's language, intellectual, physical, emotional, and social development.

Spitz (1945, 1946) examined the developmental quotients of infants at the beginning and the end of their first year with regard to social class and experience. Spitz compared a group of urban children (mother absent) with three other groups with the mother present: Professional, Peasant, and Unmarried Delinquents. Children in the mother-absent group showed the greatest decline in developmental quotient, dropping from 124 in their 1st through 4th months, to 72 in the 9th through 12th months.

Goldfarb (1945) reported similar results in a series of studies. He compared a group of 15 children who had spent their first 3 years in an institution to 15 controls who had not spent time in an institution. Mean IQ score of the Institution group was 72, compared to 95 for the Control group. Social maturity, as measured on the *Vineland Social Maturity Scale* (Doll, 1935), was 79 for the Institution group, compared to 98 for the Control group. In examining factors such as ability to keep rules, guilt in breaking rules, and capacity for relationships, the author found that only 2 or 3 of the 15 children in the institution group had positive ratings. This highlights the dramatic effects of institutional care on cognition, social skills, and adaptive behavior.

Much of the early research on the effects of institutionalization emphasized maternal deprivation as the contributing factor. In the 1960s, divergent lines of research drawn from Harlow's animal research with primates (Harlow, 1958; Harlow & Harlow, 1966; Harlow & Suomi, 1970) and from work with children in institutions and long-term hospitalizations (Bowlby, 1951, 1953) concluded that a mother (or mother figure) is essential for normal infant development.

In 1961, Casler pointed out that, in addition to maternal deprivation, other factors such as reduced handling, reduced opportunities for interaction, and overall decreased stimulation characterized institutionalization. Casler (1961, 1968) stated that the damage to infant development previously reported to be due to maternal deprivation was the result of insufficient perceptual stimulation. Infants in institutions do not have a consistent mother (or mother figure) to provide touch and movement experiences that are critical for emotional and physical growth and development.

Provence and Lipton (1962) compared the development of 75 institutionalized infants with 75 infants raised in families and, as their colleagues had seen, found that institutionalized children exhibited delays in motor development, social skills, language development, and discovery of the body. These authors also found that the longer the institutionalization, the lower the developmental quotient.

Provence and Lipton (1962) reported that the institutional environment was sensory deprived and that institutionalized infants had limited sensory experiences. For example, infants received feedings in their cribs with a propped bottle, so they missed the opportunity for the touch, smell, position sense, and sight provided by a primary caregiver during feeding time. Provence and Lipton emphasized that the concept of maternal care includes stimulation, particularly tactile and kinesthetic. These authors suggested that sensory stimulation is important in building a repertoire of experiences from which an individual can organize and interpret external stimulation to produce voluntary actions. They commented on the babies' passivity in a variety of areas, including feeding and play, and concluded that an infant who does not have adequate nurturing is often apathetic and does not enter into or initiate playful interactions with others.

In a review of research, Ainsworth (1965) suggested that the most detrimental aspect of institutionalization is the lack of handling and interaction with a mother figure, which results in the child growing unresponsive to the toys provided.

Thus, two factors appear to contribute to the delays in development and problems in play that institutionalized children demonstrate: an environment deprived of adequate stimulation and a lack of a significant person who rejoices in the responses of the infant/young child and encourages the infant/young child to continue to explore. In describing the evolution of play behavior, the work of Provence and Lipton (1962) highlights this relationship.

In a longitudinal study of institutionalized children, Provence and Lipton (1962) commented that "a discrepancy between maturation of the apparatus and its use in the infant's adaptation to his environment was seen in various aspects of the development of the institutionalized infants" (p. 61). They emphasized that although young infants appeared to have the capacity for interaction, they did not use this capacity as they got older. For example, they reported that until the age of 5 or 6 months, the babies would approach and grasp the toys and test materials fairly regularly, and their early reaching and grasping behaviors were normal in quality and time of appearance. However, from approximately 6 months throughout the first year, the institutionalized infants reached out for toys less frequently, and their arm movements were less smoothly coordinated. The infants showed decreased interest in toys and did not use the patterns spontaneously in a normal manner in their adaptation to the environment.

Provence and Lipton (1962) noted an increasing distortion from the age of 8 to 9 months of age onward and commented that the infants showed a low drive to approach, grasp, and manipulate toys. They stated, "The looking, banging, biting, feeling, shaking, sucking, fingering, poking, dropping and picking up again, which in the average baby become more elaborated day by day, were much less prominent in the institutionalized infants" (p. 99) and noted that "toys and other objects were rarely mouthed, sucked, or chewed" (p. 119).

The infants also showed poor modulation, and their motor system worked in "fits and starts" (Provence & Lipton, 1962, p. 63). These authors stated, "The only type of motor activity that was increased in the institutionalized infants was rocking, which appeared in most of them at five to six months and by eight months was universal" (p. 64).

In describing older infants, Provence and Lipton (1962) noted that although the infants seemed to enjoy toys, they did not express displeasure when the toys were removed, and they did not seem to prefer one toy over another. Moreover, infants did not try to recover a lost toy.

According to Provence and Lipton (1962), "What the babies missed was not the presence of the toy itself, but something that makes a toy interesting and worth while" (p. 49). They concluded that the baby needs to perceive, organize, and integrate stimuli with other experiences, and emphasized that a mother contributes to this organization: "Our data would support the view that play has its origins in the exchange between mother and infant and derives its stimulus from the relationship" (p. 83). "The mother's pleasure in the baby's activity with the toy further promotes his own pleasure in the toy" (p. 103). The authors emphasized that in order to use toys with pleasure and interest, the infant needs both the personal attachment to the mother and some opportunity to play with toys in an atmosphere where the child is not constantly asked to interact with another person.

Provence and Lipton (1962) suggested that "The multiplicity of individuals that shared in caring for the institutionalized infants resulted in a fragmentation of care and lack of constancy that are believed to make it more difficult for an infant to develop an awareness of himself and his environment" (pp. 18–19). They noted that those babies who were favorites of a nurse and who had a personal relationship were also more interested in toys.

The Importance of Touch and Movement for Growth and Development

Sensory experiences, particularly touch and movement, contribute to the growth and development of the young child. When these experiences are not available, there are significant consequences. Research with animals has permitted systematic study of the effects of rearing offspring in deprived and/or stressful environments and provides critical insights into the behavioral and neurobiological consequences of stress and deprivation.

Animal research has indicated that interacting with the human and nonhuman environment results in structural and functional changes in the brain, thereby allowing the animal to experience and interpret information from the environment more effectively (Liu et al., 1997; Sapolsky, 1997; Stein, Brailowsky, & Will, 1995). The way the brain organizes or reorganizes information reflects the developmental experiences of the animal.

In a series of studies, investigators have shown that rearing rats in enriched environments compared with deprived environments resulted in increased problem-solving behavior and also in increased thickness and weight of the cerebral cortex (Diamond, 1967; Diamond, Ingham, Johnson, Bennett, & Rosenzweig, 1976; Nyman, 1967; Rosenzweig & Bennett, 1978). The enriched environment included "toys" such as ladders, wheels, mazes, swings, and so forth. The authors found that it was important to change the toys frequently and provide the animals with novelty, or the brain changes were not as evident. The investigators also reported that depriving an animal of stimulation, either of its companions or of stimulating objects, was more detrimental to the young animal than to the adult animal, although they also reported seeing the effects of enrichment in both young and older animals.

Touch

Research with both animals and humans has found that touch and movement are critical for various aspects of development and social interaction. In studies with rats, Schanberg, Kuhn, Field, and Bartolome (1990) found that touch is critical for growth; without it, levels of growth hormones decrease and growth is stunted. This might be one of the reasons why so many children in institutions are small for their age: even with adequate nutritional intake, these children do not grow.

In a recent study, researchers found that older rats not handled when they were infants showed memory losses and less development in the hippocampus (an area of the brain known to be involved in memory) than rats who had been handled when they were infants (Meaney et al., 1990). The effects of reduced touch are long-term and long-lasting.

Recent research has helped to clarify the mechanisms underlying the importance of tactile stimulation. Maternal licking and grooming (tactile stimulation) in infant rats appear to "program" the hypothalamic-pituitary-adrenal (HPA) response to stress in the offspring, and this effect seems to persist throughout life (Liu et al., 1997). The greater the frequency of maternal licking and grooming during infancy, the lower the HPA response to stress in adulthood (Liu, et al.). Research has found that increased maternal licking and grooming triggers thyroid hormone release. This in turn activates serotonergic secretions into the hippocampus, which causes long-lasting increases in glucocorticoid receptor numbers in hippocampal neurons. Glucocorticoids exert an inhibitory, negative-feedback effect on the synthesis of hypothalamic releasing factors for adrenocorticotrophic hormone (ACTH). This in turn results in decreased hypothalamic corticotrophin-releasing hormone (CRH) and arginine vasopressin (AVP). The hippocampus helps to mediate negative-feedback inhibition of glucocorticoid, a hormone released by the adrenals during stress, by inhibiting production of CRH and AVP and reducing pituitary ACTH (Liu, et al.). Excess glucocorticoid can damage the central nervous system (CNS), and a chronic excess of glucocorticoid can accelerate the loss of certain classes of neurons during aging. Offspring of mother rats who licked and groomed the pups frequently showed less glucocorticoid secretion during a stressor and also demonstrated a faster return to baseline (Sapolsky, 1997). Tactile stimulation, derived from maternal licking and grooming, regulates pup physiology and affects CNS development.

The relationship in animals between tactile stimulation and response to stress has implications for mental health (response to stress) of children from deprived environments. It is interesting to consider this in light of the information about conditions in orphanages. Infants in such institutions are rarely handled and often spend 22 to 23 hours of every day in their cribs (Johnson & Groza, 1993). They are often fed in their cribs, with bottles propped, and care is routinized. Based on the previously described research, it is possible to hypothesize that the lack of tactile stimulation results in fewer receptors in the hippocampus. Because these receptors inhibit production of stress hormone, it is likely that the children will be more vulnerable to stress as adults. Carlson and Earls (1997) suggested that these children might have a "lifelong vulnerability to certain psychiatric disorders" (p. 424).

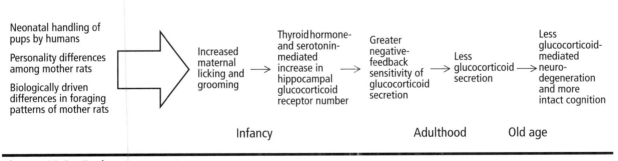

Figure 18.2. Early care counts.

Note. From "The Importance of a Well-Groomed Child," by R.M. Sapolsky, 1997, *Science, 22,* p. 1620. Copyright 1997 by the American Association for the Advancement of Science. Reprinted with permission.

Many young children in orphanages, and many of those who have been adopted from orphanages, present with sensory defensiveness. These infants do not appear to be calmed by contact comfort and often pull away or withdraw from touch. As a result, parents can feel rejected by the infants and are apt to leave the infants to their own resources, thus exacerbating the problem. A more fruitful approach to these infants might be to identify the types of touch that the infants are able to process (more often deep pressure, rather than light touch) and provide stimulation at appropriate times.

Research with monkeys has corroborated the importance of touch and movement in social and emotional development. In the course of evolution, touch has become associated with emotion and social function. The studies by Harlow and his associates (e.g., Harlow & Suomi, 1970) were the first to highlight this finding. They took infant monkeys from their mothers and raised them with artificial mothers made of wire or terrycloth. Harlow found that the monkeys responded very differently to the two types of mothers. The monkeys hugged, clung to, and climbed on the terrycloth surface and formed an attachment. Touching the terrycloth gave them the self-assurance to explore their environments and calmed them down when they were frightened. In contrast, monkeys with wire mothers did not form an attachment. Harlow concluded that comfortable touch sensations are a critical factor in the infant's emotional attachment to the mother.

Schneider (1987) compared mother-reared to nursery-reared monkeys. She found that the nursery-reared monkeys showed increased sensory reactivity, marked by a greater startle response to a loud stimulus as well as a greater response to tactile stimuli. Schneider suggested that the low stimulus input for the nursery-reared infants contributed to the high emotional reactivity. Schneider pointed out that the mother-reared infants spent the first few weeks of life clinging to their mothers, receiving tactile input from body contact and vestibular input as the mothers moved about in the environment. During the mothers' movements, the infants made adaptive responses resulting in meaningful proprioceptive feedback as well as additional vestibular input. The nursery-reared monkeys did not have the same sensorimotor experiences.

Kraemer, Ebert, Schmidt, and McKinney (1991) extended this research, examining the neurobiological concomitants of maternal deprivation. These investigators found evidence that early psychosocial experiences in monkeys affect neurotransmitter systems and that some of the changes might be permanent. Mother-deprived monkeys have decreased levels of norepinephrine (NE) in the cerebral spinal fluid, which results in a compromised brain NE system function that researchers have associated with "reduced reward, failure to attend to significant stimuli, failure to avoid stressors, altered sleep cycles, and reduced brain organizational plasticity" (p. 549).

Kraemer and colleagues (Kraemer, 1992, 1995; Kraemer et al., 1991) proposed a psychobiological theory of attachment whereby the infant acquires basic behavior-regulation systems through interactions with the caregiver and the environment in which the infant develops. In this sense, the organization and tuning of the brain function is an effect of attachment (Kraemer, 1995). Failure of the caregiver to provide an adequate model compromises the long-term regulatory capacities of the child such that the individual responds with either exaggerated or blunted behavioral and emotional responses (Kraemer, 1992). Kraemer discussed the importance of the neurobiological changes on the infant's ability to cope with future social stressors. Reite (1990) also found that touch experiences in the infant monkey were critical for the development of attachment bonds and that the development of attachment bonds in turn was important in promoting regulation of physiological and immunological systems.

Other research also verifies the effects of tactile stimulation in humans. In a meta-analysis of 19 stimulation studies, Ottenbacher and colleagues (1987) estimated that 72% of infants receiving some form of tactile stimulation showed positive effects.

In a series of studies with healthy preterm infants, Field and colleagues showed that a short-term period of tactile-kinesthetic stimulation that they referred to as massage therapy resulted in increased weight gain in the infants who received the massage protocol, compared to a control group, even though there was no difference between the groups in the average caloric intake (Field et al., 1986; Scafidi, Field, & Schanberg, 1993; Scafidi et al., 1990). Additionally, the stimulated infants performed better on developmental assessments (Field et al., 1986). Investigators also examined the effects of tactile-kinesthetic stimulation on sympathetic and adrenocortical function in preterm infants (Kuhn et al., 1991). The stimulated infants showed increased norepinephrine and epinephrine (catecholamine rise-urine sample). The authors suggested that the massage therapy facilitates the normal development of the sympathetic nervous system.

Another example of the benefits of touch is the reduction of anxiety in children and adolescents with psychiatric problems. Field et al. (1992) showed that a 5-day massage treatment produced decreases in depression and anxiety levels and lower norepinephrine stress levels. By the last day of treatment, nurses reported less fidgeting behavior as well as an improvement in affection and cooperation.

In summary, touch, particularly touch from the mother (caregiver/parent), affects the infant in a number of ways. The touching between an infant and the mother (caregiver) is essential for brain development and for the development of the mother-child bond (Ayres, 1979; Blakeslee, 1995a, 1995b). Touch sensations are an important source of emotional satisfaction for the infant. Touch is a critical component of developing intimate relationships (Royeen & Lane, 1991) and for early learning and social emotional development (Trott, Laurel, & Windeck, 1993).

Touch is also an organizer of state (level of arousal) and a means of communicating messages (e.g., "I love you") and expectations. One of the first abilities that all babies need is to be calm and regulated (Greenspan, 1995), a state that is necessary for a baby to be interested in, attentive to, and responsive to people, things, sights, sounds, and smells. The development of self-regulatory mechanisms is complex and develops as a result of physiological maturation, caregiver responsiveness, and the infant's adaptation to environmental demands (DeGangi, 1991a, 1991b). Research has indicated that as an infant or child experiences sights, sounds, and touch, he or she simultaneously registers an emotional reaction, supported by the caregiver, that helps to organize the information. These emotions then come into play in later thinking (Greenspan, 1995) and for approaching tasks (e.g., Can the world be trusted? Does it feel good? Do I want to try?).

Movement

Investigators have documented the importance of movement (vestibular) experiences, although as highlighted by Schneider (1987), who described the contact and movement experiences provided when monkey mothers carried their young, touch and movement often co-occur in the real world and are not separated. Short (1985) showed that providing vestibular stimulation enhances arousal level and alertness, visual exploratory behavior, and motor development. Studies with animals and with humans have also shown that providing vestibular stimulation reduces self-stimulatory behavior. Monkeys raised with moving wire surrogate mothers did not develop stereotyped body rocking (Mason & Berkson, 1975). They played more on their surrogates and were bolder than monkeys reared on stationary wire surrogates. As the monkeys got older, those raised on the moving surrogate mothers spent more time looking at other monkeys, and they showed less fearfulness and less impulsivity than monkeys with stationary surrogate mothers.

Studies by Schneider, Kraemer, and Suomi (1991) concurred with the findings of Mason and Berkson (1975). In the studies by Schneider et al., peer-reared infant monkeys who received extra vestibular-proprioceptive stimulation (in addition to tactile stimulation) achieved higher motor scores and responded more favorably to unfamiliar and novel situations than monkeys reared with peers but without the extra stimulation. For this study, seven monkey infants were reared with terrycloth-covered surrogates and terrycloth-covered water-filled plastic pillows that moved in response to the infants' movements. Infant monkeys in the control group were reared with stationary terrycloth-covered surrogates and terrycloth blankets. Infants receiving vestibular-proprioceptive stimulation achieved significantly higher scores on the motor and problem-solving subtests of the *Bayley Scales of Infant Development* (Bayley, 1969). They also performed better in the following situations: (a) in response to a novel environment, they spent more time climbing and exploring the environment; (b) in response to novel objects placed in their home cages, they spent significantly less time in self-mouthing and clinging behavior; and (c) in response to a fear stimulus in the home cage, they showed more play behaviors, environmental exploration, social interaction, locomotion, and jumping than infants in the nonstimulation group. Infant monkeys in the nonstimulation group were unusually fearful or anxious when faced with changes in their everyday environment. Infant monkeys in the vestibular-proprioceptive group also showed less rocking than control monkeys. Sweeney and Bascom (1995) reported a similar finding of reduced rocking and other stereotypic behaviors in Romanian institutionalized children who received comparable extra experiences (Sweeney & Bascom).

In summary, research indicates that deprivation is a significant contributor to problems in various aspects of development and that providing more optimal environments enhances functional outcomes.

Romania: Current Research

The research on children adopted from Romanian orphanages is particularly relevant because it allows investigators to examine the long-term effects of deprivation and to understand the persisting problems. It also demonstrates the extraordinary potential for recovery and the resiliency of the human spirit and of the central nervous system.

The conditions in Romanian orphanages are not unique, but the reasons why orphanages exist in Romania are unique. Ceausescu, the former dictator of Romania, wanted to increase the work force and army of Romania and mandated that women bear five or more children (Children's Health Care Collaborative Study Group, 1994). Childless families and unmarried people over the age of 25 were heavily taxed (Johnson & Groza, 1993). Scarce economic resources forced many families to give their children to Leagane (orphanages or institutions) for their guardianship and care. The death of Ceausescu in 1989 introduced the world to more than 200,000 of Romania's children in institutions (Marcovitch, Cesaroni, Roberts, & Swanson, 1995). Although childbirth is no longer mandatory and the government now permits birth control and abortions, the number of children being placed in orphanages continues, due in part to the country's poor economy.

Since 1990, people in the United States and Canada have adopted almost 10,000 children from Romania. Although families often were prepared for medical problems and developmental delays, many thought these issues would be "cured" with love and adequate nutrition. Recent research on the developmental outcomes of these children has shown that, although the majority of children do well, the effects of institutionalization are long-term, and many children have ongoing needs.

Developmental Outcomes of Romanian Children in United States and Canada

In the last 7 years, a number of studies have examined the health and development of children adopted from Romania. The earliest studies focused on the health of the children and identified many health care needs (Johnson et al., 1992). In an examination of 65 adopted children brought to the United States from Romania between 1990 and 1991, only 15% of children were physically healthy and developmentally normal. Severity of growth failure correlated directly to length of time in the orphanage system (Johnson et al.).There was a high incidence of medical problems in the institutionalized children, including intestinal parasites, Hepatitis B infection, HIV, and AIDS (infections acquired through blood transfusions administered to help failure-to-thrive babies gain weight) (Johnson et al.). Ames (1997) found that, at the time of adoption, 85% of Romanian orphans adopted in Canada placed below the 10th percentile for weight, with 59% below the 5th percentile. Rutter and colleagues (Rutter, 1998) found similar findings for Romanian children adopted by families in England.

In recent years, a number of studies have examined the developmental status of children adopted from Romania. Morison, Ames, and Chisholm (1995) compared two groups of Romanian-orphanage children adopted by individuals in Canada and the United States. The investigators grouped the children by the length of time they spent in an institution before being adopted. Parents completed two *Revised–Denver Prescreening Developmental Questionnaires* (R-DPDQ; Frankenburg, 1986), a parent report measure consisting of 105 tasks or items arranged in chronological order according to the age at which 90% of children in the *Denver Developmental Screening Test* (DDST) (Frankenburg et. al., 1975) performed them. As on the DDST, the four domains are: Personal-Social, Fine Motor Adaptive, Language, and Gross Motor. Parents rated their child as they remembered him or her when they first met in Romania. Parents then rated their child as he or she was currently, after spending approximately 11 months in their adoptive home.

In the group of 44 children who were adopted after spending at least 8 months in an orphanage, parental report on the R-DPDQ indicated that at the initial meeting, *all* children showed delays in development. Ninety-five percent showed delays in three or more areas (78% had delays in all four areas, 17% had delays in three areas) and 5% had delays in two areas. One year later, the children had made substantial gains. Only 46% still exhibited delays in three or more areas 11 months later. The length of time the child spent in an institution correlated to the number of delays the child was showing at a year postadoption and to the Gesell Developmental Quotient (DQ; Knobloch, Stevens, & Malone, 1980) that was available for those adopted children participating in early intervention programs. Parents rated the availability of toys at the time they received their child from the orphanage. As the availability of toys present for children to play with increased, the number of areas of delay on the R-DPDQ decreased and Gesell DQs increased, indicating a positive influence of toys on a child's development.

The second Romanian group in this study spent less time in an orphanage. These 26 children were adopted before they were 4 months old. Comparison of the two Romanian groups indicated less delay in the group institutionalized fewer than 4 months, although it is important to note that children in this group had spent approximately 25 months in their adoptive homes. The group institutionalized for more than 8 months had spent only approximately 11 months in their adoptive homes.

In a study titled Romanian Adoption: Parents' Dreams, Nightmares, and Realities, Marcovitch et al. (1995) reported the results of a survey completed by 105 families representing 130 children adopted from Romania to Canada. The median age at adoption was 6 months. The median present age of children was 3 years. At the time of adoption, about half the children were living in orphanages and half were living with their biological Romanian families. The investigators asked parents to identify initial problems and continuing problems. The total number of medical and developmental concerns decreased over time, although temper tantrums did not. Other difficulties that parents reported frequently included inability to attend, high activity level, distractibility, and overfriendliness.

This study also analyzed data according to the child's age at adoption (children adopted before age 2 [n=100] and after age 2 [n=30]) and according to whether children were adopted from institutions (n=71) or families (n=59). They did not consider length of time in the institution. Of the children from institutions (n=71), initially 68% had medical problems and 65% had developmental delays. Approximately 2½ years later, about half of these children continued to have problems.

Ames et al. (1992) looked at the behavior of 39 previously institutionalized children from 34 families. The median age at adoption was 18 months (range of 9 to 68 months) and the median time in an orphanage was 17 months (range 8 to 53 months). Thirty of the children were adopted before age 2, and nine were adopted after age 2. At the time of the interview, children had been in their adoptive homes for a median of 10 months (range 1 to 18 months). Parents assessed behavior problems using the *Child Behavior Checklist* (CBCL; Achenbach, 1991). Romanian children had significantly more behavior problems, including rocking, eating, and response to pain, than the comparison group of nonadopted Canadian-born children. Eighty-one percent of parents reported that their child's rocking was a behavior of concern, in contrast to 0% of the control group. Of the institutionalized group, 39% of parents reported resolution of the problem and 39% reported some improvement since time of adoption. Fifty-nine percent of parents reported difficulty with their child's eating. Some children had problems with solid food (35%), and parents reported that others ate too much and did not know when to stop (24%), compared with the control group in which 11% of parents expressed concern about feeding. Again, many parents (29%) of institutionalized children reported that the eating problems had resolved since time of adoption. Another issue that emerged frequently was pain. Although not asked, 14% of parents mentioned that their child did not report experiencing pain.

Marcovitch et al. (1997) assessed 56 Romanian orphans (adopted between January 1990 and April 1991) who were 3 to 5 years of age at the time of assessment. Children institutionalized for less than 6 months (n=37) had better outcomes on developmental measures than children with more than 6 months (n=19). Because children who were in institutions longer were also older at adoption, it was not possible to distinguish the effects of age at adoption from time in an institution. The developmental quotients for both groups were in the average range—low average for the long-term institutionalized group (X=89) and high average for the short-term institutionalized group (X=110). Similar results occurred on the *Vineland Adaptive Behavior Scales, Revised* (Sparrow, Balla, & Ciccheti, 1984) in all areas (Communication, Daily Living, Social, and Motor). In addition, the long-term institutionalized group had more behavior problems (CBCL-total). These results concurred with the follow-up studies by Ames (1997), who found that even 5 years postadoption, Romanian children adopted at older ages (i.e., older than 2 years) had lower IQ scores than Romanian children adopted at younger ages.

The results of a series of studies of Romanian children adopted in England (O'Connor & Rutter, 2000; O'Connor, Rutter, Beckett, Keaveney, & Kreppner, 2000; Rutter,

1998) were similar to those of the Canadian studies (Marcovitch et al., 1995). Research on children adopted to the U.S. are also consistent with the Canadian findings. Groza and Ileana (1996) sent surveys to 1500 U.S. families who adopted children from Romania between 1990 and 1993; 462 families responded. Children from institutions had more problems than children adopted from homes. These problems included issues in development, behavior, self-stimulation (including rocking and hitting themselves), activity level, response to environmental stimuli (over- or under-responsive), and emotional difficulty. These effects remained even after the child had been in the adoptive family for some time. Regression analyses indicated that the extent of delay related to length of time in institution.

In summary, the results of the studies on children adopted from Romania are quite consistent with reports of children in orphanages in the 1900s through the 1960s. Postinstitutionalized children have many medical and developmental problems, which often resolve or decrease with time. In general, children who have been adopted from families or have spent shorter amounts of time in an orphanage do better.

Sensory Processing

Gale Haradon, one of the first occupational therapists to work in Romania, described the effects of institutionalization on sensory integration. She concluded that the infrequency of interactions by caregivers in touching, moving, handling, speaking to, and visually stimulating the infants and young children in institutions, coupled with the lack of independent movement opportunities for the infants outside their cribs (which further limited their independent exploration and interaction with the environment), contributed to their deficiencies in the development of sensory integration and affected their behavior (Haradon, Bascom, Dragomir, & Scripcaru, 1994).

Cermak and colleagues have implemented a series of studies to examine sensory processing in children who were adopted from Romania. In the first study, the investigators mailed a Developmental History and Sensory Processing Questionnaire to approximately 400 members of a parent support group (Cermak & Daunhauer, 1997). This questionnaire included demographic data about the child, as well as questions about sensory processing and related behavior. The investigators selected these questions primarily from surveys by Occupational Therapy Associates, P.C. (1993), Dunn (1994), and a review of the literature. Items assessed sensory processing in each of the following domains: touch, movement seeks, movement avoids, vision, audition, and taste-smell. The questionnaire also included items to assess behaviors that often reflect problems in sensory processing: activity level, feeding, organization, social-emotional regulation, and sleep. Researchers found significant differences between the institutionalized group and the control group on five of the six sensory processing domains and on four of the five behavioral domains (Cermak & Daunhauer). Recent analysis using a larger sample examined the effects of length of institutionalization on sensory processing and behavior (Kadlec, 1997). In general, children with longer lengths of institutionalization showed greater difficulty (Gilbert, 1997; Kadlec, 1997; Liepprandt, 1997).

Of particular interest are some of the narrative comments included by the parents. Distractibility and attentional problems were key issues reported by parents whose children had spent substantial periods of time in orphanages. Parents frequently commented on problems in attention and organization. It is an interesting parallel that Kraemer (1995) found that motherless monkeys were especially distracted by novelty, whereas mother-reared monkeys were selective in their timing and manner of response to stimuli. The mother-reared monkeys attended to a broad array of social cues, were not overly distracted by novelty, and adapted to changes in cues needed for problem solving.

In responding to a survey sent out to families adopting children from Romania (Cermak & Daunhauer, 1997; Cermak & Groza, 1998), many parents commented on the difficulty their children had with sensory processing in the sense of touch. Comments about oversensitivity to touch were common.

> "Does not like to be hugged or kissed—it is still not natural to her. She screeches when siblings attempt to touch her. She has an aversion to children. She likes to 'bump' people with her head."

> "He gets 'like a board' at times when hugged, but other times loves to be cuddled and massaged."

> "She disliked being bathed but as with other behaviors, we felt it was because she wasn't used to it."

Whereas some parents commented on an oversensitivity to touch, other parents commented that their child didn't seem to feel pain.

> "My daughter was adopted at age 4½ from an orphanage where she lived since birth. She did not cry for the first 3 months, even when having stitches or blood tests."

> "She did not barely cry after she arrived even though she put her tooth through her lower lip."

Many parents reported a craving for proprioceptive input.

> "Thinks it's funny to fall off the bed at full speed; also likes to crash into unsuspecting people."

Oral activities (e.g., feeding and tooth brushing) were a major issue for many children with what is likely oral defensiveness, a uniformly reported characteristic.

> "It was a heartrending shock to see that my newly adopted son would not put a cracker in his mouth and gagged at the sight of any food he could not drink."

> "He doesn't like to eat. At age 2½ he couldn't tolerate a Cheerio®. Still gagged on some food at age 4. Eats only when he is starving or made to eat. He sucks on his fingers, coat, shirts, used to suck his tongue when anxious, mouthed toys until age 5."

> "She screamed and cried at getting her teeth brushed or having anything of size or texture in her mouth (she spit out all food that required chewing)."

A number of parents reported that their child also showed an oversensitivity to sound. One parent said, "He was terrified of vacuum cleaners until this past year. We suppose he's remembering some archaic medical equipment from the orphanage."

Although some children showed an oversensitivity, others showed an undersensitivity or a lack of discrimination. For example, one parent reported, "She used to stuff her mouth so full of bread that she couldn't chew it and had to take it back out."

Other parents reported changes from over- to underresponsiveness (a problem in modulation). One parent said that her son "had never had solid food, and whenever anything (e.g., cracker, crumbs, bread) touched his lips, he would gag and throw up. When he did finally start eating, he would stuff his cheek with food and keep it there for hours. We'd have to clean out his mouth when we put him to bed."

Children from orphanages appear to exhibit many indications of difficulty in sensory processing and sensory modulation. For many children, these difficulties persist over time, even after living with their adoptive families.

Prognosis

A key question therapists must ask is, To what extent is it possible to ameliorate the detrimental effects of deprivation, and if this is possible, what can be done? Several early studies have indicated that many of the effects of deprivation are reversible.

Bowlby and Ainsworth (1965) stated, "Relief from deprivation after many months of it in early infancy can result in rapid and dramatic improvement" (p. 224). Current analyses of intervention research are recognizing the adaptability of the brain and behavior throughout the entire developmental continuum (Short, 1985; Stein, Brailowski, & Will, 1995). Accordingly, even children adopted at older ages have potential for change.

Change can occur in several ways. First, it is important to improve conditions in the orphanages and institutions in an attempt to reduce the negative effects of institutionalization. Two recent studies in Romania have shown that enhancing the conditions in orphanages by providing an enriched environment can make a difference. In one study, supervisors decreased the caregiver/child ratio to one caregiver to four infants and instituted a developmental stimulation program. This enriched environment resulted in significant improvements in sensory processing for the infants (Haradon et al., 1994). In another study, Sweeney and Bascom (1995) reported that rocking diminished in the institutionalized children who participated in a developmental intervention program. However, rocking recurred during stressful or new situations and in sleep-wake transitions.

Although it is possible to improve conditions within orphanages and reduce problems, institutions are not ideal places for young children. In 1951, Bowlby concluded that it is very difficult for any institution to be "good" for infants and very young children. Bowlby has suggested that the best place for young children is in families. Thus, a second way of effecting change is through designing systems to support biological families to care for their children and, when this is not possible, to consider foster care or adoption.

Intervention

Investigators have demonstrated that enrichment of the social and physical environment results in dramatic developmental gains. However, the effects of deprivation can be long-lasting, and many children and their families require professional intervention to help ameliorate the early effects of deprivation. In discussing the potential for change, here is a continuation of Andrea's story presented at the beginning of the chapter. I have kept in touch with Andrea and her family since originally receiving the letter from her mother when Andrea was 17 months old. Andrea's mother kept a diary of her experiences and wrote,

> In looking back to the summer of 1993, I am amazed that our family survived. On August 21, 1993, I looked into those big brown eyes for the very first time. The effects of Andrea's life in the orphanage were painfully present and it almost caused our hearts to break in half. When Andrea was placed into my arms, there was no twinkle in her eyes.

Andrea's mother described the conditions in Andrea's orphanage.

> Andrea had only one red plastic block tied onto her white metal crib. I'm sure Andrea didn't even realize that it was a toy, but it did give her something else to look at other than staring at her hands. I can't imagine what

it was like for Andrea not to have anything to touch for 10 months. I can't imagine what it was like not to have anyone pick her up, or bathe her, or give her medicine when she was sick. I can't imagine what Andrea felt when I came along and said, "I am your mommy now." She obviously had no idea what in the world a mommy was. And rightly so, for Andrea didn't have a mommy to love and rock her to sleep. Andrea had to rock herself.

I wonder what Andrea felt like as she left the orphanage. She had never been outside before that day. It was as if a ball and chain had dropped off her as the plane prepared for take off. How little did I know that her chains were to imprison me for the next couple of years when I tried to resume the life that we had left behind with Juliana.

When we arrived home, Andrea was almost 11 months old and weighed 12 pounds. Her belly was grossly distended and her skinny little arms and legs stuck out of her trunk like toothpicks. Her hair was as thin as a cancer patient undergoing chemotherapy. She sucked both of her index fingers together.

Neither my husband nor I looked forward to Andrea's frequent doctor appointments, for they often yielded bad news. One neurologist, better known as Dr. Doom and Gloom, told us that Andrea's brain could be like a dried sponge that needed to be soaked with nourishment. We were functioning on overdrive and it was taking a toll on our family life. Living with Andrea had turned our lives inside out and upside down.

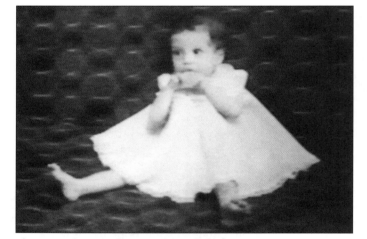

Figure 18.3. Andrea sucking her fingers.

We really needed support but we didn't find much of that from our family and friends. People couldn't see tangible problems with her. She wasn't in a wheelchair. She was gaining weight; in fact, she grew 1 inch every month that she was home during her first 6 months. She also doubled her weight during that time. Andrea's physical appearance gave a false impression that she was fine. She certainly didn't act fine to us. On one occasion, I went to my pediatrician in desperation because Andrea wasn't putting any food in her mouth. The doctor told me to leave Cheerios out and when Andrea got hungry, she would eat them. If I had taken that advice, Andrea would be dead today.

People couldn't see what we were dealing with. When we tried to explain it, many people thought we were overreacting. In Boston, Andrea received a diagnosis of sensory integration dysfunction. I wasn't even sure what it was or how to effectively deal with it. I was perplexed over how Andrea reacted to normal things that shouldn't have bothered her. Whatever touched her, repulsed her—and that was just about everything under the sun, including the sunshine or bright lights.

The pediatrician, who told me "just give Andrea love," underestimated the effects of what 10 months of maternal and sensory deprivation had on Andrea. She didn't realize that Andrea wasn't an easy child to love and that Andrea didn't necessarily want my love. No one ever told me a baby wouldn't want my love. I felt betrayed and rejected. Andrea didn't want me to touch her.

For our first year, we stayed at home to allow Andrea to adjust to her new life. We stopped going to the malls, and we never went out to dinner. We couldn't go any place where Andrea felt uncomfortable and overstimulated—and that was everywhere. We felt isolated and sad because we realized that all we wanted was a normal family life; and we had the farthest thing from it.

When Andrea was a year old, we began therapy with specialists who worked with children with sensory defensiveness. Therapists would arrive at our home at 9 in the morning. The occupational therapist came 2 hours a week; the speech and language therapist came 3 hours per week; the physical therapist came 2 hours a week; and the special educator came 1 hour a week. The therapists made my life easier by providing explanations for Andrea's actions.

Initial emphasis in occupational therapy was on parent support. Andrea's parents were strong advocates for their daughter but were at a loss to understand her behavior and felt overwhelmed by the complexity of issues. Recognizing the parents' concerns and giving them information was critical for the therapists' ability to help Andrea.

One of the first issues the therapists addressed was Andrea's refusal to eat, because this was her mother's primary concern. According to Andrea's mother,

The most serious and challenging for me was her refusal to eat. Andrea's therapist promised that someday Andrea would pick up a piece of pizza and eat it. It seemed impossible to us, but over the course of a year of intensive therapy, Andrea did enjoy eating pizza as well as a variety of other foods. Andrea learned to like macaroni and cheese and cheese doodles. Every time that we were able to include a new food into Andrea's favorite-food list, I felt a great sense of accomplishment.

Andrea's therapist introduced oral motor activities (games) that provided proprioceptive input during the day, not just at meal times, to reduce oral-motor sensitivity. For example, Andrea's father demonstrated clapping on his cheeks (deep pressure) while making a noise that would vibrate as he clapped. He then did it with Andrea, and she would imitate the noise. Other activities addressed feeding and tactile sensitivity together. For example, one activity encouraged Andrea to "paint" with whipped dessert topping on her feeding table. She would initially play with the cream using one finger. She would not put it in her own mouth but would feed her mother or father. Later, she would accept a small amount from them. Although feeding issues slowly improved, Andrea's mother said that "even at age 2, Andrea still needed to be reminded to chew her food, to swallow, to close her mouth, and to continue eating. Those tasks seem so simple as most people just take them for granted. The complexities of eating overwhelmed not only Andrea but our entire family."

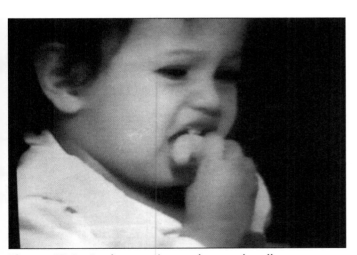

Figure 18.4. Andrea eating a cheese doodle.

Andrea's mother reported other atypical behaviors. Andrea did not seem to be able to feel pain. She would accidentally run into the wall and bang her head, and it wouldn't even bother her. Andrea would often stare at her hands and rock rhythmically instead of playing with toys. She would spin in circles several times a day for 15 to 20 minutes at a time. Andrea's mother was concerned not only because these behaviors were not productive but also because of the social implications. It "looked weird" and made Andrea appear different from her peers. The occupational therapist working with Andrea suggested a sensory diet to provide Andrea with more adaptive sensorimotor activity that would give her the vestibular input she needed. She recommended a home trampoline, swinging in playground swings, and a gymnastics program.

Andrea's mother described the changes that Andrea made from her first to her second year at home.

> I remember how happy I was the first time we made Andrea laugh. We noticed she had a wonderful smile. When she smiled, her eyes would twinkle. We were beginning to see some of her strengths, and her beauty was beginning to surface. We also discovered that Andrea had a remarkable ability to imitate. She would copy things her sister did. Actually, Andrea first bonded with her sister. I remember one evaluation in which Andrea was asked to ring a bell. I knew that Andrea had no idea what a bell was, and the concept of ringing it was even more foreign to her. Her sister went up to her and said, "Don't worry, Baby Andrea, this is a bell and this is how you ring it. Ring Ring Ring." After that demonstration, Andrea picked up the bell and rang it, wearing a proud smile for us all to see.

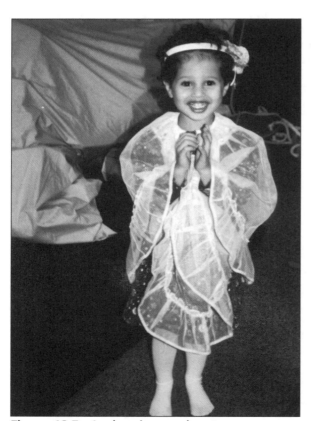

Figure 18.5. Andrea in angel costume.

During Andrea's second year with us, she started preschool. Her school report yielded wonderful news of her continuing progress. I was not accustomed to hearing such positive feedback, but it certainly gave me hope about Andrea's future. I was beginning to see a light at the end of the tunnel. We were able to go to the playground, where Andrea began to interact with other children. We were able to go on walks in the woods, down trails that were covered with crimson leaves that crinkled as we walked on them. We were able to have picnics by rolling brooks. We were beginning to feel like a normal family. We took Andrea on her first merry-go-round ride and what a thrill it was—especially for me. We were able to appreciate the simple things in life that most people take for granted. Happy faces and gleaming eyes, the kind all children should have, were now visible in both of my little girls.

Andrea taught me how to be grateful for the little things that I used to overlook. Andrea brought a different kind of love into our home and we are happy to have it. It took me several years to accept Andrea for the child she is, but now I can't imagine her any other way. She is unique and the love that I feel for her is immeasurable. I am a much wiser and kinder person today because of Andrea.

Andrea's mother concluded:

> Each child's resilience is different. Each orphanage experience is different. Each level of therapy is different. The only thing that remains the same is that most children who spend a substantial amount of time in an orphanage will need some degree of help. The children are worth saving—Andrea was. She will always be a Romanian angel to me.

Intervention Strategies and Implications of Research for Intervention

It is clear from examining the research and from working with many postinstitutionalized children that approaches to intervention must be multifaceted and interdisciplinary. Sensory integration is a critical component, but it is just one piece of the puzzle. Many children face multiple issues such as attachment, posttraumatic stress, sensory integration, language, cognitive, behavioral, and attentional concerns.

Intervention for a post-institutionalized child should begin even prior to his or her adoption. Adoption agencies must be aware of the numerous issues these children face and share this knowledge with families so that they can make informed decisions, understand their child's behavior, provide appropriate supports, and serve as advocates for their child. It is also important to provide these families with resources and professionals who are experienced in working with these children.

From an occupational therapy perspective, a primary issue facing many postinstitutionalized children is sensory defensiveness. This produces problems in relationships with parents, siblings, and peers because the children withdraw from physical contact. It also interferes with learning because many children refuse to play with toys, not liking the feel and/or the sound the toys make. Because children typically learn through playing, this avoidance of play can compound their delays even further. Sensory defensiveness interferes with activities of daily living, including bathing, hair combing, fingernail cutting, dressing, and eating. Feeding is often an issue because many children refuse solid foods. Although this relates to lack of experience for some children, it reflects oral-motor sensitivity related to sensory defensiveness for others and requires professional intervention. Other feeding problems include overstuffing the mouth, perhaps because of reduced discrimination.

Other concerns listed by a large number of parents include attention, distractibility, hyperactivity, and impulsivity. Many parents of postinstitutionalized children report that their children crave movement and proprioception. They are the "crashers" and "sensation seekers." As has been observed in other groups of children with issues in sensory integration, many of these same children show sensory defensiveness and are bothered by light touch. In her early research, Ayres (1964) reported a relationship between hyperactivity and tactile defensiveness. The relationships between sensory integration and attention, distractibility, and impulsivity need further investigation in this population.

Acknowledgments

I would like to acknowledge my family for all their support, especially my younger children, Bethany and Amanda, for sharing their "mommy time" so that I could spend time in Romania; to my husband Laird for supporting my work and holding down the fort at home; to Bill Whalen and Lucy Miller whose initial invitation to Romania in 1992 started me on this adventure; to my mentors in sensory integration, Dr. Anne Henderson and Dr. A. Jean Ayres; to Barbara Canale for sharing Andrea and her story, so that others may learn and grow; to Thais Tepper and Lois Hannon of the Parent Network for the Post-Institutionalized Child for networking parents and professionals to meet the needs of the children; to my colleagues at Boston University, Mary-Margaret Windsor, Carolyn Robinson, and our graduate students Lisa Daunhauer, Elise Gilbert, Heather Shuman, Christi Beltramo, and Geoff Reinhold who accompanied me on the 1995 trip to Romania and made the impossible possible. I extend special appreciation to Lisa Daunhauer who, upon graduation, returned to Romania as a volunteer for 6 months to continue our work. To my graduate students who have been bitten by the research bug and have collaborated with me on research, so that we can better understand the developmental and sensory integration issues: Susan Lin, Elise Gilbert, Julee Liepprandt, Lisa Daunhauer, Mary Beth Kadlec, and Kerry Dunphy. To my colleagues in Romania, particularly Dr. Veronica Draghici and family, Dr. Catalina Varlam and Ioan Varlam, Beth Bradford, Gigi Roman, and the Petrescu family, who have supported and facilitated our work and have shared their culture and their lives. I have been particularly impressed with and would like to acknowledge the work of two of my occupational therapy colleagues, Dr. Mary Schneider and Dr. Gary Kraemer. Their research at the Wisconsin Regional Primate Research Center provides critical insights into the behavioral and neurobiological consequences of stress and deprivation. Most importantly, a very special thank you to the children and their fabulous families who have shared their lives with me and helped me to grow and learn: Andrea (New York), Drue (Pennsylvania), Marc (California), Daniel (Texas), Elizabeth and Gina (New Hampshire), Elena (California), Ben (Virginia), and Charlotte (Virginia).

This chapter is dedicated in loving memory to my husband Laird.

Works Cited

Quotations on pages 387, 389, 390 from *Infants in Institutions* by S. Provence and R.C. Lipton (1962) have been reprinted with permission by International Universities Press.

References

Achenbach, T.M. (1991). *Manual for the Child Behavior Checklist/4–18 and 1991 Profile.* Burlington, VT: University of Vermont Department of Psychiatry.

Ainsworth, M.D. (1965). Further research into the adverse effects of maternal deprivation. In J. Bowlby (Ed.), *Childcare and the growth of love* (2nd ed., pp. 191–251). Baltimore: Penguin Books.

Albers, L.H., Johnson, D.E., Hostetter, M., Iverson, S., & Miller, L. (1997). Health of children adopted from the former Soviet Union and Eastern Europe. *Journal of the American Medical Association, 278,* 922–924.

Ames, E.W. (1997). *The development of Romanian orphanage children adopted to Canada.* Burnaby, British Columbia: Simon Fraser University.

Ames, E.W., Carter, M.C., Chisholm, K., Fisher, L., Gilman, L.C., Mainemer, H., McMullan, S.J., & Savoie, L.A. (1992, June). A study of Romanian orphanage children in Canada: Background, sample, and procedure. *Development of Romanian orphanage children adopted to Canada.* Symposium conducted at the Annual Convention of the Canadian Psychological Association, Quebec City, Canada.

Anderson, J.W., Johnstone, B.M., & Remley, D.T. (1999). Breast-feeding and cognitive development: A meta-analysis. *American Journal of Clinical Nutrition, 70,* 525–535.

Ayres, A.J. (1964). Tactile functions: Their relationship to hyperactive and perceptual motor behavior. *American Journal of Occupational Therapy, 18,* 6–11.

Ayres, A.J. (1979). *Sensory integration and the child.* Los Angeles: Western Psychological Services.

Bayley, N. (1969). *Bayley Scales of Infant Development.* San Antonio, TX: The Psychological Corporation.

Blakeslee, S. (1995a, August 29). In brain's early growth, timetable may be crucial. *New York Times, Science Times,* pp. C1–C3.

Blakeslee, S. (1995b, August 31). How a bad beginning can affect the brain. *New York Times,* pp. C1, C6.

Bowlby, J. (1951). *Maternal care and mental health.* Geneva, Switzerland: World Health Organization.

Bowlby, J. (1953). *Childcare and the growth of love.* Baltimore: Penguin.

Bowlby, J., & Ainsworth, M. (1965). *Child: Care, health, and development.* Baltimore: Penguin Books.

Bradley, R.H., Caldwell, B.M., Rock, S.L., & Harris, P.T. (1986). Early home environment and the development of competence: Findings from the Little Rock longitudinal study. *Children's Environments Quarterly, 3,* 10–22.

Carlson, M., & Earls, F. (1997). Psychological and neuroendocrinological sequelae of early social deprivation in institutionalized children in Romania. *Annals New York Academy of Sciences, 807,* 419–428.

Casler, L. (1961). Maternal deprivation: A critical review of the literature. *Monographs of the Society for Research in Child Development, 26*(2), 1–64.

Casler, L. (1968). Perceptual deprivation in institutional settings. In G. Newton, and S. Levine (Eds.), *Early experience and behavior* (pp. 573–626). Springfield: Charles C. Thomas.

Cermak, S., & Daunhauer, L.A. (1997). Sensory processing in the post-institutionalized child. *American Journal of Occupational Therapy, 51,* 500–507.

Cermak, S., & Groza, V. (1998). Sensory integration in post-institutionalized children: Implications for social workers. *Child and Adolescent Social Work Journal, 15*(1), 5–37.

Children's Health Care Collaborative Study Group. (1994). The causes of children's institutionalization in Romania. *Child: Care, Health and Development, 20,* 77–88.

DeGangi, G. (1991a). Part 1: Assessment of sensory, emotional, and attentional problems in regulatory disordered infants. *Infants and Young Children, 3,* 1–8.

DeGangi, G. (1991b). Part 2: Treatment of sensory, emotional, and attentional problems in regulatory disordered infants. *Infants and Young Children, 3,* 9–19.

Diamond, M.C. (1967). Extensive cortical depth measurements and neuron size increases in the cortex of environmentally enriched rats. *Journal of Comparative Neurology, 131,* 357–364.

Diamond, M.C., Ingham, C.A., Johnson, R.E., Bennett, E.L., & Rosenzweig, M.R. (1976). Effects of environment on morphology of rat cerebral cortex and hippocampus. *Journal of Neurobiology, 7,* 75–86.

Doll, E. (1935). *Vineland Social Maturity Scale.* Circle Pines, MN: American Guidance Center.

Dunn, W. (1994). Performance of typical children on the Sensory Profile: An item analysis. *American Journal of Occupational Therapy, 48*(11), 967–974.

Field, T. (1994). Caregiving environments for infants. *Children's Environments, 11*(2), 147–154.

Field, T., Morrow, C., Valdeon, C., Larson, S., Kuhn, C., & Schanberg, S. (1992). Massage reduces anxiety in child and adolescent psychiatric patients. *Journal of the American Academy of Child and Adolescent Psychiatry, 31*(1), 125–131.

Field, T., Schanberg, S.M., Scafidi, F., Bauer, C.R., Vega-Laher, N., Garcia, R., Nystrom, J., & Kuhn, C.M. (1986). Tactile-kinesthetic stimulation effects on preterm infants. *Pediatrics, 77*(5), 654–658.

Frank, D., & Zeisel, S. (1988). Failure to thrive. *Pediatric Clinics of North America, 35,* 1187–1206.

Frankenburg, W.K. (1986). *Revised Denver Prescreening Developmental Questionnaire (R-DPDQ).* Denver, CO: Denver Developmental Materials, Inc.

Frankenburg, W.K., Dodds, J., Archer, P., Bresnick, B., Maschka, P., Edelman, N., & Shapiro, H. (1975). *Denver Developmental Screening Test.* Denver, CO: Denver Developmental Materials, Inc.

Galler, J. (1993). Malnutrition and mental development. In R. Suskind & L. Lewinter-Suskind (Eds.), *Textbook of pediatric nutrition* (2nd ed., pp. 173–179). New York: Raven Press.

Galler, J., & Ross, R. (1998). Malnutrition and mental development. *POST: The Parent Network for the Post-Institutionalized Child, 20*(6), 1–8.

Gilbert, E.S. (1997). *Sensory deprivation manifested in the domain of touch in post–institutionalized children from Romania.* Unpublished master's thesis, Boston University, MA.

Goldfarb, W. (1945). Effects of psychological depth in infancy and subsequent stimulation. *American Journal of Psychiatry, 102,* 18–33.

Greenspan, S. (1995). *The challenging child.* Reading, MA: Addison Wesley.

Groza, V., & Ileana, D. (1996). A follow-up study of adopted children from Romania. *Child and Adolescent Social Work Journal, 13*(6), 541–565.

Haradon, G., Bascom, B., Dragomir, C., & Scripcaru, V. (1994). Sensory functions of institutionalized Romanian infants: A pilot study. *Occupational Therapy International, 1,* 250–260.

Harlow, H.F. (1958). The nature of love. *The American Psychologist, 13,* 673–685.

Harlow, H.F., & Harlow, M.K. (1966). Learning to love. *American Scientist, 54,* 244–272.

Harlow, H.F., & Suomi, S.J. (1970). The nature of love—Simplified. *American Psychologist, 25,* 162–168.

Johnson, A., & Groza, V. (1993). The orphaned and institutionalized children of Romania. *Journal of Emotional and Behavioral Problems, 2*(4), 49–52.

Johnson, D., Miller, L., Iverson, S., Thomas, W., Franchino, B., Dole, K., Kiernan, M., Gergieff, M., & Hostetter, M. (1992). The health of children adopted from Romania. *Journal of the American Medical Association, 268*(24), 3446–3451.

Jones, M.B. (1993). Decline of the American orphanage, 1941–1980. *Social Service Review, 67,* 459–480.

Kadlec, M.B. (1997). *Activity level, organization, and social-emotional behavior in post-institutionalized children.* Unpublished master's thesis, Boston University, MA.

Knobloch, H., Stevens, F., & Malone, F. (1980). *Gesell Developmental Schedules.* NY: The Psychological Corporation.

Kraemer, G.W. (1992). A psychobiological theory of attachment. *Behavior and Brain Sciences, 15,* 493–511.

Kraemer, G.W. (1995). Significance of social attachment in primate infants: The infant-caregiver relationship and volition. In C.R. Pryce, R.D. Martin, & D. Skuse (Eds.), *Motherhood in human and nonhuman primates, 3rd Schultz-Biegert Symposium* (pp. 152–161). Basel, Switzerland: Karger.

Kraemer, G.W., Ebert, M.H., Schmidt, D.E., & McKinney, W.T. (1991). Strangers in a strange land: A psychobiological study of mother-infant separation in rhesus monkeys. *Child Development, 62,* 548–566.

Kuhn, C., Schanberg, S., Field, T., Symanski, R., Zimmerman, E., Scafidi, F., & Roberts, J. (1991). Tactile-kinesthetic stimulation effects on sympathetic and adrenocortical function in preterm infants. *The Journal of Pediatrics, 119,* 434–440.

Latham, M. (1997). *Human nutrition in the developing world* (FAO Food and Nutrition Series, No. 29). Rome, Italy: Food and Agriculture Organization.

Liepprandt, J.A. (1997). *Sensory processing in post-institutionalized children from Romania: An analysis of the movement scale.* Unpublished master's thesis, Boston University, MA.

Liu, D., Diorio, J., Tannenbaum, B., Caldji, C., Francis, D., Freedman, A., Sharma, S., Pearson, D., Plotsky, P., & Meaney, M. (1997). Maternal care, hippocampal gluco-corticoid receptors, and hypothalamic-pituitary-adrenal responses to stress. *Science, 277,* 1659–1662.

Marcovitch, S., Cesaroni, L., Roberts, W., & Swanson, C. (1995). Romanian adoption: Parents' dreams, nightmares, and realities. *Child Welfare, 74*(5), 993–1017.

Marcovitch, S., Goldberg, S., Gold, A., Washington, J., Wasson, C., Kerkewitch, K., & Handler-Derry, M. (1997). Determinants of behavior problems in Romanian children adopted in Ontario. *International Journal of Behavioral Development, 20*(1), 17–31.

Mason, W.A., & Berkson, G. (1975). Effects of maternal mobility on the development of rocking and other behaviors in rhesus monkeys: A study with artificial mothers. *Developmental Psychobiology, 8,* 197–211.

Meaney, M., Aitken, D., Bhatnagar, S., Bodnoff, S., Mitchell, J., & Sarrieau, A. (1990). Neonatal handling and the development of the adrenocortical response to stress. In N. Gunzenhauser (Ed.), *Advances in touch: New implications for human development. Pediatric Roundtable 14* (pp. 11–22). Skill, NH: Johnson & Johnson Consumer Products.

Meyers, A., & Chawla, N. (2000, August/September). Nutrition and the social, emotional, and cognitive development of infants and young children. *Zero to Three,* 5–12.

Morison, S., Ames, E., & Chisholm, K. (1995). The development of children adopted from Romanian orphanages. *Merrill-Palmer Quarterly, 41*(4), 411–430.

Nyman, A.J. (1967). Problem solving in rats as a function of experiences at different ages. *Journal of Genetic Psychology, 110,* 31–39.

Occupational Therapy Associates, P.C. (1993). *Sensory History Checklist.* Watertown, MA: Author.

O'Connor, T.G., & Rutter, M. (2000). Attachment disorder behavior following early severe deprivation: Extension and longitudinal follow-up. *Journal of the American Academy of Child and Adolescent Psychiatry, 39*(6), 703–712.

O'Connor, T.G., Rutter, M., Beckett, C., Keaveney, L., & Kreppner, J.M. (2000). The effects of global severe privation on cognitive competence: Extension and longitudinal follow-up. *Child Development, 71*(2), 376–390.

Ottenbacher, K., Muller, L., Brandt, D., Heintzelman, A., Hojem, P., & Sharpe, P. (1987). The effectiveness of tactile stimulation as a form of early intervention: A quantitative evaluation. *Journal of Developmental and Behavioral Pediatrics, 8,* 68–76.

Perry, B.D. (1993a). Neurodevelopment and the neurophysiology of trauma I: Conceptual considerations for clinical work with maltreated children. *The Advisor, 6*(1), 1, 14–18.

Perry, B.D. (1993b). Neurodevelopment and the neurophysiology of trauma II: Conceptual considerations for clinical work with maltreated children. *The Advisor, 6*(2), 1, 14–20.

Provence, S. (1967). *Guide for the care of infants in groups.* New York: Child Welfare League.

Provence, S., & Lipton, R.C. (1962). *Infants in institutions.* New York: International Universities Press.

Reite, M. (1990). Effects of touch on the immune system. In N. Gunzenhauser (Ed.), *Advances in touch: New implications in human development. Pediatric Roundtable 14* (pp. 22–34). Skill, NJ: Johnson & Johnson Consumer Products.

Rosenzweig, M.R., & Bennett, E.L. (1978). Experimental influences on brain anatomy and brain chemistry in rodents. In G.C. Gottlieb (Ed.), *Studies on the development of behavior and the nervous system* (pp. 314–315). New York: Academic Press.

Royeen, C.B., & Lane, S.J. (1991). Tactile processing and sensory defensiveness. In A.G. Fisher, E.A. Murray, & A.C. Bundy (Eds.), *Sensory integration: Theory and practice* (pp. 108–135). Philadelphia: F.A. Davis.

Rutter, M. (1998). Developmental catch-up, and deficit, following adoption after severe global early privation. *Journal of Child Psychology and Psychiatry, 39*(4), 465–476.

Sapolsky, R.M. (1997). The importance of a well-groomed child. *Science, 277,* 1620–1621.

Scafidi, F.A., Field, T., & Schanberg, S.M. (1993). Factors that predict when preterm infants benefit most from massage therapy. *Developmental and Behavioral Pediatrics, 14*(3), 176–180.

Scafidi, F.A., Field, T., Schanberg, S., Bauer, C., Tucci, K., Roberts, J., Morrow, C., & Kuhn, C. (1990). Massage stimulates growth in preterm infants: A replication. *Infant Behavior and Development, 13,* 167–188.

Schanberg, S., Kuhn, C., Field, T., & Bartolome, J. (1990). Maternal deprivation and growth suppression. In N. Gunzenhauser (Ed.), *Advances in touch: New implications in human development. Pediatric Roundtable 14* (pp. 3–10). Skill, NJ: Johnson & Johnson Consumer Products.

Schneider, M.L. (1987). *A rhesus monkey model of human infant individual differences.* Unpublished doctoral dissertation. The University of Wisconsin, Madison.

Schneider, M., Kraemer, G., & Suomi, S. (1991). The effects of vestibular-proprioceptive stimulation on motor maturation and response to challenge in rhesus monkey infants. *The Occupational Therapy Journal of Research, 11*(3), 135–151.

Short, M. (1985). Vestibular stimulation as early experience: Historical perspectives and research implications. In K.J. Ottenbacher, & M.A. Short (Eds.), *Vestibular processing dysfunction in children* (pp. 135–152). New York: The Haworth Press.

Sigman, M., McDonald, M.A., Neumann, C., & Bwibo, N. (1991). Prediction of cognitive competence in Kenyan children from toddler nutrition, family characteristics and abilities. *Journal of Child Psychology and Psychiatry, 32,* 307–320.

Sparrow, S.S., Balla, D.A., & Cicchetti, D.V. (1984). *Vineland Adaptive Behavior Scales, Revised.* Circle Pines, MN: American Guidance Service.

Spitz, R. (1945). Hospitalism: An inquiry into the genesis of psychiatric conditions in early childhood. *The Psychoanalytic Study of the Child, 1,* 53–74.

Spitz, R. (1946). Hospitalism: A follow-up report. *The Psychoanalytic Study of the Child, 2,* 113–117.

Stein, D.G., Brailowsky, S., & Will, B. (1995). *Brain repair.* New York: Oxford University.

Sweeney, J.K., & Bascom, B.B. (1995). Motor development and self-stimulatory movement in institutionalized Romanian children. *Pediatric Physical Therapy, 7,* 124–132.

Trott, M.C., Laurel, M., & Windeck, S. (1993). *SenseAbilities, understanding sensory integration.* San Antonio, TX: Therapy Skill Builders.

Vygotsky, L.S. (1978). *Mind in society.* Cambridge, MA: Harvard University Press.

Additional Readings

Kaler, S., & Freeman, B.I. (1993). Analysis of environmental deprivation: Cognitive and social development in Romanian orphans. *Journal of Child Psychology and Psychiatry, 35,* 769–781.

Kimball, J.G. (1993). Sensory integrative frame of reference. In P. Kramer & J. Hinojosa (Eds.), *Frames of reference for pediatric occupational therapy* (pp. 87–175). Baltimore: Williams and Wilkins.

Sensory Integration and Fragile X Syndrome

Lois Hickman, M.S., OTR, FAOTA

At the close of a lecture I had given on Fragile X, I received a note from a man with Fragile X syndrome. The note said, "Thank you for telling people about us. We have a lot to teach, but we need your help. We can't do it alone."

This chapter responds to this man's plea, continuing the dialogue on Fragile X using a sensory integrative framework. Sensory integration provides a basis for understanding the nature and characteristics of this genetic disorder and for offering effective and compassionate intervention strategies.

Researchers have investigated Fragile X within scientific disciplines such as biochemistry, neurology, and the behavioral sciences and within many allied health professions such as developmental optometry, speech pathology, special education, and occupational therapy (Miller et al., 1999). Results of these investigations show that individuals who have Fragile X syndrome exhibit an extremely wide range of physical and behavioral characteristics (Hagerman, 1996). It is crucial, when interacting with these clients and their families, to consider individual differences, environmental circumstances, and the unpredictability of individual needs and personalities. It is also important to have a general understanding of the typical characteristics of Fragile X and at the same time respect the uniquenesses of each person's individuality. Because of the wide variability within this population, there can be no blanket assumptions, and there are no intervention "recipes" that address the needs of everyone with this diagnosis.

On a personal level, I have wondered what people labeled "Fragile X" share in common beyond their diagnosis. Being placed under a microscope can be quite uncomfortable. In contrast to the research that describes in detail the chromosomes and "odd" mannerisms of individuals with Fragile X, perhaps what is under the microscope—in scrutinizing Fragile X or any other disorder—is really the complexity of our own humanness. Perhaps this scrutiny magnifies and makes clear many of our own challenges, especially within our overly stimulating, overly busy, and mechanized culture. Persons whose nervous systems are generally adapting well often feel overwhelmed by the pace of today's culture. People with Fragile X feel overwhelmed most of the time (Miller et al., 1999). Their magnified reactions demonstrate just how out of balance things are for them, both within their nervous systems and in their external world. I have learned a great deal about what it means to be human from people with this syndrome, and especially what it means to be human in this culture, in the chaotic world into which we have been born and to which we are expected to adapt. A child with Fragile X captured his challenges in processing multiple sensations when he said, "There is a traffic jam in my head."

General Characteristics

Fragile X is the leading known hereditary cause of developmental disabilities, affecting approximately 1 in 1,250 males and 1 in 2,250 females in the general population (Reiss, 1996). This genetic disorder usually affects males more severely than females; however, 1 in 450 females could be carrying the gene. It occurs equally in all racial groups (Hagerman, 1996).

Geneticists have linked Fragile X syndrome with the fragile site on the X chromosome (Turner, Till, & Daniel, 1978). A very accurate pre- or postnatal DNA blood test can detect affected as well as nonaffected carriers (Feng, Lakkis, & Warren, 1995). Males and females with Fragile X syndrome can exhibit a range of physical characteristics (Hagerman et al., 1992) (Figure 19.1). These traits usually become more evident as the person approaches adolescence and adulthood (Hagerman, 1996).

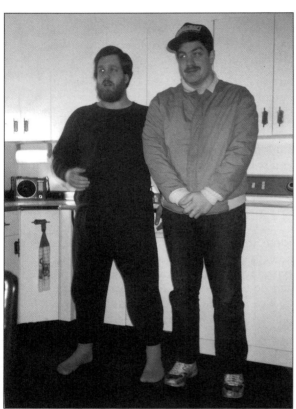

Figure 19.1. Paul and Keith are brothers with Fragile X syndrome who show typical characteristics of this genetic disorder.

Some of the characteristics of Fragile X include:

- a high incidence of otitis media in the first 6 months

- mitral valve prolapse (a benign heart condition)

- connective tissue dysplasia, evidenced by hyperextensible finger joints (fingers bend to a 90-degree or greater extension angle at the knuckle), flat feet with pronation, and looseness of thumbs, elbows, and ankles

- long, narrow face

- puffiness around the eyes and narrow palpebral fissures

- high, prominent forehead

- large or prominent ears

- strabismus, including esotropia, exotropia, and hyper-deviation

- smooth, soft skin

- macroorchidism (enlarged testicles) in adolescent and adult males

- high-arched palate, with crowding of teeth

- single palmar or simian crease

- indentation of the chest (pectum recurvatum)

- prominence of lower jaw in older males

- seizures (which usually resolve by adulthood) in about 10% of this population

In addition, the Behavioral Neurogenetics and Neuroimaging Research Center of the Kennedy Kreiger Institute has identified a variety of neurological findings revealed by magnetic resonance imaging research (Reiss, 1996):

- The vermis of the cerebellum is smaller in individuals with Fragile X than in individuals who do not have Fragile X. The vermis processes sensory information, is involved in regulation of attention and movement, and might play a role in language.

- The hippocampus, an area of the temporal lobe, tends to increase in size as the person matures. There is a related decrease in size of the superior temporal gyrus, which is important in language development.

- The caudate nucleus is larger in individuals with Fragile X than in individuals who do not have Fragile X. This region deals with eye movements, mood regulation, impulse control, and ability to adapt to changing environments.

- The lateral ventricles increase in size as the person matures. This increase, not related to hydrocephalus, occurs in other neurological conditions as well and usually reflects abnormal brain development or loss of brain tissue, with adverse effects on language development.

Investigators have correlated the severity of symptoms with the amount of protein coating in the central nervous system. Mild protein deficits occur in individuals with mild features of Fragile X syndrome, whereas more extensive protein-coating deficiency occurs in individuals with more extensive behavioral and physiological signs (Hagerman, 1996). Protein replacement therapy, which would involve protein infusion into the interior of target cells in the central nervous system, might be a viable approach in the future if researchers can resolve the immunologic complications (Ratazzi & Ianni, 1996).

Being aware of the most pertinent medical implications of this genetic disorder helps in understanding the subsequent behavioral and sensory issues that require a multifaceted approach that includes sensory integrative intervention.

General Behavioral Challenges

Individuals with Fragile X syndrome, whether male or female, exhibit varying degrees of behavioral challenges that might relate to sensory processing (Hagerman, 1996) (see the following section in this chapter, Sensory Processing Characteristics). Impulsivity, anxiety around any changes in routine, and environmental sensitivity are some of the most debilitating impairments (Miller et. al., 1999). These symptoms interact, and disturbance in any one of these sensitivities can set off a chain reaction in the others. When overstimulated, some individuals exhibit hand flapping, hand biting, or retreating to a more quiet or secluded area. If the reaction is severe, the person might have an aggressive outburst or panic attack. (However, panic attacks do not always have an obvious connection to overstimulation.) A panic attack can cause an individual to feel extremely sensitive such that he or she cannot tolerate any sound or human contact. Common environmental sensitivities include resistance to being touched or held, aversion to certain sounds or sudden noises, sensitivity to smells and visual stimuli, and fear of being out of contact with the ground.

Because males have only one X chromosome, males with Fragile X tend to exhibit greater involvement than females (Chudley & Hagerman, 1987). Both males and females demonstrate a wide variability in severity of problems, from cognition to unusual behaviors; however, most females have less physical involvement (Hagerman, 1996). Among the behaviors that individuals with Fragile X exhibit, almost all males have attention problems, along with hyperactivity and hypersensitivity to environmental stimuli (Hagerman & Cronister, 1996). Males and some females with Fragile X sometimes seek social interaction with approach-avoidance behavior, wanting to interact but then being overwhelmed by eye contact or conversation (Braden 1995, 1996; Hagerman, 1996).

Some individuals with Fragile X have the ability to remember faces, names, and details about people they meet, even after several years. In addition, playfulness and humor are natural developments when a trust relationship has grown between therapist and client. For example, a 32-year-old client likes to say, "Come on, let's play" when therapy becomes too serious. He also loves to experiment with sounds and phrases that resemble a different language, such as French, Italian, or Spanish. When I say, "I don't understand that language or a single word you're saying!" he replies with a grin, "I don't either!" A 19-year-old client told me an inside joke from his school: "Don't eat the cooks! Just eat the food!—That's my teacher's joke!"

Individuals with Fragile X are extremely and painfully shy. For example, I hadn't seen an 11-year-old boy, whom I had known since he was a toddler, for over a year. He practiced for almost an hour about how he was going to greet me. When we actually met, however, he was unable to manage even a handshake or a glance. His much-rehearsed greeting went unsaid. One young woman with more severe involvement with whom I worked was also painfully shy. She found it difficult to talk above a whisper or to lift her head during the session. However, her desire to relate socially was obvious and poignant. Although her clothes were wrinkled and her hair unkempt, she demonstrated her longing to be attractive and accepted by clutching under her arm a book on self-improvement called *Color Me Beautiful*.

All individuals with Fragile X will have behavioral challenges. The intensity of the person's reaction to the environment and to interactions with others can vary greatly and will affect all of the individual's relationships and interactions. It is important to appreciate the tremendous variability in physical, cognitive, and behavioral characteristics of individuals with Fragile X syndrome as well as their unique styles of interaction and attempts to play.

Sensory Processing Characteristics

The occupational therapist focuses on assisting people in developing independence so that they can participate meaningfully in their lives. Because persons with Fragile X syndrome demonstrate overarousal and atypical sensory processing, the therapist must contend with how these individuals respond to everything (touch, sound, smells, visual stimulation, and transitions) and everyone in the environment, and how they regulate their internal states and sensations (Miller et. al., 1999). People with Fragile X often have trouble dealing with things that most people take for granted. This is the hallmark of sensory integration as a hidden disability.

Some children who have Fragile X syndrome are afraid to move off the ground, fearful of swings or slides or of being picked up. Others need to be moving and running around constantly but move stiffly and don't have good balance if they try to move slowly and with smooth control. Others have severe defensive reactions to light touch. People with Fragile X can also exhibit a dichotomy in responsiveness to sound. A person with an almost painful aversion to certain sounds might also have a natural and acute "ear" for music. And though individuals might have impairments in social language, they sometimes have an uncannily accurate imitation of speaking and singing voices. Just as some individuals perseverate on hand flapping or rocking their bodies, others use sounds (such as "zzz") or hum when they are upset or overly excited.

Therapists can use music to advantage with these individuals to help maintain behavioral organization (Burns & Hickman, 1989; Hickman, 1997). In a summer day camp for 5- to 10-year-old children with Fragile X, music was the transitional cue between each activity. The children usually gathered in a quiet circle time with lights dimmed and calming music in the background, which gave the children an opportunity to regroup before the next activity began. These environmental factors—the definite closure of each activity, the gentle transition time allowing preparation for the next activity, and the support of the music—seemed to help the children feel more organized and able to cooperate while maintaining composure without feeling pressure.

In my own practice, I have experienced the regulatory effects that music can have in spontaneous and practical ways. On my way to do an observational visit in the high school classes of a young man with Fragile X, I was walking behind the young man. I noticed that his mincing gait and hunched posture seemed to reflect his apprehension about the impending experience of being "in the spotlight." As soon as I began humming a marching tune, his posture straightened, his stride lengthened, and he walked into his school with an air of self-confidence!

As part of a generalized sensory modulation deficit, sensitivity to smell is commonly an issue for individuals with Fragile X syndrome. Therapists frequently give this issue too little attention. Some children gag when exposed to certain smells such as strawberry, cherry, lemon, mint, chocolate, and peanut butter. Others comment that the smells are all "good!" When testing becomes too stressful, they reach for the particular aroma that is the most alerting or calming for them. Others identify all scents correctly and are so sensitive to smell that even other peoples' slight body odors cause them to become noticeably annoyed or upset. Because of this sensitivity, it is wise to avoid perfumes, scented makeup, aftershave, and deodorants when in contact with persons who have Fragile X syndrome.

Miller et al. (1999) confirmed these clinically observed sensitivities by testing electrodermal responses to noise, touch, visual, and olfactory stimuli. These investigators found that defensive sensory responses occurred across all sensory modalities and hypothesized that hyperarousal and hypersensitivity indicate an imbalance of sympathetic and parasympathetic systems.

Assessment

Behaviors and responses to environmental stresses provide valuable clues to the person's therapeutic needs. Included in an article by T.M. Stackhouse, *Sensory Integration Concepts and Fragile X Syndrome,* (1991), is a list of behaviors to observe when evaluating individuals with Fragile X syndrome.

The following questions can give additional insight into the individual's specific strengths and needs.

- Which situations at home, school, or in the community are the most stressful, and which help the person feel most accepted, calm, happy, or organized?
- Which behaviors or mannerisms are warning signs of "overload"?
- How extensive are the physiological characteristics, which can reflect the extent of neurological involvement?
- What kinds of support has the person received?
- What is important to the client and the family?
- What are their beliefs and cultural expectations?
- What does the client and the family hope to gain from your testing?

The testing situation for children with Fragile X syndrome is often a challenge. Testing might require the therapist to adapt the assessment to elicit observable behaviors. The following examples illustrate some of the adaptations and accommodations therapists can make:

- One 3-year-old boy could cooperate during a speech therapy assessment only if the occupational therapist bounced him firmly on a therapy ball between assessment items.

- A 3-year-old girl was able to focus on assessment only if she was lying prone on the therapy ball and rocked forward with deep pressure on her back and lower spine, with the test materials on the floor in front of her.

- An 8-year-old boy responded best if he could sit on a therapy ball or barrel during standardized testing. He also needed to sit with his back against the wall so that he could face the door. The examiner had to remove any extraneous items from the room to decrease distraction.

- Several children could cooperate only if they were safely under the table or sitting on the floor during the entire testing session.

- A 10-year-old girl needed to feel in control of the testing situation and "took turns" with the examiner.

- A 19-year-old young man became quite agitated midway through an occupational therapy evaluation, which was the last in a 2-day battery of tests by his team. He began biting the back of his hand. I observed, "You must get very tired of being looked at and tested so much. You must get so upset that you have to bite your hand. Let's think of some other ways that might help when things get tough." Immediately his shoulders relaxed and he breathed a big sigh. This young man had already completed the olfactory testing, and after I had acknowledged his discomfort and his hand biting, he said, "I want that smell again." He reached for the strawberry vial. During the ensuing session, various non-noxious floral and food smells helped him to stay organized. He later acknowledged his feeling of being understood in a letter he insisted on writing to me as soon as he returned home from the evaluation.

Intervention Options

Pharmacological and Optometric Interventions

Professionals have addressed the behavioral and medical challenges of Fragile X syndrome with a spectrum of drug options to control seizures, attention deficit, and panic attacks (Hagerman, 1991, 1996). Folic acid was the first medication professionals used with persons with Fragile X syndrome (Hagerman, 1996). Families reported that folic acid improved their children's attention and language and that it helped alleviate mood swings. The vitamin usually has greater results with prepubertal boys. Thought to be effective because of its effect on dopamine synthesis, folic acid supplementation can begin in early infancy, whereas physicians prescribe drugs such as clonodine, methylphenidate, dexedrine, and guanfacine only for children older than 3 years of age to control attention deficit and hyperactivity. Parents and professionals who decide to use pharmacological intervention to address the issues of anxiety, attention disorders, and panic attacks must always use medication as a complement to language, sensorimotor, family counseling, and educational support services (Hagerman, 1996; Scharfenacker, Hickman, & Braden, 1991).

Behavioral optometry has developed visual therapeutic intervention that involves awareness and control of ocular movement, then automatic ocular control. Goals and methods of intervention of the behavioral optometrist are often consistent with those of the occupational therapist (Martinez & Maino, 1993).

Sensory Integration Intervention Strategies

My own experience with children and adults with Fragile X syndrome began with one child, a 3-year-old boy whose only diagnosis had been "developmental delay." He was "untestable." The interpretation of his play behavior and reaction to the sounds, touch, and sights in his environment was that he had "dyspraxia, attention deficit, and sensory defensiveness." His balance skills and movement patterns reflected inadequate postural stability. He exhibited pronounced finger hyperextensibility and poor facial muscle tone. His speech was delayed. The little language he had was echolalic, perseverative, and often very loud. Transitions were very difficult for him. Trips to the supermarket, restaurants, or birthday parties could be overwhelming for him and extremely trying for his parents. His irritation at the feel of tags in the necks of his shirts was extreme, and his parents found that the clothes they purchased for him had to be natural fiber and couldn't be "itchy." He could tolerate only a narrow range of textures and tastes of food, not too smooth or "slimy" and not too bland.

This child's challenges spanned the realms of physical, behavioral, and language development and involved sensory modulation, discrimination, and praxis. He had difficulty with self-regulation. He began a program of occupational therapy using a sensory integrative approach combined with a speech and language program using a pragmatic speech approach. He responded very well to this type of intervention and demonstrated improvements in many of the aforementioned behaviors. A year later, a neurologist diagnosed Fragile X syndrome and was surprised at how well the child was doing compared to other children with this syndrome whom she had evaluated. In discussing her evaluation of this child with his parents, her opinion was that a major element in his progress had been the type of therapy he had received. We agreed that addressing his sensory integration issues in conjunction with his language problems had been the important variant.

Sensory integration intervention principles that Dr. A. Jean Ayres originally proposed can provide valuable insights for intervention when working with the Fragile X population (Ayres, 1972; Stackhouse, 1994, 1996). Recent neurological research based on galvanic skin reaction supports the observations made clinically that individuals with Fragile X syndrome exhibit hyperreactivity involving all sensory systems (Miller et al., 1999). Clinicians have observed that the resulting behaviors characterized by high-level sympathetic reactions lend themselves to sensory strategies for inhibition and reduction of defensive reactions (Ayres & Tickle, 1980).

In addition, a multidisciplinary approach to intervention for the child with Fragile X syndrome is important. Family-centered occupational and speech therapies in conjunction with the appropriate medical, optometric, nutritional, psychological, and educational support can address some basic needs (Windeck & Laurel, 1989).

Ideas for Therapy, Home, and the School Setting

Following are some suggestions that clinicians have found to be helpful for individuals with Fragile X syndrome.

- Provide a quiet area to which the person can retreat. Furnish this retreat with a soft mat, a favorite blanket, beanbag chairs, the person's favorite music, and other objects that help in calming.

- Reduce visual and auditory distractions. Overloading an already overloaded nervous system makes paying attention and learning more difficult for the person with Fragile X. A study carrel with an angled desk top that gives the person the option either to sit or to stand can be helpful. Posters, pictures, and charts can contribute to overstimulating clutter for individuals with Fragile X, so only those accents of information that are most necessary should be on the walls. Soft-textured and soft-colored curtains or shades might be preferable to visually overstimulating window coverings or venetian blinds.

- Carpet under tables and on chair legs can reduce noise at school as well as at home and work settings.

- Alternative seating (such as an office kneeling chair, a rocking chair, a therapy ball stabilized with an inner tube or cloth tube ring, an inflated cushion placed in the chair, or straddling a barrel or bolster) can provide helpful movement and proprioception sensations. Another possibility is to have the child sit on a doughnut-shaped water or air cushion to give a sense of boundary. These alternatives can help the person feel more centered, improve postural control, and satisfy the need to move.

- Use pleasant smells for calming and alerting. A lavender plant in a classroom, home, or work environment is one nonintrusive way to use an aroma therapeutically.

- Alternate quiet and active times. Alternate gross with fine motor activities. Use a predictable sequence or routine whenever possible, with as few transitions as possible from place to place and from person to person.

- Transitional objects are useful. For young children it could be a toy, a blanket, or a book. Muffins and cookies were the transitional objects for a 19-year-old client anticipating visiting his friends in a group home. He would become so excited about the visit that a panic attack sometimes occurred on the way to the home, and he would be as nervous as if he were going to visit strangers. He loved to cook, so the ritual of baking as well as the ritual of giving helped decrease his anxiety.

- Use music as a cue for going from one activity to another. Music can help the person develop internal control, taking the focus away from external authority. In a residential setting, clients can make group decisions in choosing music for transitions, exercise time, quiet time, mealtime, and sleep or wakeup times.

- For an adult at a work site, it is extremely important to provide predictable break times for quiet time alone, for exercise, for the appropriate oral-motor snack, or for whatever might be important in the person's sensory diet.

- Use music to introduce the next activity, to calm, or to alert (Williams & Shellenberger, 1992). Be sensitive to the kinds of sounds, beat, and melody that are most appropriate for each person. Involve clients in performing music, using their voice as an instrument. Explore sounds they can make for quality and vibration, and observe the effects on postural, oral, and motor control.

- Engage children in playful activities that provide deep pressure input and joint compression on arms, head, back, shoulders, legs, and feet, if possible. Activities such as bouncing on a therapy ball or creeping through tunnels and on textured surfaces help alleviate sensitivity to touch and improve self-regulation. Adolescents and adults sometimes enjoy structured exercise programs, therapeutic horseback riding, and hiking or climbing. Pushing book carts, vacuuming, and performing errands such as carrying bags or boxes of supplies can be part of the person's daily responsibilities and can help in self-modulation because these activities provide proprioceptive sensations.

- Chewing gum, drinking thick liquids through a straw, chewing on plastic tubing, and eating snacks with a range of textures and resistances provide oral proprioception for calming, and tastes and textures for alerting and focusing.

- Finally, whether in testing, therapy, play, school, home, or at work, it is vital to convey a true sense of respect and acceptance for the person with Fragile X.

Individuals with Fragile X syndrome will require strategies to help them with self-regulation throughout their lifetime. Such assistance will be particularly necessary when changes occur in their lives, such as a loss of a parent, and during other stressful events, such as accidents or illness. The exact strategy might require change so that it is age-appropriate. These individuals are likely to need sensory strategies for reducing anxiety when confronted with specific challenges for the rest of their lives.

Case Studies

There are many stories with countless variations involving young people with Fragile X. Personality and severity of involvement, the opportunities offered in choices of living and vocational situation, the attitude and level of acceptance within the community, and the quality of therapy the person has received are all factors that can affect outcomes. The following examples tell two very different stories. The first narrative is about Neil, whose diagnosis of Fragile X syndrome was not established until he was in his 50s. The second story is about two brothers, Dan and Tom, who benefited from intense educational and therapeutic programming.

Neil

Neil had been identified early in life as mentally retarded. As was customary for individuals his age with this type of disability, he had lived in an institution most of his life, with very little therapeutic intervention. Not until he was 50 years old was his disability diagnosed as Fragile X syndrome.

Neil was referred for an occupational therapy evaluation due to his difficulties participating in daily routines and handling social contact with others. He arrived for the evaluation wearing three layers of clothing, even though it was a very warm day. He had pulled his sleeves down over his hands, and he sat with his back pressed into a corner. He appeared to seek pressure from tugging at his clothing and from jamming himself against the wall. He had shallow breathing and poor breath support for speech. He exhibited flexion contractures of hips and knees. He shuffled his feet when ambulating, maintaining constant contact with the floor. He was unable to isolate ocular movements from total body movements so that, when asked to follow a moving object with his eyes, he moved his body as a block. He had an almost complete inability to anticipate, react, or relate to anyone or anything in other than a stereotypically fearful manner.

Neil provided an extreme example of the long-term results of lax joints, gravitational insecurity, and tactile, visual, auditory, and olfactory defensiveness. Some of these difficulties might have been prevented had therapy been available earlier in his life.

Dan and Tom

Brothers in their mid-20s, Dan and Tom lived amidst their supportive and loving extended family. They had accessed the educational and therapy opportunities available to children in the 1980s and 1990s. Together, they were a delightful pair, and the occupational therapist and speech therapist worked with them on sensory modulation, discrimination, and praxis, combining speech and occupational therapy in a variety of activities. Their therapy addressed these areas within a broader therapeutic context. For example, some of the intervention included transplanting flowers, doing light janitorial work at the clinic, and playing card games to work on math concepts as well as to have a social time at the end of each session. In fact, Dan and Tom continued into adulthood to receive occupational and speech therapies in combination with job coaching. However, as described below, Dan progressed in therapy more rapidly than his brother and was discharged when he was 28 years old. Tom needed continuing therapy into his 30s.

Dan was tall, slender, and athletic and loved participating in the Special Olympics, playing basketball, baseball, and bowling. When he played basketball, his stereotypical mannerisms, including gaze aversion, lessened. Dan ended therapy after a year, began his work as a dishwasher at a local restaurant, and continued his volunteer work, helping prepare food for the senior citizens' Meals on Wheels. He was ready to move out of his parents' home and into an apartment with a roommate. One big disappointment for Dan was due to the apprehension and fear of Little League coaches in the community who were unwilling to accept him as a scorekeeper and assistant coach, a role he would have loved and which he would have done well.

By contrast, Tom was tall, overweight, and sedentary. Tom continued to need occupational therapy, but the format changed. His challenge was to be able to stay with work assigned to him in order to develop employable skills. When he came to the office, he did light janitorial chores and alphabetized office files, for which he received a paycheck. We would often hear Tom talking aloud about his feelings, about what had happened to him that week, or about a storm that had happened a year ago that flooded his family's basement and left an indelible imprint on his memory. To hear him speak was to hear all the thoughts that ran through his mind without the typical editing that occurs for most people while speaking. He was unable to keep his thoughts to himself. Whatever came to mind, he spoke aloud.

Tom's dyspraxia became evident when he washed dishes. He had difficulty with sequencing: for example, he might pour the dish detergent into the sink, turn on the water, then wash a dish and place it in the drain (soap still on it), then put the drain stopper in the sink. It was necessary to talk him through the sequence for many weeks before the pattern became etched in his memory.

Tasks he enjoyed more than dishwashing showed steady progress. Tom had said that he would like to do office work, such as filing. Tom's first assignment, to make sure he could order items alphabetically, was to alphabetize randomly arranged cards with single letters. Next, Tom worked with cards displaying short last names (only one per alphabet letter). Gradually the task became more complex, perhaps with two identical last names but with different first names. Finally, he graduated to actual client files. Tom had two potential job skills: simple cleaning chores and filing.

As for leisure, Tom loved imitating dialects and mannerisms. He loved theater, especially Shakespeare, and he loved visiting with people. Ushering at the local Shakespearean festival in full medieval garb was one way to begin including theater as a leisure activity in his life. Volunteering at a neighborhood retirement home was another outlet for his gregarious nature.

At home, Tom was the epitome of "couch potato." He loved just sitting and watching TV at home, but at the clinic, his favorite activities involved socializing and music. From bouncing on the therapy ball to lively music, he had progressed to bouncing or rocking from side to side in time to the music, then to being part of a "rhythm band" group. After he completed his work, we would have a social musical break. He graduated to playing a beat on the drum, and as he became more able to sustain a beat, he also became creative in finding new ways to play the drum to express different animals or sounds. He'd shout, "snake," creating brushing sounds, or "rain," making a different sound on the drum with his fingertips. Another group member would match the theme, synchronizing with the piano. Students, staff, and visitors would join in, playing bells, rain sticks, or smaller drums.

The band activity provided an inroad for an exciting home program theme based on Tom's interests. First, Tom loved to watch TV. However, sitting and watching TV was not healthy. Second, Tom loved his musical/therapy ball exercise sessions at the clinic. Responding to Tom's needs and interests, we used the musical sharing times to create an exercise tape—with Tom as the star and producer—that he could play at home and exercise to with his family and friends. When Tom watched his creation for the first time, he became very quiet and said, "That's really good."

The sensory integrative framework provided the basis for all interactions with these individuals. Only after addressing the issues on modulating the social and physical environment could we move on to building more complex life skills. Comfort, safety, and routines were necessary to begin building rapport and the willingness to try something new. Therapy sessions included sensory activities that challenged existing perceptions and used sequencing, construction, and imitation within the activities that were meaningful and purposeful for these men. These individuals were then able to engage in a variety of healthy occupations within the realm of their capabilities so that they could enjoy a richer and fuller life of people and activity.

Summary

Individuals with Fragile X syndrome must have determination and willingness to reach out and interact with others. It is possible only through the respect of others for their unique processing and interaction style. It is imperative to address the intense difficulties in the areas of sensory modulation, sensory integration, and praxis for individuals with Fragile X to reach out and relate effectively and adaptively to other people and to their environment. Occupational therapy using a sensory integrative framework is in a unique position to meet this challenge. Changes in the ability to cope are possible through the pragmatic application of sensory integrative theory and an understanding of how to integrate the appropriate intervention in the person's everyday life.

Individuals with Fragile X respond to intervention based on sensory integration. There is no cure for Fragile X, but there is help, and a sensory integrative approach is a vital element. It can help persons with Fragile X syndrome develop lives that reflect who they really are beyond the labels. They are not their diagnosis. They are individuals who need assistance in finding ways to be themselves.

References

Ayres, A.J. (1972). *Sensory integration and learning disabilities.* Los Angeles: Western Psychological Services.

Ayres, A.J., & Tickle, L. (1980). Hyper-responsivity to touch and vestibular stimuli as a predictor of positive response to sensory integrative procedures by autistic children. *American Journal of Occupational Therapy, 34,* 375–381.

Braden, M. (1995, May/June). The social dilemma: Approach-avoidance. *National Fragile X Advocate, 1*(3), 1, 3–4.

Braden, M. (1996). *Fragile X: Handle with care.* Chapel Hill, NC: Avanta Media Corporation.

Burns, E., & Hickman, L. (1989). Integrated therapy in a summer camping experience for children with Fragile X syndrome. *Sensory Integration International Newsletter, 19*(1), 1–3.

Chudley, A.E., & Hagerman, R.J. (1987). Fragile X syndrome. *The Journal of Pediatrics, 110*(6), 821–831.

Feng, Y., Lakkis, D., & Warren, S.T. (1995). Quantitative comparison of FMR1 gene expression in normal and premutation alleles. *American Journal of Genetics, 56,* 101–113.

Hagerman, R.J. (1991). Medical follow-up and pharmacotherapy. In R.J. Hagerman & A.C. Silverman (Eds.), *Fragile X syndrome: Diagnosis, treatment and research* (pp. 282–310). Baltimore: Johns Hopkins University Press.

Hagerman, R.J. (1996). Physical and behavioral phenotype. In R.J. Hagerman & H.A. Cronister (Eds.), *Fragile X syndrome: Diagnosis, treatment, and research* (2nd ed., pp. 283–331). Baltimore: Johns Hopkins University Press.

Hagerman, R.J., & Cronister, A. (1996). *Fragile X syndrome: Diagnosis, treatment, and research* (2nd ed.). Baltimore: Johns Hopkins University Press.

Hagerman, R.J., Jackson, C., Amiri, K., Silverman, A. C., O'Connor, R., & Sobesky, W. (1992). Girls with Fragile X syndrome: Physical and neurocognitive status and outcomes. *Pediatrics, 89,* 395–400.

Hickman, L. (1997). From sound to story: Music encircles life and learning. *Early Childhood Connections, 3*(2), 14–20.

Martinez, S., & Maino, D. (1993). A comprehensive review of the Fragile (X) syndrome: Oculo-visual, developmental, and physical characteristics. *Journal of Behavioral Optometry, 4,* 59–63.

Miller, L.J., McIntosh, D.N., McGrath, J., Shyu, V., Lampe, M., Taylor, A. K., Tassone, F., Neitzel, K., Stackhouse, T., & Hagerman, R.J. (1999). Electrodermal responses to sensory stimuli in individuals with Fragile X: A preliminary report. *American Journal of Medical Genetics, 83*(4), 268–279.

Ratazzi, M.C., & Ianni, Y.A. (1996). Molecular approaches to therapy. In R.J. Hagerman and A. Cronister (Eds.), *Fragile X syndrome: Diagnosis, treatment, and research* (2nd ed., pp. 412–452). Baltimore: Johns Hopkins University Press.

Reiss, Z. (1996, May/June). The neuroanatomy of Fragile X syndrome. *The Fragile X Advocate, 2*(3), 2–3.

Scharfenacker, S., Hickman, L., & Braden, M. (1991). An integrated approach to intervention. In R.J. Hagerman & A.C. Silverman (Eds.), *Fragile X syndrome: Diagnosis, treatment, and research* (pp. 327–372). Baltimore: Johns Hopkins University Press.

Stackhouse, T.M. (1994). Sensory integration concepts and Fragile X syndrome. *Sensory Integration Special Interest Section Newsletter, 17*(1), 2–6.

Stackhouse, T. (1996). Sensory integration concepts and Fragile X syndrome. *The National Fragile X Foundation Educational Files, 1,* 2–3.

Turner, G., Till, R., & Daniel, A. (1978). Marker X chromosomes, mental retardation and macroorchidism [Letter to the editor]. *New England Journal of Medicine, 299,* 1472.

Williams, M.S., & Shellenberger, S. (1992). *How does your engine run: The Alert Program for self-regulation.* Albuquerque: Therapy Works.

Windeck, S.L., & Laurel, M. (1989). A theoretical framework combining speech-language therapy with sensory integration treatment. *Sensory Integration Special Interest Section Newsletter, 12,* 1–5.

Transformative Occupations and Long-Range Adaptive Responses

Erna Imperatore Blanche, Ph.D., OTR, FAOTA

> It's in the breadth of human experience that we encounter God. And . . .
> particularly it's in the realm of the senses and the beauty of art, of music,
> and of writing that (we find) . . . God. (Pat, quoted in Blanche, 1999, p. 262)

The above quote is from one of the participants in a study on play. Although Pat refers to the creation of art, he is alluding to the importance of the senses in the perception of art and the discovery of the core of who we are, what we desire, and how we create and re-create ourselves through occupations.

This chapter focuses on the role of the senses in choosing occupations that restore and challenge our sense of well-being. It is pertinent in this text because the therapist's ultimate goal is to help children develop within themselves a sense of well-being so they can move on to challenge themselves to continue developing. Helpful questions for a therapist to ask in working toward this goal are:

- How can therapists encourage children with sensory integrative deficits to expose themselves to occupations that have the potential of providing them with the sensory experiences they so desperately need?

- How do therapists prepare children for the day when intervention stops and they are independent in finding and recognizing the healing qualities of occupations?

In sensory integration, clinicians recognize that people use certain behaviors to modulate their state of arousal and often refer to these behaviors as providing a sensory diet (Wilbarger, 1995). For example, babies who are distressed calm down when fed with a bottle that provides the opportunity for sucking. School children who become overly aroused and easily distracted might run, jump, kick, bite, and push others. Adults who are distressed sometimes seek proprioceptive input through biking or smoking. However, even when therapists can identify the behaviors that help children regulate themselves during the intervention, clinicians are less proficient in finding patterns of activities that might help clients nourish their sensory needs and obtain a sense of well-being throughout their lives.

Because the relation between level of arousal, sense of well-being, and occupations is clearly observable in play, this chapter utilizes data from the author's research study on enjoyable experiences (Blanche, 1999). This chapter reviews the literature on sensation seeking and adult play as they relate to well-being and levels of arousal, describes patterns of experiences that typical individuals seek in order to nourish their sensory needs, and uses these examples to illustrate the importance of long-range planning when addressing adaptive behaviors.

Seeking Enjoyable Experiences for Their Sensory Value

There are several theories associating levels of arousal and play that support the idea that people play either to maintain an optimal level of arousal or to increase their own level of arousal. The first group of theories endorse a view of play as a behavior that "maintains an optimal flow of stimulation for the individual" (Levy, 1978, p. 137) or maintains an optimal level of arousal when the environment does not provide enough stimulation (Ellis, 1973). Optimal-level-of-arousal theories endorse a homeostatic view of arousal level in which the individual's preferred levels of arousal are intermediate. Such a person does not experience high or low levels of arousal as pleasurable; consequently these levels are not the optimal level at which the person functions (Kerr, 1994).

The second set of theories proposes explanations for the search for higher levels of arousal. Two theories—reversal theory and sensation seeking theory—explain an individual's tendency to seek high levels of arousal and sensation through engagement in specific occupations.

Reversal theory proposes that there are two equally stable preferred motivational states between which the person alternates: the telic or serious state, and the paratelic or playful state (Apter, 1992; Apter & Kerr, 1991; Kerr, 1994). A person in the telic state tends to be serious, to be planning-oriented, and to prefer low levels of felt arousal. A person in the paratelic state tends to be playful, spontaneous, and present-oriented, preferring high levels of felt arousal (Apter, 1991, 1992; Kerr, 1994). The paratelic state provides a protective, nonreal frame or a perception of safety within the boundaries of the activity. A person can stay in this protective frame as long as he or she does not perceive the impingement of the real world (Apter, 1992). In this protective, nonreal paratelic state, high levels of arousal are hedonistic (Apter, 1991; Kerr, 1994). Some persons tend to seek excitement through arousing stimulation such as loud music, bright colors, or incongruity; using fiction and narrative; or watching a horror movie. These individuals might also seek excitement by challenging themselves and/or breaking the rules. For example, activities such as rock climbing or parachuting are arousing and exciting, but individuals believe that the situation is safe. Breaking rules can also seem to be exciting, and these individuals therefore consider soccer hooliganism and participating in illegal activities as play.

Sensation seeking offers a different explanation for the search for excitement (Zuckerman, 1971, 1994). Zuckerman (1979) described sensation seeking as a trait or state defined by "the need for varied, novel, and complex sensations and experiences and the willingness to take physical, social, and financial risks for the sake of such experience" (p. 10). Sensation seeking is the tendency to seek stimulating situations that is based on an individual's biological/genetic base and simultaneously shaped by the environment (Zuckerman, 1994). Researchers view sensation seekers as seeking an optimal level of arousal through the performance of activities that might be risky or novel and sometimes provide high-intensity sensory input. According to Zuckerman (1994), the only stability in high-sensation seekers is change, such as change of job situation, marital partners, or living situation.

Over the years, Zuckerman and his colleagues have refined this theory and the scale they have used to identify sensation-seeking behaviors (Zuckerman, 1994). Zuckerman's first theoretical explanations for sensation seeking came from the theory of optimal level of arousal (1994). Recent advances in brain physiology provide more comprehensive explanations for the regulation of arousal. According to these theories, sensation seeking also relates to how sensitive the person is to stimulation, how the person processes the sensory input, and how aroused the person needs to be in order to perform optimally (Zuckerman, 1994). Theorists have come to conceptualize sensation seeking as a personality trait that affects brain physiology and originates in the interplay between genetic programs, the individual's history, and the individual's present environmental conditions (Zuckerman, 1994). Zuckerman's category of sensation seekers probably includes a large number of individuals who exhibit sensory integration deficits.

High-sensation seekers sometimes engage in what Geertz (1983) described as "deep play," "play in which the stakes are so high that it is, from this utilitarian standpoint, irrational for men to engage in it at all" (p. 54). Many of the occupations that qualify as deep play are risky, including activities such as rock climbing, bungee jumping, using drugs, and hooliganism.

Raine, Reynolds, Venables, Mednick, and Farrington (1998) also tied sensory-seeking behaviors to risky activities. Raine and colleagues proposed that there is a relationship between aggression, sensation seeking, lack of fear, and low levels of physiological arousal. He hypothesized that some children compensate for chronic low levels of arousal by behaving aggressively. These children seek novelty through interactions with others, appear fearless in that they tend to explore their environment, and approach novel stimuli independently from their mothers. In one of his studies, Raine found a correlation between sensation seeking and fearlessness at 3 years of age and a greater predisposition toward aggressive behaviors at 11 years of age. He proposed that the tendency toward aggression might have a neurological basis that relates to neurological mechanisms and levels of arousal.

In summary, reviewing the literature on sensation seeking and relating it to sensory integration suggest that among individuals who are sensation seekers or appear fearless, there are individuals with sensory integrative deficits who are trying to restore their sense of well-being. The next section describes strategies that individuals use to restore the sense of well-being.

Restorative Niches

Restorative niches are places where a person can go to regain his or her own nature or sense of self after being in a situation of stress (Little, 1998). Often these restorative niches are strategies the individual uses to generate sensory experiences that help regain but also often challenge one's sense of self or well-being. The strategies that relate to sensory processing include seeking to heighten the sense of self by increasing the sensory input and possibly engaging in high-risk activities, removing oneself from the hassles and stimulation of daily life, and temporarily increasing the level of arousal by searching for novelty. Understanding these strategies along a temporal dimension is helpful for organizing intervention.

Finding a Sense of Balance With Temporal Patterns of Occupations—Short- and Long-Term Strategies

The author's study found that people use three temporal patterns of occupations to restore their sense of balance: (1) customary, habitual activities or behaviors that the person performs frequently throughout the day, (2) activities that occupy larger temporal cycles and are memorable and meaningful in the individual's daily life, and (3) occupations that survive the passage of time and help redesign the person's life.

Customary behaviors occupy a small temporal cycle, generally lasting only a few minutes. People performing these activities are often not aware of performing them and give meaning to them as enfolded or secondary activities within larger sets of occupations. These activities often do not lead to major changes in one's lifestyle but help cope with stress for a short period. Customary activities include listening to music while driving, shooting baskets intermittently while babysitting, or socializing at work. These secondary activities are intrinsically motivated, enjoyable, and spontaneous choices that people use as restorative niches to maintain their optimal level of arousal.

A second set of strategies consists of the activities that occupy a larger temporal cycle. People look forward to performing these occupations during the day, the activities differ from the daily routines, and individuals remember these activities as pleasurable or satisfying from one day to the next. These occupations, which help people unwind, include a vast selection of activities that require removing oneself from stimulation or seeking specific types of sensory experiences, such as running, taking a catnap, walking the dog, taking a bubble bath, or meditating.

A third set of strategies encompasses occupations that endure over time, that become a unique experience in the life of a person, and that people remember as stories. Individuals often narrate these stories in the context of stressful or painful situations in life that have required transforming one's pattern of occupations. Narratives of these transitions in life become a way of gaining meaning and restoring order in one's daily round of activities, a way of redesigning one's lifestyle (Jackson, Carlson, Mandel, Zemke, & Clark, 1998).

Included in these sets of strategies are occupations that an individual might have performed accidentally on one specific occasion but that the person then repeats because of their enjoyable nature. For example, Ian, who has run the New York marathon for the last 11 years, reported that he went running one day when his father was dying in the hospital. Ian described this occupation in the following way:

> I run the New York marathon every year and I started the year my dad was in the hospital and he was dying, and it seemed like the only release that would sort of handle all the amount of feelings and stress and everything that I was feeling was to go out and start running. It's like "Forrest Gump." When he started running, it was the same thing, and I decided to run the marathon. That was two weeks after my dad died and then I just kept running marathons every year. (Ian, quoted in Blanche, 1999, p. 246)

This person used running as a restorative niche where he could regain his own sense of self. Over time, running became part of his routine and helped him cope with the loss of his father. Most probably, running also supplied the necessary sensory nourishment that initially helped him regain a momentary sense of well-being and then became a lifetime occupation.

Another young man, an avid rock climber, reported having a troubled childhood. He recalled that when he has young, his parents took him to see a Tarzan movie. When he came home, he tied a rope from the banisters and swung from it until the rope became untied and he crashed on the floor. He remembered this activity for a long time. Later, when he was going through difficult teenage years, a friend took him rock climbing. He saw rock climbing as helping him get his life back on track and continued this activity throughout his life. In this case, the sensory experience derived from swinging on a rope was memorable, and he later repeated it through rock climbing.

Others have turned occasional restorative pursuits into full-time occupations. For example, a rock-climbing instructor and a yoga instructor both worked in several businesses before they decided to become instructors. During the time they were in other business, life was difficult or did not make much sense. Throughout that period, both performed these pleasurable occupations at first as restorative niches and later as full-time businesses.

Fanchiang (1996) noted a similar process in an individual with sensory integrative dysfunctions who tended to engage in "thrill-seeking" activities such as skateboarding, bike riding, and running during his childhood, then in risky and socially unacceptable "hell-raising" activities such as vandalism and making bombs during his adolescence. The individual described these necessary activities as "adrenaline surges" and not as impulsive acts. During these activities (which he called "a charge"), he felt extreme physical exhaustion and a sense of power. In adulthood, he discovered that the occupation of giving massages allowed him to release some of the energy and nourished his sensory needs.

Analysis of Occupations as Restorative Niches

Analysis of pleasurable activities according to their nature uncovers the following strategies individuals utilize to regain a sense of well-being:

- reduction of sensory overload by engaging in restorative, calming activities
- exposure to new information by participating in novel experiences
- increase in self-awareness by engaging in challenging, stimulating, and often dangerous activities that heighten the individuals' awareness of themselves

This chapter focuses on only those activities with an association to the use of sensory experiences to obtain an optimal state of arousal.

Restoration by Removing Sensory Overload

People often enjoy activities during which they can relax by removing themselves from a situation or by reducing the number of activities in which they are engaged. For example, one participant in the author's study reported that one of the most pleasurable activities he performed during the day was driving. When questioned further, he explained that he had an extremely busy schedule. During the day, he often had multiple phone calls he needed to attend to simultaneously, and driving was a time to unwind and be away from the daily hassles. In addition, driving gave him the freedom to go to places where he could unwind. He recounted that, during the day, he sometimes stopped everything and drove himself to the shore, where he sat and watched the boats. He described this occupation as something that gave him peace and helped him put things into perspective. He nurtured this activity even further by buying an antique convertible car, which made driving fun.

Another participant described the sensory experiences produced by mundane activities such as gardening and washing the car as calming or organizing. She explained that washing the car and gardening gave her sensory experiences that she could not describe fully. Performing these activities allowed her to unwind and think about other things or not think at all.

Participants often reported "unwinding activities" to be less physically or mentally active than what they did during the rest of the day. In addition, the participants often described these activities in reference to the sensory experience they derived from doing the activities. These occupations required decreasing external demands, changing one's focus, and gaining control over oneself, or "centering." The activities often were simple, mundane tasks such as sitting on the couch, putting one's feet up, and looking at the mail for about 20 minutes; having a pedicure or a massage; washing the car; watering the garden; or taking a "catnap." The participants considered these activities necessary to their being able to continue with their daily hassles.

Seeking Novelty: A Sense of Adventure

Some people engage in activities that are prompted by novelty or a desire to experience a new aspect of the world or an activity. These individuals describe new events and new information as "energizing." Novel experiences include being exposed to something to which one is not usually exposed, such as experiencing beauty in nature, taking a random walk in an unknown city, having a philosophical conversation, or gauging rare coins. Individuals can derive the experience of adventure from an activity that requires physical, intellectual, or spiritual exploration.

Seeking novelty might relate to the childhood urge to explore. Berlyne (1969), Hutt (1978), and Day (1981) all proposed a play typology with two types of play: diversive play and exploratory play. Diversive play is initiated by boredom or a decrease in the level of arousal, has the characteristics of being aimless, is disrupted easily, is fun and relaxed, and has pleasure as its goal (Day, 1981). In comparison, exploratory play is initiated by novelty, uncertainty, and curiosity (Day, 1981). The adult's search for newness and adventure has some of the characteristics of exploratory play but is not prompted by the environment. Instead, this search arises from the person's curiosity or desire to find novelty and uncertainty and could be initiated by boredom.

This information relates to sensory processing disorders because there are many children who seem to seek novelty in order to stay focused and interested in a task. In the author's study, adults reported engaging in simultaneous occupations at least 50% of the time. The experiential qualities of the secondary (or surplus) occupation differed from the primary (or main) occupation in that secondary occupations included more of the characteristics of play; that is, they were more intrinsically motivated, energizing, and pleasurable. These secondary activities also helped people embellish their daily routine. Clinicians often notice that some individuals with attention deficits fidget and may become disruptive. However, in light of the research on secondary occupations, the tendency of the child with attention deficits to engage in other occupations and become disruptive might be suggestive of boredom and a tendency to seek novelty by engaging in more than one occupation at a time. Clinicians then can help the client develop the ability to engage successfully in simultaneous occupations.

Stretching Oneself to the Limits: Seeking Stimulation and Heightened Self-Awareness

Some people perform occupations they consider enjoyable because these activities lead to an increased sense of self physically, intellectually, or spiritually. These occupations require intense focus and deep immersion in them. For example, one individual described playing the piano as an activity that provided a sense of relief. He believed that during his engagement in music, he learned something about himself and felt released, calm, and able to breathe.

Some individuals described occupations (including mystical/religious experiences such as yoga, attending a religious service, and meditation) as intense and providing a heightened sense of self. For others, the use of illicit drugs produced these experiences, and for still others, activities providing specific intense sensory input supplied these experiences. In this last group, people seemed to seek specific types of sensory input to release tension and to gain a sense of heightened self-awareness. For example, Herman, a lawyer, played tennis once a week, and Paloma, who was learning aerobatics from her husband, flew an airplane every weekend. Herman described the activity as necessary to release tension. Paloma considered aerobatics necessary because it made her feel like her body was her own. Others described such activities as "getting a rush," "climbing a mountain," or "the closest one could get to God" (Blanche, 1999, p. 224). In the author's study on play, activities that heightened self-awareness were intense activities that the participants often characterized as exciting, stressful, and energizing, such as teaching, yoga, aerobatics, acting, painting, rock climbing, performing surgery, and creating music. Interestingly, these activities simultaneously require high levels of energy and are energizing.

Seeking Novelty and Heightened Self-Awareness: Taking Risks

Some people tended to seek experiences that coupled intense sensations with novelty. This combination of experiences was sometimes physically or emotionally risky. These risks included an element of adventure and heightened self-awareness, and individuals undertook these risks in a variety of circumstances and contexts. They apparently sought the intensity of an experience regardless of the cost involved.

The author's study identified two types of risky occupations. One category of risk included individuals' challenging their skills to the point of not being aware that they might be entering a dangerous situation. In other cases, individuals took risks apparently to seek a certain type of experience and awareness regardless of the consequences. In this second category, the activity was not necessarily skilled, and at the same time, the person appeared to be fully aware of the risk he or she was taking. People described as sensation seekers (Zuckerman, 1994) sometimes engage in these activities that do not require specific skill development. Because of the element of chance and the high risk involved in these nonskilled occupations, the term *Russian roulette* accurately describes these activities.

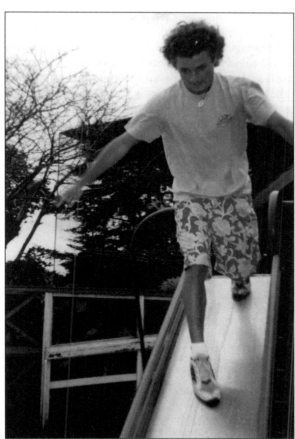

Figure 20.1. A search for novelty and sensory input leads this adolescent to perform risky activities.

One participant in the author's study, a skilled personal-watercraft driver named Tom, gave an example of a risky occupation that required mastery and consequently made it safer. Tom liked playing tricks on others when driving on the lake. One morning, he decided to splash someone sitting in the sun on a houseboat. Overestimating his skill, he took the risk of approaching the boat at a high speed to do the splashing. He challenged his skills, adding more adventure to his occupation. However, his skill was not sufficient to prevent him from having an accident when he lost control of the vehicle. Tom described his tendency to seek risks in the following way:

> I'm one of those guys that says "Wow, today is another day. Let's see what we can make of it because if I die tonight at least I can say I had a good day" . . . you know, I've seen the risks. I've seen what happens when people fall and break. It's like I know that when I go there that I could come home with a cast. I could come home with a bunch of scrapes and bumps and bruises. Or I could not come home at all. (Tom, quoted in Blanche, 1999, p. 254)

A search for novelty and a need to increase the feeling of risk involved in the activity seem to have contributed to the performance of risky occupations. These risky occupations included performing novel physical activities or pushing the limits of mastered occupations to obtain a sense of adventure. Some of the hazardous activities included risky sexual encounters, illicit drug use, hooliganism, and loitering. These occupations or behaviors provided the necessary sensory experiences but didn't require any mastery or skill development. For example, one participant in this study described an occasion on which he chose to jump from a very high rock into a stream; not knowing how much water it carried to protect him. Other participants described the use of drugs or vandalizing in earlier periods in their lives. Interestingly, later in life they had found occupations such as dancing, piloting, driving an ambulance, and rock climbing that provided them with large amounts of vestibular and proprioceptive input in a safe manner.

Understanding patterns of activities as restorative niches along a temporal continuum can help practitioners facilitate the client's ability to find his or her own restorative niche.

Clinical Application: Constructing a Lifestyle as an Adaptive Behavior/Response

Ayres (1979) defined adaptive responses as "appropriate action(s) in which the individual responds successfully to some environmental demand" (p. 181). Ayres added the term "adaptive behavior" (1984) and differentiated between lower- and higher-level adaptive behaviors according to their complexity. A less complex adaptive response implies that the environment imposes itself on the individual, whereas in a more complex adaptive behavior, the individual initiates the interaction when he or she recognizes an invitation from the environment to act on it.

Helping clients to become autonomous in crafting their own menu of activities that restore and/or challenge their sense of well-being is, in reality, the promotion of long-term adaptive behaviors that ultimately lead to a healthy life. Health is "the possession of a repertoire of skills that enables people to achieve their vital goals in their own environment" (Yerxa, 1998, p. 412). Promoting health requires supporting the individual's development of a repertoire of skills that will enable the person to recognize the healing potential offered by some activities in the environment. Long-term goals leading to health through adaptive behaviors need to include assisting individuals to develop repertoires of occupations that help them maintain their optimal level of arousal, provide a sense of well-being, and enable them to achieve their goals in society.

By studying the way people find their restorative niches and healthy patterns of occupations, clinicians can find a blueprint for helping clients to develop a menu or a repertoire of nourishing occupations. Developing such a repertoire requires consideration of the characteristics of the experience, the nature of the occupations, and the temporal aspect of activities.

The characteristics of occupations that provide a sense of well-being include being enjoyable, intrinsically motivated, and oriented toward the process rather than the product. Consequently, it is necessary to consider these characteristics when looking for occupations that will be nourishing for the client.

Second, it is important to analyze the nature of occupations the client needs by asking the following questions:

- What type of enjoyable and satisfying experiences is the client seeking?

- Does the client seek restorative niches that reduce the input in the environment, novel activities that increase the person's sense of adventure in the environment, or intense activities that heighten the sense of self?

- If the person is attempting to heighten his or her sense of self, how does the individual need to obtain that sense—through physical activity and somatosensory input, religious/mystical activities, intense auditory input, illicit activities, or some other type of occupations?

- Does the client engage in risky occupations?

  Do these activities appear to be prompted exclusively by a search for sensory experiences, or are they prompted by a search for experiences that include sensory as well as cognitive aspects?

- If the client engages in risky or illicit occupations, what type of sensory input is the person seeking, and is it possible to replace these activities with skilled and acceptable activities that provide the same experience?

Third, the menu needs to consider the temporal cycles of occupations. By addressing different temporal cycles, therapists can create a more varied menu of activities, including those that individuals can perform often during the day, once per day or week, and seasonally. In the author's study, a common theme among participants who later initiated a transition toward redesigning their lifestyle was finding an occupation that served initially as a restorative niche and subsequently as a daily endeavor. In the clinic, therapists can explore the existence of experiences the client might have performed once or twice but remember later. Memorable activities might have become meaningful because of their sensory value, and by asking older clients about them, the clinician can identify occupations that could serve as restorative niches. These occupations might provide clues about possible choices of profession or nourishing recreational activities.

Analyzing the form, function, and meaning of occupations also comes into play in considering the temporal aspects and nature of occupations (Clark, Wood, & Larson, 1998).

- *Form* refers to the observable aspects of occupations (direct observation of behavior). For children with Autistic Disorder, observations of stereotypic behaviors such as rocking or running contribute to an understanding of the restorative niches that these individuals utilize to regain balance. In sensory integration, clinicians often observe the form of occupations and draw conclusions about their function as a coping strategy in the child's daily life.

- *Function* refers to the ways in which occupation serves adaptation. The focus is on relationship of occupation to health, well-being, daily functioning, stress management, and development of mastery (Clark et al., 1998). In sensory integration, function often refers to the functional value that specific activities have in the life of a child. Clinicians interpret avoidance of specific activities and repetition of others as serving a coping function for the child. For example, children with developmental disabilities and sensory integrative difficulties compensate for their difficulties by avoiding activities that the children perceive as difficult to master. In turn, avoiding these activities increases children's functional limitations (Blanche, 1998).

  On the other hand, choosing activities for their intrinsic value might serve the function of nurturing the person's sensory needs, consequently the individual repeats the activity and it becomes part of the person's repertoire. Chapter 10 of this text, Praxis and Organization of Behavior in Space and Time, describes some of the difficulties children have with organizing their actions and how they might avoid certain situations and utilize social strategies to cope with the environmental demands.

- *Meaning* refers to the significance of occupation within the context of real lives and their culture. Occupations become meaningful because they are the vehicles through which people can express emotion. Using narrative, therapists can gain an understanding of the child's trajectory and determine whether sensory experiences serve a balancing function in the meaningful themes that weave through the child's choice of occupations.

Sense of self emerges out of daily experiences and how these experiences link to a meaningful life. For example, individuals who engage in sports might eventually see themselves as athletic and include this view of self into their narrative. Children with sensory integrative disorders sometimes see themselves as not being able to perform many activities and then incorporate this more negative self-appraisal into their view of self.

Children with sensory integrative dysfunctions also tend to seek large amounts of input in unsafe ways and might constitute a large percentage of Zuckerman's (1994) category of sensation seekers, or Raine et al.'s (1998) sensory seekers who later became aggressive. It is then imperative for occupational therapists to find the menu that will provide sensory experiences without the client's engaging in risky or violent occupations. For example, the child who seeks large amounts of proprioceptive input might benefit from rock climbing, mountaineering, or kickboxing. The child who habituates sooner and requires constant novelty to maintain interest and the level of arousal might benefit from daily schedules that are stimulating and enjoyable or activities that provide uneven and assorted input, such as engaging in simultaneous occupations (see Table 20.1).

People who need novelty and/or stimulation in the environment are more prone to engage in risky occupations and may need to develop skills early on so they have a menu of safe activities that will provide them with the necessary experiences. For example, scooters, skateboards, and bikes provide alternate means of transportation and exercise, and mountaineering, piloting, and driving an unusual car can take a person to different places and thereby increase novelty.

Table 20.1. The Relationship Between Sensory Needs and Occupational Patterns of Performance

Sensory Need/Behavior
- Maintaining interest and attention by creating opportunities for novelty by incorporating secondary activities in the daily routine (e.g., fidgeting, doodling, daydreaming, listening to music, clowning around)
- Coping with sense of becoming overwhelmed by input in the environment by withdrawing
- Increasing organization of self and sense of self by searching for intense physical activity and sensory experiences (e.g., running, crashing, twirling, rocking, climbing on trees, dangling from balconies, sliding down the banister)

Daily Activities
- Daily schedules that include novelty and multiple and diverse interests (e.g., dressing up for dinner, going to restaurants the person hasn't visited, playing the stock market, surfing the Internet, taking classes on nontraditional topics such as bellydancing,)
- Driving to the beach, park, or other secluded area
- Taking a bubble bath
- Meditating
- Running, dancing, biking, skating, playing the drums, listening to loud music, kick boxing, soccer

Long-Range Occupations
- Planning vacations to places that the person has not visited before
- Sightseeing
- Vacations in secluded places
- Attending rock concerts, participating in tournaments of intense sports, participating in marathons, rock climbing, bungee jumping

Children with sensory integration deficits often derive meaning from the sensory input provided by occupations. The meaning of the occupation contributes to the person's repeating that occupation over time so it becomes part of a particular lifestyle or helps construct that lifestyle. In this text, the term *lifestyle construction,* as borrowed from Bateson (1989), refers to a more ad hoc process that might even happen unintentionally as the individual moves through life. Individuals with sensory integration dysfunctions often tend to fall accidentally into activities that nourish their sensory needs; therefore the term *lifestyle construction* may capture more accurately the essence of the process in this population.

It is appropriate to conclude this chapter with a quote from Linda, the mother of a child with Autistic Disorder who was a participant in the author's study. Linda's friends and associates often disapproved of her because she allowed her child to have fun and be himself rather than providing a structure to facilitate his development. Linda preferred to allow him to be happy and play the way he liked playing—climbing stairs, opening and slamming doors, and running. Scotty, her son, appeared content. She said:

> Scotty doesn't have like all that much appropriate toy play. So, he's real easily bored. So, he wants to go out, too. What I try to do on those days, is like, you know, give him something like nourishment for his soul. I take him to the botanical garden and let him run outside. And these are things he likes. (Linda, quoted in Blanche, 1999, p. 258)

In following his lead, Linda provided Scotty not only with the *sensory* nourishment but also, as she called it, *"nourishment for his soul."*

Acknowledgment

The author would like to acknowledge Diane Parham for her assistance in developing these ideas during the dissertation process.

Works Cited

Quotations on pages 423, 426, and 429 from *Play and Process: The Experience of Play in the Life of the Adult* by E. I. Blanche (1999) have been reprinted with permission from Erna I. Blanche.

References

Apter, M. (1991). A structural phenomenology of play. In J. Kerr & J. Apter (Eds.), *Adult play: A reversal theory approach* (pp. 13–30). Amsterdam: Swets & Zeitlinger B.V.

Apter, M. (1992). *The dangerous edge: The psychology of excitement.* New York: The Free Press.

Apter, M., & Kerr, J. (1991). The nature, function and value of play. In J. Kerr & M. Apter (Eds.), *Adult play: A reversal theory approach* (pp. 163–176). Amsterdam: Swets & Zeitlinger B.V.

Ayres, A.J. (1979). *Sensory integration and the child.* Los Angeles, CA: Western Psychological Services.

Ayres, A.J. (1984). *Adaptive behavior as a therapeutic process.* Unpublished manuscript.

This chapter is based on the doctoral dissertation entitled *Play and process: The experience of play in the life of the adult* by Erna Imperatore Blanche, accepted in fulfillment of a doctoral degree in Occupational Science at the University of Southern California.

Bateson, M.C. (1989). *Composing a life*. New York: Penguin Books.

Berlyne, D.E. (1969). Laughter, humor and play. In G. Lindsey & E. Aronson (Eds.), *The handbook of social psychology: Vol. 3* (pp. 795–851). Reading, MA: Addison-Wesley.

Blanche, E.I. (1998). The impact of sensory processing on early child development. In K.N. Inamura (Ed.), *Sensory integration in early intervention* (pp. 1–42). Tucson, AZ: Therapy Skill Builders.

Blanche, E.I. (1999). *Play and process: The experience of play in the life of the adult.* Ann Arbor, MI: UMI.

Clark, F., Wood, W., & Larson, E. (1998). Occupational science: Occupational therapy's legacy for the 21st century. In M. Neistadt & E. Crepeau (Eds.), *Willard and Spackman's occupational therapy* (9th ed., pp. 13–21). Philadelphia: J.B. Lippincott.

Day, H.I. (1981). Play: A ludic behavior. In H.I. Day (Ed.), *Advances in intrinsic motivation and aesthetics* (pp. 225–250). New York: Plenum Press.

Ellis, M.J. (1973). *Why people play.* Englewood Cliffs, NJ: Prentice-Hall.

Fanchiang, S. (1996). The other side of the coin: Growing up with a learning disability. *American Journal of Occupational Therapy, 50,* 277–285.

Geertz, C (1983). Deep play: Notes on the Balinese cockfight. In J.C. Harris & R.J. Park (Eds.), *Play, games, and sports in cultural context* (pp. 39–78). Champaign, IL: Human Kinetics. (Reprinted from *Daedalus,* Winter 1972, *101,* 1–37)

Jackson, J., Carlson, M., Mandel, D., Zemke, R., & Clark, F. (1998). Occupations in lifestyle redesign: The well elderly study occupational therapy program. *American Journal of Occupational Therapy, 52*(2), 326–336.

Hutt, C. (1978). Exploration and play in children. In D. Muller-Schwarze (Ed.), *Evolution of play behavior* (pp. 328–348). Stroudsburg, PA: Dowden, Huchinson & Ross.

Kerr, J. (1994). *Understanding soccer hooliganism.* Buckingham, England: Open University Press.

Levy, J. (1978). Play and the future: A time for renaissance. In *Play behavior* (pp. 183–190). New York: John Wiley & Sons.

Little, B. (1998, March). *Personal projects and occupational science: On the bearable lightness of well-being.* Paper presented at the Occupational Science Symposium XI, Play: Occupation for a lifetime, University of Southern California Department of Occupational Science and Occupational Therapy, Los Angeles, CA.

Raine, A., Reynolds, C., Venables, P., Mednick, S., & Farrington, D. (1998). Fearlessness, stimulation-seeking, and large body size at age 3 years as early predispositions to childhood aggression at age 11 years. *Archives of General Psychiatry, 55*(8), 745–751.

Wilbarger, P. (1995). The sensory diet: Activity programs based on sensory processing theory. *Sensory Integration Special Interest Section Newsletter, 18*(2), 1–4.

Yerxa, E.J. (1998). Health and the human spirit for occupation. *American Journal of Occupational Therapy, 52,* 412–418.

Zuckerman, M. (1971). Dimensions of sensation seeking. *Journal of Consulting and Clinical Psychology, 36*(1), 45–52.

Zuckerman, M. (1979). *Sensation seeking: Beyond the optimal level of arousal.* Hillsdale, NJ: Erlbaum.

Zuckerman, M. (1994). *Behavioral expressions and biosocial bases of sensation seeking.* Cambridge, England: Cambridge University Press.

Additional Readings

Apter, M. (1989). *Reversal theory: Motivation, emotion and personality*. London: Routledge.

Apter, M. (1993). Phenomenological frames and the paradoxes of experience. In J.H. Kerr, S. Murgatroyd, & M.J. Apter (Eds.), *Advances in reversal theory* (pp. 27–40). Amsterdam: Swets & Zeitlinger B.V.

Berlyne, D.E. (1960). *Conflict, arousal, and curiosity*. New York: McGraw-Hill.

Clark, F., & Larson, E. (1993). Developing an academic discipline: The science of occupation. In H. Hopkins & H. Smith (Eds.), *Willard and Spackman's occupational therapy* (8th ed., pp. 44–55). Philadelphia: J.B. Lippincott.

Kerr, J., & Apter, M. (1991). *Adult play: A reversal theory approach*. Amsterdam: Swets & Zeitlinger B.V.

Zuckerman, M. (1984). Experience and desire: A new format for sensation seeking scales. *Journal of Behavioural Assessment, 6*(2), 101–114.